In Silico Drug Discovery and Design

Theory, Methods, Challenges, and Applications

In Silico Drug Discovery and Design

Theory, Methods, Challenges, and Applications

Edited by **Claudio N. Cavasotto**

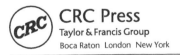

CRC Press
Taylor & Francis Group
Boca Raton London New York

CRC Press is an imprint of the
Taylor & Francis Group, an **informa** business

CRC Press
Taylor & Francis Group
6000 Broken Sound Parkway NW, Suite 300
Boca Raton, FL 33487-2742

First issued in paperback 2017

© 2016 by Taylor & Francis Group, LLC
CRC Press is an imprint of Taylor & Francis Group, an Informa business

No claim to original U.S. Government works

ISBN-13: 978-1-4822-1783-4 (hbk)
ISBN-13: 978-1-138-74758-6 (pbk)

Library of Congress Cataloging-in-Publication Data

In silico drug discovery and design : theory, methods, challenges, and applications /
    editor, Claudio N. Cavasotto.
    p. ; cm.
    Includes bibliographical references and index.
    ISBN 978-1-4822-1783-4 (hardcover : alk. paper)
    I. Cavasotto, Claudio N., editor.
    [DNLM: 1. Drug Discovery--methods. 2. Models, Molecular. 3. Small Molecule
Libraries--chemistry. QV 745]

    RS420
    615.1'9--dc23   2015007701

Visit the Taylor & Francis Web site at
http://www.taylorandfrancis.com

and the CRC Press Web site at
http://www.crcpress.com

Contents

Section I Theory, Methods, and Applications

Section II   Advanced Techniques

Section III   Challenges

Preface

In silico methods are today a solidly established key component in early drug lead discovery (Jorgensen 2009). A plethora of computational tools are routinely used to identify and select therapeutic relevant targets, study the molecular basis of ligand–protein interactions, structurally characterize binding sites, develop target-specific compound libraries, model target proteins, identify hits by ligand- and structure-based virtual screening, estimate binding free energy, and optimize lead compounds, all of which can be used to rationalize and increase the efficiency, speed, and cost-effectiveness of the drug discovery process.

The ever-increasing availability, and decreasing cost of computational power, algorithmic and software development, and the large number of web servers have contributed to the success of computational drug lead discovery. However, it should be acknowledged that progress in some areas seems to have slowed down, and rethinking and innovation both in terms of the perspective of the problem as well as in the computational tools themselves are still needed. Moreover, Peter Goodford's perspectives after the "3D Molecular Structure and Drug Action" meeting in Erice, Italy, in 1989, on where the field should go, may sound surprisingly current (Van Drie 2007).

It is reasonable to think that more accurate and reliable methods would surely help to overcome the stagnation in the number of approved drugs in recent years, especially if *in silico* discovery and optimization of high-affinity ligands is coupled with druggability assessments early in the drug discovery process. In particular, a deeper understanding of the forces governing macromolecular interaction, a more accurate estimation of the enthalpic and entropic contributions to ligand binding, and accounting for protein dynamics should have a strong impact in computer-aided drug design.

It should, however, be noted that the ease of access of computational tools in drug design (programs, databases, web servers) has also come at a price. Too often, programs have become black-boxes, where the user has little or almost no knowledge of the underlying physical basis of the methods used, which clearly compromises the understanding and interpretation of the results thus obtained. In several published studies, the use of methods outside their range of application casts serious doubts as to whether meaningful results could indeed be obtained. It would be possible, for example, that docking hits could be experimentally validated, while the ligand–receptor interaction pattern is not accurately described: good results would be obtained, though not for the right reasons, which would clearly jeopardize lead optimization efforts.

These facts led me to consider a volume that provides a comprehensive, unified, and in-depth overview of current methodological strategies in computer-aided drug discovery and design. Its main aims are to introduce the theoretical framework and algorithms, discuss the range of validity, strengths and limitations of each methodology, and present applications to real world problems in the drug discovery arena. Special emphasis has been given to the emerging and most pressing methodological challenges in *in silico* drug discovery and design. This approach should clearly facilitate a better interpretation of the simulation results, and should give the reader the adequate background to face the current challenges of the field.

This book is divided into three sections. Section I titled, "Theory, Methods, and Applications," presents the core methodology used in computational drug discovery, together with selected applications in Chapters 1 through 9. Chapters 1 and 2 set the tone by addressing the physical basis of ligand binding, and the force field representation of biomolecular systems. Chapter 3 discusses the concepts of chemical library representation and design, fragment libraries, drug-likeness, and filtering.

Chapters 4 through 7 cover the major *in silico* drug discovery methods: ligand-based chemical library screening, pharmacophore modeling and screening, and ligand–protein docking. Chapter 4 introduces the concepts of chemical space and molecular similarity in the context of structure–activity relationships (SARs) and hit identification, discusses the advantages and limitations of ligand-based methods, while also providing some recent examples from the literature. Chapter 5 describes the techniques of pharmacophore model generation, validation, virtual screening using various software, also including the specific requirements for those tasks. Due to its importance in characterizing ligand–protein interactions, and in structure-based virtual screening and lead optimization, two chapters are devoted to ligand–protein docking: Chapter 6 introduces the topic, focusing on binding mode prediction rather than hit discovery or ranking. Chapter 7, instead, introduces ligand docking in the context of virtual screening, describing the general workflow and the basic steps of this technique, and also reporting successful applications of docking-based virtual screening in drug discovery.

Three-dimensional protein structures have multiple uses in the computer-aided drug design scenario. Whenever experimental structures are not available, *in silico* characterized structures play a key role in drug discovery. In Chapter 8, the theoretical framework of homology or comparative modeling is presented, the individual steps of the entire process are discussed, and the use of homology models in structure-based drug discovery is reviewed, with a special focus on G protein-coupled receptors (GPCRs).

Implicit solvent methods for studying macromolecular interaction are described in Chapter 9. The theoretical foundations are presented, together with the practical aspects of their application in the context of ligand–receptor interaction, focusing on the Poisson–Boltzmann and generalized Born methods in the framework of molecular mechanics; the limitations of classical force field–based implicit solvent models are also discussed, and recent applications of quantum mechanics–based calculations in structure-based drug design are discussed together with their advantages, progresses, and limitations. Chapter 9 lays the ground for the application of generalized Born methods for rescoring in docking-based virtual screening (Chapter 11).

Section II titled "Advanced Techniques" (Chapters 10 through 14) presents the theory, algorithms, and applications of those methods which either require a more skilled theoretical background, or their use is not as common or established compared to methods from Section I. Chapter 10 introduces the topic of druggability prediction, critically important to expand the target space beyond current limits, and from there toward the notion of the cellular "pocketome" and predictive polypharmacology.

The strengths and limitations of methods for postprocessing hits from structure-based virtual screening are presented in Chapter 11; these techniques have emerged as important computational approaches in structure-based lead optimization, since they provide for congeneric molecules superior correlations with experimental binding data than the traditional high-throughput docking scores. Free-energy calculations, presented in Chapter 12, represent a more accurate way to calculate ligand-binding free energies; this approach is not suited for evaluating binding affinities of large chemical databases of small molecules, but is rather invaluable in lead optimization scenarios, where accurate free-energy calculations are sought; this chapter provides the statistical mechanical basis of these methods, a description of available techniques, and discusses advantages and shortcomings of various approaches; future directions of free-energy calculations in the context of drug design are outlined. Chapter 13 is dedicated to molecular mechanics/coarse-grain approaches for structural prediction, a still not-too-explored avenue in drug discovery.

The general background, methodologies, and applications of small molecular fragments, instead of larger whole molecules, in virtual screening are presented in Chapter 14, highlighting that fragment screening not only improves hit rates but could offer a more balanced property profile for lead candidates developed from fragments; case studies are presented, including those targeting GPCRs.

Section III titled "Challenges," (Chapters 15 through 18) introduces the reader to the most pressing issues, where advances are sought to improve the performance and/or predictability of *in silico* methods in drug discovery and design. In Chapter 15 the role of water molecules and hydration properties in modeling ligand–protein interaction is presented, including the consideration of explicit water molecules in biomolecular interfaces, the description of methods to distinguish between bound and displaceable water molecules in the binding site of protein–ligand complexes, and applications of incorporating explicit water molecules in the context of drug design.

A major challenge, accounting for protein flexibility in structure-based drug discovery, is presented in Chapter 16, discussing the trade-off between incorporating protein degrees of freedom and computational affordability, depicting the most common approaches used by docking programs to incorporate ligand and/or protein flexibility, exploring the use of molecular dynamics techniques to sample the conformational space of a target protein, and presenting real case examples.

The emerging challenge of targeting protein–protein interaction sites as pharmaceutical targets is thoroughly discussed in Chapter 17; the field is introduced, *in silico* tools and databases that can aid in the design of low molecular weight protein–protein interface modulators are described, key challenges are discussed, and finally, how *in silico* methods can be used and combined with experimental information to identify those modulators is illustrated.

Early-phase drug discovery has traditionally focused on optimizing drug-binding affinity, overlooking drug-binding kinetics; however, mounting evidence suggests that considering drug-binding kinetics early in the drug discovery process may increase the odds of success. Chapter 18 presents recent views on how drug-binding kinetics could impact drug discovery, introducing fast and approximate computational methods for aiding the design of drug candidates with favorable binding kinetics.

Throughout the book, particular attention has been paid to outline the theoretical basis of the described methods, thus providing the necessary background to avoid a "black-box" approach. In each self-contained chapter, the methodology is presented together with the latest developments and applications, and the challenges that lie ahead. This book constitutes both a desktop reference for academic and industrial researchers in the field, and a textbook for students in the area of molecular modeling and drug discovery.

I express my deep gratitude to all the contributors to this book, for their commitment, hard work, and outstanding chapters. I am grateful to my colleague Dr. Mario Rossi for insightful discussions. And finally, I thank Michael Slaughter from CRC Press/Taylor & Francis for his invitation to edit this book, and for his support throughout this project.

References

Jorgensen, W. L. 2009. Efficient drug lead discovery and optimization. *Acc. Chem. Res.* 42(6): 724–733.

Van Drie, J. H. 2007. Computer-aided drug design: The next 20 years. *J. Comput. Aided Mol. Des.* 21(10–11): 591–601.

Editor

Claudio N. Cavasotto, PhD, earned his MSc and PhD in physics from the University of Buenos Aires. He conducted his postdoctoral training at The Scripps Research Institute after which in 2002 he moved to MolSoft LLC, La Jolla, California, as senior research scientist, where he remained until 2007.

Dr. Cavasotto was then assistant and associate professor in the School of Biomedical Informatics at the University of Texas Health Science Center at Houston. In 2012, he moved to the Biomedicine Research Institute of Buenos Aires—Partner Institute of the Max Planck Society, where he is head of computational chemistry and drug design. His research interests are primarily biomolecular simulation, computer-aided drug discovery, and cheminformatics. His group develops and applies computational methods to study molecular interactions in biological systems, and to design molecules that modulate targets of pharmaceutical relevance.

Contributors

Ruben A. Abagyan
Skaggs School of Pharmacy and
    Pharmaceutical Sciences
University of California
San Diego, California

Muhammad Akram
Institute of Pharmacy/
    Pharmaceutical Chemistry
and
Center for Molecular Biosciences
    Innsbruck (CMBI)
University of Innsbruck
Innsbruck, Austria

Rainer Bomblies
Physics Department T38
Technical University Munich
Garching, Germany

Josep M. Campanera
Departament de Fisicoquímica
and
Institut de Biomedicina (IBUB)
Universitat de Barcelona
Barcelona, Spain

Paolo Carloni
Computational Biomedicine (IAS-5/
    INM-9)
Institute for Neuroscience and
    Medicine
and
Institute for Advanced Simulation
Forschungszentrum Jülich
    GmbH
and
Computational Biophysics
German Research School for
    Simulation Sciences GmbH
Jülich, Germany

Claudio N. Cavasotto
Biomedicine Research Institute
    of Buenos Aires—CONICET—
Partner Institute of the Max
    Planck Society
Buenos Aires, Argentina

Antonella Ciancetta
Department of Pharmaceutical and
    Pharmacological Sciences
University of Padova
Padova, Italy

Álvaro Cortés-Cabrera
Department of Biomedical
    Sciences
Alcalá University
Madrid, Spain

Pietro Cozzini
Molecular Modeling Lab
Department of Food Chemistry
University of Parma
Parma, Italy

Luca Dellafiora
Molecular Modeling Lab
Department of Food Chemistry
University of Parma
Parma, Italy

Federico Gago
Department of Biomedical
    Sciences
Alcalá University
Madrid, Spain

Alfonso T. García-Sosa
Institute of Chemistry
University of Tartu
Tartu, Estonia

Tiziana Ginex
Molecular Modeling Lab
Department of Food Chemistry
University of Parma
Parma, Italy

Alejandro Giorgetti
Computational Biophysics
German Research School for
    Simulation Sciences and
    Computational Biomedicine
Institute for Advanced Simulation
    IAS-5
and
Institute of Neuroscience and
    Medicine INM-9
Forschungszentrum Jülich
Jülich, Germany

and

Department of Biotechnology
University of Verona
Verona, Italy

Cristiano R. W. Guimarães
Department of Research,
    Development and Innovation
Aché Laboratórios Farmacêuticos
São Paulo, Brazil

Teresa Kaserer
Institute of Pharmacy/
    Pharmaceutical Chemistry
and
Center for Molecular Biosciences
    Innsbruck (CMBI)
University of Innsbruck
Innsbruck, Austria

György Miklós Keserű
Research Centre for Natural Sciences
Budapest, Hungary

Melaine A. Kuenemann
INSERM
Université Paris Diderot
Paris, France

David Lagorce
INSERM
Université Paris Diderot
Paris, France

Manuel Luitz
Physics Department T38
Technical University Munich
Garching, Germany

F. Javier Luque
Departament de Fisicoquímica
and
Institut de Biomedicina (IBUB)
Universitat de Barcelona
Barcelona, Spain

Alexander D. MacKerell, Jr.
Department of Pharmaceutical
    Sciences
School of Pharmacy
Computer Aided Drug Design
    Center
University of Maryland
Baltimore, Maryland

Gergely Makara
ComInnex Inc.
Budapest, Hungary

Maria A. Miteva
INSERM
Université Paris Diderot
Paris, France

Stefano Moro
Department of Pharmaceutical and
    Pharmacological Sciences
University of Padova
Padova, Italy

Antonio Morreale
REPSOL Technology Center
Madrid, Spain

Pedro A. Sánchez Murcia
Department of Biomedical Sciences
Alcalá University
Madrid, Spain

Francesco Musiani
Scuola Internazionale Superiore di
    Studi Avanzati (SISSA/ISAS)
Trieste, Italy

Damián Palomba
Biomedicine Research Institute
    of Buenos Aires—CONICET—
    Partner Institute of the Max
    Planck Society
Buenos Aires, Argentina

Daniela Schuster
Institute of Pharmacy/
    Pharmaceutical Chemistry
and
Center for Molecular Biosciences
    Innsbruck (CMBI)
University of Innsbruck
Innsbruck, Austria

Thomas Simonson
Laboratoire de Biochimie
Department of Biology
Ecole Polytechnique
Palaiseau, France

Meagan C. Small
Department of Pharmaceutical
    Sciences
School of Pharmacy
Computer Aided Drug Design
    Center
University of Maryland
Baltimore, Maryland

Christoph A. Sotriffer
Institute of Pharmacy and Food
    Chemistry
University of Würzburg
Würzburg, Germany

Olivier Sperandio
INSERM
Université Paris Diderot
Paris, France

Francesca Spyrakis
Department of Life Science
University of Modena and Reggio
    Emilia
Modena, Italy

Bryn Taylor
Skaggs School of Pharmacy and
    Pharmaceutical Sciences
University of California
San Diego, California

Márton Vass
Gedeon Richter Plc.
Budapest, Hungary

Hugo O. Villar
Altoris, Inc.
San Diego, California

Bruno O. Villoutreix
INSERM
Université Paris Diderot
Paris, France

Chung F. Wong
Department of Chemistry and
    Biochemistry
and
Center for Nanoscience
University of Missouri-Saint Louis
St. Louis, Missouri

Martin Zacharias
Physics Department T38
Technical University Munich
Garching, Germany

William Zamora
Departament de Fisicoquímica
Institut de Biomedicina (IBUB)
Universitat de Barcelona
Barcelona, Spain

Section I

Theory, Methods, and Applications

1

The Physical Basis of Ligand Binding

Thomas Simonson

CONTENTS

1.1 Introduction

Noncovalent binding among molecules, such as enzymes/substrates, ligands/receptors, or proteins/nucleic acids, is an important element of the biochemistry and information flow in cells (Böhm and Schneider, 2003, Gohlke, 2012, Pawson, 1995). Specificity is needed to preserve the correctness of the biochemical pathways and the integrity of the information. Binding affinity and specificity are often provided by noncovalent interactions among neighboring chemical groups, through hydrogen bonds, salt bridges, tight packing of complementary molecular surfaces, and hydrophobic forces mediated by solvent, although longer-range electrostatic interactions also play a role, particularly in the formation of encounter complexes (Fersht, 1999, Israelachvili, 1992, Jeffrey, 1997, Saenger, 1984).

In the crowded cellular environment, the number and variety of binding partners enormous, ranging from small ions to large cellular machines. With drug design as a goal, our scope is more limited, but still enormous. Even small, drug-like molecules can have complex energy surfaces, with polar, nonpolar, and polarizable groups, hard and soft degrees of freedom, multiple protonation states, possibly co-bound ions, all of which can reorganize on binding. They must recognize dynamic, fluctuating, macromolecular targets, displace water molecules, and compete with a host of other molecules. In addition, to engineer small ligands that interfere with protein/protein or protein/RNA complexes, we should understand the forces that govern such large complexes.

Only a few of these topics are covered, briefly, in this introductory chapter; various other aspects are covered in the remaining chapters. We focus on small molecule solvation and binding, mostly in the framework of the equilibrium thermodynamics of dilute solutions. In reality, the cell is crowded, stochastic, chemically open, and out of equilibrium. Nevertheless, this is the most basic and important framework with which to start an analysis of biological ligand binding, not only because it is relevant for the *in vitro* biochemistry that goes on in drug design, but also because the *in vitro* picture very often carries over in a qualitative or quantitative way to the cell.

Many of the concepts presented are general, and can be applied to any macromolecular receptor. However, RNA and DNA have some specific properties as receptors, including a high density of ionic phosphate groups, a corresponding ion cloud, their particular tertiary organization, and the high flexibility of some weakly structured RNAs. These aspects are not detailed; only for proteins do we sometimes go into specifics and detailed examples. This is partly due to space, and partly due to the prime importance of proteins as drug targets until now.

We assume a basic knowledge of molecular modeling and statistical mechanics. When we discuss molecular interactions, we treat the solutes and solvent at about the same level of theory as a molecular mechanics force field, using classical mechanics. We do not develop force field modeling, which is covered in Chapter 2, but we speak of atomic charges, point polarizabilities, van der Waals interactions, and so on. In contrast, we do not have the space or the need to discuss the shape of orbitals, spin states, tunneling, or other quantum effects.

We begin by discussing the definition of the bound state, the concept of chemical potential, and the law of mass action. Next, we discuss contributions to the binding free energy that are specifically associated with the solute degrees of freedom: external rotations/translations and internal vibrations. We then turn to effects associated more specifically with aqueous solvent. To isolate some of the free energy contributions more clearly, we introduce a multistep binding path, where the ligand is first uncharged, then moved into the binding site, and then recharged. This allows us to separate (mostly) the discussion of electrostatic and hydrophobic effects. We also consider the displacement of water molecules from the binding pocket. Next, we discuss the separate enthalpic and entropic components of the binding free energy and their correlation or compensation. Finally, we discuss the role of conformational selection (CS) and induced fit (IF). Closely related topics that are taken up in more detail in later chapters include the many roles of solvent, receptor flexibility, and the kinetics of binding.

1.2 Defining the Bound State

To study receptor/ligand binding theoretically, one must partition the conformational space into "bound" and "unbound" states (Gallicchio and Levy, 2011, Jorgensen et al., 1988). There is no unique way to do this, but in practical situations there is often a natural choice. Thus, conformations where the ligand is within a well-defined binding pocket would be labeled "bound."[*] In some cases, the binding pocket will correspond to a deep energy well, so that ligand conformations near the boundary of the pocket will have high energies and low statistical weights. Thus, they will not contribute much to the thermodynamic properties, such as the binding constant, which will be robust with respect to the exact definition of the pocket (Gallicchio and Levy, 2011). In addition, when the binding of two similar ligands to a receptor is compared, there will be some cancellation of the boundary region contributions of each ligand. Even if two definitions of the binding site volume differ by a factor of two, the two definitions of the binding free energy would typically differ by $kT \log 2$, just 0.4 kcal/mol at room temperature (where kT is the thermal energy). Such a change is not too important for a nanomolar binder at micromolar doses (a few grams in the bloodstream).

When simulations are compared to experiments, the problem is slightly different. The experiments measure a physical signal, such as heat release or optical energy absorption, and we should consider which conformations contribute to the experimental signal and use them as the basis for comparison. The most direct approach is to compute the physical signal directly from a simulation. Signals that can be directly modeled include NMR chemical shifts, pK_a shifts for protonation of a reporter group, fluorescence spectra,

---

[*] Here, a conformation is defined by the positions of all the atoms in the system, including the overall translation and rotation of the ligand relative to the receptor.

shifts in vibrational infrared bands, and so on. If the experimental signal is a local one, like a transfer of magnetization to a specific group in the binding site, then the full range of spectroscopically active conformations can be sampled in a molecular dynamics simulation, albeit with obvious limitations (imperfect force field and sampling). In general, modeling of the physical signal itself is not perfectly accurate, introducing further errors and uncertainty.

Other experimental techniques give a more global signal, like equilibrium dialysis or titration calorimetry. With these signals, minor binding sites can also contribute, including nonspecific sites located on the receptor surface. In theory, *all* the conformations may contribute, even ones where the ligand is separated from the receptor (Mihailescu and Gilson, 2004). Separating the contribution of specific and nonspecific binding modes is not straightforward. In practice, the simulation will (usually) not try to sample all possible conformations, but will focus on one or a few local regions and binding modes, and neglect the others. Furthermore, a signal like heat release usually cannot be modeled directly, and we must adopt a different route, computing the binding free energy for one or a few specific sites. This is the most common approach in free energy simulations. As mentioned, the results will often be robust with respect to the precise delimitation of the binding pocket(s); for more details, see a recent review (Gallicchio and Levy, 2011).

1.3 Chemical Potentials and Mass Action

The thermodynamic quantity that governs binding equilibria in solution is the free energy per molecule, or chemical potential (Fowler and Guggenheim, 1939, Hill, 1962, Landau and Lifschitz, 1980)

$$\mu_X = \frac{\partial G}{\partial n_X} = -kT \frac{\partial \log Q}{\partial n_X} \tag{1.1}$$

where X is a component of the solution (solvent, ligand L, receptor R, or complex RL), G is the Gibbs free energy, Q the partition function, n_X the number of molecules, and kT the thermal energy. We assume for now that X is not ionic. In what follows, we do not distinguish between Gibbs and Helmholtz free energies (NpT vs. NVT ensemble), because they differ by a negligible pV term (about 0.0005 kcal/mol for a volume change corresponding to a single water molecule at atmospheric pressure). If the solution is dilute with respect to X, μ_X has a simple, logarithmic dependence on concentration

$$\mu_X = v_X(p,T) + kT \log \frac{[X]}{[S]} = \mu_X^\circ(p,T) + kT \log \frac{[X]}{[X]^\circ} \tag{1.2}$$

where $[S]$ is the solvent concentration, p is the pressure, v_X is concentration-independent, and the superscript "o" indicates a "standard" reference state, arbitrary except that it must also be dilute (or "ideal-dilute," see below). For the binding free energy, if we choose $[R]^\circ = [L]^\circ = [RL]^\circ \overset{\text{def}}{=} C^\circ$ for simplicity, we have

$$\Delta G = \mu_{RL} - \mu_L - \mu_R = \Delta G^\circ + kT \log \frac{C^\circ [RL]}{[R][L]} \tag{1.3}$$

The concentration dependence arises from the loss of translational entropy upon binding.

In Equation 1.3, the free energy is defined for a peculiar equilibrium state, where the concentrations are held fixed through some kind of constraints. If the constraints are removed, the system relaxes into a more usual equilibrium. Being at a minimum, the free energy is stationary with respect to small fluctuations in the concentrations, like those produced by a single binding event. Therefore, the reaction free energy $\mu_{RL}^{eq} - \mu_L^{eq} - \mu_R^{eq} = 0$, which gives

$$\Delta G^\circ = -kT \log \frac{C^\circ [RL]_{eq}}{[R]_{eq}[L]_{eq}} \overset{\text{def}}{=} -kT \log C^\circ K_{eq}(p, T) \tag{1.4}$$

where K_{eq} is the equilibrium constant. Equation 1.4 is known as the law of mass action. It allows us to convert free energies into concentrations, and vice versa.

It is worth a small additional effort to see just how general are Equations 1.2 through 1.4. A very concise derivation can be found in Section 9.87 of Landau and Lifschitz (1980).* Remarkably, the only assumptions in this derivation are infinite dilution, nonionic solutes, and the validity of classical statistical mechanics. The derivation holds if the solute is not dilute but inter-solute interactions are absent, as in the usual 1 M "ideal-dilute" standard state (Ben Naim, 1973).

Biochemical applications routinely involve ionic ligands and/or receptors, so it is essential to generalize Equations 1.2 through 1.4 to this case. With an ionic solute, the derivation above* breaks down: solute/solute interactions occur at large distances, the environment of any particular solute is no longer uniform, and the free energy $\delta G(n, N)$ depends on the details of the solute positions. Thus, each anion lowers its free energy by preferentially surrounding itself by cations, and vice versa, and this alters the form of the chemical

---

* Suppose we add n molecules of a nonionic solute X to a large collection of N solvent molecules. At very high dilution, the solute molecules do not interact, and the free energy changes from the pure solvent value by $\delta G(n, N) = n\alpha(p, T, N) + kT \log n! \approx nkT \log((n/e)e^{\alpha/kT})$, where α is an unknown function and we use Stirling's approximation for $n!$. The $n!$ term appears because the n solute molecules are indistinguishable, which introduces a factor $1/n!$ into the partition function (Fowler and Guggenheim, 1939). δG must be a first-order homogeneous function of n and N, so that $e^{\alpha/kT}$ has the form $f(p,T)/N$. Taking $\mu_X = \partial \delta G/\partial n$ gives Equation 1.2.

potential. Fortunately, Debye–Hückel theory generalizes Equation 1.2 in a way that is exact in the limit of infinite dilution. A detailed proof is given by Hill (1962) (more general than the original one (Fowler and Guggenheim, 1939)). For monovalent ions in aqueous solution, Debye–Hückel theory is accurately verified for concentrations up to 100 mM or so, close to physiological ionic strength.

For simplicity, we consider a neutral pair of solutes X, Y that form a monovalent 1:1 salt, with $[X] = [Y]$. To generalize the form of μ_X, we add a second concentration term to Equation 1.2

$$\mu_X = \mu_X^\circ(p,T) + kT \log \frac{[X]}{C^\circ} + kT \log \gamma_X([X],p,T) \tag{1.5}$$

and similarly for Y; γ_X is known as the activity coefficient. Debye and Hückel showed that at infinite dilution, γ_X has a very simple concentration dependence

$$kT \log \gamma_X([X],p,T) \sim \frac{q_X^2}{2\varepsilon} \kappa, \quad \text{when } \kappa \to 0 \tag{1.6}$$

where q_X is the charge of X, ε is the solvent dielectric constant, and κ is the ionic strength.

$$\kappa^2 = \frac{4\pi}{kT\varepsilon}(q_X^2 \rho_X + q_Y^2 \rho_Y) \tag{1.7}$$

We have written κ in a general form, not limited to a monovalent salt; ρ_X is the number density of X. Thus, for ionic solutes, there is an additional, square-root, concentration dependence in the chemical potential μ_X. But as the ion concentrations approach 0, the activity coefficients approach 1, so the law of mass action (Equation 1.4) is still rigorously valid in this limit.

The magnitude of activity coefficients at finite ion concentrations can be illustrated by an Mg^{2+}:phosphate^{2-} salt at a concentration of 13.3 mM (one ion of each type in a $50 \times 50 \times 50$ Å^3 simulation box). The Debye–Hückel free energy is $2kT \log \gamma_X = -0.83$ kcal/mol. This is very small compared to the excess chemical potential (or solvation free energy) of each ion, around -400 kcal/mol. While Debye–Hückel theory is only qualitative at physiological ionic strength, it can always be checked or improved by computing chemical potentials directly with rigorous simulations (Lin et al., 2014, Simonson, 2001); for details, see the free energy simulation Chapter 12 in this book or a recent review (Lin et al., 2014). Salt effects in biomolecular solutions are often studied using Poisson–Boltzmann theory, which contains essentially the same physics as Debye–Hückel (Baker, 2004, Hill, 1962). Our goal above was more basic, however, to generalize the law of mass action.

Deviations from the ideal chemical potential and Equation 1.4 occur for both ionic and nonionic solutes when concentrations increase. In the most general situation where two species mix at arbitrary concentrations, the mathematical form of μ_X is very complex, and requires integral equation theories and numerical solutions (Hill, 1962, Roux and Simonson, 1999). Extensive work has been done to develop approximate theories for various situations, such as regular mixtures and polymer solutions (Flory, 1953, Fowler and Guggenheim, 1939). A subject of current interest is cellular crowding and its effect on biomolecular structure, stability, and binding (Dhar et al., 2010, Feig and Sugita, 2012). These topics are (arguably) less relevant to drug design and beyond the scope of this chapter.

We conclude with an obvious comment that in biochemical systems, the solvent is not dilute. Water concentration is close to 55.5 M, and so the ideal form (Equation 1.2) of the chemical potential is invalid. If water is the ligand in a binding reaction, special care is needed (Roux et al., 1996). Choosing a 1 M ideal-dilute standard state for the solvent is not useful. Rather, the usual choice of standard chemical potential for the aqueous solvent is the chemical potential of pure water at the same temperature and pressure (Landau and Lifschitz, 1980), and the standard water/receptor binding free energy is $\Delta G^\circ = -kT \log[RW]_{eq}/[R]_{eq}$. We discuss water binding/release in more detail below.

1.4 Free Energy Contributions Associated with Solute Motions

We noted above that loss of solute translation entropy leads to a distinct, concentration-dependent term in the binding free energy. In fact, the solute partition function and chemical potential contain several contributions associated with its overall translation, which are all independent of the solvent and separable from the other contributions (Fowler and Guggenheim, 1939, Hill, 1962, Tidor and Karplus, 1994). Overall rotation also leads to distinct contributions that are largely independent of the solvent (in the dilute limit). Finally, contributions from intrasolute motions are usually divided into two categories: (i) vibrational terms associated with oscillations within an energy basin and (ii) conformational terms associated with degrees of freedom that have several distinct energy basins (Fowler and Guggenheim, 1939). To simplify the analysis of the free energy contributions associated with solute motions, we first introduce the concept of potential of mean force (PMF) for the solute X.

1.4.1 Integrating Out the Solvent: The PMF

The idea here is to integrate the solvent degrees of freedom out of the partition function, so that we are left with an explicit dependence on the solute structure, but not on the solvent, which contributes implicitly (Roux and Simonson, 1999). This will isolate the solute coordinates more clearly in view of the following analysis. Our rearrangement of the partition function does not require any approximation. Indeed, we can always write the potential energy function U as a function of the solute and solvent coordinate vectors, **X** and **Y**:

$$U(\mathbf{X}, \mathbf{Y}) = U_u(\mathbf{X}) + U_{uv}(\mathbf{X}, \mathbf{Y}) + U_v(\mathbf{Y}) \tag{1.8}$$

X includes the six external translation and rotation coordinates of the solute. The configurational partition function for the whole system then has the form:

$$Q = \int d\mathbf{X} d\mathbf{Y}\, e^{-[U_u(\mathbf{X}) + U_{vv}(\mathbf{Y}) + U_{uv}(\mathbf{X}, \mathbf{Y})]/kT} \stackrel{\text{def}}{=} \int d\mathbf{X}\, e^{-W(\mathbf{X})/kT} \tag{1.9}$$

$W(\mathbf{X})$ is called the potential of mean force, or PMF (Roux and Simonson, 1999). It can be interpreted by noting that $\delta W = W - U_u$ is the free energy to transfer the solute from vacuum into solvent when it is held fixed in the conformation **X**. For a sufficiently dilute, homogeneous, isotropic solution, this free energy is independent of the location we choose within the container (neglecting boundary effects) and the solute orientation, and so W only depends on the internal coordinates of the solute.

The PMF concept by itself does not introduce any approximations, and the partition function Q in Equation 1.9 is still exact, as long as W is the exact PMF. However, it is also common to replace the exact PMF by approximate ones, such as ones provided by dielectric theory or integral equation theory (Roux and Simonson, 1999). These approximate methods are covered in Chapter 9.

1.4.2 Solute Translations and Rotations

To isolate contributions related to solute translation, let $Q_X^{\text{trans}} = (q_X^{\text{trans}})^{n_X} / n_X!$ be the contribution to the partition function that arises from overall translations of the n_X solute molecules, including the $n_X!$ factor for their possible permutations. We have (Fowler and Guggenheim, 1939; Tidor and Karplus, 1994)

$$q_X^{\text{trans}} = \frac{V(2\pi m_X kT)^{3/2}}{h^3} \tag{1.10}$$

$$\mu_X^{\text{trans}} = -kT \frac{\partial \log Q_X^{\text{trans}}}{\partial n_X} = \frac{3}{2}kT - kT\left[\frac{3}{2} + \frac{3}{2}\log\left(\frac{2\pi m_X kT}{h^2}\right) - \log \rho_X\right] \tag{1.11}$$

Here, V is the volume, m_X the solute mass, h Planck's constant, and ρ_X the number density of X. The factor $h(2\pi m_X kT)^{-1/2}$ is the thermal de Broglie wavelength Λ, and so q_X^{trans} is dimensionless. The second term in μ_X^{trans}, within brackets, is the entropic term. It contains the concentration term seen above (Equation 1.2, since $\rho_X \propto [X]$). The first term in μ_X^{trans} is the mean kinetic energy associated with center of mass motion. The solute structure appears only through log m_X, as an entropic contribution (related to the width of its velocity distribution). We emphasize that V is the total volume (Fowler and Guggenheim, 1939, Hill, 1962), not a reduced or "free" volume considered to be "outside" the solvent molecules. Indeed, we just saw that the PMF $W(\mathbf{X})$ does not depend on the solute center of mass coordinates. Therefore, these give rise to the same factor V in the partition function (Equation 1.9) as in the gas phase, independent of the nature or structure of the solvent.

Rotational kinetic energy and entropy are also largely or entirely separable and independent of the solvent. A simple and general model is the "rigid rotor harmonic oscillator" (RRHO) model, where the internal degrees of the solute are assumed to be stiff, so that they vibrate harmonically and are independent of the external rotational degrees of freedom (Finkelstein and Janin, 1989, Fowler and Guggenheim, 1939, Hill, 1962, Tidor and Karplus, 1994). This will be accurately verified for small, rigid solutes and ligands. Even for large (but structured) solutes like folded proteins or RNAs, although the internal motions are by no means harmonic, we can still assume they are roughly separable from the overall rotation. In fact, this assumption is implicit in simulations where the orientation of a solute is restrained (e.g., a protein with some of its atoms tethered by harmonic restraints). Integrating over the three rotational degrees of freedom and their conjugate momenta, we obtain the rotational contribution to the solute partition function and chemical potential (Fowler and Guggenheim, 1939, Hill, 1962, Tidor and Karplus, 1994) as

$$q_X^{rot} = 8\pi^2 \frac{(2\pi kT)^{3/2}}{h^3}(I_1 I_2 I_3)^{1/2} \tag{1.12}$$

$$\mu_X^{rot} = \frac{3}{2}kT - kT\left[\frac{3}{2} + \frac{1}{2}\log(I_1 I_2 I_3) + \log\left(8\pi^2\frac{(2\pi kT)^{3/2}}{h^3}\right) - \log(\sigma)\right] \tag{1.13}$$

where the I_i are the principle moments of inertia of the solute and σ is a symmetry number (=1 if X has no symmetry). The factor $8\pi^2$ comes from the orientational degeneracy of the energy (giving a 4π solid angle and another 2π angle). Again, there is a mean kinetic energy of $kT/2$ for each rotation angle. The solute structure appears only in the entropy, through $\log(I_1 I_2 I_3)$, where the I_i are computed for the mean solute structure. The RRHO model was originally used for the gas phase, but in fact it carries over to dilute solutions, with no additional assumptions. Indeed, in a dilute, isotropic solution, the solvation free energy $\delta W(\mathbf{X})$ (Equation 1.9) does not depend on orientation, and the angular degeneracy of the energy is maintained. Thus, experimental rotational entropies in solution are very close to the gas phase estimates (Mammen et al., 1998; Searle and Williams, 1992). Illustrative values for this and the other terms in Equations 1.11 and 1.13 are given in Table 1.1.

1.4.3 Solute Vibrations and Conformational Changes

The internal solute vibrations contribute a third set of terms. They are usually described with a Gaussian fluctuation model, also known as the quasiharmonic model (Edholm and Berendsen, 1984, Gohlke et al., 2003, Karplus and Kushick, 1981), as it generalizes the normal mode theory of simple, rigid molecules (Wilson et al., 1955). With normal mode theory, the potential energy is assumed to have a single, harmonic well, and the system behaves like a collection of independent harmonic oscillators, whose enthalpy and entropy are known (Fowler and Guggenheim, 1939, Hill, 1962, Tidor and Karplus, 1994). With the quasiharmonic model, we begin without any assumptions about the potential energy surface. We compute the atomic fluctuations from a molecular dynamics simulation, which can use a realistic energy function and solvent environment. Specifically, we compute the atomic displacement covariance matrix C, where $C_{ij} = \langle \delta x_i \delta x_j \rangle$; δx_i represents the displacement of the atomic coordinate x_i from its mean position, and the brackets represent a time average. Only after this do we introduce the assumption that the motions are harmonic. We determine the matrix H of force constants that would lead to the observed covariances, *if* the solute dynamics were harmonic, from the relation (Edholm and Berendsen, 1984, Karplus and Kushick, 1981) $H = kT\,C^{-1}$. Finally, we diagonalize a mass-weighted version of H to obtain the corresponding "quasiharmonic" vibrational modes and their enthalpy and entropy (Baron et al., 2009, Harpole and Sharp, 2011). Notice that for a given variance, the assumption of Gaussian fluctuations is the one that gives the maximum entropy, leading to some amount of systematic bias (Harpole and Sharp, 2011).

A single vibrational mode, of frequency v and treated quantum mechanically, contributes to the partition function and chemical potential according to (Fowler and Guggenheim, 1939, Hill, 1962, Tidor and Karplus, 1994):

$$q_X^{\text{vib}}(v) = \frac{e^{hv/2kT}}{e^{hv/kT} - 1} \tag{1.14}$$

$$\mu_X^{\text{vib}}(v) = \left[\frac{1}{2}hv + \frac{hv}{e^{hv/kT} - 1}\right] - \left[\frac{hv}{e^{hv/kT} - 1} - kT\log(1 - e^{-hv/kT})\right] \tag{1.15}$$

$$\approx kT - kT\left[1 - \log\frac{hv}{kT}\right], \quad \text{when } hv \ll kT \tag{1.16}$$

TABLE 1.1

Entropy and Binding Entropy Contributions for Selected Molecules and Complexes

Reference	System (mass[a])	Transl.	Rotat.	vibr./conf.[b]	Method
Finkelstein and Janin (1989)	Naphthalene (128)	-10.2	-7.8	-3.9	RRHO + experiment
Finkelstein and Janin (1989)	BPTI (6500)	-13.8	-15.0	-600	RRHO + normal modes
Finkelstein and Janin (1989)	BPTI/trypsin[c]	6.9	7.2–9.0	–	Equation 1.22; υ, α guessed
Tidor and Karplus (1994)	Insulin (5990)	-12.8	-14.0	-1561	RRHO + normal modes
Tidor and Karplus (1994)	Insulin/insulin	12.1	13.3	-5.1	RRHO + normal modes
Harpole and Sharp (2011)	Biotin (244)	–	–	-13.2	Equation 1.18 + QH theory
Harpole and Sharp (2011)	Biotin/streptavidin	10.6		2.6[d]	Equation 1.18 + QH theory
Luo and Sharp (2002)	Biotin/streptavidin	4.3	4.2	3.5[d]	Quasiharmonic (QH)
Luo and Sharp (2002)	Inhibitor/FAB (781)	4.3	5.0	0.0	Quasiharmonic
Luo and Sharp (2002)	NMA/NMA (75)	2.4	0.8	1.0[d]	Quasiharmonic
Murray and Verdonk (2002)	Inhibitor/stromelysin (282)	3.4			Fragment joining model
Murray and Verdonk (2002)	Inhibitor/avidin (214)	6.9			Fragment joining model
Murray and Verdonk (2002)	Inhibitor/vancomycin (742)	5.1			Fragment joining model
Fowler and Guggenheim (1939)	10/100 cm^{-1} oscillator			-4.4/-0.3	Normal mode theory
Dunitz (1994)	Water → ice	2.4			Experiment
Dunitz (1994)	Water → inorganic salt	1.4–2.3			Experiment
Huggins et al. (2011)	Water → protein surface	-0.5–2.4			MD + theory

Free energy contributions $-TS$ in kcal/mol. 1 M standard state, room temperature.

a For complexes, we give the molar mass of the smaller partner.

b Vibrational and/or conformational contributions.

c For complexes, we report the contributions to the binding free energy. A positive value opposes binding.

d These values arise from torsion angles that are trapped in a single well upon binding.

The enthalpy and entropy terms in $\mu_X^{vib}(v)$ are given separately, in brackets. The first enthalpy term, $hv/2$, is the zero-point energy. When $hv = kT$, we are in the classical mechanical regime, and the enthalpy becomes kT (half kinetic and half potential energy). At 300 K, we have $kT = 0.596$ kcal/mol $\equiv 208.4$ cm^{-1}. Conversely, for a frequency of 100 cm^{-1} (3.0 ps^{-1}), $hv = 0.286$ kcal/mol $\approx (1/2)$ kT; and the classical form is already quite accurate, giving an entropy term of +1.033 kcal/mol, just 0.006 kcal/mol below the quantum value. When $hv \equiv 10$ cm^{-1} (0.30 ps^{-1}), the entropy term is 4.4 kcal/mol. A small protein in vacuum typically has several hundred normal modes in the range 0–100 cm^{-1} (Simonson and Perahia, 1996; Tidor and Karplus, 1994); however, the quasi-harmonic frequencies in solution are significantly lower (Baron et al., 2009, Gohlke et al., 2003, Harpole and Sharp, 2011, Simonson and Perahia, 1996).

For torsional degrees of freedom with multiple energy wells, the Gaussian or quasiharmonic picture is incorrect. Thus, for ethane, there are three distinct energy wells. While each well can be approximated locally by a parabola, the resulting vibrational partition functions for the three wells should be added up. This adds a term $k \log 3$ to the entropy, and $-kT \log 3 \approx -0.65$ kcal/mol to the free energy, representing a conformational contribution. For a linear saturated hydrocarbon molecule, there will also be three energy wells for each torsion angle, which will still be roughly, though no longer exactly equivalent, giving a −0.65 kcal/mol free energy gain for each successive C–C bond. Deviations from this simple picture arise if the energy wells become more heterogeneous. The torsion angles can also become interdependent, so that the number of effectively independent energy wells is lowered. Several empirical estimates of the entropy term $-TS$ associated with a rotatable bond ranging from −0.4 to −1.1 kcal/mol (Page and Jencks, 1971, Searle and Williams, 1992); empirical scoring functions often use values between −0.3 and −0.7 kcal/mol (Böhm, 1998, Head et al., 1996, Murray and Verdonk, 2002).

To express the contribution of multiple energy wells and conformations formally, it is helpful to integrate out the solvent degrees of freedom, as above (Equation 1.9), and write the free energy or the entropy as an integral over the remaining, $3N$ solute coordinates $\mathbf{X} = (r_1, \ldots, r_N)$:

$$\exp(-\Delta S/k) \propto \int \exp[-\beta W(\mathbf{X})]dr_1 \cdots dr_N \qquad (1.17)$$

Here, ΔS is the excess entropy compared to the pure solvent and $W(\mathbf{X})$ is the PMF for the solute. The integral in Equation 1.17 can be decomposed into a sum over all the solute energy wells that are thought to be significantly populated.

Another way to express the contribution of multiple conformations is obtained by rearranging Equation 1.17 and summing explicitly over the n solute conformations

$$S = \sum_i p_i S_i - k \sum_i p_i \log p_i \qquad (1.18)$$

where p_i is the occupancy of conformation i and S_i is the entropy when the solute is restricted to be in conformation i. In Equation 1.17, $e^{-\Delta S/k}$ is written as a configuration space volume, with each volume element $dr_1 \cdots dr_N$ weighted exponentially by the energy. The more spread out is $e^{-\beta W}$, the larger the entropy. In Equation 1.18, the energy weighting is less obvious but the disorder due to the multiple wells is clearly isolated (the log 3 term for ethane). Real solutes are usually too complex to solve analytically. Nevertheless, the principles above are general, and Equations 1.17 and 1.18 can be a basis to help interpret experiments or simulations.

1.4.4 Contributions to the Binding Free Energy

The effects analyzed above should now be considered in the context of the binding reaction, $L + R \rightarrow RL$, and the standard binding free energy, ΔG°. We consider first the six center of mass translations of $R + L$. Upon binding, they are replaced by three center of mass coordinates of the RL complex, and three internal coordinates. Rewriting the chemical potential μ_X^{trans} (Equation 1.11) in the standard state

$$\mu_X^{trans,\circ} = -kT \log\left[\left(\frac{2\pi m_X kT}{h^2} \right)^{3/2} V^\circ \right] \tag{1.19}$$

we see that the contribution to ΔG° is

$$\Delta G^\circ_{trans} = +kT \log\left[\left(\frac{2\pi m_{red} kT}{h^2} \right)^{3/2} V^\circ \right] \tag{1.20}$$

where $m_{red} = (1/m_L + 1/m_R)^{-1}$ is the reduced mass. If $m_L \ll m_R$, then $m_{red} \approx m_L$; it is as if the lost translations belonged entirely to the ligand. The three lost rotations contribute

$$\Delta G^\circ_{rot} = +kT \log\left[8\pi^2 \frac{(2\pi kT)^{3/2}}{h^3} \left(\frac{I_1^R I_2^R I_3^R I_1^L I_2^L I_3^L}{I_1^{RL} I_2^{RL} I_3^{RL}} \right)^{1/2} \right] \tag{1.21}$$

Upon RL binding, the rotational and translational degrees of freedom are of course not lost completely: rather, they are converted into vibrational degrees of freedom for the RL complex (Finkelstein and Janin, 1989, Hill, 1962, Karplus and Janin, 1999, Tidor and Karplus, 1994). Thus, the thermal energies in Equations 1.11 and 1.13 are present in the complex as normal mode thermal energies (Fowler and Guggenheim, 1939, Tidor and Karplus, 1994), with the same magnitude ($kT/2$ each), and so they do not contribute to

$\Delta G°$. For the lost translation and rotation entropy, there are also compensating terms in the bound state. One approach is to distinguish, within the *RL* complex, the external translations and rotations of the ligand, and view them as roughly separable from the other degrees of freedom. Thus, Finkelstein and Janin proposed that for a bound ligand, the RRHO model could still be applied, but replacing the angular integral $8\pi^2$ and volume $V°$ available to the free ligand in the standard state by an angular integral α^3 and a volume υ available to the bound ligand within its binding site. With this model, the mass- and I_i-dependent terms in ΔG_{trans}, ΔG_{rot} cancel out and we are left with entropy losses upon binding that do not have any explicit dependence on molecular weight (Finkelstein and Janin, 1989, Gallicchio and Levy, 2011, Murray and Verdonk, 2002):

$$\Delta G_{trans}° = -kT \log\left(\frac{\upsilon}{V°}\right); \qquad \Delta G_{rot}° = -kT \log\left(\frac{\alpha^3}{8\pi^2}\right) \tag{1.22}$$

With the 1 M ideal standard state, $V° = 1661 \text{ Å}^3 = (11.84 \text{ Å})^3$. If the bound ligand has residual center of mass motion on the order of 1 Å (benzene bound to a lysozyme mutant (Hermans and Wang, 1997)), the translation entropy penalty for standard state binding is then about 4.4 kcal/mol. This is the same entropy carried by a 10 cm^{-1} harmonic oscillator. With residual ligand rotation of $\alpha = \pi/10$ (benzene/lysozyme (Hermans and Wang, 1997)), the rotation entropy penalty is 4.6 kcal/mol. Residual motions in the same range were found for several protein/ligand complexes (Harpole and Sharp, 2011).

A well-known strategy for ligand design is to reduce entropy in the unbound state by freezing some of the internal degrees of freedom, by cyclization or cross-linking (Page and Jencks, 1971) (which can also increase binding specificity). To be successful, the method should target degrees of freedom that can explore several conformers in the unbound state, but become largely frozen in the bound state. Indeed, such degrees of freedom help stabilize the unbound state entropically, and therefore oppose binding. If their flexibility is eliminated, the binding entropy should become more favorable. At the same time, the chemical modifications should not disrupt the favorable ligand/receptor interactions in the bound state.

An extreme variant of this strategy is to create a single ligand by linking two smaller fragments, which bind to two nearby sites on a receptor, in a "divalent" manner (Shuker et al., 1996). By assembling two fragments into one molecule, the loss of translational entropy is reduced (loss of three, not six coordinates), while the binding interactions of each fragment can hopefully be preserved (Jencks, 1981, Murray and Verdonk, 2002), so that the binding affinity of the single ligand is greater than the sum of the fragment affinities. This strategy is illustrated by several successful examples (Erlanson et al., 2003, Rao et al., 1998, Shuker et al., 1996, Zhou and Gilson, 2009). A detailed analysis of six published examples (Murray and Verdonk, 2002) showed that the unfavorable contribution to binding due to loss of the rigid body entropy was 3.4–6.9 kcal/mol. While this is a large effect, it is smaller than the rigid body free energy in the unbound state, because it includes the compensating effect of residual motions in the bound state.

The tradeoff between motions and entropy in the unbound and bound states is just one example of the compensation effects that occur in ligand binding and design. A related effect is the enthalpy/entropy compensation that occurs when one introduces a strong, new interaction in a receptor/ligand complex, for example, by adding a new polar group. The gain of enthalpy produced by the new interaction can be offset by a loss of entropy, if the new interaction tightens the complex and reduces the extent of bound ligand motion (reduced υ, α in Equation 1.22). Enthalpy/entropy compensation in molecular recognition has been reviewed recently (Baron and McCammon, 2013, Chodera and Mobley, 2013) and is discussed below.

1.5 Aqueous Solvent: Electrostatic Aspects

So far, the solvent has appeared implicitly, through the PMF (W in Equations 1.9, 1.17), where it alters the effective energy surface experienced by the solutes. More explicitly, aqueous solvent plays multiple roles in ligand binding: filling the binding pocket when the ligand is unbound, interacting with both partners in their bound and unbound states, shielding their charges, driving hydrophobic groups together, and competing for counterions and protons. These effects are all related to the polar character of the water molecule and its tendency to form strong hydrogen bonds with polar solutes and other water molecules (Eisenberg and Kauzmann, 1969). The polarity of water can be measured, for example, by its gas phase dipole moment, 1.85 Debyes (increasing to about 2.8 D in solution (Mahoney and Jorgensen, 2000, Ren and Ponder, 2003)), its gas phase dimerization energy, −5.4 kcal/mol, its heat of vaporization, 10.5 kcal/mol, or its static dielectric constant at room temperature and pressure, about 80 (relative to the vacuum permittivity) (Eisenberg and Kauzmann, 1969, Mahoney and Jorgensen, 2000, Ren and Ponder, 2003). The static dielectric constant is one parameter that characterizes water in the context of simple dielectric continuum models (Gilson and Honig, 1988, Knight and Brooks, 2011, Kollman et al., 2000, Simonson, 2007).

To help identify the main solvent effects, we introduce a pathway that decomposes the binding reaction into simpler steps (Gilson and Honig, 1988, Simonson, 2007). We assume the ligand and receptor are each characterized by a set of atomic partial charges, and possibly inducible dipoles (Lopes et al., 2007). Some force field models include permanent dipoles and quadrupoles on the solute atoms (Ponder et al., 2010); for our discussion, these can

Step IV: restore ligand charges

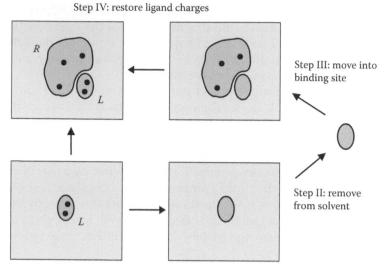

Step III: move into binding site

Step II: remove from solvent

Step I: remove ligand charges

FIGURE 1.1
Multi-step pathway for a ligand *L* binding to a receptor *R*.

be seen as small additional groups of charges (e.g., two for each permanent dipole). In addition, we assume the solute and solvent atoms interact through Lennard-Jones (van der Waals) interactions, as in molecular mechanics models. These ingredients are known to provide a good approximation to the molecular interactions, as detailed in Chapter 2.

We use the pathway shown in Figure 1.1. It starts from the unbound state. Step I switches off the ligand charges; Step II switches off the attractive, dispersion interactions and any inducible dipoles, leaving an empty, ligand-shaped cavity, then removes the cavity from the bulk solvent; Step III reintroduces it in the binding pocket, then reintroduces the dispersion interactions and inducible dipoles. Finally, Step IV reintroduces the ligand permanent charges. Notice that any inducible dipole in the solute has an interaction energy with each solvent molecule that decreases as $1/r^6$ (where r is their separation distance) and is weakly directional. Therefore, we group it in Steps II and III along with the dispersion interactions. We consider first the steps that are primarily electrostatic, I and IV, and we use the concepts of continuum electrostatics as a guide. The other steps are discussed next, in relation to hydrophobic effects (II), or a mixture of effects (III).

1.5.1 Ligand Uncharging in Solution

Step I removes the partial charges q_i originally on each ligand atom. This is equivalent to inserting the opposite charges, $-q_i$, and analogous to other processes where a solute is (un)charged in solution: (de)protonation, or changing the atomic charges to model the transformation of one ligand into another. For small, drug-like solutes, the intrasolute interactions are fairly straightforward to model and compute, and will cancel to a first approximation when we recharge the ligand in Step IV. The solvent behavior is more complex, with two distinct free energy contributions. The solvent is initially organized to interact with any ligand polar groups through hydrogen bonds and longer-range dipole interactions. When we introduce the new charges $-q_i$, they interact with (or "couple to") this "preorganized" solvent; each new, perturbing charge $-q_i$ contributes a term $-q_i \langle V_i \rangle$ to the free energy, where $\langle V_i \rangle$ is the mean electrostatic potential produced by the solvent on atom i when the ligand is fully charged (the initial state). As the new charges are inserted, the solvent adapts or reorganizes, becoming polarized by the new charges; this leads to a second free energy term: the reorganization or relaxation free energy (Aqvist and Hansson, 1996, Hummer et al., 1995, Marcus, 1996, Simonson et al., 1999). Aqueous solvent can be expected to respond to the new charges as a linear medium, to a very good first approximation (Aqvist and Hansson, 1996, Hummer et al., 1995). This means that the reaction field and potential that develop are proportional to the new charges. The corresponding, reorganization free energy then depends quadratically on the perturbing charges (Aqvist and Hansson, 1996, Hummer et al., 1995, Marcus, 1996, Simonson et al., 1999).

In the case of a very small ionic solute, the sodium ion, the electrostatic potential on the ion varies from about −200 kcal/mol/e (8.7 eV) to +9 kcal/mol/e when the ion is uncharged (Lin et al., 2014), for an uncharging free energy of about +94 kcal/mol. While the precise potential and free energy values depend on the simulation method and certain conventions (Hummer et al., 1997, Lin et al., 2014), the trends are general. The assumption of linear solvent response for this case leads to a free energy error of about 4 kcal/mol, or 4%. For protonation of an aspartate sidechain analogue, the free energy is about 60 kcal/mol, and the linear response assumption gives an error of about 3 kcal/mol, or 5% (Lin et al., 2014). The deviations in both cases can be understood as an effect of dielectric saturation: the solvent cannot respond quite as strongly to a large charge as to a small one, so the free energy departs slightly from a quadratic charge dependence.

The behavior above can be understood qualitatively by a dielectric continuum model (Simonson and Brünger, 1994, Sitkoff et al., 1994); see Chapter 9. In particular, viewing the solute as a low dielectric body makes it clear that completely nonpolar groups on the ligand, like methyl substituents, can still have an effect on the charging free energy, by increasing the volume of the low dielectric region and moving high dielectric solvent away from other, polar groups. An example is given by chloride addition on the D ring of the tetracycline antibiotic (Aleksandrov et al., 2009). This makes the ligand less hydrophilic, facilitating its desolvation (see Step II below) and its binding to the Tet repressor protein by 0.8 kcal/mol. However, when the chloride is added next to an amino substituent, it also facilitates desolvation by a second mechanism, reducing the favorable interactions of water with the amino group. This effect was quantified specifically using simulations; it contributes an additional 0.3 kcal/mol to desolvation and binding (Aleksandrov et al., 2009).

After Step I, our ligand is uncharged but may contain polarizable centers and inducible dipoles. The interaction energy between a permanent dipole p, such as water's, and a polarizable particle has the form

$$U(r,\theta) = -\frac{\alpha p^2}{2r^6}(3\cos^2\theta + 1) \tag{1.23}$$

where r is the separation, θ the angle between the water dipole and the separation axis, p the water dipole, and α the polarizability. With $p = 2.8$ D (water), $\alpha = 2.5$ Å^3 (ammonium or methane), r in Å, and averaging over θ, we have $\langle U \rangle_\theta = -353/r^6$ kcal/mol. For $r = 2.9$ Å, $\langle U \rangle_\theta = -0.6$ kcal/mol, the thermal energy, and $U(\theta = 0) - U(\theta = \pi/2) = 1.2 \langle U \rangle_\theta = -0.7$ kcal/mol. Thus, the inducible dipoles weakly favor orientations where the water molecules in the first solvation shell have their dipoles oriented radially, directly toward the solute or directly away from it. The same picture is obtained by viewing the solute as a dielectric body with a dielectric constant that captures its electronic polarizability (around 2, dielectric constant and atomic polarizabilities being related by the Clausius–Mossotti relation (Fröhlich, 1949)).

1.5.2 Ligand Uncharging in the Binding Pocket

Our final Step IV reintroduces the charges onto the ligand within the binding pocket; it is equivalent to discuss the reverse step: ligand uncharging. Compared to the solution Step I, the environment is now heterogeneous, with receptor groups that are more or less polar and rigid, and solvent molecules that may differ in several respects from those in the bulk. For example, their valence electrons may be less polarized, giving a weaker molecular dipole moment, and they may not have as much freedom to reorient in response to nearby charges, like those of the ligand. Nevertheless, the overall picture is similar: the solvent and polar groups on the receptor are initially organized to interact with the ligand's polar groups, generating a mean potential throughout the ligand. When we introduce the canceling charges $-q_i$, each one couples to the mean potential and contributes a term $-q_i \langle V_i \rangle$ to the free energy. In addition, the environment reorganizes in response to the new charges, producing a reaction potential that is at least roughly proportional to the new charges. This gives a reorganization free energy that depends quadratically on the perturbing charges. Again, this behavior is the one that would be predicted by a simple dielectric continuum model. Compared to Step I, a major difference is that the dielectric response in the binding pocket is heterogeneous and anisotropic, with the solvent being more polarizable than the receptor, whether protein or RNA. Another major difference is that the solvent polarization now has an additional effect: it shields and reduces the receptor/ligand electrostatic interactions. The shielding is greater for exposed binding pockets, and smaller for more buried or dryer pockets. Compared to Step I, a third major difference is that the precise polarizability of the receptor is much harder to predict than that of the solvent environment in Step I, and will vary from one receptor to another (Archontis et al., 2001, Schutz and Warshel, 2001, Simonson, 2003, Simonson and Perahia, 1995). This is reflected by the range of solute dielectric constant(s) used in continuum models (Kollman et al., 2000, Simonson, 2007).

1.6 Aqueous Solvent: Nonpolar or Hydrophobic Effects

Our binding pathway (Figure 1.1) includes a step to form or delete a cavity in water (Step II), which we discuss in the general context of hydrophobic effects. This is a broad and complex area, studied for decades (Ben-Naim, 1980, Chandler, 2005, Chothia, 1974, Pratt and Pohorille, 2002, Tanford, 1980). It has benefited in recent years from theoretical breakthroughs and the increasing capabilities of computer simulations (Chandler, 2005, Gallicchio et al., 2000, Hummer et al., 1996, Lum et al., 1999, Pratt and Pohorille, 2002, Rajamani et al., 2005, Raschke et al., 2001). Nonpolar groups like alkanes form interactions with water molecules that are much weaker than water/ water interactions, and so the two do not readily mix at room temperature. This leads to a water-mediated clustering of hydrophobic groups. For example, solvent contributes about −0.5 kcal/mol to the association free energy of two methanes in water at their optimal separation of about 4 Å, at room temperature (Jorgensen et al., 1988, Sobolewski et al., 2007). However, the details depend strongly on the size and shape of the nonpolar solute or, more generally, of the water/hydrophobe interface. Thus, interfaces of a few nanometer square behave differently from small alkanes in water, which differ from small water clusters in a liquid alkane (Rasaiah et al., 2008).

For a small alkane molecule at room temperature and pressure, transfer into water from a less polar, nonassociated liquid like heptane or cyclohexane is associated with three effects that are considered a signature: the standard transfer free energy is unfavorable (Figure 1.2), there is an entropy penalty, and a large increase in heat capacity. In the solvent, the water molecules lining the solute have fewer hydrogen-bonding partners; this does not actually lead to a net loss of hydrogen bonds for small solutes; rather, the water molecules rearrange slightly to "straddle" the solute and form hydrogen bonds around it (Sobolewski et al., 2007). The reduced number of such hydrogen-bonding arrangements leads to the entropy penalty. Such water-cage structures around the solute, although highly dynamic and by no means rigid, are

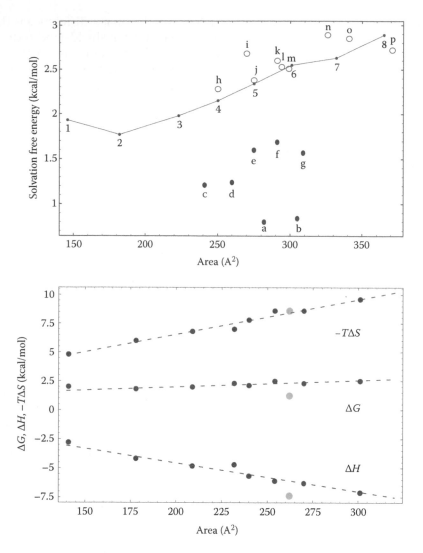

FIGURE 1.2

Top: Vapor to water transfer free energies for saturated hydrocarbons as a function of accessible surface area. (From A. Ben-Naim and Y. Marcus. 1984. *J. Chem. Phys.*, 81:2016–2027.). Standard states are 1 M ideal gas and solution phases. Linear alkanes (small dots) are labeled by the number of carbons. Cyclic compounds (large dots) are: a = cyclooctane, b = cycloheptane, c = cyclopentane, d = cyclohexane, e = methylcyclopentane, f = methylcyclohexane, g = *cis*-1,2-dimethylcyclohexane. Branched compounds (circles) are: h = isobutane, i = neopentane, j = isopentane, k = neohexane, l = isohexane, m = 3-methylpentane, n = 2,4-dimethylpentane, o = isooctane, p = 2,2,5-tri-methylhexane. *Bottom:* Transfer free energies, enthalpies and entropies for a subset of the molecules, both linear (black dots) and cyclic (cyclohexane, gray dots). (From E. Gallicchio, M. M. Kubo, and R. M. Levy. 2000. *J. Phys. Chem. B*, 104:6271–6285.). Dashed lines are linear fits, excluding methane and cyclohexane.

reminiscent of the old iceberg model of Frank and Evans (1945). In contrast, for a large water/hydrophobe interface, above 1 nm^2, the qualitative behavior is different: the mean number of hydrogen bonds is reduced for the interface waters (by almost 1), there is dewetting of the hydrophobic surface, the free energy penalty to form the interface is dominated by enthalpy, and the interfacial entropy is actually positive (favorable) (Ashbaugh, 2009, Chandler, 2005, Rajamani et al., 2005).

The cavity Step II in our binding pathway is closely analogous to the transfer of a nonpolar molecule, not from hexane or heptane, but from the gas phase. Within Step II, we can distinguish further the formation of an empty cavity, and the insertion of the attractive dispersion interactions. These two steps have been studied separately (Chandler, 2005, Gallicchio et al., 2000, Hummer et al., 1996, Pratt and Pohorille, 2002). The free energy to form an empty cavity measures the probability for the cavity to appear transiently through a spontaneous fluctuation in the solvent (Chandler, 2005, Hummer et al., 1996, Pratt and Pohorille, 2002), which becomes less likely as the cavity size increases. For cavities shaped like alkanes with 2–8 carbons, this free energy scales approximately with the surface area. More generally, Mobley et al. showed recently that for 504 small, neutral, organic molecules, the cavity free energy scales accurately with surface area (Mobley et al., 2009). The contribution of the dispersion interactions is also highly correlated with surface area, but the sum of the two is much smaller, and does not correlate as well with surface area, as illustrated by the solvation free energy differences between linear and cyclic alkanes (Gallicchio et al., 2000, Simonson and Brünger, 1994).

Another very general contribution to the cavity free energy is the so-called excluded volume effect: it is entropically unfavorable to exclude solvent molecules from a cavity volume. Lee and colleagues (1985, 1991) pointed out that this entropic penalty also contributes to solute aggregation and is especially large when the solvent molecules are small, like water molecules. Indeed, for a small solvent, the volume exclusion affects a greater number of solvent molecules and thus more degrees of freedom. The magnitude of this contribution to the hydrophobic effect has been controversial, but it appears to be significantly smaller than the more "classic" effect described above: the entropy reduction due to restrictions on the hydrogen bond network close to a water/hydrophobe interface (Lazaridis, 2001).

The cavity and dispersion contributions to our cavity Step II are dominated, respectively, by entropy and enthalpy. Thus, the free energy to solvate small alkanes arises from large and compensating enthalpic and entropic contributions, which both scale approximately with the surface area (Gallicchio et al., 2000) (Figure 1.2). The compensation is highlighted by the proportionality coefficients γ between the surface area and the transfer-free energies for vapor $\rightarrow$ water and cyclohexane $\rightarrow$ water transfer, which are very different: $\gamma_{v \rightarrow w} \approx 6$ cal/mol/Å^2 and $\gamma_{c \rightarrow w} \approx 25$ cal/mol/Å^2 (Gallicchio et al., 2000, Simonson and Brünger, 1994). These coefficients can be seen as atomic surface tensions. The $\gamma_{v \rightarrow w}$ value is smaller, because the unfavorable transfer entropy is counterbalanced by the favorable solute/solvent dispersion interactions. In contrast, for cyclohexane → water transfer, the dispersion interactions roughly cancel out between the two endpoints and one is left with the bare entropic penalty. Thus, for Step II overall, the entropic cost to form the empty cavity is largely (though not entirely!) compensated by a strengthening of the water/water interactions and especially by establishing the attractive solute/solvent dispersion interactions. The net effect is an entropic penalty for hydrophobic solvation. We expect that these alkane trends carry over to the artificially uncharged, ligand-shaped "molecules" that we produce in Step I of our pathway, as verified for the 504 solutes of Mobley et al. (2009).

A peculiarity of our multistep pathway is that it assigns a hydrophobic contribution to polar substituents, like the tetracycline D ring amino group, mentioned above. Indeed, once the ligand is uncharged, all its groups contribute to the hydrophobic Step II, including the ones that were originally polar. However, the hydrophobic contribution from an amino or hydroxyl group is expected to be significantly smaller than its total, predominantly electrostatic contribution. Thus, hydroxyl groups added to several tetracycline positions contributed about 2.5 kcal/mol overall to the ligand-binding free energy, mainly through an electrostatic effect (Aleksandrov et al., 2009).

In many applications, we are interested in comparing one or more pairs (L, L') of similar ligands, like the modified tetracyclines. Suppose L' has an additional hydrophobic group, a methyl, say. The analysis above allows us to estimate its a priori effect on solvation and binding: roughly proportional to its surface area. Indeed, to apply the analysis above, we can extend our pathway: uncharge each ligand, remove it to vacuum, then recharge it. If necessary, we can move each ligand into a binding site by doing analogous steps in reverse, to obtain a binding free energy difference $\Delta\Delta G$.

There are obviously other, simpler pathways for ligand desolvation and binding. One is to desolvate each ligand without uncharging it. Another is to change L into L' directly and alchemically, both in solution and in the binding site, as is common with MD simulations (Aleksandrov et al., 2010, Jorgensen, 2003). All these methods would give the same free energy result, $\Delta\Delta G$, yielding the same measure of a methyl substituent's effect on solvation and/or binding. However, the multistep pathway assigns a (small) hydrophobic contribution to the polar substituents as well, whereas the more direct pathways do not (Boresch et al., 1994). This is a choice of convention that should be kept in mind but does not change the physics of binding. In the same way, more detailed, semiempirical models have been extensively developed for small molecule solvation (Almlof et al., 2007, Cramer and Truhlar, 2008, Ferrara et al., 2004, Knight and Brooks III, 2011, Liu et al., 2010), as well as fully empirical, QSAR models (Duffy and Jorgensen, 2000, Oliferenko et al., 2009). The most successful models confirm the importance of size, shape, and substituent polarity for solvation, but characterize them through somewhat different parameters and free energy components.

1.7 Aqueous Solvent: Displacing Water from the Binding Pocket

Step III in our binding pathway is the formation of a ligand-shaped cavity in the binding pocket, complete with dispersion interactions and possibly inducible dipoles. Water molecules that initially occupied the pocket are expelled into bulk solvent. In fact, displacing waters from binding sites has emerged as a general strategy for ligand optimization (Barillari et al., 2007, Ladbury, 1996, Lam et al., 1994, Michel et al., 2009, Yang et al., 2013). Water displacement has several effects. First, the receptor groups (respectively, ligand groups) in the pocket form van der Waals interactions with the ligand (receptor) atoms instead of with solvent, while the displaced waters now form van der Waals interactions with other waters. There will be significant cancellation for this exchange, whose extent will vary depending on the receptor/ligand contacts. For protein/ligand complexes with very good steric complementarity, the van der Waals interactions in the complex will more than offset those in the unbound state, since the density of nonhydrogen atoms in a protein is higher than in solvent ($1/18 \, \text{Å}^{-3}$ vs. $1/30 \, \text{Å}^{-3}$; Michael Schaefer, personal communication). This aspect is not discussed further. Second, instead of high dielectric water, the ligand volume in the pocket is now filled with a low dielectric, nonpolar, ligand analogue, modifying the electric field and potential. Third, the waters from the pocket are expelled into the bulk, where they experience a more polar and less confined environment. We discuss first the effect on the electrostatic interactions in the pocket; next, we discuss the effects on the expelled waters. All these aspects are covered in more detail in Chapter 9.

1.7.1 Cavity Formation in the Binding Pocket: Electrostatic Aspects

In Step III, we open up a ligand-shaped cavity in the binding pocket. This has two important effects on the receptor/solvent and receptor/receptor electrostatic interactions. First, it removes solvent from the polar groups lining the pocket, giving a desolvation free energy that will increase with the size of the ligand cavity. Second, the solvent removed from the pocket is no longer available to shield the electrostatic interactions *within* the receptor. Thus, intrareceptor salt bridges or hydrogen bonds close to the ligand will typically be strengthened. Both these effects can be quantified using simulations. They can be readily estimated with a continuum model, although their magnitude will depend on model parameters, especially the receptor dielectric constant. For example, when a cavity shaped like aspartate was opened up in the binding site of aspartyl-tRNA synthetase and some of its mutants, the free energy increase was between 1 and 7 kcal/mol, depending on the mutant (using a protein *and* a cavity dielectric constant of 4); individual ionized sidechains in the binding pocket incurred desolvation penalties of about 1–3 kcal/mol (Archontis et al., 2001). The reduced dielectric shielding of the interactions between these sidechains changed the free energy by a smaller amount, about −0.5 kcal/mol (respectively, +0.5 kcal/mol) for a pair with opposite (equal) signs. For a larger ligand cavity, these effects would be somewhat larger.

1.7.2 Cavity Formation in the Binding Pocket: Displacing Water

A strongly bound water molecule can be seen as a "ligand." Extending a lead compound to fill the water's position and displace it into the bulk is then roughly analogous to the merging of two ligands into one (Michel et al., 2009). Merging or linking ligands that bind to neighboring positions is usually done in the hope of reducing the entropic cost of binding, as discussed above. In the bulk, water has a 55.5 M concentration; its chemical potential does not obey the dilute form (Equation 1.2), and there is no simple way to separate its entropy into translation and rotation components. However, the total standard solution entropy of liquid water is known experimentally: 16.7 cal/mol/K at 298 K (Dunitz, 1994). That of ice at its freezing temperature is 9.9 cal/mol/K. In hydrated inorganic salts like $ZnSO_4$ or $MgCl_2$, each water contributes an amount similar to ice, around 9–12 cal/mol/K (Dunitz, 1994). Thus, the entropy gain for transfer of a highly ordered crystal water into bulk solution is about 8 cal/mol/K at most, for a maximum free energy gain of about 2.4 kcal/mol. Notice that the liquid phase entropy is much smaller than the gas phase value: for liquid → gas transfer under standard conditions, $-T\Delta S_{l\to g}^{\circ} = -3.7$ kcal/mol (Baron et al., 2008, Ben-Naim and Marcus, 1984) (while $\Delta H_{l\to g}^{\circ} = +10$ kcal/mol and $\Delta G_{l\to g}^{\circ} = +6.3$ kcal/mol).

Binding entropies in the same range, 0–2.4 kcal/mol were obtained recently for nine hydration sites at the surface of a protein (plus one negative value, −0.5 kcal/mol) (Huggins et al., 2011), using simulations and the approximate Inhomogeneous Fluid Solvation Theory of Lazaridis (Lazaridis, 1998, Li and Lazaridis, 2006). A value of 2.9 kcal/mol was obtained for a completely buried water in HIV protease (Li and Lazaridis, 2003, 2006). All these examples hopefully represent the most typical entropy range associated with displacing ordered waters from a binding pocket. In general, we expect that the waters close to hydrophobic or ionic sites, or those in a very narrow binding pocket will be near the top of the range, while water molecules close to neutral polar groups, or in more open pockets will be nearer the bottom.

Finally, displacing waters from a completely buried, polar or nonpolar cavity within a protein represents an interesting special case (Baron et al., 2008, Collins et al., 2005, Rasaiah et al., 2008, Yin et al., 2010, Young et al., 2010). The equilibrium concentration of water in nonpolar solvents is low (another form of the hydrophobic effect): one water molecule per $(100 \text{ Å})^3$ for cyclohexane in equilibrium with water vapor (Wolfenden and Radzicka, 1994). In a similar way, nonpolar cavities in proteins can be partly or completely dry, and therefore provide a preformed cavity for ligand binding.

1.8 Enthalpy, Entropy, and Their Compensation

Although the binding free energy determines the equilibrium binding constant, its separate enthalpic and entropic components provide important additional information. Together, the binding free energy, enthalpy, and entropy are sometimes referred to as the thermodynamic signature of binding. When optimizing a ligand, a rule of thumb is that "binding opposes motion": we may introduce groups to form new interactions, only to find that the gain in binding enthalpy is erased because the new complex is tighter and has a lower entropy (Lafont et al., 2007). This is an example of enthalpy/entropy compensation, a general issue for ligand design (Baron and McCammon, 2013, Chodera and Mobley, 2013, Dunitz, 1995, Gallicchio and Levy, 1998, Gilli et al., 1994, Olsson et al., 2011, Sharp, 2001). We refer to it as H/S compensation. For biochemical binding reactions, the measured enthalpy and entropy are usually larger than the free energy, which implies a certain level of compensation. A question is whether the observed compensation is due to measurement errors, whether it is real but due to the limited experimental window (only small $\Delta\Delta G$ values can be measured) (Chodera and Mobley, 2013), or whether it is a general feature of biochemical solutes and aqueous solvent, or of noncovalent binding in general.

Dunitz pointed out that biochemical reactions are usually not too far from equilibrium; they are often reversible, and have a significant bound population at biological concentrations. This means that the reaction free energy is not far from zero, which corresponds to perfect H/S cancellation (Dunitz, 1995). The experimental binding free energy range is illustrated by the BindingDB database (Liu et al., 2007), which contains data for over 0.6 million protein/ligand complexes. They include natural complexes and also many engineered ligands or inhibitors, which are typically designed to have high affinities. The subset of data from isothermal titration calorimetry (ITC) has standard binding free energies mostly in the range from 0 to –15 kcal/mol. IC50 values and inhibition constants span comparable ranges (Gohlke and Klebe, 2002, Liu et al., 2007). This is much less than the range of binding enthalpies and entropies. For example, a large subset of the BindingDB ITC data spanned a ΔG range of 15, whereas ΔH and $-T\Delta S$ spanned ranges about 3 times larger, over 45 kcal/mol (Chodera and Mobley, 2013, Olsson et al., 2011).

Several authors have pointed out that experimental binding enthalpies and entropies can have correlated errors, particularly values deduced from van t'Hoff plots (Chodera and Mobley, 2013, Olsson et al., 2011); this leads to H/S values that appear to be compensating. Random errors, combined with a limited affinity range, can also lead to the appearance of H/S compensation (Chodera and Mobley, 2013, Olsson et al., 2011, Sharp, 2001). In general, ΔH and ΔS are derivatives of ΔG and are usually obtained with lower precision. Thus, experimental H/S components and reports of compensation should be viewed with caution. Nevertheless, for the BindingDB ITC dataset, statistical analysis showed that random errors could not fully explain the apparent H/S compensation, and a significant, genuine compensation is present (Olsson et al., 2011). For 674 ligand modifications and 32 proteins, 68% were compensated to more than 10% (i.e., enthalpy cancels over 10% of the entropy and vice versa); 22% were compensated to more than 80%. This was double the apparent compensation expected from random errors. The H/S correlation was similar to a model created with an intrinsic correlation of −0.91. H/S reinforcement was rare. Here, the compensation was characterized for series of ligands binding to a single protein, which reduces the effect of the random errors (Olsson et al., 2011), compared to pooling the proteins together.

Several physical mechanisms have been proposed to explain H/S compensation, including some already discussed above. The simplest idea is that a deeper energy well, for an RL complex, will also be narrower, leading to reduced vibrational entropy (Dunitz, 1995, Ford, 2005). As a toy model that roughly mimics weak gas phase associations, we might assume the bound system has one or two energy wells, with harmonic vibrations in each well. With this model, H/S compensation occurs if the force constant within the lowest energy well increases with well depth (Ford, 2005). While this may be true for specific systems, such a correlation between well depth and well width is not obvious in general.

A second idea is that H/S compensation is mediated by solvent. Jencks, and Lumry and Rajender have suggested compensation was a fundamental property of processes occurring in water (Jencks, 1986, Lumry and Rajender, 1970). Indeed, we saw above that solvation of a nonpolar solute leads to a form of strong compensation, with waters near the solute forming new and slightly stronger hydrogen bonds among themselves, to replace the ones lost due to the solute volume. Toy models have been studied where each water molecule can exchange between states with different numbers of hydrogen bonds, and a formal connection to H/S compensation was made (Grunwald and Steel, 1995, Lee and Graziano, 1996). A related, and very general quantity that characterizes the tradeoff between solvent/solute and solvent/solvent interactions is the solvent reorganization energy: the change in the solvent/solvent interaction energy when the solute is introduced. Yu and Karplus showed that for a dilute solution, the solvent reorganization energy contributes to the solvation energy and entropy, but cancels out of the free energy (Yu and Karplus, 1988). This leads to H/S compensation for solvation, but also for RL binding (since the binding in solution can be carried out by desolvating R and L separately, binding in the gas phase, then resolvating the complex; the reorganization terms for the solvation processes will all cancel out from the binding free energy). Another very general analysis was done by Qian and Hopfield (1996), who considered an arbitrary change in the energy function, which leads to enthalpy and entropy changes ΔH and ΔS. They identified a term that appears in ΔH and exactly cancels the entropy term $-T\Delta S$. These sources of compensation are valid for any solute and solvent. Although they are too general to give specific guidelines, they point ways for further analyses of specific systems (Gallicchio and Levy, 1998), for example by computing reorganization energies from simulations or theories like Inhomogeneous Fluid Solvation Theory (Lazaridis, 1998).

1.9 Conformational Selection and Induced Fit

Before any discussion of fluctuations and dynamics, it is a good idea to recall that proteins and large, structured RNAs fold into specific structures that are preorganized for function. To appreciate the importance of preorganization for processes like enzyme catalysis or electron transfer, one can compare the structures of oxidized and reduced cytochrome c, for example (rms difference of just 0.4 Å), or the magnitude of dielectric relaxation in an enzyme active site (rather limited) vs. aqueous solvent ($\approx$10 times greater) (Archontis et al., 2001). Indeed, a certain active site rigidity is needed to establish a free energy difference between transition state and ground state binding (Robertson, 2005), the essence of enzyme catalysis. Thus, the old lock-and-key paradigm for binding is still a good pedagogical approximation.

Of course, real locks fluctuate (on molecular length scales), and so do biomolecules. Thus, ligand binding is always accompanied by some amount of intramolecular rearrangement of the partners. These rearrangements can be small or large; they can affect the bound/unbound endpoints and/or the binding pathway and kinetics. Thus, in the very first protein crystal structures, hemoglobin and myoglobin, the need for structural fluctuations was evident for oxygen to reach its binding site: access is "gated" by protein fluctuations (Case and Karplus, 1979). The rearrangements upon ligand binding can be structural shifts, like loop or domain closure, or they can take the form of disorder/order transitions, like loop or sidechain ordering. Another possibility is the rearrangement of protonation states associated with ligand binding (Onufriev and Alexov, 2013). While proton binding is perhaps not exactly a conformational rearrangement, it can certainly be viewed as a "structural" rearrangement, since it modifies the solute charge distribution. Ligand-induced proton binding and release are the main source of the pH-dependence of the binding affinity, whose importance is strikingly illustrated by the Bohr effect in hemoglobin (Perutz, 1990) and by pH-induced viral uncoating (Chiu et al., 1997).

In recent years, structural rearrangements upon binding have usually been discussed in terms of "induced fit" (IF) or "conformational selection" (CS) (Baron and McCammon, 2013, Boehr et al., 2009, Grant et al., 2010, Zavodsky and Hajdu, 2012). With IF (Koshland, 1958), the receptor rearranges *after* the ligand has become partly or fully bound. With CS, the rearrangements occur before binding, and the ligand simply selects a conformation that preexisted—albeit with a low occupancy, and pins it in place. CS was proposed as a mechanism for hemoglobin as early as 1965, as part of the Monod–Wyman–Changeux theory (Changeux, 2012, Szabo and Karplus, 1972) and, independently, by Eigen and Straub (Zavodsky and Hajdu, 2012). In statistical physics, the concept is distinctly older: the "fluctuation-dissipation" theorem shows that the response of a system to a perturbation (such as ligand binding) can be understood from its fluctuations in the absence of the perturbation (Landau and Lifschitz, 1980). This is the basis of linear response theory, which is widely used in biochemistry, for example, for protein electrostatics and ligand binding (Aqvist et al., 2002, Levy et al., 1991, Simonson, 2013, Simonson et al., 2002).

The IF and CS limits correspond to two different pathways for the binding reaction, which interconnect identical endpoints, as schematized in Figure 1.3. Which picture, if any, is most correct depends on which pathway is most commonly followed, and this can be quantified by defining a flux along each pathway (Hammes et al., 2009). In some cases, IF is an obvious requirement, because receptor groups have to move after the ligand binds (loop closure) (Sullivan and Holyoak, 2008); in others, kinetic measurements can rule out IF (Cai and Zhou, 2011, Vogt and Di Cera, 2012, 2013). CS was shown to be compatible with a wider range of kinetic behaviors, and thus harder to rule out (Vogt and Di Cera, 2012, 2013). However, both CS and IF are simplified models. In general, the binding reaction is more complex, with a series of conformational rearrangements occurring, some before and some after binding. The most general framework for these effects is to consider the full set of conformations available to each partner, and the redistribution of occupancies that occurs along the binding reaction path. Equivalently, one can consider the way in which each partner alters the energy landscape of the other as they come together (Cai and Zhou, 2011). In general, there can be an ensemble of pathways that carry a significant flux (Hammes et al., 2009, Karplus, 2000, Khavrutskii et al., 2009, Yang et al., 2009), and each of them can have a CS or IF character or both. Thus, it is not surprising that several

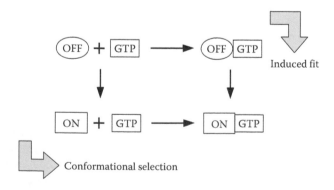

FIGURE 1.3
Induced fit vs. conformational selection. The ligand here is GTP and the receptor can be in an "OFF" or "ON" conformation.

systems have been described as displaying both CS and IF (Bucher et al., 2011, Peters and de Groot, 2012, Wlodarski and Zagrovic, 2009).

Notice that above, we used a different, multistep pathway (Figure 1.1), not to discuss the binding kinetics but to decompose the binding free energy into simpler components. Although this is not the kinetically realistic pathway, it should include the same structural rearrangements between the bound/unbound states. They can occur at different points along our pathway. For example, the receptor undergoes dielectric relaxation in response to the ligand charges (step IV); with a continuum electrostatic description, the solutes' relaxation would be determined by their shape and dielectric constants and take the form of induced charge and polarization (Baker, 2004). The receptor can also rearrange when the van der Waals interactions between ligands are introduced (Step III). For example, nearby sidechains or nucleic acid bases can become ordered. Overall, the multistep pathway imposes a specific order of events, which is chosen for convenience in the free energy decomposition, and does not imply that CS or IF is more relevant kinetically for any given system.

1.10 Allostery and Linkage

An essential requirement in the cell is to combine and process information from multiple channels, building up networks for signaling, energy transduction, or metabolism. This means that many biomolecules must bind more than one partner, sometimes sequentially (e.g., the respiratory chain) but often simultaneously and cooperatively (Perutz, 1990, Szabo and Karplus, 1972, Wyman and Gill, 1990). Crosstalk between two ligands that bind the same biomolecule is referred to either as linkage (Wyman and Gill, 1990) or allostery, a term coined by Jacques Monod 50 years ago (Changeux, 2012). "Allo-" refers to the case where the ligands are not in close contact, but communicate over a certain distance. The most common mechanism for allostery is for one ligand to select or induce a conformational change that affects a second, distant binding site. A classic example is hemoglobin, where oxygen binding changes the heme structure, and leads to a shift in helix packing and overall tertiary structure (Changeux, 2012, Perutz, 1990). Another example is the induction of gene regulators like the Tet repressor, which binds tetracycline 20 Å away from the protein/DNA interface, triggering the pendulum motion of a long helix and DNA unbinding (Aleksandrov et al., 2008, Orth et al., 2000). Finally, GTPases and ATPases commonly change from an inactive (or OFF) to an active (ON) conformation in response to GTP/ATP binding, where the ON conformation is competent to bind a second, downstream partner (Levinson et al., 2006, Myasnikov et al., 2005, Vetter and Wittinghofer, 2001).

When two ligands X, Y bind to different sites on the same receptor R, linkage occurs if they influence each other's binding constant. It manifests itself when we compare the free energies $\Delta G(X)$, $\Delta G(Y)$ to bind each ligand separately and the free energy $\Delta G(X, Y)$ to bind them simultaneously. If the difference $\Delta G_{XY} = \Delta G(X, Y) - \Delta G(X) - \Delta G(Y)$ is nonzero, there is linkage, or coupling between the ligands. A negative ΔG_{XY} (respectively, positive) indicates cooperative (anticooperative) binding. Linkage can be "homotropic" (X and Y are the same species) or heterotropic (X and Y are different species). ΔG_{XY} is also the free energy for the reaction $XR + YR \leftrightharpoons R + XRY$. A negative value means the system favors the right-hand state, $R + XRY$. If the X, Y binding sites are nearby, linkage can arise from their direct interactions (two protons binding to a diacid, for example). But cooperativity and linkage between distant sites—allostery—is of course common, without any direct X–Y interaction. The mathematical treatment is usually developed for the special case of a symmetrical receptor where the binding sites on different subunits are independent (Perutz, 1990, Wyman and Gill, 1990). Cooperativity is found to arise whenever there are two conformations (R and T, say), with different binding affinities for one or both ligands: $\Delta G_R(X) \neq \Delta G_T(X)$ and/or $\Delta G_R(Y) \neq \Delta G_T(Y)$ (Perutz, 1990, Wyman and Gill, 1990). X and Y can be as small as two oxygen molecules targeting hemoglobin, or they can be as complex as a tRNA and a ribosomal subunit, brought together by a translational GTPase (Johnson, 2009).

Allostery is of particular interest for drug design, since it implies that more than one site can be targeted for inhibitor or antagonist binding. What is more, the existence of a large, delocalized, conformational transition implies that still other sites can be targeted, to block the transition and trap the system, either in its initial conformation or in an intermediate conformation along the transition path. This includes sites that form transiently during the transition; such transient sites have been successfully targeted in a few cases and represent CS by an inhibitor (Berneman et al., 2013, Laine et al., 2010, Lee and Craik, 2009, Tzeng and Kalodimos, 2013). Conformational trapping of kinases and ATPases/GTPases in an inactive, OFF state is an established therapeutic strategy (Johnson, 2009, Liu and Gray, 2006, Weisberg et al., 2007). For this reason, we conclude by discussing briefly ligand binding by a kinase or ATPase, as an example of issues that can arise with CS (Hauryliuk et al., 2008, Simonson and Satpati, 2012).

We consider a protein K that can switch between two conformations, called ON and OFF, with two ligands that compete for the same binding site. For a kinase or ATPase, we can assume the ligands are ATP and ADP (referred to jointly as ANP); the ON but not the OFF conformation is active for binding a second partner, and ATP has a greater tendency than ADP to stabilize the ON conformation and activate K. We characterize the ATP preference of each state by the binding free energy differences: $\Delta\Delta G_{ON} = \Delta G_{ON}(ATP) - \Delta G_{ON}$ (ADP), and similarly for OFF. We characterize the ligand preference of each state by the free energy differences: $\Delta\Delta G_{ATP} = \Delta G_{ATP}(ON) - \Delta G_{ATP}(OFF)$, and similarly for ADP. The overall specificity can be characterized by the triple free energy difference

$$\Delta\Delta\Delta G = \Delta\Delta G_{ATP} - \Delta\Delta G_{ADP} = \Delta\Delta G_{ON} - \Delta\Delta G_{OFF} \leq 0 \qquad (1.24)$$

$\Delta\Delta\Delta G$ is negative by definition of the ON/OFF states; a large magnitude indicates a large ATPase specificity. For example, if ON and OFF both have large preferences for their respective nucleotides, $\Delta\Delta G_{ON}$ is large and negative, while $\Delta\Delta G_{OFF}$ is large and positive, so that $\Delta\Delta\Delta G$ is large and negative. Notice however that $\Delta\Delta G_{ON}$ and $\Delta\Delta G_{OFF}$ can sometimes have the same sign; such ATPases are considered "non-classical" (Hauryliuk et al., 2008). For example, both states may prefer to bind ATP, as long as $\Delta\Delta\Delta G \leq 0$.

We can express the overall ATP/ADP binding free energy difference $\Delta\Delta G_{bind} = \Delta G_{bind}(ATP) - \Delta G_{bind}(ADP)$ as a function of the values above. Denoting $G(ON{:}ANP)$, $G(OFF{:}ANP)$ the free energies of the ON/OFF complexes, we have (Simonson, 2001)

$$e^{-\beta\Delta G_{bind}(ANP)} = \frac{e^{-\beta G(ON:ANP)} + e^{-\beta G(OFF:ANP)}}{e^{-\beta G(ON)} + e^{-\beta G(OFF)}} e^{\beta G(ANP)} \qquad (1.25)$$

$$e^{-\beta\Delta\Delta G_{bind}} = e^{-\beta\Delta\Delta G_{ON}} \frac{e^{-\beta x(ATP)} + 1}{e^{-\beta x(ADP)} + 1} = e^{-\beta\Delta\Delta G_{OFF}} \frac{e^{+\beta x(ATP)} + 1}{e^{+\beta x(ADP)} + 1} \qquad (1.26)$$

where $x(ANP) = G(ON{:}ANP) - G(OFF{:}ANP)$. Noticing that $x(ATP) - x(ADP) = \Delta\Delta\Delta G \leq 0$, we see that $\Delta\Delta G_{bind}$ is intermediate between the ON and OFF values:

$$\Delta\Delta G_{ON} \leq \Delta\Delta G_{bind} \leq \Delta\Delta G_{OFF} \qquad (1.27)$$

The complexity of this formalism and the many free energies involved underline the care that is needed in applications and the difficulty of an exhaustive analysis of any given kinase, whether computational or experimental. The complexity increases further if we consider multiple phosphorylation states, one or more inhibitors, and binding to more than one kinase. Indeed, an essential issue is inhibitor promiscuity, cross-binding to any target paralogues, and the resulting side effects. One important route is to engineer inhibitors that act by stabilizing the inactive kinase conformation, like the anticancer drug imatinib (Liu and Gray, 2006). In this case, different ON/OFF populations for different kinases will produce binding specificity. Binding specificity for a particular kinase K, compared to another kinase K′, will be achieved if the free energies of the OFF states are sufficiently different, even if the inhibitor binding sites are conserved and make the same contacts (Aleksandrov and Simonson, 2010). The inhibitor will bind preferentially to the kinase with the most stable OFF conformation, say K. Interestingly, the K/K′ binding free energy difference will actually report on the ON/OFF free energy difference in apo-K′ (and different inhibitors will report the same value) (Aleksandrov and Simonson, 2010).

1.11 Conclusions

It is an exciting time to study molecular recognition and ligand design. Computers and simulation models have reached the point where small proteins can be folded in the computer and ligands can bind and unbind spontaneously in a timeframe accessible to simulations (Borhani and Shaw, 2012, Karplus and McCammon, 2002, Lindorff-Larsen et al., 2011, Shan et al., 2011). Thus, computer-aided design can now rely on a spectrum of methods that range from simple empirical models all the way up to detailed simulations with chemical accuracy. Synergy between experiment and simulations is more important than ever. At the same time, theoretical concepts and models are essential to interpret both simulations and experiments, and to understand them in a way that is firmly grounded in fundamental physical principles. We have recalled some of those principles above, through a combination of basic thermodynamics, toy models, simple experimental model systems, and selected examples of biomolecules. The references were necessarily incomplete, but hopefully point the way to many classic books and papers and many specialized analyses for further study. We leave it to our colleagues of the subsequent chapters to do the rest.

Acknowledgments

I am grateful to Michael Schaefer (Novartis) and Georgios Archontis (University of Cyprus) for careful reading and comments, and to Benoit Roux (University of Chicago) for insightful discussion.

References

A. Aleksandrov and T. Simonson. 2010. Molecular dynamics simulations show that conformational selection governs the binding preferences of imatinib for several tyrosine kinases. *J. Biol. Chem.*, 285:13807–13815.

A. Aleksandrov, L. Schuldt, W. Hinrichs, and T. Simonson. 2008. Tet repressor induction by tetracycline: A molecular dynamics, continuum electrostatics, and crystallographic study. *J. Mol. Biol.*, 378:896–910.

A. Aleksandrov, L. Schuldt, W. Hinrichs, and T. Simonson. 2009. Tetracycline–Tet Repressor binding specificity: Insights from experiments and simulations. *Biophys. J.*, 97:2829–2838.

A. Aleksandrov, D. Thompson, and T. Simonson. 2010. Alchemical free energy simulations for biological complexes: Powerful but temperamental... *J. Mol. Recognit.*, 23:117–127.

M. Almlof, J. Carlsson, and J. Aqvist. 2007. Improving the accuracy of the linear interaction energy method for solvation free energies. *J. Chem. Theory Comput.*, 3:2162–2175.

J. Aqvist and T. Hansson. 1996. On the validity of electrostatic linear response in polar solvents. *J. Phys. Chem.*, 100:9512–9521.

J. Aqvist, V. B. Luzhkov, and B. O. Brandsdal. 2002. Ligand binding affinities from MD simulations. *Acc. Chem. Res.*, 35:358–365.

G. Archontis, T. Simonson, and M. Karplus. 2001. Binding free energies and free energy components from molecular dynamics and Poisson–Boltzmann calculations. Application to amino acid recognition by aspartyl-tRNA synthetase. *J. Mol. Biol.*, 306:307–327.

H. S. Ashbaugh. 2009. Entropy crossover from molecular to macroscopic cavity hydration. *Chem. Phys. Lett.*, 477:109–111.

N. A. Baker. 2004. Poisson–Boltzmann methods for biomolecular electrostatics. *Methods Enzym.*, 383:94.

C. Barillari, J. Taylor, R. Viner, and J. W. Essex. 2007. Classification of water molecules in protein binding sites. *J. Am. Chem. Soc.*, 129:2577–2587.

R. Baron and J. A. McCammon. 2013. Molecular recognition and ligand association. *Ann. Rev. Phys. Chem.*, 64:151–175.

R. Baron, P. Setny, and J. A. McCammon. 2008. Hydrophobic association and volume-confined water molecules. In H. Gohlke, editor, *Protein–Ligand Interactions*, pp. 145–170. Academic Press, New York.

R. Baron, P. H. Hünenberger, and J. A. McCammon. 2009. Absolute single-molecule entropies from quasi-harmonic analysis of microsecond molecular dynamics: Correction terms and convergence properties. *J. Chem. Theory Comput.*, 5:3150–3160.

A. Ben-Naim. 1973. Standard thermodynamics of transfer. Uses and misuses. *J. Phys. Chem.*, 82:792–803.

A. Ben-Naim. 1980. *Hydrophobic Interactions*. Plenum Press, New York.

A. Ben-Naim and Y. Marcus. 1984. Solvation thermodynamics of nonionic solutes. *J. Chem. Phys.*, 81:2016–2027.

A. Berneman, L. Montout, S. Goyard, N. Chamond, A. Cosson, S. d'Archivio et al. 2013. Combined approaches for drug design points the way to novel proline racemase inhibitor candidates to fight Chagas' disease. *PLoS One*, 8:e60955.

D. D. Boehr, R. Nussinov, and P. E. Wright. 2009. The role of conformational ensembles in biomolecular recognition. *Nat. Chem. Biol.*, 5:789–796.

H. J. Böhm. 1998. Prediction of binding constants of protein ligands: A fast method for the prioritization of hits obtained from *de novo* design or 3D database search programs. *J. Comp. Aided Mol. Des.*, 12:309–323.

H. J. Böhm and G. Schneider. 2003. *Protein–Ligand Interactions: From Molecular Recognition to Drug Design*. Wiley-VCH, Weinheim, Germany.

S. Boresch, G. Archontis, and M. Karplus. 1994. Free energy simulations: The meaning of the individual contributions from a component analysis. *Proteins*, 20:25–33.

D. W. Borhani and D. E. Shaw. 2012. The future of molecular dynamics simulations in drug discovery. *J. Comp. Aided Mol. Des.*, 26:15–26.

D. Bucher, B. J. Grant, and J. A. McCammon. 2011. Induced fit or conformational selection and mechanism underlie specificity in noncovalent interactions with ubiquitin? The role of the semi-closed state in the maltose binding protein. *Biochemistry*, 50:10530–10539.

L. Cai and H. X. Zhou. 2011. Theory and simulation on the kinetics of protein-ligand binding coupled to conformational change. *J. Chem. Phys.*, 134:105101.

D. A. Case and M. Karplus. 1979. Dynamics of ligand binding to heme proteins. *J. Mol. Biol.*, 132:343–368.

D. Chandler. 2005. Interfaces and the driving force of hydrophobic assembly. *Nature*, 437:640–647.

J. P. Changeux. 2012. Allostery and the Monod–Wyman–Changeux model after 50 years. *Ann. Rev. Biochem.*, 41:103–133.

W. Chiu, R. M. Burnett, and R. L. Garcea. 1997. *Structural Biology of Viruses*. Oxford University Press, Oxford.

J. D. Chodera and D. L. Mobley. 2013. Entropy–enthalpy compensation: Role and ramifications in biomolecular ligand recognition and design. *Ann. Rev. Biochem.*, 42:121–142.

C. Chothia. 1974. Hydrophobic bonding and accessible surface area in proteins. *Nature*, 248:338–339.

M. D. Collins, G. Hummer, M. L. Quillin, B. W. Matthews, and S. M. Gruner. 2005. Cooperative water filling of a nonpolar protein cavity observed by high-pressure crystallography and simulation. *Proc. Natl. Acad. Sci. USA*, 102:16668–16671.

C. J. Cramer and D. G. Truhlar. 2008. A universal approach to solvation modeling. *Acc. Chem. Res.*, 41:760–768.

A. Dhar, A. Samiotakis, S. Ebbinghaus, L. Nienhaus, D. Homouz, M. Gruebele, and M. S. Cheung. 2010. Structure, function, and folding of phosphoglycerate kinase are strongly perturbed by macromolecular crowding. *Proc. Natl. Acad. Sci. USA*, 107:17586–17591.

E. Duffy and W. L. Jorgensen. 2000. Prediction of properties from simulations: Free energies of solvation in hexadecane, octanol, and water. *J. Am. Chem. Soc.*, 122:2878–2888.

J. D. Dunitz. 1994. The entropic cost of bound water in crystals and biomolecules. *Science*, 264:670.

J. D. Dunitz. 1995. Win some, lose some: Enthalpy–entropy compensation in weak intermolecular interactions. *Curr. Biol.*, 2:709–712.

O. Edholm and H. Berendsen. 1984. Entropy estimation from simulations of non-diffusive systems. *Mol. Phys.*, 51:1011–1020.

D. Eisenberg and W. Kauzmann. 1969. *The Structure and Properties of Water*. Clarendon Press, Oxford.

D. A. Erlanson, J. W. Lam, C. Wiesmann, T. N. Luong, R. L. Simmons, W. L. DeLano et al. 2003. *In situ* assembly of enzyme inhibitors using extended tethering. *Nat. Biotech.*, 21:308–314.

M. Feig and Y. Sugita. 2012. Variable interactions between protein crowders and biomolecular solutes are important in understanding cellular crowding. *J. Phys. Chem. B*, 116:599–605.

P. Ferrara, H. Gohlke, D. J. Price, G. Klebe, and C. L. Brooks. 2004. Assessing scoring functions for protein–ligand interactions. *J. Med. Chem.*, 47:3032–3047.

A. Fersht. 1999. *Structure and Mechanism in Protein Science: A Guide to Enzyme Catalysis and Protein Folding.* Freeman, New York.

A. V. Finkelstein and J. Janin. 1989. The price of lost freedom: Entropy of bimolecular complex formation. *Prot. Eng.*, 3:1–3.

P. J. Flory. 1953. *Principles of Polymer Chemistry.* Cornell University Press, Ithaca, New York.

D. M. Ford. 2005. Enthalpy–entropy compensation is not a general feature of weak association. *J. Am. Chem. Soc.*, 127:16167–16170.

R. H. Fowler and E. A. Guggenheim. 1939. *Statistical Thermodynamics.* Cambridge University Press, Cambridge, United Kingdom.

H. Frank and M. Evans. 1945. Free volume and entropy in condensed systems III. Entropy in binary liquid mixtures; partial molal entropy in dilute solutions; structure and thermodynamics in aqueous electrolytes. *J. Chem. Phys.*, 13:507–532.

H. Fröhlich. 1949. *Theory of Dielectrics.* Clarendon Press, Oxford.

E. Gallicchio and R. M. Levy. 1998. Entropy–enthalpy compensation in solvation and ligand binding revisited. *J. Am. Chem. Soc.*, 120:4526–4527.

E. Gallicchio and R. M. Levy. 2011. Recent theoretical and computational advances for modeling protein-ligand binding affinities. *Adv. Prot. Chem. Struct. Biol.*, 85:27–80.

E. Gallicchio, M. M. Kubo, and R. M. Levy. 2000. Enthalpy–entropy and cavity decomposition of alkane hydration free energies: Numerical results and implications for theories of hydrophobic hydration. *J. Phys. Chem. B*, 104:6271–6285.

P. Gilli, V. Ferretti, G. Gilli, and P. A. Borea. 1994. Enthalpy–entropy compensation in drug-receptor binding. *J. Phys. Chem.*, 98:1515–1518.

M. Gilson and B. Honig. 1988. Calculation of the total electrostatic energy of a macromolecular system: Solvation energies, binding energies, and conformational analysis. *Proteins*, 4:7–18.

H. Gohlke. 2012. *Protein–Ligand Interactions.* Wiley-VCH, Weinheim, Germany.

H. Gohlke and G. Klebe. 2002. Approaches to the description and prediction of the binding affinity of small molecule ligands to macromolecular receptors. *Ang. Chem. Int. Ed.*, 41:2645–2676.

H. Gohlke, C. Kiel, and D. A. Case. 2003. Insight into protein–protein binding by binding free energy calculation and free energy decomposition for the Ras–Raf and Ras–RalGDS complexes. *J. Mol. Biol.*, 330:891–913.

B. J. Grant, A. A. Gorfe, and J. A. McCammon. 2010. Large conformational changes in proteins: Signalling and other functions. *Curr. Opin. Struct. Biol.*, 20:142–147.

E. Grunwald and C. Steel. 1995. Solvent reorganization and thermodynamic enthalpy–entropy compensation. *J. Am. Chem. Soc.*, 117:5687–5692.

G. G. Hammes, Y. C. Chang, and T. G. Oas. 2009. Conformational selection or induced fit: A flux description of reaction mechanism. *Proc. Natl. Acad. Sci. USA*, 106:13,737–13,741.

K. W. Harpole and K. A. Sharp. 2011. Calculation of configurational entropy with a Boltzmann-quasiharmonic model: The origin of high-affinity protein–ligand binding. *J. Phys. Chem. B*, 115:9461–9472.

V. Hauryliuk, S. Hansson, and M. Ehrenberg. 2008. Cofactor dependent conformational switching of GTPases. *Biophys. J.*, 95:1704–1715.

R. D. Head, M. L. Smythe, T. I. Oprea, C. L. Waller, S. M. Green, and G. R. Marshall. 1996. Validate: A new method for the receptor-based prediction of binding affinities of novel ligands. *J. Am. Chem. Soc.*, 118:3959–3969.

J. Hermans and L. Wang. 1997. Inclusion of loss of translational and rotational freedom in theoretical estimates of free energies of binding. Application to a complex of benzene and mutant T4 lysozyme. *J. Am. Chem. Soc.*, 119:2702–2714.

T. Hill. 1962. *Introduction to Statistical Thermodynamics*. Addison-Wesley, Reading, Massachusetts.

D. J. Huggins, M. Marsh, and M. C. Payne. 2011. Thermodynamic properties of water molecules at a protein–ligand interaction surface. *J. Chem. Theory Comput.*, 7:3514–3522.

G. Hummer, L. Pratt, and A. Garcia. 1995. Hydration free energy of water. *J. Phys. Chem.*, 99: 14188–14194.

G. Hummer, S. Garde, A. E. Garcia, A. Pohorille, and L. R. Pratt. 1996. An information theory model of hydrophobic interactions. *Proc. Natl. Acad. Sci. USA*, 93:8951–8955.

G. Hummer, L. Pratt, A. Garcia, B. J. Berne, and S. W. Rick. 1997. Electrostatic potentials and free energies of solvation of polar and charged molecules. *J. Phys. Chem. B*, 101:3017–3020.

J. Israelachvili. 1992. *Intermolecular and Surface Forces*. Academic Press, London.

G. A. Jeffrey. 1997. *An Introduction to Hydrogen Bonding*. Oxford University Press, London.

W. P. Jencks. 1981. On the attribution and additivity of binding free energies. *Proc. Natl. Acad. Sci. USA*, 78:4046–4050.

W. P. Jencks. 1986. *Catalysis in Chemistry and Enzymology*. Dover, New York.

L. N. Johnson. 2009. Protein kinase inhibitors: Contributions from structure to clinical compounds. *Quart. Rev. Biophys.*, 42:1–40.

W. Jorgensen, K. Buckner, S. Boudon, and J. Tirado-Rives. 1988. Efficient computation of absolute free energies of binding by computer simulations. Application to the methane dimer in water. *J. Chem. Phys.*, 89:3742–3746.

W. L. Jorgensen. 2003. The many roles of computation in drug discovery. *Science*, 303:1813–1818.

M. Karplus. 2000. Aspects of protein reaction dynamics: Deviations from simple behavior. *J. Phys. Chem. B*, 104:11–27.

M. Karplus and J. Janin. 1999. Comment on 'the entropy cost of protein association'. *Prot. Eng.*, 12:185–186.

M. Karplus and J. N. Kushick. 1981. Method for estimating the configurational entropy of macro-molecules. *Macromolecules*, 14:325–332.

M. Karplus and J. A. McCammon. 2002. Molecular dynamics simulations of biomolecules. *Nat. Struct. Mol. Biol.*, 9:646–651.

I. V. Khavrutskii, B. Grant, S. S. Taylor, and J. A. McCammon. 2009. A transition path ensemble study reveals a linchpin role for Mg^{2+} during rate-limiting ADP release from protein kinase A. *Biochemistry*, 48:11532–11545.

J. L. Knight and C. L. Brooks III. 2011. Surveying implicit solvent models for estimating small molecule absolute hydration energies. *J. Comput. Chem.*, 32:2909–2922.

P. A. Kollman, I. Massova, C. Reyes, B. Kuhn, S. Huo, L. Chong et al. 2000. Calculating structures and free energies of complex molecules: Combining molecular mechanics and continuum models. *Acc. Chem. Res.*, 33:889–897.

D. E. Koshland. 1958. Application of a theory of enzyme specificity to protein synthesis. *Proc. Natl. Acad. Sci. USA*, 44:98–104.

J. E. Ladbury. 1996. Just add water! The effect of water on the specificity of protein–ligand binding sites and its potential application to drug design. *Chem. Biol.*, 3:973–980.

V. Lafont, A. A. Armstrong, H. Ohtaka, Y. Kiso, L. M. Amzel, and E. Freire. 2007. Compensating enthalpic and entropic changes hinder binding affinity optimization. *Chem. Biol. Drug Des.*, 69:413–422.

E. Laine, C. Goncalves, J. C. Karst, A. Lesnard, S. Rault, W. Tang et al. 2010. Use of allostery to identify inhibitors of calmodulin-induced activation of Bacillus anthracis edema factor. *Proc. Natl. Acad. Sci. USA*, 107:11,277–11,282.

P. Y. S. Lam, P. K. Jadhav, C. J. Eyermann, C. N. Hodge, Y. Ru, L. T. Bacheler et al. 1994. Rational design of potent, bioavailable, nonpeptide cyclic ureas as HIV protease inhibitors. *Science*, 263:380–384.

L. Landau and E. Lifschitz. 1980. *Statistical Mechanics*. Pergamon Press, New York.

T. Lazaridis. 1998. Inhomogeneous fluid approach to solvation thermodynamics. 1. Theory. *J. Phys. Chem. B*, 102:3531–3541.

T. Lazaridis. 2001. Solvent size vs cohesive energy as the origin of hydrophobicity. *Acc. Chem. Res.*, 34:931–937.

B. K. Lee. 1985. The physical origin of the low solubility of nonpolar solutes in water. *Biopolymers*, 24:813–823.

B. K. Lee. 1991. Solvent reorganization contribution to the transfer thermodynamics of small nonpolar molecules. *Biopolymers*, 31:993–1008.

B. K. Lee and G. Graziano. 1996. A two-state model of hydrophobic hydration that produces compensating enthalpy and entropy changes. *J. Am. Chem. Soc.*, 118:5163–5168.

G. M. Lee and C. S. Craik. 2009. Trapping moving targets with small molecules. *Science*, 324:213–215.

N. M. Levinson, O. Kuchment, K. Shen, M. A. Young, M. Koldobskiy, M. Karplus et al. 2006. A Src-like inactive conformation in the Abl tyrosine kinase domain. *PLoS Biol.*, 4:753–767.

R. Levy, M. Belhadj, and D. Kitchen. 1991. Gaussian fluctuation formula for electrostatic free energy changes. *J. Chem. Phys.*, 95:3627–3633.

Z. Li and T. Lazaridis. 2003. Thermodynamic contributions of the ordered water molecule in HIV-1 protease. *J. Am. Chem. Soc.*, 125:6636–6637.

Z. Li and T. Lazaridis. 2006. Thermodynamics of buried water clusters at a protein-ligand binding interface. *J. Phys. Chem. B*, 110:1464–1475.

Y. L. Lin, A. Aleksandrov, T. Simonson, and B. Roux. 2014. Electrostatic free energy computations for solutions and proteins. *J. Chem. Theory Comput.*, 10:2690–2709.

K. Lindorff-Larsen, S. Piana, R. O. Dror, and D. E. Shaw. 2011. How fast-folding proteins fold. *Science*, 334:517–520.

J. Liu, C. P. Kelly, A. C. Goren, A. V. Marenich, C. J. Cramer, D. G. Truhlar, and C. G. Zhan. 2010. Free energies of solvation with surface, volume, and local electrostatic effects and atomic surface tensions to represent the first solvation shell. *J. Chem. Theory Comput.*, 6:1109–1117.

T. Liu, Y. Lin, X. Wen, R. N. Jorissen, and M. K. Gilson. 2007. BindingDB: A web-accessible database of experimentally determined protein–ligand binding affinities. *Nucl. Acids Res.*, 35:D198–201.

Y. Liu and N. S. Gray. 2006. Rational design of inhibitors that bind to inactive kinase conformations. *Nat. Chem. Biol.*, 2:358–364.

P. E. M. Lopes, G. Lamoureux, B. Roux, and A. D. MacKerell Jr. 2007. Polarizable empirical force field for aromatic compounds based on the classical Drude oscillator. *J. Phys. Chem. B*, 111:2873–2885.

K. Lum, D. Chandler, and J. D. Weeks. 1999. Hydrophobicity at small and large length scales. *J. Phys. Chem. B*, 103:4570–4577.

R. Lumry and S. Rajender. 1970. Enthalpy–entropy compensation phenomena in water solutions of proteins and small molecules: A ubiquitous property of water. *Biopolymers*, 9:1125–1127.

H. Luo and K. A. Sharp. 2002. On the calculation of absolute macromolecular binding free energies. *Proc. Natl. Acad. Sci. USA*, 99:10399–10404.

M. W. Mahoney and W. L. Jorgensen. 2000. A five-site model for liquid water and the reproduction of the density anomaly by rigid, non-polarizable potential functions. *J. Chem. Phys.*, 112:8910–8922.

M. Mammen, E. I. Shakhnovich, J. M. Deutch, and G. M. Whitesides. 1998. Estimating the entropic cost of self-assembly of multiparticle hydrogen-bonded aggregates based on the cyanuric acid-melamine lattice. *J. Org. Chem.*, 63:3821–3830.

R. Marcus. 1996. Electron transfer reactions in chemistry: Theory and experiment. In D. S. Bendall, editor, *Protein Electron Transfer*, pp. 249–272. BIOS Scientific Publishers, Oxford.

J. Michel, J. Tirado-Rives, and W. L. Jorgensen. 2009. Energetics of displacing water molecules from protein binding sites: Consequences for ligand optimization. *J. Am. Chem. Soc.*, 131:15403–15411.

M. Mihailescu and M. K. Gilson. 2004. On the theory of noncovalent binding. *Biophys. J.*, 87:23–36.

D. L. Mobley, C. I. Bayly, M. D. Cooper, M. R. Shirts, and K. A. Dill. 2009. Small molecule hydration free energies in explicit solvent: An extensive test of fixed-charge atomistic simulations. *J. Chem. Theory Comput.*, 5:350–358.

C. W. Murray and M. L. Verdonk. 2002. The consequences of translational and rotational entropy lost by small molecules upon binding to proteins. *J. Comp. Aided Mol. Des.*, 16:741–753.

A. G. Myasnikov, S. Marzi, A. Simonetti, A. M. Giuliodori, C. O Gualerzi, G. Yusupova et al. 2005. Conformational transition of initiation factor 2 from the GTP- to GDP-bound state visualized on the ribosome. *Nat. Struct. Mol. Biol.*, 12:1145–1149.

P. V. Oliferenko, A. A. Oliferenko, G. Poda, V. A. Palyulin, N. S. Zefirov, and A. R. Katritzky. 2009. New developments in hydrogen bonding acidity and basicity of small organic molecules for the prediction of physical and ADMET properties. Part 2. The universal solvation equation. *J Chem. Inf. Model.*, 49:634–646.

T. S. G. Olsson, J. E. Ladbury, W. R. Pitt, and M. A. Williams. 2011. Extent of enthalpy–entropy compensation in protein–ligand interactions. *Prot. Sci.*, 20:1607–1618.

A. V. Onufriev and E. Alexov. 2013. Protonation and pK changes in protein-ligand binding. *Quart. Rev. Biophys.*, 46:181–209.

P. Orth, D. Schnappinger, W. Hillen, W. Saenger, and W. Hinrichs. 2000. Structural basis of gene regulation by the tetracycline inducible Tet repressor-operator system. *Nat. Struct. Mol. Biol.*, 7:215–219.

M. I. Page and W. P. Jencks. 1971. Entropic contributions to rate accelerations in enzymic and intramolecular reactions and the chelate effect. *Proc. Natl. Acad. Sci. USA*, 68:1678–1683.

T. Pawson. 1995. Protein modules and signalling networks. *Nature*, 373:573–580.

M. Perutz. 1990. *Mechanisms of Cooperativity and Allosteric Regulation in Proteins.* Cambridge University Press, Cambridge.

J. H. Peters and B. L. de Groot. 2012. Ubiquitin dynamics in complexes reveal molecular recognition mechanisms beyond induced fit and conformational. *PLoS Comp. Biol.*, 8:e1002704.

J. W. Ponder, C. J. Wu, P. Y. Ren, V. S. Pande, J. D. Chodera, M. J. Schnieders et al. 2010. The current status of the AMOEBA polarizable force field. *J. Phys. Chem. B*, 114:2549–2564.

L. R. Pratt and A. Pohorille. 2002. Hydrophobic effects and modeling of biophysical aqueous solution interfaces. *Chem. Rev.*, 102:2671–2691.

H. Qian and J. J. Hopfield. 1996. Entropy–enthalpy compensation: Perturbation and relaxation in thermodynamic systems. *J. Chem. Phys.*, 105:9292–9298.

S. Rajamani, T. M. Truskett, and S. Garde. 2005. Hydrophobic hydration from large to small length-scales: Understanding and manipulating the crossover. *Proc. Natl. Acad. Sci. USA*, 102:9475–9480.

J. Rao, J. Lahiri, L. Isaacs, R. M. Weis, and G. M. Whitesides. 1998. A trivalent system from vancomycin: D-Ala–D-Ala with higher affinity than avidin–biotin. *Science*, 280:708–711.

J. C. Rasaiah, S. Garde, and G. Hummer. 2008. Water in nonpolar confinement: From nanotubes to proteins and beyond. *Ann. Rev. Phys. Chem.*, 59:713–740.

T. M. Raschke, J. Tsai, and M. Levitt. 2001. Quantification of the hydrophobic interaction by simulations of the aggregation of small hydrophobic solutes in water. *Proc. Natl. Acad. Sci. USA*, 98:5965–5969.

P. Ren and J. Ponder. 2003. Polarizable atomic multipole water model for molecular mechanics simulation. *J. Phys. Chem. B*, 107:5933–5947.

J. G. Robertson. 2005. Mechanistic basis of enzyme-targeted drugs. *Biochemistry*, 44:5561–5571.

B. Roux and T. Simonson. 1999. Implicit solvent models. *Biophys. Chem.*, 78:1–20.

B. Roux, M. Nina, R. Pomes, and J. Smith. 1996. Thermodynamic stability of water molecules in the Bacteriorhodopsin proton channel: A molecular dynamics and free energy perturbation study. *Biophys. J.*, 71:670–681.

W. Saenger. 1984. *Principles of Nucleic Acid Structure.* Springer, New York.

C. N. Schutz and A Warshel. 2001. What are the dielectric 'constants' of proteins and how to validate electrostatic models? *Proteins*, 44:400–417.

M. S. Searle and D. H. Williams. 1992. The cost of conformational order: Entropy changes in molecular associations. *J. Am. Chem. Soc.*, 114:10690–10697.

Y. Shan, E. Kim, M. P. Eastwood, R. O. Dror, M. A. Seeliger, and D. E. Shaw. 2011. How does a drug molecule find its target binding site? *J. Am. Chem. Soc.*, 133:9181–9183.

K. A. Sharp. 2001. Entropy–enthalpy compensation: Fact or artefact? *Prot. Sci.*, 10:661–667.

S. B. Shuker, P. J. Hajduk, R. P. Meadows, and S. W. Fesik. 1996. Discovering high-affinity ligands for proteins: SAR by NMR. *Science*, 274:1531–1534.

T. Simonson. 2001. Free energy calculations. In O. Becker, A. D. Mackerell Jr., B. Roux, and M. Watanabe, editors, *Computational Biochemistry & Biophysics*, chapter 9. Marcel Dekker, New York.

T. Simonson. 2003. Electrostatics and dynamics of proteins. *Rep. Progr. Phys.*, 66:737–787.

T. Simonson. 2007. Free energy calculations: Approximate methods for biological macromolecules. In C. Chipot and A. Pohorille, editors, *Free Energy Calculations: Theory and Applications in Chemistry and Biology*, chapter 12. Springer, New York.

T. Simonson. 2013. Protein:ligand recognition: Simple models for electrostatic effects. *Curr. Pharma. Des.*, 19:4241–4256.

T. Simonson and A. T. Brünger. 1994. Solvation free energies estimated from macroscopic continuum theory: An accuracy assessment. *J. Phys. Chem.*, 98:4683–4694.

T. Simonson and D. Perahia. 1995. Internal and interfacial dielectric properties of cytochrome c from molecular dynamics simulations in aqueous solution. *Proc. Natl. Acad. Sci. USA*, 92:1082–1086.

T. Simonson and D. Perahia. 1996. Charge screening in proteins: A molecular dynamics study of cytochrome c. *Farad. Disc.*, 103:71–90.

T. Simonson and P. Satpati. 2012. Nucleotide recognition by the initiation factor aIF5B: Free energy simulations of a neo-classical GTPase. *Proteins*, 80:2742–2757.

T. Simonson, G. Archontis, and M. Karplus. 1999. A Poisson–Boltzmann study of charge insertion in an enzyme active site: The effect of dielectric relaxation. *J. Phys. Chem. B*, 103:6142–6156.

T. Simonson, G. Archontis, and M. Karplus. 2002. Free energy simulations come of age: The protein–ligand recognition problem. *Acc. Chem. Res.*, 35:430–437.

D. Sitkoff, K. Sharp, and B. Honig. 1994. Accurate calculation of hydration free energies using macroscopic solvent models. *J. Phys. Chem.*, 98:1978–1988.

E. Sobolewski, M. Makowski, C. Czaplewski, A. Liwo, S. Oldziej, and H. A. Scheraga. 2007. Potential of mean force of hydrophobic association: Dependence on solute size. *J. Phys. Chem. B*, 111:10765–10774.

S. M. Sullivan and T. Holyoak. 2008. Enzymes with gate-lidded active sites must operate by an induced fit mechanism instead of conformational selection. *Proc. Natl. Acad. Sci. USA*, 105:13829–13834.

A. Szabo and M. Karplus. 1972. Mathematical model for structure-function relations in hemoglobin. *J. Mol. Biol.*, 72:163–197.

C. Tanford. 1980. *The Hydrophobic Effect*. John Wiley and Sons, New York.

B. Tidor and M. Karplus. 1994. The contribution of vibrational entropy to molecular association: The dimerization of insulin. *J. Mol. Biol.*, 238:405–414.

S.-R. Tzeng and C. G. Kalodimos. 2013. Allosteric inhibition through suppression of transient conformational states. *Nat. Chem. Biol.*, 9:462.

I. R. Vetter and A. Wittinghofer. 2001. The guanine nucleotide-binding switch in three dimensions. *Science*, 294:1299–1304.

A. D. Vogt and E. Di Cera. 2012. Conformational selection or induced fit? A critical appraisal of the kinetic mechanism. *Biochemistry*, 51:5894–5902.

A. D. Vogt and E. Di Cera. 2013. Conformational selection is a dominant mechanism of ligand binding. *Biochemistry*, 52:5723–5729.

E. Weisberg, P. W. Manley, S. W. Cowan-Jacob, A. Hochhaus, and J. D. Griffith. 2007. Second generation inhibitors of BCR-ABL for the treatment of imatinib-resistant chronic myeloid leukemia. *Nat. Rev. Cancer*, 7:345–357.

E. B. Wilson, J. C. Decius, and P. C. Cross. 1955. *Molecular Vibrations. The Theory of Infrared and Raman Vibrational Spectra*. McGraw-Hill, New York.

T. Wlodarski and B. Zagrovic. 2009. Conformational selection and induced fit mechanism underlie specificity in noncovalent interactions with ubiquitin. *Proc. Natl. Acad. Sci. USA*, 106:19346–19351.

R. Wolfenden and A. Radzicka. 1994. On the probability of finding a water molecule in a nonpolar cavity. *Science*, 265:936–937.

J. Wyman and S. J. Gill. 1990. *Binding and Linkage*. University Science Books, Mill Valley, USA.

S. Yang, N. K. Banavali, and B. Roux. 2009. Mapping the conformational transition in Src activation by cumulating the information from multiple molecular dynamics trajectories. *Proc. Natl. Acad. Sci. USA*, 106:3776–3781.

Y. Yang, F. C. Lightstone, and S. E. Wong. 2013. Approaches to efficiently estimate solvation and explicit water energetics in ligand binding: The use of WaterMap. *Exp. Opin. Drug Disc.*, 8:277–287.

H. Yin, G. Feng, G. M. Clore, G. Hummer, and J. Rasaiah. 2010. Water in the polar and nonpolar cavities of the protein interleukin-1β. *J. Phys. Chem. B*, 114:16,290–16,297.

T. Young, L. Hua, R. Abel, R. Friesner, and B. J. Berne. 2010. Dewetting transitions in protein cavities. *Proteins*, 78:1856–1869.

H. A. Yu and M. Karplus. 1988. A thermodynamic analysis of solvation. *J. Chem. Phys.*, 89:2366–2379.

P. Zavodsky and I. Hajdu. 2012. Evolution of the concept of conformational dynamics of enzyme functions over half a century: A personal view. *Biopolymers*, 99:263–269.

H. X. Zhou and M. K. Gilson. 2009. Theory of free energy and entropy in noncovalent binding. *Chem. Rev.*, 109:4092–4107.

2

Force-Field Representation of Biomolecular Systems

Meagan C. Small and Alexander D. MacKerell, Jr.

CONTENTS

2.1 Potential Energy Function

2.1.1 Functional Form of the Potential Energy Function

A force field (FF) is the potential energy function and the collection of parameters that have been optimized for use in that potential energy function. The function and parameters are used together to evaluate the potential energies and forces of molecules in a simulation. In general, a potential energy function comprises bonded terms that describe the bond, valence angle, dihedral or torsion angle, and, in some cases, out-of-plane torsion (or improper dihedral angle) contributions to the potential energy and forces, and nonbonded terms that describe the electrostatics and van der Waals' (VDW) contributions. FFs vary based on the form of the potential energy function that is employed, but the most widely used in CADD is shown in Equation 2.1. This general form is used in AMBER (Cornell et al., 1995), CHARMM (MacKerell, 1998), OPLS (Jorgensen and Tirado-Rives, 1988), and GROMOS (van Gunsteren and Berendsen, 1987), and is known as a Class I FF.

$$U(\vec{R}) = \sum_{\text{bonds}} K_b(b - b_0)^2 + \sum_{\text{angles}} K_\theta(\theta - \theta_0)^2 + \sum_{\text{dihedrals}} K_\chi(1 + \cos(\eta\chi - \delta))$$

$$+ \sum_{\text{impropers}} K_{\text{imp}}(\varphi - \varphi_0)^2$$

$$+ \sum_{\text{nonbond}} \left(\varepsilon_{ij} \left[\left(\frac{R_{\text{min},ij}}{r_{ij}} \right)^{12} - \left(\frac{R_{\text{min},ij}}{r_{ij}} \right)^6 \right] + \frac{q_i q_j}{\varepsilon r_{ij}} \right) \qquad (2.1)$$

Equation 2.1 may be broken down into terms describing the parameters in the model and the three-dimensional (3D) structure, R, of the molecules. For a generic molecule, as schematically shown in Figure 2.1, the 3D structure may be considered in terms of the bond lengths, b; valence angles, θ; dihedral angles, χ; out-of-plane torsion angles, φ; and distances between atoms i and j, r_{ij}. These terms may come from a crystal or NMR structure or from a molecular model. The remaining terms in Equation 2.1 are force-field parameters, which may be separated into the bonded (internal/intramolecular terms) or nonbonded (external/intermolecular/interaction terms) contributions. The

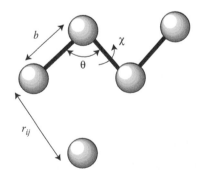

FIGURE 2.1
Cartoon representation of a generic molecule, where b represents the bond length between two atoms, θ represents the angle between three atoms, χ is the dihedral angle between four atoms, and r_{ij} is the intermolecular distance between two atoms.

energy function and parameters combined with the 3D structure of the molecule allow determination of the potential energy and forces.

Parameters are unique for different types of atoms so that the simple, computationally efficient function shown in Equation 2.1 can be used for a wide range of chemical entities. For example, parameters for the C–C bond in ethane differ from the C=C bond in ethene. Since the two types of carbons have their own parameters (namely equilibrium bond length and bond force constant), the energy and forces for the two molecules can be calculated using Equation 2.1. The simplicity of the classical potential energy function not only makes large-scale simulations computationally accessible, but also exhibits a high degree of accuracy for biomolecules given an appropriately optimized collection of parameters (MacKerell, 2004).

As seen in Equation 2.1, the bond and valence angle contributions to the potential energy are calculated using a harmonic functional form, which assumes values oscillating relatively close to equilibrium. For most simulations of biomolecules, harmonic treatment is appropriate because the simulations are performed at room temperature and do not include breaking or formation of bonds, thus their conformations remain close to their equilibrium values. The associated parameters include the bond force constant, K_b, and equilibrium bond length, b_0, and the valence angle force constant, K_θ, and equilibrium valence angle, θ_0. The potential energy due to rotation about bonds (or torsions), Figure 2.1, is computed through the dihedral angle term. As rotation is through 360° and oscillates between a range of values, the mathematical form is a cosine function, in which the dihedral force constant, K_χ, is the amplitude indicating the barrier to rotation; the multiplicity, n, is the periodicity dictating the number of cycles of rotation per 360°; and the phase angle, δ, is the constant controlling the location of the maxima of the energy surface. In most FFs, the phase angle is kept at 0° or 180° to maintain symmetry as required to apply the parameters to diastereomers. However, the option of using other values for the phase is available in most programs (Blondel and Karplus, 1996). For rotation about the C–C bond in ethane from the aforementioned example, the multiplicity $n = 3$ and the rotations generate two low energy staggered conformations and a high energy eclipsed conformation. The dihedral energy about an individual bond may be described by more than one dihedral term by summing the cosine functions into a Fourier series (Equation 2.1) that is useful in reproducing, for example, a target quantum mechanical (QM) dihedral potential energy surface (PES). The potential energy associated with out-of-plane torsions (or improper angles) is also calculated harmonically and its parameters include an improper angle force constant, K_{imp}, and equilibrium improper angle, φ_0. The existence of the improper angle term is primarily to maintain planarity and prevent inversion of the molecule's chirality, especially in FFs that do not explicitly contain all hydrogen atoms (e.g., the CHARMM Param19 FF) (Neria et al., 1996).

The nonbonded terms in Equation 2.1 represent the most important contributions to the potential energy and include the VDW and electrostatic interaction energy. For both the VDW and electrostatic interaction energies, the interactions between atoms covalently bonded to each other or separated by two covalent bonds (i.e., 1,2 and 1,3 interactions, respectively) are ignored. In most FFs, the VDW contribution to the potential energy is calculated using a Lennard-Jones 6-12 function (LJ 6-12, Equation 2.1), though alternative terms have been used (see below). In the LJ 6-12 function, the repulsive term is a "hard" wall potential of $1/r^{12}$, enforcing Pauli's exclusion principle that electron clouds cannot overlap and the attractive term is $1/r^6$, which approximates the London dispersion energy. The interaction parameters ε_{ij} and $R_{\min,ij}$ describe the Lennard-Jones well depth and the minimum interaction distance between two atoms i and j, respectively. The well depth is a measure of how favorable the London dispersion force is between the atoms, while the minimum interaction distance is dependent on the VDW radius of the atoms. Generally, ε_i and $R_{\min,i}$ are obtained for individual atom types (such as for the carbon and hydrogen atom types of ethane), then combined according to a set of combining rules to yield the pairwise ε_{ij} and $R_{\min,ij}$. The combining rules vary among FFs as the arithmetic mean or the geometric mean. These differences, along with other considerations (see below), make it inappropriate to mix parameters between FFs. For pairwise interactions that are not described well by the use of standard combination rules, atom-pair specific (NBFIX) LJ parameters can be applied (Baker et al., 2010).

The electrostatic contribution to the potential energy is evaluated using Coulomb's law. In additive, pairwise FFs, the electrostatic parameters include the partial atomic charges of the atoms, q. In FFs that explicitly treat electronic polarizability, additional terms to treat the atomic polarizability are included, as discussed below. When applying Coulomb's law with an explicit solvent representation, the dielectric constant ε is set equal to 1. However, there are a wide range of approximations, referred to as implicit solvent models, to avoid the use of explicit solvent thereby offering significant savings in computational costs. A number of recent reviews have addressed these models (Feig and Brooks, 2004; Roux and Simonson, 1999).

2.1.2 Extensions to the Classical Potential Energy Function

When selecting an FF to use, the system under study and the desired outcomes must be taken into consideration. In certain cases, a more complex form of the potential energy function may be desired. These are known as Class II FFs. Historically, owing to limited computer resources as well as increasing difficulty in optimization of the parameters in these FFs made expanded treatment of the potential energy function difficult. Extensions of the potential energy function can be made to either the bonded or nonbonded terms, which are described below. A recent review describes advances in potential energy models in more detail (Demerdash et al., 2014).

2.1.2.1 Bonded Terms

The harmonic form of the bond potential energy is less accurate for molecular geometries far from equilibrium, which can be accounted for using the Morse potential (Equation 2.2) that includes bond breaking and bond dissociation energy. Bond stretching asymmetry can be treated using cubic and quartic extension terms. Linear molecules such as hydrogen cyanide and carbon dioxide are better treated with a cosine functional form for the angular potential energy rather than the harmonic valence angle terms (Mayo et al., 1990; Rappe et al., 1992). Cross terms that relate the interdependence of the bonds, angles, and dihedrals to each other can also be used. For instance, the conformational properties associated with correlation of two adjacent dihedrals can be treated using a grid-based dihedral energy correction map (CMAP), used mostly to enhance the conformational properties of protein backbone dihedrals φ and ψ (Best et al., 2012; MacKerell et al., 2004a,b; Ren and Ponder, 2002). Recently, CMAP in conjunction with Hamiltonian Replica Exchange has been used to improve conformational sampling of peptides and carbohydrates (Mallajosyula et al., 2013; Mallajosyula and MacKerell, 2011; Patel et al., 2015). While these enhancements more accurately treat the change in energy with intramolecular geometry, for the most part the Class I additive potential energy function is satisfactory for CADD.

$$U(\text{bond}) = D_e \left(1 - e^{-\sqrt{(K_b/2D_e)}(b - b_0)}\right)^2 \tag{2.2}$$

2.1.2.2 Nonbonded Terms

Improvements to the accuracy of the potential energy function can also be achieved via higher-order nonbonded functions. Nonbonded terms represent the most important contribution to the potential energy because electrostatics and VDW terms dominate interactions dictating the structure and dynamics of biopolymers as well as ligand–protein interactions and related phenomena. They are also most computationally expensive to calculate, and nonbonded terms of a higher level of accuracy can quickly become cost-prohibitive due to the $N \times N/2$ calculations required, where N is the number of particles in the system. Concerning the VDW interactions, in most cases, the LJ 6-12 term is sufficient to treat biomolecules, but given interatomic distances r_{ij} smaller than $R_{\min,ij}$ the energy increase is overestimated as r decreases (Halgren, 1992). Modified potentials have sought to "soften" the repulsive part of the VDW contribution using a ninth-order repulsive term (LJ 6-9) or modifying the functional form as in the Buckingham potential (or Exp-6 potential; Buckingham, 1938), which treats the repulsion as an exponential that gives a more gradual increase in energy as r decreases (White, 1997). Additionally, the buffered 14-7 potential (Halgren, 1992) uses buffering constants that modulate the repulsive and attractive terms of the LJ potential and is the functional form of the VDW potential energy employed in the Merck molecular force field (MMFF) (Halgren, 1999), with a variation of that function used in the polarizable AMOEBA FF (Ponder et al., 2010; Ren and Ponder, 2002; Shi et al., 2013).

The inclusion of higher-order terms for the electrostatic interactions warrants a more extensive discussion than the previous potential energy terms. A majority of FFs utilize Coulomb's law as in Equation 2.1. Partial atomic charges on each atom are static and the contribution of the electrostatic interactions to the potential is the sum of all of the pairwise Columbic interactions (excluding 1,2 and 1,3 interactions). Hence, this is known as the additive model. Additive FFs do not capture the contributions of polarizability explicitly. This is a major drawback because the electron distribution of a molecule is influenced by the surrounding environment. Thus, models that include the explicit treatment of polarization have been the subject of ongoing work for over 30 years (Warshel and Levitt, 1976). To overcome the fixed charged approximation in additive FFs, polarization is treated in a mean-field way by adjusting the partial atomic charges to overestimate the gas phase molecular dipoles and hence the electrostatic interactions of the molecule in aqueous systems are approximated. While including polarizability implicitly has fortuitously shown good agreement between condensed phase and experimental molar volumes and heats of vaporization (Fox and Kollman, 1998; Gough, 1992; Jorgensen, 1986; Jorgensen et al., 1996; MacKerell and Karplus, 1991) as well as solvation free energies (Chen et al., 2002; Kaminski et al., 1994; Rizzo and Jorgensen, 1999; Yin and MacKerell, 1998), there is room for improvement for biomolecules (Shirts et al., 2003). Indeed, recent advances in polarizable FFs are now yielding improvements in a range of systems (Chowdary et al., 2013; He et al., 2013; Jiao et al., 2008, 2009; Lopes et al., 2013; Ponder et al., 2010; Savelyev and MacKerell, 2014; Shi et al., 2012; Zhang et al., 2012).

Explicit treatment of polarizability introduces a new term into the potential energy function, U_{polar} (Lopes, P.E.M. et al. 2009; Rick and Stuart, 2002). The polarizability needed to determine U_{polar} may be calculated using induced dipoles (Bernardo et al., 1994; Caldwell et al., 1990; Dang, 1998; Sprik and Klein, 1988; Wallqvist and Berne, 1993), fluctuating charges (Asensio et al., 2000; Bryce et al., 1998; Llanta et al., 2001; Patel and Brooks, 2003; Rick and Berne, 1996; Rick et al., 1995; Yoshii et al., 2000), and the classical Drude oscillator (Kunz and van Gunsteren, 2009; Lopes, P.E. et al. 2009; van Maaren and van der Spoel, 2001). In the induced dipole model, the functional form of U_{polar} is based on introducing an induced dipole onto each atom in addition to the partial atomic charge. This is performed in the AMOEBA polarizable FF, in addition to treatment of the static contribution to the electrostatics with a multipole expansion out to quadrapoles (Ponder et al., 2010; Ren and Ponder, 2002; Shi et al., 2013). Fluctuating charge models are based on allowing the partial atomic charges to fluctuate in response to the electric field. The polarization energy is related to the absolute (Mulliken) electronegativity (Iczkowski and Margrave, 1961; Mulliken, 1934) and the hardness of the atom (Parr and Pearson, 1983), which themselves are dependent on the electron affinity and ionization potential of an atom. Although their names imply a change in the number of electrons, in the context of chemical polarization these are the measures of how likely the electronic distribution is polarized and are easier to understand in terms of two atoms.

Models based on the classical Drude oscillator (Anisimov et al., 2005; Lamoureux et al., 2003; Yu et al., 2003) (also known as Shell or charge-on-spring models) account for polarization by introducing a massless, partially charged Drude particle that is harmonically attached to the nucleus of the parent atom. The atomic polarizability is simply the Drude charge squared divided by the force constant on the harmonic term between the Drude particle and the atomic core. In practice, the charge on the atom and the Drude particle are corrected to account for the partial atomic charge on the atom. Thus, for a fixed set of atomic positions, the Drude particles can relax in the surrounding electric field yielding the polarization response. This relaxation can be performed via energy minimization, which is equivalent to a self-consistent field calculation, although computationally efficient methods are used to treat the Drude particles in MD simulations, as discussed in the following section.

2.2 FF Parametrization

The usefulness of an FF in target-based drug design is based on the availability of parameters for the target molecule, typically a protein, and the ligands under study. These aspects of the FF must be compatible with each other, which is based on their parameters being optimized using a consistent approach. Such an approach has been taken with different components of the CHARMM additive FF. In the remainder of this section, we give an overview of the parameter optimization approach for model compounds representative of biomolecules and of the range of functional groups in drug-like molecules. This will be followed by an overview of the additional optimization steps required for macromolecules focusing on the recent update of the CHARMM36 protein FF (Best et al., 2012; MacKerell et al., 2004a,b).

2.2.1 Parameter Optimization for Model Compounds

Optimization of an FF follows the general steps in Figure 2.2; a more detailed overview of the parameter optimization process in the context of the CHARMM additive model may be obtained elsewhere (Vanommeslaeghe et al., 2010). To illustrate this procedure, we use histidine as an example. In Step 1, histidine, which is treated in its dipeptide form (i.e., N-acetyl, C-methylamide), is broken down into two model compounds: N-methyl acetamide (NMA) for the backbone and 4-methylimidazole (MIMI) for the side chain (Figure 2.3a). To generate target data (Step 2), we utilize experimental

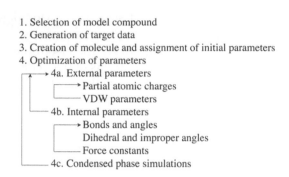

1. Selection of model compound
2. Generation of target data
3. Creation of molecule and assignment of initial parameters
4. Optimization of parameters
   - 4a. External parameters
     - Partial atomic charges
     - VDW parameters
   - 4b. Internal parameters
     - Bonds and angles
     - Dihedral and improper angles
     - Force constants
   - 4c. Condensed phase simulations

FIGURE 2.2
Flowchart representing the steps in the optimization of a force field.

data such as crystal structures and condensed phase properties, which we supplement with QM data. QM calculations include minimized NMA and MIMI structures and vibrational spectra, as well as supramolecular data for water or dimer interactions. In Step 3, the topology is created and initial parameters are assigned as illustrated in the example CHARMM topology in Figure 2.3b. The MIMI topology entry contains the atom names and types, partial atomic charges, connectivity information, and, in special cases, specific improper terms.

Once the topology information is in place, the appropriate parameters must be identified. There are a number of available algorithms that can assign initial guess parameters by analogy and are compatible with the existing FFs (Krieger et al., 2002; Malde et al., 2011; Miller et al., 2008; Ribiero et al., 2008; Schuttelkopf and van Aalten, 2004; Vanommeslaeghe and MacKerell, 2012; Vanommeslaeghe et al., 2012; Wang et al., 2006; Zoete et al., 2011). These include the ParamChem/CHARMM General Force Field (CGenFF) engine (Vanommeslaeghe and MacKerell, 2012; Vanommeslaeghe et al., 2012) and MATCH (Yesselman et al., 2012), both of which may be used with the CHARMM additive FFs. When performing this task manually, the program CHARMM (Brooks et al., 2009) automatically identifies the missing parameters during the structure generation process. With the topology built and initial parameters assigned, the partial atomic charges and VDW parameters are then optimized as in Step 4a. Water interactions for NMA and MIMI (Figure 2.3c) provide interaction energies and geometries that are used to adjust the partial atomic charges until good agreement with the QM supramolecular distances and energies is observed. VDW parameters are optimized using gas and condensed phase simulations of NMA and MIMI to target molar volumes and heats of vaporization (Yin and MacKerell, 1998). Alternatively, crystal- or hydration-free energies as well as QM data may be used for VDW parameter optimization, which may be considered the most difficult aspect of the parameter optimization process. However, in the majority of cases VDW parameters may be directly transferred from known molecules without additional optimization.

(a)

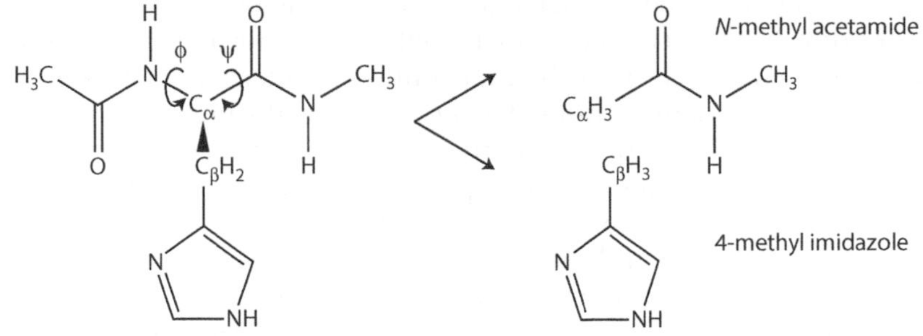

(b)

RESI MIMI   0.00

ATOM NDI NR1 -0.36
ATOM HDI H   -0.32
ATOM CG   CPH1 0.05
ATOM CB   CT3 -0.18
ATOM HB1 HA3   0.09
ATOM HB2 HA3   0.09
ATOM HB3 HA3   0.09
ATOM NE2 NR2 -0.70
ATOM CD2 CPH1 0.22
ATOM HD2 HR3   0.10
ATOM CE1 CPH2 0.25
ATOM HE1 HR1   0.13

BOND NE2 CE1 ND1 CG   CE1 ND1
BOND ND1 HD1 CD2 HD2 CE1 HE1
BOND CG CB   NE2 CE1 CD2 CG
BOND CB HB1   CB HB2   CB HB3

IMPH ND1 CG CE1 HD1
IMPH CD2 CG NE2 HD2
IMPH CE1 ND1 CE2 HE1

(c)

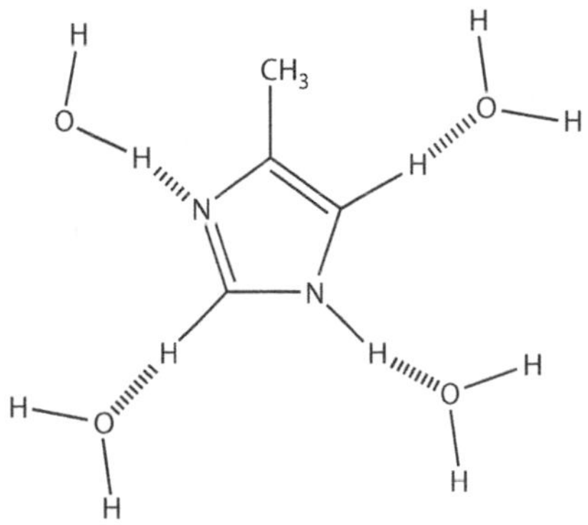

FIGURE 2.3
(a) Model compounds for the Parametrization of a histidine dipeptide. The dipeptide can be broken down into the backbone represented by *N*-methyl acetamide (NMA) and the sidechain represented by 4-methylimidazole (MIMI). The Cα hydrogen is omitted for clarity. After Parametrization of the two models compounds, they are connected and the covalent linkage between Cα and Cβ as well as the φ, ψ dihedral angles are optimized. (b) An example CHARMM topology for the model compound MIMI. It contains the atom names and types, partial atomic charges, connectivity information, and specific improper terms acting on the hydrogens. (c) Interactions between water and MIMI are used to obtain the supramolecular target data for optimization of the partial atomic charges. Note that while four waters are shown in the figure, the water–MIMI interactions are each evaluated individually.

Once the external parameters have been optimized, the bonded parameters are adjusted (Step 4b). Bond and angle equilibrium values are adjusted until good agreement with geometries from QM calculations or surveys of the Cambridge crystallographic database (Allen et al., 1979) is achieved. The bond and angle force constants are parameterized by comparing to experimental and QM vibrational spectra. Vibrational spectra in CHARMM may be analyzed using the MOLVIB module (Kuczera et al., 1993), which creates a potential energy distribution (PED) matrix (Pulay et al., 1979) that breaks down each frequency into its contributing normal modes and allows straightforward analysis of the contribution of internal degrees of freedom to the spectra. Dihedral parameters are optimized against vibrational spectra and, for the "softer" degrees of freedom (e.g., rotation about single bonds), using PESs for rotations around specific bonds. PESs are typically determined for torsions involving only nonhydrogen atoms, with the dihedral parameters adjusted until the molecular mechanical (MM) PES agrees with the QM surface. In addition, dihedrals associated with terminal hydroxyl or sulfhydryl groups are also often optimized. Typically, the phase for each dihedral angle is limited to either 0° or 180°, with the focus of optimization on the force constant and multiplicity, with additional dihedral terms added to the Fourier series as necessary. For example, the dihedral Fourier series for the peptide bond typically includes the expected twofold term ($n = 2$) to treat the double-bond character of the amide bond, with a onefold term included to fine tune the relative energies of the *cis* versus *trans* states of the peptide bond.

At this point, the first round of parameter optimization is completed. To check whether the changes to the bonded terms have affected our external parameters, it is necessary to loop over Step 4 again and determine whether the deviations are within the defined convergence criteria. For instance, in the CGenFF (Vanommeslaeghe et al., 2010), deviations for the bond and valence angles of 0.03 Å and 3° from the QM target data, respectively, are acceptable while differences of 5% or less between the QM and MM vibrational frequencies are ideal. The final step in the Parametrization of histidine is to connect the model compounds and optimize the parameters that are involved in the linkages; for instance, the Cα–Cβ bond and φ, ψ dihedrals as noted in Figure 2.3a. For the latter, the QM target data for dipeptides serves as a useful model for optimizing the backbone dihedrals (MacKerell et al., 2004a,b).

As a final note on Parametrization, it is important that parameters from different FFs should not be combined due to the treatment of the VDW and electrostatic terms. For example, OPLS and CHARMM partial atomic charges are targeted to water interactions with the compound obtained at the HF/6-31G* level of theory while charges in AMBER are fit to restrained electrostatic potentials (RESPs) (Bayly et al., 1993) of the same QM level. This leads to variations in the charge distributions between the FFs, which may impact the nature of the atomistic interactions of the molecule with its surroundings (Chen et al., 2002). Additionally, for the LJ combining rules CHARMM and AMBER use the geometric mean for epsilon and arithmetic mean for R_{min}, while OPLS uses the geometric mean for both (Jorgensen and Tirado-Rives, 1988). OPLS also defines the radius, sigma, where the LJ energy between two atoms is zero, whereas the R_{min} in CHARMM and AMBER is where the LJ energy is at its minimum. FFs also use different scaling factors for 1,4 nonbonded interactions (Jorgensen and Tirado-Rives, 1988; Weiner et al., 1984).

2.2.2 Additional Optimization for Biomolecular FFs

Once the model compounds have been parameterized, they are compiled into an FF. Following our example of histidine, the dipeptides of all the amino and imino acids are combined to yield a protein FF. At this stage it is crucial to validate the quality of the protein FF using condensed phase simulations of peptide and proteins for which experimental data are available. When necessary, further optimization is performed to balance local and global macromolecular properties. For instance, additional optimization (Best et al., 2012; MacKerell et al., 2004a,b) of the CHARMM22 protein FF (MacKerell et al., 1998) was undertaken to reduce the relative population of π helix that was observed in longer simulations (Feig et al., 2003). First, the alanine, glycine, and proline dipeptides were used as model systems to refine the parameters for the φ, ψ backbone dihedrals based on QM data. The φ, ψ backbone distributions were improved by introducing a new φ, ψ dihedral cross term to the potential energy function that is a grid-based energy CMAP (MacKerell et al., 2004a,b) that allows for near ideal reproduction of dipeptide QM energy surfaces. Then, additional adjustments were performed to fine tune the conformational sampling, yielding the CHARMM22-CMAP protein FF in 2004 (MacKerell et al., 2004a,b). Subsequently, additional optimization was undertaken to correct the overstabilization of helices leading to CHARMM36 (Best et al., 2012; MacKerell et al., 2004a,b). CHARMM36 refines the CMAP by further adjusting the Ala dipeptide CMAP surface targeting the conformational sampling of the $(Ala)_5$, GB1, and CH_3-$(AAQAA)_3$-NH_2 peptides in aqueous solution. In addition, higher level QM calculations on the glycine and proline dipeptides were used to define their CMAP terms. Additional optimization of CHARMM36 involved the dihedral parameters associated with the χ_1, χ_2 sidechain torsions. This optimization targeted both QM data, NMR data, and χ_1, χ_2 distributions from a survey of the protein databank (Berman et al., 2000). The parameters were then validated using simulations of test proteins in crystal, aqueous, and denaturing environments. This effort illustrated that longer simulations are required to guide refinements of FF parameters and that additional optimization leads to improved representation of biomolecules by an FF.

2.3 Classes of Biomolecular FFs

FFs vary in the numerical approximations and target data used in their development as discussed above. They are often designed targeting a subset of molecules. In this section, the major FFs available for biomolecular simulations will be briefly discussed with particular emphasis given to the CHARMM, AMBER, OPLS, and to a lesser extent the GROMOS FF. Additional

FFs will be presented as they relate to the biomolecules. This summary is not intended to be a thorough review on all of the available biomolecular FFs. For that, the reader is referred to additional articles (Fadda and Woods, 2010; French and Johnson, 2011; Guvench and MacKerell, 2008; MacKerell, 2004; Ponder and Case, 2003).

2.3.1 Protein FFs

The first molecular dynamics (MD) simulation of a biological macromolecule was a protein (McCammon et al., 1977), and proteins continue to be the most studied biological molecules to date for *in silico* drug design. The AMBER (Cornell et al., 1995; Duan et al., 2003; Hornak et al., 2006; Kollman, 1996; Wang et al., 2000), CHARMM (MacKerell et al., 1998, 2004a,b), and OPLS (Jorgensen et al., 1996; Kaminski et al., 2001) protein FFs are all-atom, while GROMOS (Oostenbrink et al., 2004; Schmid et al., 2011; Schuler et al., 2001; Soares et al., 2005; van Gunsteren et al., 1996) incorporates the hydrogens into the parent heavy atoms (united atom), with the exception of polar hydrogens. These are discussed in great detail in a comprehensive protein FF review by Ponder and Case (2003).

In general, all the aforementioned FFs tend to reproduce experimental 3D structures of proteins (Price and Brooks, 2002). CHARMM and AMBER were optimized to reproduce the QM data and experimental data based on surveys of crystallographic databases on model compounds representative of proteins. OPLS uses the internal parameters from AMBER (ff94) (Cornell et al., 1995), from which selective torsions are optimized using the QM data (Jorgensen et al., 1996; Kaminski et al., 2001). For the LJ parameters, all of the FFs use condensed phase simulations. While CHARMM and AMBER use the TIP3P water model (Jorgensen et al., 1983), OPLS was parameterized to work primarily with TIP3P (Jorgensen et al., 1983), though it has been used with TIP4P (Jorgensen et al., 1983) and related models (Berendsen et al., 1981, 1987; Horn et al., 2004; Jorgensen, 1986; Jorgensen et al., 1983). GROMOS is typically used with the SPC model (Berendsen et al., 1981).

One of the considerations in FF development is that the data used during the Parametrization process can bias the results. Therefore, the user must critically analyze the outcomes of FF simulations to determine whether particular interactions may be artifacts of FF bias. In a comparison of OPLS, AMBER, GROMOS, and CHARMM (Feig et al., 2003), it was found that the relative energy barrier between the α and π helix state was underestimated compared to high-level QM calculations by 1 to 2 kcal/mol. Thus, in many FF simulations of proteins, the relative population of the π helix was higher than expected. This observation led to the creation of the CMAP terms in CHARMM (MacKerell et al., 2004a,b) as discussed above. Similarly, FFs have been found to be either too helical or not helical enough (Best et al., 2008). The CHARMM36 protein FF has addressed this by targeting the aqueous phase conformational sampling of multiple peptides, as discussed above. With the

AMBER FF, a number of variants have been developed (e.g., ff96 [Kollman, 1996], ff99 [Wang et al., 2000], AmberGS [Garcia and Sanbonmatsu, 2002], Amber03 [Duan et al., 2003], Amber03* [Best and Hummer, 2009], ff99SB [Hornak et al., 2006], ff99SB* [Best and Hummer, 2009], ff99SB-ildn [Lindorff-Larsen et al., 2010], ff99SBnmr1 [Li and Bruschweiler, 2010]) with the more recent FFs being better behaved with respect to polypeptides in solution, as with CHARMM36. Limitations in all the protein FFs have become evident because of the growing computational resources and longer simulation times for biomolecules; these observations ultimately lead to improvements in the models over time.

2.3.2 Nucleic Acid FFs

Early on, the charged nature of the nucleic acid backbone made optimization of nucleic acid FFs a challenge (MacKerell, 2001, 2004). Simulations using the early nucleic acid FFs such as AMBER (Weiner and Kollman, 1981), CHARMM (Nilsson and Karplus, 1986), and GROMOS (van Gunsteren and Berendsen, 1987) achieved mediocre success due to the stability of oligonucleotides. The use of appropriate truncation methods (Norberg and Nilsson, 2000) and particle mesh Ewald to treat long-range electrostatics (Darden et al., 1993) later allowed for longer, stable MD simulations to be performed (MacKerell, 1997; Norberg and Nilsson, 1996). Updates to the AMBER and CHARMM nucleic acid FFs yielded AMBER (ff94) (Cornell et al., 1995) and CHARMM22 (MacKerell et al., 1995). These were subsequently updated to AMBER (ff99) (Cheatham et al., 1999) and CHARMM27 (Foloppe and MacKerell, 2000; MacKerell and Banavali, 2000) that were developed to improve the sugar pucker and equilibrium between the A and B canonical forms, respectively. Notably, CHARMM27 was a full reoptimization of the CHARMM22 nucleic acid FF to balance the energetics of the model compounds based on the QM data with the conformational properties of duplex DNA in solution, while AMBER (ff99) updated the torsion parameters pertaining to the sugar pucker. Most recently, updates have been made to CHARMM27 to better treat the 2'OH group on RNA and the equilibrium between the BI and BII DNA states, leading to CHARMM36 (Denning et al., 2011; Hart et al., 2012). At the present time, the most recommended AMBER nucleic acid FF is ff99bsc0 (Perez et al., 2007) for canonical DNA and RNA, which is a refinement of ff99 intended to correct overpopulation of the γ = trans state. For noncanonical RNA, the ff99bsc0χ_{OL} which involves adjustments of the glycosidic linkage parameters is recommended (Zgarbova et al., 2011).

Another nucleic acid FF of note is the Bristol–Myers–Squibb (BMS) nucleic acid FF (Langley, 1998). BMS uses the internal parameters from CHARMM27 for the nucleobases and CHARMm/Quanta (a commercial CHARMM FF by Accelrys, Inc.) for the sugar and phosphate backbone internal parameters. To date, the BMS FF has not seen wide use, in part, due to it not being compatible with a wider range of biomolecules.

One caveat of FFs, as mentioned in the previous section, is that the target data can bias the results from a simulation. For instance, the extent to which the above FFs utilize the QM target data for the larger model compounds and experimental structures for DNA/RNA duplexes varies. The BMS nucleic acid FF uses mostly the experimental nucleic acid structures as obtained from the nucleic acid database (NDB) (Berman et al., 1992; Coimbatore Narayanan et al., 2014). For this reason, simulations done with the BMS FF tend to have a predominantly B form of DNA. CHARMM27/36 uses both the A and B form structures from the NDB and the QM conformational energies of larger model compounds. Hence, the model yields an improved equilibrium between A and B form DNA. The most recent CHARMM36, in fact, is optimized to yield an equilibrium between the BI and BII states of DNA as well as properly treating the equilibrium between A and B form DNA. AMBER (ff94) did not use experimental duplex DNA/RNA structures during Parametrization, though AMBER (ff99) revision did incorporate this into the optimization of the final dihedrals. Still, it was found that AMBER (ff99) led ultimately to degradation of the B form, leading to the most recent variant of the AMBER FF (ff99bsc0) that addresses B form stabilization using high-level QM calculations of larger model compounds that are more representative of nucleotides. For noncanonical structures, ff99bsc0 has been noted to lead to incorrect loop geometries and other structural inconsistencies (Cheatham and Case, 2013), which have led to χ modifications introduced in the χOL variant (Zgarbova et al., 2011) and ff99χ (Yildirim et al., 2010).

2.3.3 Carbohydrate FFs

The Parametrization of sugar FFs has been challenging for two reasons. First, there are many types of monosaccharides and, second, the chemical nature of sugars makes it challenging to balance the inter- and intramolecular hydrogen bonding that occurs via the sugar hydroxyls in water. For polysaccharides, this effect is amplified by the different types of glycosidic linkages as well as the α and β anomers. The two most used FFs for sugars are the AMBER GLYCAM (Kirschner et al., 2008, 2012; Kirschner and Woods, 2001; Woods et al., 1995) and CHARMM carbohydrate (Guvench et al., 2008, 2009; Hatcher et al., 2009a,b; Raman et al., 2010) FFs. The original AMBER GLYCAM_93 (Woods et al., 1995) was optimized for model compounds derived from tetrahydrofuran. Partial atomic charges were fit to RESP maps. In the most recent GLYCAM06 (Kirschner et al., 2008, 2012), problems with solvation and diffusion rates were overcome. The FF was optimized to generate a transferable set of parameters that were not specific to one type of monosaccharide using a large training and test set of molecules from a diverse group of chemical families. A recent update to the GLYCAM06 FF has been developed for lipopolysaccharide membranes (Kirschner et al., 2012).

Another complication in FF-based simulations of carbohydrates is that a carbohydrate FF must be compatible with the existing protein and lipid

FFs, because carbohydrates involved in recognition are generally covalently attached to lipids or proteins. Therefore, simulations are done using combinations of carbohydrate and lipid/protein parameters. While GLYCAM06 is general enough to study a diverse set of biomolecules such as proteins, nucleic acids, lipids, and small molecules, there are some inconsistencies with the AMBER protein FF because the 1,4 scaling factor of 1/1.2 is excluded in GLYCAM06, potentially leading to altered conformational energies. The CHARMM carbohydrate FFs are designed specifically to be compatible with the remainder of the additive CHARMM biomolecular FF. The advantage is that when heterogeneous systems are to be studied, glycoprotein or glycolipid simulations can be performed using parameters that have been specifically optimized for each biomolecule, including 1–4 interactions between the different biomolecules, while maximizing the accuracy of the interactions between each class of biomolecule. Presently, the CHARMM carbohydrate FFs have been optimized for hexopyranose monosaccharides (Guvench et al., 2008), furanoses (Hatcher et al., 2009a,b), acyclic polyalcohols (Hatcher et al., 2009a,b), as well as glycosidic linkages between hexopyranoses (Guvench et al., 2009) and furanoses (Raman et al., 2010). Other carbohydrate FFs include OPLS (Kony et al., 2002) and GROMOS (Hansen and Hunenberger, 2011; Lins and Hunenberger, 2005), though these are not discussed in detail here and the reader is referred to a comprehensive review (Fadda and Woods, 2010).

2.3.4 Lipid FFs

Lipid FFs have been difficult to optimize because accurate treatment of the gel–liquid phase properties of the bilayer is challenging. The most widely used FFs for membrane simulations are the all-atom CHARMM FF (Feller and MacKerell, 2000; Klauda et al., 2005a,b, 2010; Yin and MacKerell, 1998) and to a lesser extent the united-atom OPLS-UA (Ulmschneider and Ulmschneider, 2009) and GROMOS96 (van Gunsteren et al., 1996) FFs, and the coarse-grained MARTINI FF (Marrink et al., 2007). Among these, the CHARMM lipid FF is the most popular mainly because it was the only all-atom FF highly optimized specifically for lipid molecules. The general AMBER FF (GAFF) (Wang et al., 2004) has also been used for lipid simulations. Though not specifically optimized for lipids, simulations on various membranes using GAFF have shown that it yields reasonable agreement with certain experimental values, namely membrane thickness, area per lipid, and deuterium order parameters (Jojart and Martinek, 2007; Rosso and Gould, 2008; Siu et al., 2008). However, the level of agreement was achieved only after application of a surface tension to the interface (e.g., to obtain the correct surface area/head group) and that agreement tended to be limited to a few properties. A more recent AMBER lipid FF named LIPID11 was developed using GAFF parameters that were refined for the phospholipid tails and headgroups (Skjevik et al., 2012).

United-atom FFs are popular for lipid simulations mainly due to their computational efficiency. The most commonly used united-atom FF is the GROMOS96 FF (van Gunsteren et al., 1996), which in this context refers to the original 43A1 FF and its derivatives. The VDW parameters in 43A1 were optimized targeting condensed phase properties of alkanes (Daura et al., 1998), then the hydrocarbon chains were updated (Berger et al., 1997) by adjusting the LJ parameters to target pentadecane properties. Subsequent updates (Chiu et al., 2009; Poger et al., 2010) have focused on improving bilayers, though most of these are derived from the 43A1 (Schuler et al., 2001) parameter set.

The CHARMM27 lipid FF (Feller and MacKerell, 2000; Klauda et al., 2005a, b; Yin and MacKerell, 1998) was a reoptimization of the original CHARMM22 lipid FF (Schlenkrich et al., 1996). The torsional parameters for the aliphatic groups were optimized to high-level QM target data for butane and hexane and the phosphate headgroups were optimized in the context of the lipids and nucleic acids since the phosphate is common to both. The most recent CHARMM36 (Klauda et al., 2010) FF is the recommended CHARMM lipid FF. It addresses two major drawbacks of CHARMM27, as well as other lipid FFs, which are the need for an applied surface tension to prevent bilayer shrinkage and the limited reproduction of deuterium order parameters. These issues have been addressed by optimizing the partial atomic charges of the headgroup and select torsional parameters for the headgroup and glycerol linker. Results show that simulations of select lipid bilayers using the CHARMM36 lipid FF result in stable liquid crystalline bilayers, as judged by the correct surface area/head group (Klauda et al., 2010), which is of great importance in studying membrane proteins using *in silico* drug design methods that often include lipids, proteins, and drug-like molecules along with water and ions.

2.3.5 Small Molecule FFs

Development of a small molecular FF that can cover the vastness of the chemical universe is challenging. A few of the most widely used FFs specifically parameterized for small drug-like molecule in condensed phase include CHARMM's CGenFF (Vanommeslaeghe et al., 2010), Merck's MMFF (Halgren, 1996a,b,c), and AMBER's GAFF (Wang et al., 2004). All three FFs utilize the same basic optimization scheme, which was discussed in Section 2.1. MMFF was developed with condensed phase protein–ligand simulations in mind, however, the ability of the FF to accurately reproduce condensed phase properties, including structural features of proteins, is limited. This is due to the lack of optimization of parameters for proteins as compared to specific biomolecular FFs. Furthermore, because it uses a different functional form for the potential energy function than that shown in Equation 2.1, combining it with a more specific biomolecular FF such as CHARMM will most likely result in inaccurate interaction energies due to differences in the way nonbonded interactions are treated. GAFF overcomes this obstacle since it was parameterized to be used with the existing AMBER FF. Similarly, CGenFF was optimized to be compatible with the existing CHARMM FFs. Ultimately, this is advantageous due to wide variety of biomolecules represented by the additive CHARMM FF, allowing the biomolecular portion of the system to be treated using parameters specifically optimized for the biomolecule of interest, while the small molecule can be treated using CGenFF. In fact, because all of the CHARMM FFs are optimized in a similar fashion, calculation of the nonbonded terms is expected to be reasonably accurate and balanced, which is crucial in computer-aided drug design.

There are a number of automated parameter assignment engines available for selected small molecule FFs (Krieger et al., 2002; Malde et al., 2011; Miller et al., 2008; Ribiero et al., 2008; Schuttelkopf and van Aalten, 2004; Vanommeslaeghe and MacKerell, 2012; Vanommeslaeghe et al., 2012; Wang et al., 2006; Yesselman et al., 2012; Zoete et al., 2011). AnteChamber (Wang et al., 2006) was designed for use with GAFF and generates AMBER topologies. It assigns bonded parameters by analogy from GAFF and partial atomic charges based on Mulliken charges first calculated at the AM1 level and then corrected to RESP-like charges using bond charge correction parameters derived from a training set of molecules (Jakalian et al., 2000, 2002). Alternatively, AnteChamber can also utilize user-supplied Gaussian output files to generate actual RESP charges with QM calculations done at the HF/6-31G* level of theory to maintain compatibility with GAFF parameters. ParamChem (Vanommeslaeghe and MacKerell, 2012; Vanommeslaeghe et al., 2012) is an engine designed for use with CGenFF and generates CHARMM topologies. Bonded parameters are assigned by analogy to CGenFF parameters, while charges are assigned using a bond charge increment scheme optimized targeting the partial atomic charges of a training set of model compounds. This scheme is loosely based on MMFF's charge assignment implementation and is a more modular approach to the assignment of partial atomic charges (Halgren, 1996a,b,c). MATCH (Yesselman et al., 2012) is also available to generate CHARMM topologies and parameters by analogy. The key feature of MATCH is that it represents each molecule as a graphical tree that it uses to make comparisons between molecules in order to obtain a set of parameters for a novel compound. Other parameter assignment engines include ATB (Malde et al., 2011) and PRODRG (Schuttelkopf and van Aalten, 2004) for GROMOS, SwissParam (Zoete et al., 2011) for CHARMM and MMFF, YASARA (Krieger et al., 2002) for GAFF, and GENRTF (Miller et al., 2008) for CHARMM.

2.3.6 Polarizable FFs

The Parametrization of FFs that treat polarizability is an active area in FF development. Reviews of polarizable FFs have been published elsewhere (Lopes, P.E. et al., 2009; Lopes, P.E.M. et al. 2009; Rick and Stuart, 2002). The inclusion of polarizability into the potential energy function was discussed in Section 1.2.2. Adding to that, implementation of polarizable FFs will be briefly discussed for the CHARMM Drude (Lopes et al., 2013; Savelyev and MacKerell, 2014) and AMOEBA (Ponder et al., 2010; Ren and Ponder, 2002; Shi et al., 2013) polarizable FFs. The CHARMM Drude polarizable FF is a product of work in this laboratory in collaboration with Roux and coworkers, and Parametrization of it has required significant effort and time, dating back over 10 years (Lamoureux et al., 2003). Since then, major progress has been made and at this time lipid (Chowdary et al., 2013), protein (Lopes et al., 2013), and nucleic acid (Savelyev and MacKerell, 2014) parameters are available, with parameters also available for a subset of carbohydrates, including polyalcohols (He et al., 2013) and hexapyranoses (Patel et al., 2015). The implementation of the Drude FF in CHARMM overcomes the demand of treating the Drude particles via self-consistent field calculations in MD simulations by instead treating them as classical dynamic variables in the context of an extended Lagrangian formalism (Lamoureux and Roux, 2003). In practice, this is achieved by assigning a small mass (0.4 AMU) to the Drude particle from the parent atom and applying specific thermostats to the real versus the virtual Drude particles. The AMOEBA (Ren and Ponder, 2002; Shi et al., 2013) FF is based on atomic multipoles and induced dipoles and is available for proteins (Shi et al., 2013) and general organic molecules (Shi et al., 2011). Each atomic center comprises a partial charge, dipole vector, and quadrapole tensor. MD simulations with AMOEBA are computationally demanding, although the recent development of a water model utilizing a direct polarization approximation (iAMOEBA) (Wang et al., 2013a) partially overcomes this issue. However, such treatment represents a significant approximation whereby the induced dipoles do not relax with respect to each other as compared to the more rigorous use of an extended Lagrangian, which mimics the SCF regimen (Martyna et al., 1996; Sprik and Klein, 1988; Tuckerman and Martyna, 2000). While water models that reproduce a range of experimental properties may be obtained, recently using the ForceBalance method (Wang et al., 2013b), it remains to be seen whether neglecting mutual polarization will result in the same accuracy for the presence of solutes, including ions and biomolecules.

2.4 Applications of FFs to Drug Design

FF-based simulations are an important part of *in silico* drug design. Simulations are used to generate an ensemble of protein and/or drug conformations that represent the dynamics of the molecule in solution, from which thermodynamic or conformational properties are measured. A prime example is the calculation of absolute and relative free energies of binding using free energy perturbation methods (Kollman, 1993; Straatsma and McCammon, 1992) among a variety of other methods (Jorgensen, 2004; Shim and MacKerell, 2011; Shirts et al., 2003; Sliwoski et al., 2014; Zhong and MacKerell, 2007). In the remainder of this section, emphasis will be placed on two methodologies developed in this laboratory: conformationally sampled pharmacophore (CSP) and site-identification by ligand competitive saturation (SILCS).

2.4.1 Conformationally Sampled Pharmacophore (CSP)

CSP is a pharmacophore-based method in which ensembles of ligand conformations are generated using MD simulations from which probability distributions are calculated for select distances and angles in the molecule (i.e., pharmacophore features) (Bernard et al., 2003). Analyses are then performed to correlate the biological activity of the ligand with the CSP pharmacophoric features. The method may be used qualitatively to identify biologically important geometric features as well as quantitatively to predict the activity of other ligands. Notably, physical properties of ligands may be readily incorporated into CSP models. In an approach such as CSP, the utility of the method is based on the accurate treatment of conformational sampling by the ligands, a property directly related to the FF used in the MD simulations.

CSP has been applied in this laboratory to three important classes of ligands: opioids, bile acids, and antibiotics. For the opioid receptor δ (Bernard et al., 2003, 2005, 2007), CSP was applied to develop a model able to distinguish agonists from antagonists, while the CSP model applied to μ receptor ligands (Shim et al., 2012) provided a comprehensive structure–activity relationship explaining how ligand modification altered activity. Notable was the use of CSP to facilitate the design of an opioid that acts as both a mu agonist and a delta antagonist, thereby having a decreased tolerance profile. The application of CSP-SAR to bile acid transporters yielded a model that indicated that ligands with higher intramolecular hydrogen bonding were more active against human apical sodium-dependent bile acid transporter (hASBT) due to increased hydrophobicity (Rais et al., 2010). Interestingly, the model also predicted that dianionic bile acid conjugates can achieve high binding affinities using a molecular switch controlled by the location of a carboxyl group that is involved in intramolecular hydrogen bonding. Recently, CSP was applied to analogs of the antibiotic telithromycin to show that removal of methyl groups from the antibiotic ring reduced activity compared to telithromycin by increasing the conformational flexibility of the analog (Velvadapu et al., 2011, 2012; Wagh et al., 2012).

2.4.2 Site-Identification by Ligand Competitive Saturation (SILCS)

The final application that will be discussed in this chapter is the SILCS method (Guvench and MacKerell, 2009; Raman et al., 2011, 2013). SILCS harnesses the power of FF-based simulations to map the functional group affinities of a protein or any other macromolecule, an approach that has been used in other laboratories for individual ligands (Bakan et al., 2012; Ben-Shimon and Eisenstein, 2010; Brenke et al., 2009; Halgren, 2007; Lexa and Carlson, 2011; Miranker and Karplus, 1991; Tan et al., 2012; Wang and Yang, 2011), thereby incorporating macromolecule flexibility and solvation into the maps. This is achieved by first performing a number of parallel MD simulations of the protein in a box of explicit water with ~0.25–1 M fragments. The fragments are a diverse set of small molecules selected such that they capture the chemical features common to drugs, namely hydrophobic and hydrogen bonding groups, including both charged and neutral species. During the simulations, the fragments interact with all regions on the protein, thus allowing the generation of 3D probability maps (FragMaps), which are normalized with respect to the fragments in solution alone and converted to free energies (called grid-free energies, GFEs). The 3D distribution of GFE FragMaps identifies regions of the protein, including occluded pockets (Lakkaraju et al., 2014) that bind fragments favorably, as well as regions where specific fragment types are not favored. Notably, the normalization procedure leads to the FragMaps including the energetic penalty for ligand desolvation, and since the fragments must compete with water on the protein, it also accounts for the energetic penalty required to compete with water solvating the protein. Thus, the approach inherently includes the information in water-mapping methods, such as WaterMap (Abel et al., 2008; Young et al., 2007), while also identifying the types of functional groups that can successfully interact with different regions of the protein surface. In addition, the binding affinity of ligands may be estimated based on the ligand-based GFE (LGFE).

Initial studies from this laboratory using SILCS involved the use of two fragments (Tier I SILCS): benzene to represent aromatic groups and propane to represent aliphatic groups, with water used to represent hydrogen bond donor and acceptor (Guvench and MacKerell, 2009; Raman et al., 2011). More recently, the number of fragments was expanded to include benzene, propane, formamide, acetaldehyde, acetate, methylammonium, and methanol, which is referred to a Tier II SILCS (Raman et al., 2013). Benzene and propane again represent aromatic and aliphatic groups, respectively, while formamide, acetaldehyde, and methanol represent neutral hydrogen bond donors (via their polar hydrogens) and acceptors (via their oxygens). Methylammonium and acetate are included to represent charged hydrogen bond donors and acceptors, respectively. In addition, imidazole can be included to represent a heterocycle as well as both an additional neutral donor and acceptor. Although Tier I SILCS showed that the crystallographic binding modes of ligands for a diverse set of proteins could be reproduced even with a simple set of drug-like fragments, it also indicated that the simple set of fragments that is used limited the ability to correctly rank LGFE scores for protein ligands (Guvench and MacKerell, 2009; Raman et al., 2011). This, along with the need to map the functional requirements for specific types of hydrogen bonding groups, stimulated the use of more specific fragment types. Importantly, the presence of chemically distinct hydrogen bonding fragments in SILCS is advantageous because the fragments compete with each other and with water, such that the resulting FragMaps include the energetic cost of the displacement of water, as mentioned above. It was shown that the Tier II SILCS fragment maps are also able to identify the classes of protein–ligand interactions that are observed in crystal structures (Raman et al., 2013). With respect to quantitative ranking of ligands, it was shown that the use of an ensemble of ligand conformations leads to significant improvements. Notable in that study was the use of the FragMap LGFE scores in conjunction with Monte-Carlo sampling to generate ensembles of ligand conformations. Such an approach essentially represents the use of the SILCS method for ligand docking. Toward this end, a SILCS pharmacophore-based database screening protocol has been presented and shown to yield improved enrichment rates in three test proteins (Yu et al., 2014). Future extensions of the SILCS method may involve the use of different types a functional groups, a process that will be facilitated by the availability of parameters for the molecules of interest, as may be obtained from CGenFF.

2.5 Conclusion

In silico drug design is an important part of the drug development process. The use of computational methods saves time, money, and resources, and can be a useful tool when experimental evidence is difficult to obtain or lacking. In Section 2.1, the potential energy functions were presented and the terms contributing to the energy function were described. Section 2.2 detailed how biomolecular FFs are optimized, while Section 2.3 discussed the various classes of biomolecular FFs. Finally, in Section 2.4, two novel approaches to drug design were discussed: CSP and SILCS. These methods rely on FF-based simulations and hence are a good representation of the application of FFs in combination with molecular simulations to drug design.

Acknowledgments

This work was supported by the NIH (AI080968 and GM070855), a fellowship of the University of Maryland, School of Pharmacy Department of Pharmaceutical Sciences and the University of Maryland Computer-Aided Drug Design Center.

Conflict of Interest

ADM is co-founder and Chief Scientific Officer of SilcsBio LLC.

References

Abel, R., T. Young, R. Farid, B.J. Berne, and R.A. Friesner. 2008. Role of the active-site solvent in the thermodynamics of factor Xa ligand binding. *J. Am. Chem. Soc.* 130(9):2817–2831.

Allen, F.H., S. Bellard, M.D. Brice et al. 1979. The Cambridge crystallographic data centre: Computer-based search, retrieval, analysis and display of information. *Acta Cryst. B* 35(10):2331–2339.

Anisimov, V.M., G. Lamoureux, I.V. Vorobyov, N. Huang, B. Roux, and A.D. MacKerell, Jr. 2005. Determination of electrostatic parameters for a polarizable force field based on the classical Drude oscillator. *J. Chem. Theory Comput.* 1(1):153–168.

Asensio, J.L., F.J. Canada, X.H. Chen, N. Khan, D.R. Mootoo, and J. Jimenez-Barbero. 2000. Conformational differences between O- and C-glycosides: The alpha-O-Man-(1->1)-beta-Gal/alpha-C-Man-(1->1)-beta-Gal case—A decisive demonstration of the importance of the exo-anomeric effect on the conformation of glycosides. *Chem. Eur. J.* 6(6):1035–1041.

Bakan, A., N. Nevins, A.S. Lakdawala, and I. Bahar. 2012. Druggability assessment of allosteric proteins by dynamics simulations in the presence of probe molecules. *J. Chem. Theory Comput.* 8(7):2435–2447.

Baker, C.M., P.E. Lopes, X. Zhu, B. Roux, and A.D. MacKerell, Jr. 2010. Accurate calculation of hydration free energies using pair-specific Lennard-Jones parameters in the CHARMM drude polarizable force field. *J. Chem. Theory Comput.* 6(4):1181–1198.

Bayly, C.I., P. Cieplak, W.D. Cornell, and P.A. Kollman. 1993. A well-behaved electrostatic potential based method using charge restraints for deriving atomic charges: The RESP model. *J. Phys. Chem.* 97(40):10269–10280.

Ben-Shimon, A. and M. Eisenstein. 2010. Computational mapping of anchoring spots on protein surfaces. *J. Mol. Biol.* 402(1):259–277.

Berendsen, H.J.C., J.P.M. Postma, W.F. van Gunsteren, and J. Hermans. 1981. Interaction models for water in relation to protein hydration. In: *Intermolecular Forces*, B. Pullman. (ed.), Dordrecht, Holland: Reidel Publishing Co.

Berendsen, H.J.C., J.R. Grigera, and T. Straatsma. 1987. The missing term in effective pair potentials. *J. Phys. Chem.* 91(24):6269–6271.

Berger, O., O. Edholm, and F. Jahnig. 1997. Molecular dynamics simulations of a fluid bilayer of dipalmitoylphosphatidylcholine at full hydration, constant pressure, and constant temperature. *Biophys. J.* 72(5):2002–2013.

Berman, H.M., J. Westbrook, Z. Feng et al. 2000. The protein data bank. *Nucl. Acids Res.* 28(1):235–242.

Berman, H.M., W.K. Olson, D.L. Beveridge et al. 1992. The nucleic acid database: A comprehensive relational database of the three-dimensional structures of nucleic acids. *Biophys. J.* 63(3):751–759.

Bernard, D., A. Coop, and A.D. MacKerell, Jr. 2003. 2D conformationally sampled pharmacophore: A ligand-based pharmacophore to differentiate delta opioid agonists from antagonists. *J. Am. Chem. Soc.* 125(10):3101–3107.

Bernard, D., A. Coop, and A.D. MacKerell, Jr. 2005. Conformationally sampled pharmacophore for peptidic delta opioid ligands. *J. Med. Chem.* 48(24):7773–7780.

Bernard, D., A. Coop, and A.D. MacKerell, Jr. 2007. Quantitative conformationally sampled pharmacophore for δ opioid ligands: Reevaluation of hydrophobic moieties essential for biological activity. *J. Med. Chem.* 50(8):1799–1809.

Bernardo, D.N., Y. Ding, K. Krogh-Jespersen, and R.M. Levy. 1994. An anisotropic polarizable water model: Incorporation of all-atom polarizabilities into molecular mechanics force fields. *J. Phys. Chem.* 98(15):4180–4187.

Best, R.B. and G. Hummer. 2009. Optimized molecular dynamics force fields applied to helix-coil transition of polypeptides. *J. Phys. Chem. B* 113(26):9004–9015.

Best, R.B., N.V. Buchete, and G. Hummer. 2008. Are current molecular dynamics force fields too helical? *Biophys. J.* 95(1):L07–L09.

Best, R.B., X. Zhu, J. Shim et al. 2012. Optimization of the additive CHARMM all-atom protein force field targeting improved sampling of the backbone phi, psi and side-chain chi(1) and chi(2) dihedral angles. *J. Chem. Theory Comput.* 8(9):3257–3273.

Blondel, A. and M. Karplus. 1996. New formulation for derivatives of torsion angles and improper torsion angles in molecular mechanics: Elimination of singularities. *J. Comput. Chem.* 17:1132–1141.

Brenke, R., D. Kozakov, G.Y. Chuang et al. 2009. Fragment-based identification of druggable "hot spots" of proteins using Fourier doman correlation techniques. *Bioinformatics* 25(5):621–627.

Brooks, B.R., C.L. Brooks III, A.D. MacKerell, Jr. et al. 2009. CHARMM: The biomolecular simulation program. *J. Comput. Chem.* 30(10):1545–1614.

Bryce, R.A., M.A. Vincent, N.O.J. Malcolm, I.H. Hillier, and N.A. Burton. 1998. Cooperative effects in the structure of fluoride water clusters: Ab initio hybrid quantum mechanical/molecular mechanical model incorporating polarizable fluctuating charge solvent. *J. Chem. Phys.* 109:3077–3085.

Buckingham, R.A. 1938. The classical equation of state of gaseous helium, neon and argon. *Proc. Roy. Soc. of Lond. Ser. Math. Phys. Sci.* 168:264–283.

Caldwell, J., L.X. Dang, and P.A. Kollman. 1990. Implementation of nonadditive intermolecular potentials by use of molecular dynamics: Development of a water–water potential and water–ion cluster interactions. *J. Am. Chem. Soc.* 112(25):9144–9147.

Cheatham, T.E., III and D.A. Case. 2013. Twenty-five years of nucleic acid simulations. *Biopolymers* 99(12):969–977.

Cheatham, T.E., III, P. Cieplak, and P.A. Kollman. 1999. A modified version of the Cornell et al. force field with improved sugar pucker phases and helical repeat. *J. Biomol. Struct. Dyn.* 16(4):845–861.

Chen, I.J., D. Yin, and A.D. MacKerell, Jr. 2002. Combined ab initio/empirical approach for optimization of Lennard-Jones parameters for polar-neutral compounds. *J. Comput. Chem.* 23(2):199–213.

Chiu, S.-W., S.A. Pandit, H.L. Scott, and E. Jakobsson. 2009. An improved united atom force field for simulation of mixed lipid bilayers. *J. Phys. Chem. B* 113(9):2748–2763.

Chowdary, J., E. Harder, P.E.M. Lopes, L. Huang, A.D. MacKerell, Jr., and B. Roux. 2013. A polarizable force field of dipalmitoylphosphatidylcholine based on the classical drude model for molecular dynamics simulations of lipids. *J. Phys. Chem. B* 117(31):9142–9160.

Coimbatore Narayanan, B., J. Westbrook, S. Ghosh et al. 2014. The nucleic acid database: New features and capabilities. *Nucl. Acids Res.* 42(1):D114–D122.

Cornell, W.D., P. Cieplak, C.I. Bayly et al. 1995. A second generation force field for the simulation of proteins, nucleic acids, and organic molecules. *J. Am. Chem. Soc.* 117(19):5179–5197.

Dang, L.X. 1998. Importance of polarization effects in modeling hydrogen bond in water using classical molecular dynamics techniques. *J. Phys. Chem. B* 102(3):620–624.

Darden, T., D. York, and L. Pedersen. 1993. Particle mesh Ewald: An N*log(N) method for Ewald sums in large systems. *J. Chem. Phys.* 98(12):10089–10092.

Daura, X., A.E. Mark, and W.F. van Gunsteren. 1998. Parametrization of aliphatic CHn united atoms of GROMOS96 force field. *J. Comput. Chem.* 19(5):535–547.

Demerdash, O., E.-H. Yap, and T. Head-Gordon. 2014. Advanced potential energy surfaces for condensed phase simulations. *Annu. Rev. Phys. Chem.* 65:149–174.

Denning, E.J., U.D. Priyakumar, L. Nilsson, and A.D. Mackerell, Jr. 2011. Impact of 2′-hydroxyl sampling on the conformational properties of RNA: Update of the CHARMM all-atom additive force field for RNA. *J. Comput. Chem.* 32(9):1929–1943.

Duan, Y., C. Wu, S. Chowdhury et al. 2003. A point-charge force field for molecular mechanics simulations of proteins based on condensed-phase quantum mechanical calculations. *J. Comput. Chem.* 24(16):1999–2012.

Fadda, E. and R.J. Woods. 2010. Molecular simulations of carbohydrates and protein–carbohydrate interactions: Motivation, issues and prospects. *Drug Discov. Today* 15(15–16):596–609.

Feig, M., A.D. MacKerell, Jr., and C.L. Brooks, III. 2003. Force field influence on the observation of π-helical protein structures in molecular dynamics simulations. *J. Phys. Chem. B* 107(12):2831–2836.

Feig, M. and C.L. Brooks, III. 2004. Recent advances in the development and application of implicit solvent models in biomolecular simulations. *Curr. Opin. Struct. Biol.* 14(2):217–224.

Feller, S.E. and A.D. MacKerell, Jr. 2000. An improved empirical potential energy function for molecular simulations of phospholipids. *J. Phys. Chem. B* 104(31):7510–7515.

Foloppe, N. and A.D. MacKerell, Jr. 2000. All-atom empirical force field for nucleic acids: (1) Parameter optimization based on small molecule and condensed phase macromolecular target data. *J. Comput. Chem.* 21:86–104.

Fox, T. and P.A. Kollman. 1998. Application of the RESP methodology in the parametrization of organic solvents. *J. Phys. Chem. B* 102(41):8070–8079.

French, A.D. and G.P. Johnson. 2011. Computerized molecular modeling of carbohydrates. *Methods Mol. Biol.* 715:21–42.

Garcia, A.E. and K.Y. Sanbonmatsu. 2002. Alpha-helical stabilization by side chain shielding of backbone hydrogen bonds. *Proc. Natl. Acad. Sci. USA* 99(5):2782–2787.

Gough, C.A., S.E. DeBolt, and P.A. Kollman. 1992. Derivation of fluorine and hydrogen atom parameters using liquid simulations. *J. Comput. Chem.* 13(8):963–970.

GROMOS 86: Groningen Molecular Simulation Program Package. University of Groningen, Groningen, The Netherlands.

Guvench, O. and A.D. MacKerell, Jr. 2008. Comparison of protein force fields for molecular dynamics simulations. *Methods Mol. Biol.* 443:63–88.

Guvench, O. and A.D. MacKerell, Jr. 2009. Computational fragment-based binding site identification by ligand competitive saturation. *PLoS Comput. Biol.* 5(7):e1000435.

Guvench, O., E.R. Hatcher, R.M. Venable, R.W. Pastor, and A.D. Mackerell. 2009. CHARMM additive all-atom force field for glycosidic linkages between hexopyranoses. *J. Chem. Theory Comput.* 5(9):2353–2370.

Guvench, O., S.N. Greene, G. Kamath et al. 2008. Additive empirical force field for hexopyranose monosaccharides. *J. Comput. Chem.* 29(15):2543–2564.

Halgren, T.A. 1992. Representation of van der Waals (vdW) Interactions in molecular mechanics force fields: Potential form, combination rules, and vdW parameters. *J. Am. Chem. Soc.* 114(20):7827–7843.

Halgren, T.A. 1996a. Merck molecular force field. I. Basis, form, scope, Parametrization, and performance of MMFF94. *J. Comput. Chem.* 17(5–6):490–519.

Halgren, T.A. 1996b. Merck molecular force field. II. MMFF94 van der Waals and electrostatic parameters for intermolecular interactions. *J. Comput. Chem.* 17(5–6):520–552.

Halgren, T.A. 1996c. Merck molecular force field. V. Extension of MMFF94 using experimental data, additional computational data, and empirical rules. *J. Comput. Chem.* 17(5 & 6):616–641.

Halgren, T.A. 1999. MMFF VII. Characterization of MMFF94, MMFF94s, and other widely available force fields for conformational energies and for intermolecular-interaction energies and geometries. *J. Comput. Chem.* 20(7):730–748.

Halgren, T.A. 2007. New method for fast and accurate binding site identification analysis. *Chem. Biol. Drug Des.* 69(2):146–148.

Hansen, H.S. and P.H. Hunenberger. 2011. A reoptimized GROMOS force field for hexopyranose-based carbohydrates accounting for the relative free energies of ring conformers, anomers, epimers, hydroxymethyl rotamers, and glycosidic linkage conformers. *J. Comput. Chem.* 32(6):998–1032.

Hart, K., N. Foloppe, C.M. Baker, E.J. Denning, L. Nilsson, and A.D. Mackerell, Jr. 2012. Optimization of the CHARMM additive force field for DNA: Improved treatment of the BI/BII conformational equilibrium. *J. Chem. Theory Comput.* 8(1):348–362.

Hatcher, E., O. Guvench, and A.D. MacKerell, Jr. 2009a. CHARMM additive all-atom force field for acyclic polyalcohols, acyclic carbohydrates and inositol. *J. Chem. Theory Comput.* 5(5):1315–1327.

Hatcher, E., O. Guvench, and A.D. MacKerell, Jr. 2009b. CHARMM additive all-atom force field for aldopentofuranoses, methyl-aldopentofuranosides, and fructofuranose. *J. Phys. Chem. B* 113(37):12466–12476.

He, X., P.E. Lopes, and A.D. MacKerell, Jr. 2013. Polarizable empirical force field for acyclic polyalcohols based on the classical drude oscillator. *Biopolymers* 99(10):724–738.

Horn, H.W., W.C. Swope, J.W. Pitera et al. 2004. Development of an improved four-site water model for biomolecular simulations: TIP4P-EW. *J. Chem. Phys.* 120(20):9665–9678.

Hornak, V., R. Abel, A. Okur, B. Strockbine, A. Roitberg, and C. Simmerling. 2006. Comparison of multiple Amber force fields and development of improved protein backbone parameters. *Proteins* 65(3):712–725.

Iczkowski, R.P. and J.L. Margrave. 1961. Electronegativity. *J. Am. Chem. Soc.* 83(17):3547–3551.

Jakalian, A., B.L. Bush, D.B. Jack, and C.I. Bayly. 2000. Fast, efficient generation of high-quality atomic charges. AM1-BCC model: 1. Method. *J. Comput. Chem.* 21(2):132–146.

Jakalian, A., D.B. Jack, and C.I. Bayly. 2002. Fast, efficient generation of high-quality atomic charges. AM1-BCC model: II. Parametrization and validation. *J. Comput. Chem.* 23(16):1623–1641.

Jiao, D., J. Zhang, R.E. Duke, G. Li, M.J. Schnieders, and P. Ren. 2009. Trypsin-ligand binding free energies from explicit and implicit solvent simulations with polarizable potential. *J. Comput. Chem.* 30(11):1701–1711.

Jiao, D., P.A. Golubkov, T.A. Darden, and P. Ren. 2008. Calculation of protein-ligand binding free energy by using a polarizable potential. *Proc. Natl. Acad. Sci. USA* 105(17):6290–6295.

Jojart, B. and T.A. Martinek. 2007. Performance of the general amber force field in modeling aqueous POPC membrane bilayers. *J. Comput. Chem.* 28(12):2051–2058.

Jorgensen, W.L. 1986. Optimized intermolecular potential functions for liquid alcohols. *J. Phys. Chem.* 90(7):1276–1284.

Jorgensen, W.L. 2004. The many roles of computation in drug discovery. *Science* 303(5665):1813–1818.

Jorgensen, W.L., D.S. Maxwell, and J. Tirado-Rives. 1996. Development and testing of the OPLS all-atom force field on conformational energetics and properties of organic liquids. *J. Am. Chem. Soc.* 118(45):11225–11236.

Jorgensen, W.L., J. Chandrasekhar, J.D. Madura, R.W. Impey, and M.L. Klein. 1983. Comparison of simple potential functions for simulating liquid water. *J. Chem. Phys.* 79:926–936.

Jorgensen, W.L. and J. Tirado-Rives. 1988. The OPLS potential function for proteins. Energy minimizations for crystals of cyclic peptides and crambin. *J. Am. Chem. Soc.* 110(6):1657–1666.

Kaminski, G., E.M. Duffy, T. Matsui, and W.L. Jorgensen. 1994. Free energies of hydration and pure liquid properties of hydrocarbons from the OPLS all-atom model. *J. Phys. Chem.* 98(49):13077–13082.

Kaminski, G., R.A. Friesner, J. Tirado-Rives, and W.L. Jorgensen. 2001. Evaluation and reparametrization of the OPLS-AA force field for proteins via comparison with accurate quantum chemical calculations on peptides. *J. Phys. Chem. B* 105(28):6474–6487.

Kirschner, K.N., A.B. Yongye, S.M. Tschampel et al. 2008. GLYCAM06: A generalizable biomolecular force field. Carbohydrates. *J. Comput. Chem.* 29(4):622–655.

Kirschner, K.N., R.D. Lins, A. Maass, and T.A. Soares. 2012. A glycam-based force field for simulations of lipopolysaccharide membranes: Parametrization and validation. *J. Chem. Theory Comput.* 8(11):4719–4731.

Kirschner, K.N. and R.J. Woods. 2001. Solvent interactions determine carbohydrate conformation. *Proc. Natl. Acad. Sci. USA* 98(19):10541–10545.

Klauda, J.B., B.R. Brooks, A.D. MacKerell, Jr., R.M. Venable, and R.W. Pastor. 2005a. An ab initio study on the torsional surface of alkanes and its effect on molecular simulations of alkanes and a DPPC bilayer. *J. Phys. Chem. B* 109(11):5300–5311.

Klauda, J.B., R.M. Venable, J.A. Freites et al. 2010. Update of the CHARMM all-atom additive force field for lipids: Validation on six lipid types. *J. Phys. Chem. B* 114(23):7830–7843.

Klauda, J.B., R.W. Pastor, and B.R. Brooks. 2005b. Adjacent gauche stabilization in linear alkanes: Implications for polymer models and conformational analysis. *J. Phys. Chem. B* 109(33):15684–15686.

Kollman, P.A. 1993. Free energy calculations: Applications to chemical and biochemical phenomena. *Chem. Rev.* 93(7):2395–2417.

Kollman, P.A. 1996. Advances and continuing challenges in achieving realistic and predictive simulations of the properties of organic and biological molecules. *Acc. Chem. Res.* 29(10):461–469.

Kony, D., W. Damm, S. Stoll, and W.F. Van Gunsteren. 2002. An improved OPLS-AA force field for carbohydrates. *J. Comput. Chem.* 23(15):1416–1429.

Krieger, E., G. Koraimann, and G. Vriend. 2002. Increasing the precision of comparative models with YASARA NOVA-a self-parameterizing force field. *Proteins: Structure, Function, and Genetics* 47(3):393–402.

Kuczera, K., J.K. Wiorkiewicz, and M. Karplus. 1993. MOLVIB: Program for the Analysis of Molecular Vibrations, CHARMM, Harvard University.

Kunz, A.-P.E. and W.F. van Gunsteren. 2009. Development of a nonlinear classical polarization model for liquid water and aqueous solution: COS/D. *J. Phys. Chem. A* 113(43):11570–11579.

Lakkaraju, S.K., E.P. Raman, W. Yu, and A.D. MacKerell, Jr. 2014. Sampling of organic solutes in aqueous and heterogeneous environments using oscillating excess chemical potentials in grand canonical-like Monte Carlo-molecular dynamics simulations. *J. Chem. Theory Comput.* 10(6):2281–2290.

Lamoureux, G., A.D. MacKerell, Jr., and B. Roux. 2003. A simple polarizable model of water based on classical Drude oscillators. *J. Chem. Phys.* 119(10):5185–5197.

Lamoureux, G. and B. Roux. 2003. Modeling induced polarization with drude oscillators: Theory and molecular dynamics simulation algorithm. *J. Chem. Phys.* 119(6):3025–3039.

Langley, D.R. 1998. Molecular dynamics simulations of environment and sequence dependent DNA conformation: The development of the BMS nucleic acid force field and comparison with experimental results. *J. Biomol. Struct. Dyn.* 16(3):487–509.

Lexa, K.W. and H.A. Carlson. 2011. Full protein flexibility is essential for proper hot-spot mapping. *J. Am. Chem. Soc.* 133(2):200–202.

Li, D.-W. and R. Bruschweiler. 2010. NMR-based protein potentials. *Angew. Chem. Int. Ed. Engl.* 49(38):6778–6780.

Lindorff-Larsen, K., S. Piana, K. Palmo et al. 2010. Improved side-chain torsion potentials for the Amber ff99SB protein force field. *Proteins* 78(8):1950–1958.

Lins, R.D. and P.H. Hunenberger. 2005. A new GROMOS force field for hexopyranose-based carbohydrates. *J. Comput. Chem.* 26(13):1400–1412.

Llanta, E., K. Ando, and R. Rey. 2001. Fluctuating charge study of polarization effects in chlorinated organic liquids. *J. Phys. Chem. B* 105(32):7783–7791.

Lopes, P.E., B. Roux, and A.D. MacKerell, Jr. 2009. Molecular modeling and dynamics studies with explicit inclusion of electronic polarizability. Theory and applications. *Theor. Chem. Acc.* 124(1–2):11–28.

Lopes, P.E., J. Huang, J. Shim et al. 2013. Force field for peptides and proteins based on the classical drude oscillator. *J. Chem. Theory Comput.* 9(12):5430–5449.

Lopes, P.E.M, E. Harder, B. Roux, and A.D. MacKerell, Jr. 2009. Formalisms for the explicit inclusion of electronic polarizability in molecular modeling and dynamics studies. In: *Multiscale Quantum Models for Biocatalysis: Modern Techniques and Applications*, D. York and T.-S. Lee (eds.); in the series, *Challenges and Advances in Computational Chemistry and Physics*, Vol. 7, J. Leszczynski (ed.), Springer Dordrecht Heidelberg, London, New York, pp. 219–218, ISBN: 978-1-4020-9955-7.

MacKerell, A.D., Jr. 1997. Influence of magnesium ions on duplex DNA structural, dynamic, and solvation properties. *J. Phys. Chem. B* 101(4):646–650.

MacKerell, A.D., Jr. 1998. Protein force fields. In: *Encyclopedia of Computational Chemistry*, P.v.R. Schleyer, N.L. Allinger, T. Clark et al. (eds.), Chichester: John Wiley & Sons.

MacKerell, A.D., Jr. 2001. Atomistic models and force fields. In: *Computational Biochemistry and Biophysics*, O.M. Becker, A.D. MacKerell, Jr., B. Roux, and M. Watanabe (eds.), New York: Marcel Dekker, Inc.

MacKerell, A.D., Jr. 2004. Empirical force fields for biological macromolecules: Overview and issues. *J. Comput. Chem.* 25(13):1584–1604.

MacKerell, A.D., Jr., D. Bashford, M. Bellott et al. 1998. All-atom empirical potential for molecular modeling and dynamics studies of proteins. *J. Phys. Chem. B* 102(18):3586–3616.

MacKerell, A.D., Jr., J. Wiórkiewicz-Kuczera, and M. Karplus. 1995. An all-atom empirical energy function for the simulation of nucleic acids. *J. Am. Chem. Soc.* 117(48):11946–11975.

MacKerell, A.D., Jr., M. Feig, and C.L. Brooks, III. 2004a. Extending the treatment of backbone energetics in protein force fields: Limitations of gas-phase quantum mechanics in reproducing protein conformational distributions in molecular dynamics simulations. *J. Comput. Chem.* 25(11):1400–1415.

MacKerell, A.D., Jr., M. Feig, and C.L. Brooks, III. 2004b. Improved treatment of the protein backbone in empirical force fields. *J. Am. Chem. Soc.* 126(3):698–699.

MacKerell, A.D., Jr. and M. Karplus. 1991. Importance of attractive van der Waals contribution in empirical energy function models for the heat of vaporization of polar liquids. *J. Phys. Chem.* 95(26):10559–10560.

MacKerell, A.D., Jr. and N.K. Banavali. 2000. All-atom empirical force field for nucleic acids: II. Application to molecular dynamics simulations of DNA and RNA in solution. *J. Comput. Chem.* 21(2):105–120.

Malde, A.K., L. Zuo, M. Breeze et al. 2011. An automated force field topology builder (ATB) and repository: Version 1.0. *J. Chem. Theory Comput.* 7(12):4026–4037.

Mallajosyula, S.S. and A.D. MacKerell, Jr. 2011. Influence of solvent and intramolecular hydrogen bonding on the conformational properties of o-linked glycopeptides. *J. Phys. Chem. B* 115(38):11215–11229.

Mallajosyula, S.S., K.M. Adams, J.J. Barchi, and A.D. MacKerell, Jr. 2013. Conformational determinants of the activity of antiproliferative factor glycopeptide. *J. Chem. Inf. Model.* 53(5):1127–1137.

Marrink, S.J., H.J. Risselada, S. Yefimov, D.P. Tieleman, and A.H. de Vries. 2007. The MARTINI force field: Coarse grained model for biomolecular simulations. *J. Phys. Chem. B* 111(27):7812–7824.

Martyna, G.J., M.E. Tuckerman, D.J. Tobias, and M.L. Klein. 1996. Explicit reversible integrators for extended systems dynamics. *Mol. Phys.* 87(5):1117–1157.

Mayo, S.L., B.D. Olafson, and W.A. Goddard, III. 1990. DREIDING: A generic force field for molecular simulations. *J. Phys. Chem.* 94(26):8897–8909.

McCammon, J.A., B.R. Gelin, and M. Karplus. 1977. Dynamics of folded proteins. *Nature* 267(5612):585–590.

Miller, B.T., R.P. Singh, J.B. Klauda, M. Hodoscek, B.R. Brooks, and H.L. Woodcock, III. 2008. CHARMMing: A new, flexible web portal for CHARMM. *J. Chem. Inf. Model.* 48(9):1920–1929.

Miranker, A. and M. Karplus. 1991. Functionality maps of binding sites: A multiple copy simultaneous search method. *Proteins* 11(1):29–34.

MOLVIB: Program for the Analysis of Molecular Vibrations. CHARMM, Harvard University.

Mulliken, R.S. 1934. A new electroaffinity scale; together with data on valence states and on valence ionization potentials and electron affinities. *J. Chem. Phys.* 2:782–793.

Neria, E., S. Fischer, and M. Karplus. 1996. Simulation of activation free energies in molecular systems. *J. Chem. Phys.* 105:1902–1919.

Nilsson, L. and M. Karplus. 1986. Empirical energy functions for energy minimization and dynamics of nucleic acids. *J. Comput. Chem.* 7(5):591–616.

Norberg, J. and L. Nilsson. 1996. Constant pressure molecular dynamics simulations of hte dodecamers: d(GCGCGCGCGCGC)2 and r(GCGCGCGCGCGC)2. *J. Chem. Phys.* 104(15):6052–6057.

Norberg, J. and L. Nilsson 2000. On the truncation of long-range electrostatics in DNA. *Biophys. J.* 79(3):1537–1553.

Oostenbrink, C., A. Villa, A.E. Mark, and W.F. van Gunsteren. 2004. A biomolecular force field based on the free enthalpy of hydration and solvation: The GROMOS force-field parameter sets 53A5 and 53A6. *J. Comput. Chem.* 25(13):1656–1676.

Parr, R.G. and R.G. Pearson. 1983. Absolute hardness: Companion parameter to absolute electronegativity. *J. Am. Chem. Soc.* 105(26):7512–7516.

Patel, D., X. He, and A.D. MacKerell, Jr. 2015. Polarizable empirical force field for hexopyranose monosaccharides based on the classical drude oscillator. *J. Phys. Chem. B* 119: 637–652. Doi:10.1021/jp412696m.

Patel, S. and C.L. Brooks, III. 2003. CHARMM fluctuating charge force field for proteins: I Parametrization and application to bulk organic liquid simulations. *J. Comput. Chem.* 25(1):1–15.

Perez, A., I. Marchan, D. Svozil et al. 2007. Refinement of the AMBER force field for nucleic acids: Improving the description of alpha/gamma conformers. *Biophys. J.* 92(11):3817–3829.

Poger, D., W.F. van Gunsteren, and A.E. Mark. 2010. A new force field for simulating phosphatidylcholine bilayers. *J. Comput. Chem.* 31(6):1117–1125.

Ponder, J.W., C. Wu, P. Ren et al. 2010. Current status of the AMOEBA polarizable force field. *J. Phys. Chem. B* 114(8):2549–2564.

Ponder, J.W. and D.A. Case. 2003. Force fields for protein simulations. *Adv. Protein Chem.* 66:27–85.

Price, D.J. and C.L. Brooks, III. 2002. Modern protein force fields behave comparably in molecular dynamics simulations. *J. Comput. Chem.* 23(11):1045–1057.

Pulay, P., G. Fogarasi, F. Pang, and J.E. Boggs. 1979. Systematic ab initio gradient calculation of molecular geometries, force constants, and dipole moment derivatives. *J. Am. Chem. Soc.* 101(10):2550–2560.

Rais, R., C. Acharya, G. Tririya, A.D. MacKerell, Jr., and J.E. Polli. 2010. Molecular switch controlling the binding of anionic bile acid conjugates to human apical sodium-dependent bile acid transporter. *J. Med. Chem.* 53(13):4749–4760.

Raman, E.P., O. Guvench, and A.D. MacKerell, Jr. 2010. CHARMM additive all-atom force field for glycosidic linkages in carbohydrates involving furanoses. *J. Phys. Chem. B* 114(40):12981–12994.

Raman, E.P., W. Yu, O. Guvench, and A.D. Mackerell. 2011. Reproducing crystal binding modes of ligand functional groups using Site-Identification by Ligand Competitive Saturation (SILCS) simulations. *J. Chem. Inf. Model.* 51(4):877–896.

Raman, E.P., W. Yu, S.K. Lakkaraju, and A.D. Mackerell, Jr. 2013. Inclusion of multiple fragment types in the Site Identification by Ligand Competitive Saturation (SILCS) approach. *J. Chem. Inf. Model.* 53(12):3384–3398.

Rappe, A.K., C.J. Casewit, K.S. Colwel, W.A. Goddard, III, and W.M. Skiff. 1992. UFF, a full periodic table force field for molecular mechanics and molecular dynamics simulations. *J. Am. Chem. Soc.* 114(25):10024–10035.

Ren, P. and J.W. Ponder. 2002. Consistent treatment of inter- and intramolecular polarization in molecular mechanics calculations. *J. Comput. Chem.* 23(16):1497–1506.

Ribiero, A.A.S.T., B.A.C. Horta, and R.B. de Alencastro. 2008. MKTOP: A program for automatic construction of molecular topologies. *J. Braz. Chem. Soc.* 19:1433–1435.

Rick, S.W. and B.J. Berne. 1996. Dynamical fluctuating charge force fields: The aqueous solvation of amides. *J. Am. Chem. Soc.* 118(3):672–679.

Rick, S.W. and S.J. Stuart. 2002. Potentials and algorithms for incorporating polarizability in computer simulations. *Rev. Comp. Chem.* 18:89–146.

Rick, S.W., S.J. Stuart, J.S. Bader, and B.J. Berne. 1995. Fluctuating charge force fields for aqueous solutions. *Stud. Phys. Theor. Chem.* 83:31–40.

Rizzo, R.C. and W.L. Jorgensen. 1999. OPLS all-atom model for amines: Resolution of the amine hydration problem. *J. Am. Chem. Soc.* 121(20):4827–4836.

Rosso, L. and I.R. Gould. 2008. Structure and dynamics of phospholipid bilayers using recently developed general all-atom force fields. *J. Comput. Chem.* 29(1):24–37.

Roux, B. and T. Simonson. 1999. Implicit solvent models. *Biophys. Chem.* 78(1–2):1–20.

Savelyev, A. and A.D. MacKerell, Jr. 2014. All-atom polarizable force field for DNA based on the classical drude oscillator model. *J. Comput. Chem.* 35(16):1219–1239.

Schlenkrich, M., J. Brinkman, A.D. MacKerell, Jr., and M. Karplus. 1996. An empirical potential energy function for phospholipids: Criteria for parameter optimization and applications. In: *Membrane Structure and Dynamics*, K.M. Merz, and B. Roux (eds.), Boston: Birkhauser.

Schmid, N., A.P. Eichenberger, A. Choutko et al. 2011. Definition and testing of the GROMOS force-field versions 54A7 and 54B7. *Eur. Biophys. J.* 40(7):843–856.

Schuler, L.D., X. Daura, and W.F. van Gunsteren. 2001. An improved GROMOS96 force field for aliphatic hydrocarbons in the condensed phase. *J. Comput. Chem.* 22(11):1205–1218.

Schuttelkopf, A.W. and D.M. van Aalten. 2004. PRODRG: A tool for high-throughput crystallography of protein-ligand complexes. *Acta Crystallogr. D Biol. Crystallogr.* 6(8):1355–1363.

Shi, Y., C. Wu, J.W. Ponder, and P. Ren. 2011. Investigation of multipole electrostatics in hydration free energy calculations. *J. Comput. Chem.* 32(5):967–977.

Shi, Y., C.Z. Zhu, S.F. Martin, and P. Ren. 2012. Probing the effect of conformational constraint on phosphorylated ligand binding to an SH2 domain using polarizable force field simulations. *J. Phys. Chem. B* 116(5):1716–1727.

Shi, Y., Z. Xia, J. Zhang et al. 2013. The polarizable atomic multipole-based AMOEBA force field for proteins. *J. Chem. Theory Comput.* 9(9):4046–4063.

Shim, J., A. Coop, and A.D. MacKerell, Jr. 2012. Consensus 3D model of mu-opioid receptor ligand efficacy based on a quantitative conformationally sampled pharmacophore. *J. Phys. Chem. B* 115(22):7487–7496.

Shim, J. and A.D. MacKerell, Jr. 2011. Computational ligand-based rational design: Role of conformational sampling and force fields in model development. *Med. Chem. Commun.* 2(5):356–370.

Shirts, M.R., J.W. Pitera, W.C. Swope, and V.S. Pande. 2003. Extremely precise free energy calculations of amino acid side chain analogs: Comparison of common molecular mechanics force fields for proteins. *J. Chem. Phys.* 119(11):5740–5761.

Siu, S.W.I., R. Vacha, P. Jungwirth, and R.A. Bockman. 2008. Biomolecular simulations of membranes: Physical properties from different force fields. *J. Chem. Phys.* 128(12):125103.

Skjevik, A.A., B.D. Madej, R.C. Walker, and K. Teigen. 2012. LIPID11: A modular framework for lipid simulations using amber. *J. Phys. Chem. B* 116(36):11124–11136.

Sliwoski, G., S. Kothiwale, J. Meiler, and E.W. Lowe, Jr. 2014. Computational methods in drug discovery. *Pharmacol. Rev.* 66(1):334–395.

Soares, T.A., P.H. Hunenberger, M.A. Kastenholz et al. 2005. An improved nucleic acid parameter set for the GROMOS force field. *J. Comput. Chem.* 26(7):725–737.

Sprik, M. and M.L. Klein. 1988. A polarizable model for water using distributed charge sites. *J. Chem. Phys.* 89(12):7556–7560.

Straatsma, T.P. and J.A. McCammon. 1992. Computational alchemy. *Annu. Rev. Phys. Chem.* 43:407–435.

Tan, Y.S., P. Sledz, S. Lang et al. 2012. Using ligand-mapping simulations to design a ligand selectively targeting a cryptic surface pocket of polo-like kinase I. *Angew. Chem. Int. Ed. Engl.* 51(40):10078–10081.

Tuckerman, M.E. and G.J. Martyna. 2000. Understanding modern molecular dynamics: Techniques and applications. *J. Phys. Chem. B* 104(2):159–178.

Ulmschneider, J.P. and M.B. Ulmschneider. 2009. United atom lipid parameters for combination with the optimized potentials for liquid simulations all-atom force field. *J. Chem. Theory Comput.* 5(7):1803–1813.

van Gunsteren, W.F. and H.J.C. Berendsen. 1987. *Groningen Molecular Simulation (GROMOS) Library Manual*, Biomos, Groningen, The Netherlands, pp. 1–221.

van Gunsteren, W.F., S.R. Billeter, A.A. Eising et al. 1996. *Biomolecular Simulation: The GROMOS96 Manual and User Guide*. Zürich: BIOMOS b.v.

van Maaren, P.J. and D. van der Spoel. 2001. Molecular dynamics simulations of water within novel shell-model potentials. *J. Phys. Chem. B* 105(13):2618–2626.

Vanommeslaeghe, K. and A.D. MacKerell, Jr. 2012. Automation of the CHARMM General Force Field (CGenFF) I: Bond perception and atom typing. *J. Chem. Inf. Model.* 52(12):3144–3154.

Vanommeslaeghe, K., E. Hatcher, C. Acharya et al. 2010. CHARMM general force field: A force field for drug-like molecules compatible with the CHARMM all-atom additive biological force fields. *J. Comput. Chem.* 31(4):671–690.

Vanommeslaeghe, K., E.P. Raman, and A.D. MacKerell, Jr. 2012. Automation of the CHARMM General Force Field (CGenFF) II: Assignment of bonded parameters and partial atomic charges. *J. Chem. Inf. Model.* 52(12):3155–3168.

Velvadapu, V., I. Glassford, M. Lee et al. 2012. Desmethyl macrolides: Synthesis and evaluation of 4,10-didesmethyl telithromycin. *ACS Med. Chem. Lett.* 3(3):211–215.

Velvadapu, V., T. Paul, B. Wagh et al. 2011. Desmethyl macrolide analogues to address antibiotic resistance: Total synthesis and biological evaluation of 4,8,10-tridesmethyl telithromycin. *ACS Med. Chem. Lett.* 2(1):68–72.

Wagh, B., T. Paul, I. Glassford et al. 2012. Desmethyl macrolides: Synthesis and evaluation of 4,8-didesmethyl telithromycin. *ACS Med. Chem. Lett.* 3(12):1013–1018.

Wallqvist, A. and B.J. Berne. 1993. Effective potentials for liquid water using polarizable and nonpolarizable models. *J. Phys. Chem.* 97(51):13841–13851.

Wang, J., P. Cieplak, and P.A. Kollman. 2000. How well does a restrained electrostatic potential (RESP) model perform in calculating conformational energies of organic and biological molecules? *J. Comput. Chem.* 21(12):1049–1074.

Wang, J., R.M. Wolf, J.W. Caldwell, P.A. Kollman, and D.A. Case. 2004. Development and testing of a general Amber force field. *J. Comput. Chem.* 25(9):1157–1174.

Wang, J., W. Wang, P.A. Kollman, and D.A. Case. 2006. Automatic atom type and bond type perception in molecular mechanical calculations. *J. Mol. Graph. Model.* 25(2):247–260.

Wang, L.-P., T. Head-Gordon, J.W. Ponder et al. 2013a. Systematic improvement of a classical molecular model of water. *J. Phys. Chem. B* 117(34):9956–9972.

Wang, L.-P., J. Chen, and T.Van Voorhis. 2013b. Systematic parametrization of polarizable force fields from quantum chemistry data. *J. Chem. Theory Comput.* 9(1):452–460.

Wang, S. and C.-Y. Yang. 2011. Hydrophobic binding hot spots of Bcl-xL protein-protein interfaces by cosolvent molecular dynamics simulations. *ACS Med. Chem. Lett.* 2(4):280–284.

Warshel, A. and M. Levitt. 1976. Theoretical studies of enzymatic reactions: Dielectric, electrostatic, and steric stabilization of the carbonium ion in the reaction of lysozyme. *J. Mol. Biol.* 103(2):227–249.

Weiner, P.K. and P.A. Kollman. 1981. AMBER: Assisted Model Building with Energy Refinement. A general program for modeling molecules and their interactions. *J. Comput. Chem.* 2(3):287–303.

Weiner, S.J., P.A. Kollman, D.A. Case et al. 1984. A new force field for molecular mechanical simulation of nucleic acids and proteins. *J. Am. Chem. Soc.* 106(3):765–784.

White, D.N.J. 1997. A computationally efficient alternative to the Buckingham potential for molecular mechanics calculations. *J. Comput. Aided Mol. Des.* 11(5):517–521.

Woods, R.J., R.A. Dwek, C.J. Edge, and B. Fraser-Reid. 1995. Molecular mechanical and molecular dynamical simulations of glycoproteins and oligosaccharides. 1. GLYCAM_93 parameter development. *J. Phys. Chem.* 99:3832–3846.

Yesselman, J.D., D.J. Price, J.L. Knight, and C.L. Brooks, III. 2012. MATCH: An atom-typing toolset for molecular mechanics force fields. *J. Comput. Chem.* 33(2):189–202.

Yildirim, I., H.A. Stern, S.D. Kennedy, J.D. Tubbs, and D.H. Turner. 2010. ReParametrization of RNA chi torsion parameters for the AMBER force field and comparison to NMR spectra for cytidine and uridine. *J. Chem. Theory Comput.* 6(5):1520–1531.

Yin, D. and A.D. MacKerell, Jr. 1998. Combined ab initio/empirical approach for optimization of lennard-jones parameters. *J. Comput. Chem.* 19(3):334–338.

Yoshii, N., R. Miyauchi, S. Miura, and S. Okazaki. 2000. A molecular-dynamics study of the equation of state of water using a fluctuating-charge model. *Chem. Phys. Lett.* 317(3–5):414–420.

Young, T., R. Abel, B. Kim, B.J. Berne, and R.A. Friesner. 2007. Motifs for molecular recognition exploiting hydrophobic enclosure in protein-ligand binding. *Proc. Natl. Acad. Sci. USA* 104(3):808–813.

Yu, H., T. Hansson, and W.F. Van Gunsteren. 2003. Development of a simple, self-consistent polarizable model for liquid water. *J. Chem. Phys.* 118(1):221–234.

Yu, W., S.K. Lakkaraju, E.P. Raman, and A.D. MacKerell, Jr. 2014. Site-identification by ligand competitive saturation (SILCS) assisted pharmacophore modeling. *J. Comput. Aided Mol. Des.* 28(5):491–507.

Zgarbova, M., M. Otyepka, J. Sponer et al. 2011. Refinement of the Cornell et al. nucleic acids force field based on reference quantum chemical calculations of glycosidic torsion profiles. *J. Chem. Theory Comput.* 7(9):2886–2902.

Zhang, J., W. Yang, J.P. Piquemal, and P. Ren. 2012. Modeling structural coordination and ligand binding in zinc proteins with a polarizable potential. *J. Chem. Theory Comput.* 8(4):1314–1324.

Zhong, S. and A.D. MacKerell, Jr. 2007. Binding response: A descriptor for selecting ligand binding site on protein surfaces. *J. Chem. Inf. Model.* 47(6):2303–2315.

Zoete, V., M.A. Cuendet, A. Grosdidier, and O. Michielin. 2011. SwissParam: A fast force field generation tool for small organic molecules. *J. Comput. Chem.* 32(11):2359–2368.

3

Library Design, Chemical Space, and Drug Likeness

Hugo O. Villar

CONTENTS

3.1 Introduction

High-throughput screening is a well-established method that dominates the discovery of compounds that can become clinical candidates. A critical factor for its success has been the assembly of an adequate chemical collection, geared to produce multiple high-quality hits with efficient use of resources (Bakken et al., 2012). Library design should not be viewed as an entirely creative process. The term design is used to convey the idea of purpose, planning, and intention in assembling a chemical collection for use. The design process will vary with the intended use of the collection, which may include not only commercially available or easy-to-synthesize compounds, but also virtual collections of structures.

Chemical libraries are also part of virtual screening, which is the base for computational techniques in lead discovery and optimization. Other techniques rely on the design of a chemical library as well, including structure-based and fragment-based drug design. Library design concepts have been adapted to other parts of the chemical industry, in areas as diverse as material sciences (Rajan, 2008) or agrochemicals (Lindell et al., 2009). Our focus will remain on the discovery of pharmacological agents.

Practically, library design refers to the methods used for selecting compounds from an available pool or a virtual collection to maximize the likelihood of identifying chemical series with improved prospects to satisfy their intended purpose, quickly and cost-effectively. A series of methods are applied successively to reduce the vast number of possibilities that chemistry offers (Villar and Koehler, 2000) while retaining a number of compounds capable of yielding a solid starting point for research and development. The compound selection process will follow different paths depending on the intended use of the library, and for some technologies and target classes where there is little information about ligands, these libraries could be large, while for other techniques such as fragment-based design, they could be relatively small. The more we know about the intended use of the collection, the more stringently we can define the library and increase its likelihood of success, though not always reduce its size.

We summarize in the following the technologies used in library design. We start discussing the use of filters used to eject compounds from a chemical collection, either because of unsuitability for their purpose—because we intend to focus its use in a particular region of the druggable genome (Overington et al., 2006)—or to apply it to a specific lead discovery technique. Filters are complemented with sampling techniques that aim to identify a subset of compounds that represent the characteristics of a much larger collection. This is usually done, because after the application of all reasonable filters, the number of chemicals that would be possible to screen would be significantly larger than those that can reasonably be acquired or managed. Finally, we discuss the problem of completeness of a screening file and some of the methods used to bring it closer to completeness. The importance of the topic has spurred for a large body of research on its many facets. We do not intend to have a comprehensive review, but we provide some solid pointers to each of these subjects with a particular emphasis on topics that are logical next steps in its evolution.

3.2 Chemical Collections: Commercial Libraries, Virtual Libraries, and Combinatorial Library Enumeration

When discussing the ensemble of all organic molecules that would be possible to generate, it is common to define the challenge in terms of chemical space (Dobson, 2004). The concept of chemical space evokes the idea of a geographical map, and it is used to determine the distribution of molecules according to their properties. The map is hyper-dimensional, and it is created by assigning dimensions to a series of molecular properties. Each molecule, represented by a vector of its molecular properties in the hyperspace selected, corresponds to a point in property space. The properties used to define that hyperspace vary greatly with the intended purpose of the library or with the stage of library design. The selection of properties is one of the key issues in library design as it defines the perspective we will adopt to analyze chemical space. As thousands of molecular descriptors exist, any combination of these properties may be used to define a property space with hundreds of different dimensions, as it will be discussed below. The distribution of the points is dependent on the properties selected, and therefore, there is no unique chemical space. The ambiguity of the concept should then be transparent. The use of positional information within the space can be judged by proximity among points (compounds) and the preferred occupancy of that space can be used to enrich a library with the desired activity or property (Reymond and Awale, 2012).

While chemical space can be quite large and populated theoretically by extremely large numbers of compounds (Villar and Koehler, 2000), in practice the largest chemical files available are of the order of a few million compounds. In fact, only a tiny fraction of all possible chemical entities has been explored. Most compound vendors provide lists of chemicals in easy-to-access form. Some websites provide aggregation of the different vendor catalogs (Saxena and Prathipati, 2006) that are freely accessible.

In addition to the aggregation of catalogs from multiple vendors, databases of chemicals that can potentially be synthesized, typically via parallel or combinatorial synthesis, can be generated. For a given chemical reaction and a list of chemicals capable of undergoing such reaction, the resulting chemicals can be enumerated (Leach et al., 1999). The automated enumeration can take place by simply using an open valence (i.e., clipping the molecule) at the reactive group and generating the combination of all complementary open valences in the reacting groups. This method is quite simple and rapid, but knows no chemistry. The issue is in generating the lists of reactive groups and their positions of attachment to a scaffold or linkage among pairs. The alternative approach is the reaction transform approach (Pirok et al., 2006). The software takes as input the list of reagents and applies the transformation to generate the product. *In silico,* these lists of prophetic compounds can reach into tens of millions, which also pales in comparison to the overall number of chemicals that are potentially available.

The enumeration of virtual libraries continues to evolve aiming toward knowledge-based systems where the reaction is encoded in vectors that encompass the changes that take place during a chemical transformation as descriptors that are gained in the products and those lost from the reactants (Patel et al., 2009). The heart of the system for enumeration is quickly becoming the design of reaction libraries (Pirok et al., 2006).

The result of the enumerated libraries or the aggregations of commercial vendor catalogs are lists of chemicals. Not all these chemicals would be suitable for the intended purpose as therapeutic agents or even starting points for medicinal chemistry. Compounds that do not meet the criteria for use ought to be culled from the libraries. In the end, virtual collections or commercially available compounds will always be larger than the resources available to screen them. Consequently, methods that allow us to prioritize compounds of interest are of great importance in the planning of a library for screening. These topics will be covered in the coming sections.

Once a chemical file of interest is generated, the most common next step is to filter it to eject compounds that are unsuitable for the intended purpose (Bologa and Oprea, 2012). We would remove highly reactive chemicals or compounds that do not jive with our current understanding of what makes a compound a drug, including those unlikely to achieve adequate distribution, prone to solubility issues, and so on.

3.3 Filters

The source of the chemicals for any screening exercise can be in-house synthesis, including library synthesis, and corporate collections, accumulated through time. These compounds are supplemented with samples acquired from commercial vendors or strategic collaborations developed to enrich the existing collections. Addition of new chemicals to a screening library is typically preceded by the use of a series of filters aimed to remove compounds that are clearly unsuitable for their purpose as drug candidates, as shown in Figure 3.1.

3.3.1 Grossly Unsuitable Chemicals: Structural Screening

Pharmaceutical companies have developed lists of structural features that are reactive or have been shown to be problematic. These exclusion lists are dependent on internal biases that companies or their medicinal chemists may have. Mapping hit promiscuity from historical primary HTS data provides an avenue to objectively identify the troublesome functional groups (Pearce et al., 2006). The undesirable functional groups go beyond simple reactive groups and many times cannot be identified by simple exclusion of predefined lists. Lists of excluded features in one instance have been reported to top 540 separate structural features (Bakken et al., 2012). Compounds can be excluded from an initial scanning of the file for a variety of reasons, including idiosyncratic ones such as interference with the primary assay used for screening or lack of sufficient solubility in the screening conditions (Di and Kerns, 2006). At times, exclusions are the result of past screening, where such

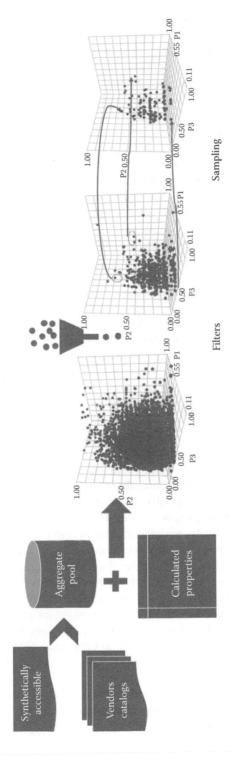

FIGURE 3.1

Simplified schematic of the library design process. Library design begins by assembling the lists of chemicals that are potentially available, either from vendors or libraries of compounds that could be synthesized. Once the chemical files are merged to create an aggregate pool, or we use one available, depending on our goals in assembling the library and the techniques to be used for lead discovery. Filters are then applied to remove compounds unlikely to succeed based on their physicochemical properties or predictions from some virtual screening model. The filters could be to bias the collection for compounds that are likely to interact with a family of targets of interest. The resulting library could be larger than the number of compounds that can be acquired, and therefore some sampling method, such as clustering, should be used to select a representative sample.

compounds have been reported to be active in many disparate assays (Baell and Holloway, 2010).

There is consensus among chemoinformatics professionals that smaller and simpler chemicals constitute a better starting point for medicinal chemistry work. The consensus seems to emerge from a convergence of simplicity of the chemistry work and, as we will discuss in the following section, requirements for good absorption, distribution, metabolism, and excretion (ADME) properties (Bologa and Oprea, 2012). This concept may be starting to change as new biological process such as protein–protein interactions need to be disrupted, which seems to require larger molecules (Buchwald, 2010).

The filters in general constitute a good starting point for most library generation exercises, but the ultimate use of the chemical should be kept in mind when planning which filters should be applied. Compounds capable of binding covalently or compounds that can be quickly metabolized can be useful as prodrugs, which can make the scientist reconsider the filters applied. The approach to be followed to optimize the compounds should be a factor as reactive compounds can be used in fragment-based drug design (Yang et al., 2009). Filters that are applied in the hope of having a greater chance of oral availability should be reconsidered for certain therapeutic classes, where parenteral administration would be the mode of administration for the drug or if the compounds will be CNS active drugs where additional filters may be appropriate. At all times the library design process should be mindful of the endpoint.

3.3.2 Considerations of Drug Likeness—ADME

As discussed earlier, chemical space is quite large due to the number of properties that are relevant to the drug discovery and development process. Fortunately, not every combination of molecular properties are promising if the goal is to identify a clinical candidate. At least in terms of the potential number of compounds, the biologically relevant chemical space is only a fraction of the complete chemical space. A drug is really the result of a complex interplay among bioactivity, toxicity, chemical and metabolic stability, and several other factors that few compounds can satisfy. This observation provides another way to filter out compounds. Certain compounds fall outside the typical range of properties that have been observed in drugs. Filtering out those compounds that do not share similarities with bioactive compounds can be a useful way to focus the library toward its intended purpose, resulting in files of drug-like compounds. From early on, the focus of the drug-like concept has been the physicochemical properties that most (not all) orally available drugs share, but in some cases, certain functional groups were also deemed unlikely to succeed as drugs.

The most commonly cited and widely used criteria for drug-likeness are simple ranges of physicochemical properties, such as the "rule of 5" (Lipinski et al., 2001). The rules were derived by using a 90 percentile rule for all of four properties observed in orally available drugs. Molecular weight less than 500, an octanol water partition coefficient calculated using the Hansch and Leo approach should be in a range of −5 to 5; the number of hydrogen bond donors calculated simply as the sum of the number of oxygens and nitrogens with a hydrogen attached should be <5; the sum of oxygens and nitrogens without hydrogen attached should be <10. There are numerous caveats that apply to these coarse rules that should be remembered when applying them. First, the properties are calculated in a very specific manner. Except the molecular weight, all other properties have been calculated with specific assumptions. Second, the analysis is carried out looking for orally available compounds and there are some significant differences between oral drugs and other classes (Vieth et al., 2004). More accurately, the rule of 5 should be regarded as quick rules for oral availability rather than drug likeness. Third, the rules were derived from marketed drugs, while the libraries to be used in screening aim to identify lead compounds or reasonable starting points for medicinal chemistry. Fourth, the analysis was retrospective, and for novel targets, they might be inadequate. The purpose of library is to provide a lead compound that could be optimized into a clinical candidate. Lead-like compounds as opposed to drug-like ones may follow a different distribution of physicochemical properties. Some rules for a valuable lead have been put forward: the molecular weight should be in the 200–350 molecular weight, cLogP in the 1–3 units range and not more than a single charge, because medicinal chemist add complexity to the scaffolds as they seek to improve the pharmacological profile (Rishton, 2008).

Beyond the rule of 5, other physicochemical parameters have also been found to be of importance to define drug-like character. Two parameters, the number of rotatable bonds, which should remain under 10, and total polar surface area equal to or less than 140 $Å^2$ (Veber et al., 2002) have been consistently used as desirable physicochemical characteristics.

Over the time the rule of 5 has been regarded as overly lax; and for orally available drugs, the parameters observed tend to be in a narrower range. For example, the number of hydrogen bond donors should be <3.

Using sets of physicochemical properties, libraries may be tailored for different purposes. The cost per well of screening and the numerous possible uses of the high throughput technology makes it necessary to focus on areas of the chemical space that have high value for drug discovery (Duffy et al., 2012). Virtual screening using different models developed for the prediction of pharmacokinetic parameters have been in use for over a decade (Oprea and Matter, 2004). From water solubility prediction, to blood–brain barrier permeability for libraries used for central nervous system (CNS) targets, models can potentially be applied to the design of a screening library. The efficiency and success of preselection will clearly depend on the goodness of the models used and their range of applicability.

Even when building libraries that could be used for any pharmaceutical target, so far, pharmaceutical research has focused on a relatively small fraction of the genome, in what has been dubbed the druggable genome. As our searches expand toward new classes of therapeutic agents, the criteria for "drug-like" will have to be updated. Strict adherence to fixed rules derived in what is known may hinder pharmaceutical discovery in the long run. There is significant interest in tools to assess the druggability of a target that is how amenable it is to an interaction with a small molecule that may result in eliciting a pharmaceutical response. Fueled in part by the continuing explosion in available protein crystal structures, structure-based druggability assessment can become a component of target selection (Fauman et al., 2011). The problem is quite complex, since crystallographic data do not capture the dynamic effects that accompany binding in particular for challenging target classes. The next frontier will be in the development of similar methods to assess druggability by antibodies, peptides, and other biologics and make a determination whether small molecules should be pursued for a given target family or other therapeutic agents should be pursued.

3.4 Targeted Focused Libraries

The emphasis on screening libraries that can be applicable to any druggable target has declined in favor of libraries that can be applied to specific target families (Villar and Hansen, 2009). Beyond the cost advantage of screening smaller libraries, they are more controllable in terms of quality and purity. A library is described as focused when compounds selected into the library are optimized with respect to at least one target property (Ebalunode et al., 2011)

The use of computational techniques to reduce the size of screening libraries by focusing them on specific targets or target families can be approached in different ways. The most common approach has been to focus the library on certain popular target classes (Orry et al., 2006). Virtual screening techniques can be used to bias compound selection toward specific target families. In general, virtual screening can be any computational technology that can be used to evaluate a large number of structures (which might have already been filtered for drug-likeness) to be studied in biological assays (Bologa and Oprea, 2012). The use of physicochemical descriptors to narrow or filter the drug-like space even further to those properties shared by known ligands of a protein superfamily are the simpler technical approaches. For example for kinases, a study suggests that compounds tend to be heavier, more flexible, and have a higher polar surface while retaining high hydrophobicity overall compared to chemicals in other biological databases (Singh et al., 2012).

Rational selection of compounds from commercial libraries of already synthesized compounds prevails in the industry and academic work (Ebalunode et al., 2011). Structure-based and ligand-based methods provide the two basic approaches for virtual screening toward building-focused libraries for screening. The use of traditional computational tools such as predictive quantitative structure–activity relationship (QSAR) models and pharmacophore models, based on alignments or solely based on shape and/or electrostatics, has been reported to be useful in the design of small screening libraries with varying degrees of success. To apply these techniques, a few ligands should be known for the target or related targets that can help in biasing the library design process.

As more structural information about the targets becomes available, structure-based virtual screening can also be used to design libraries. In the absence of direct structural information, a chemogenomics approach that incorporates sequence and mutagenesis data has been used as well (Harris et al., 2011). As datasets of compounds and target structures become larger, new challenges emerge in the use of virtual screening (Heikamp and Bajorath, 2013). Higher throughput may result in lower accuracy, which may make virtual screening more suitable for the design of libraries as opposed to the identification of individual compounds. The added need for speed also entails the development of faster methods for virtual screening and a move toward pharmacophore-based approaches or hybrid approaches that may take into account the explicit characteristics of the interaction between the ligand and the protein, but reduce them to the form of a filter for screening or pharmacophore type fingerprint (Deng et al., 2006).

3.5 Fragment Libraries

The use of fragment-based drug discovery (FBDD) has become an alternative strategy to high-throughput screening to identify lead compounds. The techniques have proven to be quite successful for the pharmaceutical research, with several examples of compounds at different stages of clinical evaluation and some compounds discovered using the approach in the market. Targets that traditionally were deemed intractable have been successfully approached with these techniques (Baker, 2013). The use of physical methods for screening able to detect weak binding compounds, such as NMR, allowed the screening of very low molecular weight compounds and the detection of weak binders. The combination that results with structure-based design techniques allowed the linkage of these low molecular weight compounds (dubbed fragments) in way that resulted in compounds that spanned more of the target binding site, displaying a larger number of interactions with the target that resulted in affinities in the range of good quality lead compounds. Extensive reviews are available on the scope and techniques used for FBDD (Rognan, 2012; Joseph-McCarthy et al., 2014).

FBDD relies on the use of libraries for screening. Since the objective is to identify compounds that could be linked to others to generate the lead compounds, these fragments should have physical properties that when summed to the other fragments to which it will be connected will be in the range acceptable for drug-like molecules. This reasoning led to act by analogy to the Rule of 5 and create for fragments the Rule of 3 that states that the fragments should have molecular weight <300, cLogP lower than or equal to 3, and hydrogen bond donor and acceptor counts should each be lower than 3. In parallel with the developments of regular screening libraries, additional criteria based on polar surface area and number of rotatable bond have also been added (Hajduk and Greer, 2007). A retrospective analysis of successful projects in FBDD revealed that the average number of heavy atoms (nonhydrogen atoms) in a scaffold was approximately 18, to which 11 more were added to generate the lead (Orita et al., 2009). Concepts such as ligand efficiency, defined as the binding energy per heavy atom, are particularly important for FBDD, where each atom should be made to count toward increased activity. Otherwise, very large molecules could be the result and unlikely to satisfy the criteria of druggability for a lead compound. The use of ligand efficiency and other generalized parameters (Bembenek et al., 2009) seem to correlate with the success in finding a viable lead compound from FBDD.

Other considerations are important when dealing with very low molecular weight compounds, which could be primarily used as reactants and therefore blocking reactive groups may be necessary (Schuffenhauer et al., 2005), unless the technique used explicitly involves the use of reactive groups such as the linkage of thiols to form disulphide bonds when the molecules are in close proximity (Erlanson et al., 2004; Buck and Wells, 2005).

Beyond physical properties, there have been studies aimed at computationally fragmenting molecules of interest to identify the building blocks of bioactive compounds. Initially, removal of acyclic bonds led to the first attempt in this direction (Rognan, 2012). The question posed by this approach is to what extent the fragments identified represent intrinsic biases of chemist or chemical tractability. Moreover, the fragments found in this way tend to be simple aromatic. The work has evolved to recognize that high-quality interactions cannot be found if the fragments used are simple skeletons with limited complexity in terms of functional groups or substituents (Wilde and Link, 2013).

The design of fragment libraries for screening continues to attract significant attention as its specific characteristics will be dependent on the intended use. A convergence of techniques is likely to emerge that may lead to redefining the challenge of designing small molecular weight collections. An interesting example is the design of fragment libraries for specific target classes based on a knowledge base of protein structural environments annotated with the small molecule substructures they bind (Tang and Altman, 2014).

While experimental approaches to FBDD have only been possible for about a decade, the idea is not new as *de novo* synthesis based on computational techniques has been available in different forms for much longer. The multiple copy simultaneous search can be considered a precursor of other entirely computational techniques (Caflisch et al., 1993). Other strategies for *de novo* ligand design such as LUDI (Bohm, 1992), GROW (Moon and Howe, 1991), or GrowMol (Bohacek et al., 1999) can be reasonably viewed as *in silico* fragment-based design.

3.6 Diversity Selection

After applying the different types of filters discussed to any large collection, there will remain a larger number of chemicals than what it would be possible to make or acquire. The library design problem then becomes one of selecting a smaller sample that retains the characteristics of the larger collection. The issue introduces the question of how we retain the characteristics of the larger sample, and what retaining the characteristics of the larger sample means. This last question requires us to analyze the possible ways in which we can characterize a chemical collection. The answer has usually been that we want to use a set of properties that represent such collection. Molecules in the collection are correlated with molecular properties or descriptors. The properties are numeric in nature, and could be binary, integers, or real, but in the end the result is a vector whose elements are the different descriptors selected. There is an alternative to going from molecules to properties to analyze their diversity. Scaffold or chemotype analysis has been an alternative used in chemoinformatics for the classification of molecules and their subsetting. In these approaches, molecules are items that can be decomposed into elements (substructures), lending it to categorical analysis. The issue of how a much larger collection can be represented by a smaller sample in a defined chemical space is a mathematical one. Classification techniques and clustering in particular can provide an answer as discussed below.

3.6.1 Property-Based Subset Selection

The reduction of molecules to their properties, thus defining a chemical space and representative sample selection based on the use of classification techniques such as clustering methods, has been the most widely used strategy in library design (Gillet, 2008). The use of techniques to select a representative sample and avoid repetition of chemical classes was implemented before the use of drug-like filters or target-biased library design. This topic has been extensively reviewed (Schnur, 2008; Villar and Hansen, 2009; Lisurek et al., 2010; Ebalunode et al., 2011).

Essentially, two components are needed to pick a nonredundant subset from a chemical collection that could be added to an existing library. First, the molecular descriptors are used to define chemical space. Second, a methodology is needed to select a representative sample from that chemical space. An extensive review of the different aspects of this topic has been published (Gorse, 2006) a few years back, but it provides a good overview of what has been tried in the field.

Topological indices, fingerprint-based descriptors generated from connectivity tables, physicochemical properties, and fingerprints based on pharmacophoric elements available to the molecule are among a myriad properties to be used. Until a recent study by Koutsoukas et al. (2014), there had been sporadic effort in determining best practices by comparing techniques. When aiming to determine which properties provided the most adequate coverage of the bioactive space, several important points emerged that could lead to better criteria for compound selection. The study evaluated a number of different classes of molecular descriptors, including fingerprint-based descriptors, pharmacophore-based descriptors, physicochemical descriptors that can be evaluated from the 2D representation of the molecule, and connectivity-based descriptors. Descriptors based on atom topology (i.e., fingerprint-based descriptors and pharmacophore-based descriptors) correlated well in rank-ordering compounds, in bioactivity both within and between descriptor types. However, shape-based descriptors showed weak correlation with the other descriptors utilized in this study, demonstrating significantly different behavior.

Bayesian affinity fingerprints (Nguyen et al., 2013) were found to be marginally superior to other types of fingerprints when the number of bioactive classes retrieved was examined. Bayesian affinity fingerprints are the computational equivalent of affinity fingerprints (Kauvar et al., 1995, 1998; Kauvar and Villar, 1998; Beroza et al., 2002), determined based on the pattern of binding affinity against a reference panel of proteins, which showed statistical independence among them. Conceptually, the use of docking scores as molecular properties similar to Bayesian affinity fingerprints had already been proposed, for diversity selection (Briem and Kuntz, 1996; Koehler and Villar, 2000).

Fingerprints based on atom topology were used quite often initially. These fingerprints that simply indicated presence or absence of functional groups or atom type provided the initial impetus to the field. Nowadays, the most frequently used fingerprints are those based on the Morgan concepts where for a fixed topological distance, the atom types are recorded for every atom in the molecule (Morgan, 1965). Extended-connectivity fingerprints (ECFP) (Rogers and Hahn, 2010) can be very rapidly calculated; they are not predefined and can represent an essentially infinite number of different molecular features (including stereochemical information); their features represent the presence of particular substructures, allowing easier interpretation of analysis results; and the ECFP algorithm can be tailored to generate different types of circular fingerprints, optimized for different uses. This class of fingerprints was also found to be quite effective when looking for coverage of different pharmacological classes in chemical space (Nguyen et al., 2013).

The methods used to select a subset of representative compounds from the chemical space have been centered on the use of clustering techniques for the most part (Pascual et al., 2003). The most significant challenge with the diverse clustering methods is that they are not suitable for large chemical collections. In particular, Ward's hierarchical clustering methods have been identified to have superior performance in its class. The Jarvis-Patrick clustering technique was used often, but the method generates very large and very small clusters, as well as a large number of singletons, which has reduced its use. K-means, where the number of clusters wanted is predetermined, has also been used. When using clustering, compounds are selected from the center of each cluster or as close to its centroid as possible. Dissimilarity-based selection provides an alternative to clustering. The collection is grown by identifying the most dissimilar compound to the ones already selected. The Max–Min algorithm is commonly employed in this class, but many others can be used as well (Eckert and Bajorath, 2007).

Clustering and dissimilarity algorithms require some metric for similarity or dissimilarity that needs to be implemented as a distance or a discriminant. The Tanimoto coefficient (Willett, 2006) has been widely used and continues to be used as a similarity index for binary variables, despite its well-documented size bias (Dixon and Koehler, 1999). Several other metrics beyond Tanimoto have been developed and implemented (Willett, 2006). For continuous variables, the Euclidean distances are commonly used, but other distances have also been employed to determine molecular similarity.

A final topic that should be given consideration is the issue of space dimensionality. Simply adding molecular properties does not add information about the set. A lower dimensionality chemical space is preferable, as it simplifies all diversity analysis tasks, as long as the property set embodies the information needed for selection. There are numerous dimensionality-reducing techniques that have been employed over time from principal components analysis to Kohonen self-organizing maps (Eckert and Bajorath, 2007; Akella and DeCaprio, 2010).

The topic of compound selection is a complex one. There are many aspects to be considered, with a convergence of multiple areas of research. Clearly, chemical space is vast and the selection of descriptors for that space can be approached from different perspectives. This is an active area of research because there is still no consensus on best practices, and new techniques continue to emerge.

3.6.2 Scaffold-Based Diversity Analysis

An area of emphasis that continues to gain momentum in diversity analysis is scaffold or chemotype diversity (Gillet, 2008). Scaffold typically refers to a common core structure that characterizes a group of molecules (Hu et al., 2011). A chemotype is a more generic form and may refer to pendent groups as well as central cores. The initial direction was to focus on molecular frameworks (Bemis and Murcko, 1996), but advances in the development of methods for scaffold perception have greatly expanded the initial analysis (Villar et al., 2007; Villar and Hansen, 2009).

The use of chemotype analysis and privileged substructures is conceptually easier to follow than fingerprint or property-based techniques. Molecular scaffold analysis and privileged structures are gaining interest as a means of data analysis (Hu et al., 2011). Chemotype analysis has been used to define subsets of compounds for screening, and applied to the retrieval of dihydrofolate reductase (DHFR) inhibitors from a chemical library. The use of chemotype-based subsets greatly increased the enrichment of the library (Johnson et al., 2009). The use of chemotype analysis also reveals that certain substructures are found more frequently in bioactive compounds. Even after accounting for prevalence in a library certain substructures appear to enrich for bioactivity, as well as others are seldom found in bioactive compounds. Privileged chemotypes should be taken into account as libraries are designed (Klekota and Roth, 2008).

The use of scaffold or chemotype analysis allows the utilization of concepts derived over time, with very simple implementations. Inclusion of privileged structures (Klekota and Roth, 2008) or compounds with scaffolds found in natural products (Yongye et al., 2012) in the library design efforts can easily be achieved by scaffold analysis.

Some rules that aim at increasing the likelihood of finding lead compounds can be expressed in terms of scaffold frequency or abundance. For example, in a library that frequently results in lead compounds has been shown to include 50–100 chemicals (Nilakantan et al., 2002) for each cyclic system. Scaffold analysis can be easily implemented with a chemotype analysis perspective.

The use of chemotype coverage is enticing, because it is chemically intuitive. Chemotypic coverage is effective and can facilitate secondary evaluation (Johnson et al., 2009). As software becomes available for scaffold analysis, the use of these techniques is likely to become more extended given their conceptual simplicity.

3.6.3 Design for Sequential Screening

Sequential or iterative screening provides another avenue to identify hit compounds. Here again, the types of techniques to be used in the selection of a screening library will be varied based on the type of assays and the nature of the target.

Typically, FBDD is an iterative approach. In general, the process would involve the screening of a single compound set and use the results to inform the subsequent steps. Iterative approaches are not in line with the work flows followed by most groups working on lead discovery that prefer the screening of a larger collection in a single step. Another level of complexity in library design can be added with iterative approaches that are feasible for lead identification (Beroza et al., 2002; Kéri and Székelyhidi, 2005).

Some technologies rely on the use of follow-on libraries after an initial round of screening. The TRAP technology went through a diversified chemical set based on affinity fingerprints (Beroza et al., 2002). This was followed by screening compounds with similar affinity fingerprints, rather than relying on chemical similarity to validate an initial hit or identify additional hits. The aim of sequential or iterative screening has been to reduce the number of compounds to be screened, so that they can be used to identify leads in phenotypic screens or other cumbersome assays systems. The basic tenant is that at each round of screening, the hypothesis can be refined and compounds that are more likely to succeed can be identified.

Sequential screening was also applied based on chemoinformatics analysis and the use of clustering techniques (Engels et al., 2000). Automated systems that would suggest new compounds for screening based on the existing hits, even if weak, were implemented. The major issue with the sequential or iterative approach was that it runs in counter to the use of high-throughput screening, where large collections are screened in a single step to identify hits in an assay followed by confirmatory screens and subsequent secondary assays. Sequential screening meant that assays would be run in batches.

The use of phenotypic assays and other more complex screening set-ups bring an opportunity to use iterative screening technologies, where a small set of compounds is screened to identify ligands of interest based on a number of possible techniques, and which are followed by additional compounds (Matheny et al., 2013). In some cases, the phenotypic assays are used to identify a compound with the desired characteristics, which is used to identify a molecular target that is then used for screening.

3.7 Library Completeness

Chemical libraries for screening are built in stages over time. The vast number of chemicals that can be acquired or potentially made is incomprehensibly large (Villar and Koehler, 2000) even when constrains of drug likeness are imposed. The completeness of a chemical library can be tied to the portion of chemical space that is druggable (Fauman et al., 2011).

For any representation of chemical space chosen, there is still the potential that the collection available is incomplete. For chemical libraries that will be used against a variety of targets, it is not possible to have biases in the properties of potential hits beyond the general characteristics of druggability. Therefore, the druggable space should be broadly and completely covered with chemicals. This requires that we examine our chemical collection and search for holes in the space, those are compounds with properties that are not represented in the library available.

The development of algorithms to fill in gaps in the property space has been developed for quite some time, including methods that take into account constrains imposed because of the intended use of those chemicals (Koehler et al., 1999; Koehler and Villar, 2000).

The methods typically aim to find some similarity metric between an existing library and a second collection used from where compounds will be added, using fingerprints and a minimization technique such as simulated annealing (An et al., 2012).

Chemical space by any acceptable definition will be sparsely populated regarding the size of the collection and therefore techniques to add compounds to a screening library, virtual, physical, or prophetic, will play a significant role in the design and maintenance of the collection.

3.8 Final Remarks

The use of computational techniques to select a subset of chemicals that can be used for screening purposes is an important component of the current process for lead discovery. The actual protocols to be followed to build library that delivers high-quality hits vary significantly with the intended use of the library and the screening techniques available. The number of techniques and algorithms that have been described in the literature have been developed largely by analogies, without too much effort going into determining best practices. The evaluation and comparison of techniques is still lacking.

There is also an evolution as to what constitute druggable targets (Makley and Gestwicki, 2013), with an expansion in the types of processes that researchers aim to alter for drug discovery purposes. Library design will have to effectively service these new classes of targets, which will imply a change in our understanding of the chemicals that should be part of a screening library and the methods that are used to bias chemical collections for drug discovery.

References

Akella, L. B. and D. DeCaprio. 2010. Cheminformatics approaches to analyze diversity in compound screening libraries. *Curr. Opin. Chem. Biol.* 14(3): 325–330.

An, Y., W. Sherman, and S. L. Dixon. 2012. Hole filling and library optimization: Application to commercially available fragment libraries. *Bioorg. Med. Chem.* 20(18): 5379–5387.

Baell, J. B. and G. A. Holloway. 2010. New substructure filters for removal of pan assay interference compounds (PAINS) from screening libraries and for their exclusion in bioassays. *J. Med. Chem.* 53(7): 2719–2740.

Baker, M. 2013. Fragment-based lead discovery grows up. *Nat. Rev. Drug Disc.* 12(1): 5–7.

Bakken, G. A., A. S. Bell, M. Boehm et al. 2012. Shaping a screening file for maximal lead discovery efficiency and effectiveness: Elimination of molecular redundancy. *J. Chem. Inf. Mod.* 52(11): 2937–2949.

Bembenek, S. D., B. A. Tounge, and C. H. Reynolds. 2009. Ligand efficiency and fragment-based drug discovery. *Drug Discov. Today* 14(5–6): 278–283.

Bemis, G. W. and M. A. Murcko. 1996. The properties of known drugs. 1. Molecular frameworks. *J. Med. Chem.* 39(15): 2887–2893.

Beroza, P., H. O. Villar, M. M. Wick et al. 2002. Chemoproteomics as a basis for postgenomic drug discovery. *Drug Disc. Today* 7(15): 807–814.

Bohacek, R., C. Mcmartin, P. Glunz et al. 1999. GrowMol, a *de Novo* computer program, and its application to thermolysin and pepsin: Results of the design and synthesis of a novel inhibitor. *Inst. Math. Appl.* 108: 103–114.

Bohm, H. J. 1992. The computer-program Ludi—A new method for the Denovo design of enzyme-inhibitors. *J. Comput.-Aided Mol. Des.* 6(1): 61–78.

Bologa, C. G. and T. I. Oprea. 2012. Bioinformatics and drug discovery. *Meth. Mol. Biol.* 910: 125–143.

Briem, H. and I. D. Kuntz. 1996. Molecular similarity based on DOCK-generated fingerprints. *J. Med. Chem.* 39(17): 3401–3408.

Buchwald, P. 2010. Small-molecule protein-protein interaction inhibitors: Therapeutic potential in light of molecular size, chemical space, and ligand binding efficiency considerations. *IUBMB Life* 62(10): 724–731.

Buck, E. and J. A. Wells. 2005. Disulfide trapping to localize small-molecule agonists and antagonists for a G protein-coupled receptor. *Proc. Natl. Acad. Sci. USA* 102(8): 2719–2724.

Caflisch, A., A. Miranker, and M. Karplus. 1993. Multiple copy simultaneous search and construction of ligands in binding sites: Application to inhibitors of HIV-1 aspartic proteinase. *J. Med. Chem.* 36(15): 2142–2167.

Deng, Z., C. Chuaqui, and J. Singh. 2006. Knowledge-based design of target-focused libraries using protein–ligand interaction constraints. *J. Med. Chem.* 49(2): 490–500.

Di, L. and E. H. Kerns. 2006. Biological assay challenges from compound solubility: Strategies for bioassay optimization. *Drug Disc. Today* 11(9–10): 446–451.

Dixon, S. L. and R. T. Koehler. 1999. The hidden component of size in two-dimensional fragment descriptors: Side effects on sampling in bioactive libraries. *J. Med. Chem.* 42(15): 2887–2900.

Dobson, C. M. 2004. Chemical space and biology. *Nature* 432(7019): 824–828.

Duffy, B. C., L. Zhu, H. Decornez, and D. B. Kitchen. 2012. Early phase drug discovery: Cheminformatics and computational techniques in identifying lead series. *Bioorg. Med. Chem.* 20(18): 5324–5342.

Ebalunode, J. O., W. Zheng, and A. Tropsha. 2011. Chemical library design. *Methods Mol. Biol.* 685: 111–133.

Eckert, H. and J. Bajorath. 2007. Molecular similarity analysis in virtual screening: Foundations, limitations and novel approaches. *Drug Disc. Today* 12(5–6): 225–233.

Engels, M. F. M., T. Thielemans, D. Verbinnen et al. 2000. {CerBeruS:} A system supporting the sequential screening process. *J. Chem. Inf. Model.* 40(2): 241–245.

Erlanson, D. A., J. A. Wells, and A. C. Braisted. 2004. Tethering: Fragment-based drug discovery. *Ann. Rev. Biophys. Biomol. Struct.* 33(2004): 199–223.

Fauman, E. B., B. K. Rai, and E. S. Huang. 2011. Structure-based druggability assessment—Identifying suitable targets for small molecule therapeutics. *Curr. Opin. Chem. Biol.* 15(4): 463–468.

Gillet, V. 2008. New directions in library design and analysis. *Curr. Opin. Chem. Biol.* 12(3): 372–378.

Gorse, A. D. 2006. Diversity in medicinal chemistry space. *Curr. Top. Med. Chem.* 6(1): 3–18.

Hajduk, P. J. and J. Greer. 2007. A decade of fragment-based drug design: Strategic advances and lessons learned. *Nat. Rev. Drug Disc.* 6(3): 211–219.

Harris, C. J., R. D. Hill, D. W. Sheppard et al. 2011. The design and application of target-focused compound libraries. *Comb. Chem. High Throughput Screen.* 14(6): 521–531.

Heikamp, K. and J. Bajorath. 2013. The future of virtual compound screening. *Chem. Biol. Drug Des.* 81(1): 33–40.

Hu, Y., D. Stumpfe, and J. Bajorath. 2011. Lessons learned from molecular scaffold analysis. *J. Chem. Inf. Model.* 51(8): 1742–1753.

Johnson, M., V. Shanmugasundaram, G. Bundy et al. 2009. Chemotypic coverage: A new basis for constructing screening sublibraries. *J. Chem. Inf. Model.* 49(3): 531–542.

Joseph-McCarthy, D., A. J. Campbell, G. Kern et al. 2014. Fragment-based lead discovery and design. *J. Chem. Inf. Model.* 54(3): 693–704.

Kauvar, L. M., D. L. Higgins, H. O. Villar et al. 1995. Predicting ligand binding to proteins by affinity fingerprinting. *Chem. Biol.* 2(2): 107–118.

Kauvar, L. M. and H. O. Villar. 1998. Deciphering cryptic similarities in protein binding sites. *Curr. Opin. Biotech.* 9(4): 390–394.

Kauvar, L. M., H. O. Villar, J. R. Sportsman et al. 1998. Protein affinity map of chemical space. *J. Chromat. B* 715(1): 93–102.

Kéri, G. and Z. Székelyhidi. 2005. Drug discovery in the kinase inhibitory field using the nested chemical library™ technology. *Assay Drug Dev. Technol.* 3(5): 543–551.

Klekota, J. and F. P. Roth. 2008. Chemical substructures that enrich for biological activity. *Bioinformatics* 24(21): 2518–2525.

Koehler, R. T. and H. O. Villar. 2000. Statistical relationships among docking scores for different protein binding sites. *J. Comput. Aided Mol. Des.* 14(1): 23–37.

Koehler, R. T., S. L. Dixon, and H. O. Villar. 1999. LASSOO: A generalized directed diversity approach to the design and enrichment of chemical libraries. *J. Med. Chem.* 42(22): 4695–4704.

Koutsoukas, A., S. Paricharak, W. R. J. D. Galloway et al. 2014. How diverse are diversity assessment methods? A comparative analysis and benchmarking of molecular descriptor space. *J. Chem. Inf. Model.* 54(1): 230–242.

Leach, A. R., J. Bradshaw, D. V. Green et al. 1999. Implementation of a system for reagent selection and library enumeration, profiling, and design. *J. Chem. Inf. Comp. Sci.* 39(6): 1161–1172.

Lindell, S. D., L. C. Pattenden, and J. Shannon. 2009. Combinatorial chemistry in the agrosciences. *Bioorg. Med. Chem.* 17(12): 4035–4046.

Lipinski, C. A., F. Lombardo, B. W. Dominy et al. 2001. Experimental and computational approaches to estimate solubility and permeability in drug discovery and development settings. *Adv. Drug Deliv. Rev.* 46(1–3): 3–26.

Lisurek, M., B. Rupp, J. Wichard et al. 2010. Design of chemical libraries with potentially bioactive molecules applying a maximum common substructure concept. *Mol. Divers.* 14(2): 401–408.

Makley, L. N. and J. E. Gestwicki. 2013. Expanding the number of druggable targets: Non-enzymes and protein–protein interactions. *Chem. Biol. Drug Des.* 81(1): 22–32.

Matheny, C. J., M. C. Wei, M. C. Bassik et al. 2013. Next-generation NAMPT inhibitors identified by sequential high-throughput phenotypic chemical and functional genomic screens. *Chem. Biol.* 20(11): 1352–1363.

Moon, J. B. and W. J. Howe. 1991. Computer design of bioactive molecules: A method for receptor-based *de novo* ligand design. *Proteins* 11(4): 314–328.

Morgan, H. L. 1965. The generation of a unique machine description for chemical structures—A technique developed at chemical abstracts service. *J. Chem. Doc.* 5(2): 107–112.

Nguyen, H. P., A. Koutsoukas, F. M. Fauzi et al. 2013. Diversity selection of compounds based on "Protein Affinity Fingerprints" improves sampling of bioactive chemical space. *Chem. Biol. Drug Des.* 82(3): 252–266.

Nilakantan, R., F. Immermann, and K. Haraki. 2002. A novel approach to combinatorial library design. *Comb. Chem. High Throughput Screen.* 5(2): 105–110.

Oprea, T. I. and H. Matter. 2004. Integrating virtual screening in lead discovery. *Curr. Opin. Chem. Biol.* 8(4): 349–358.

Orita, M., K. Ohno, and T. Niimi. 2009. Two "Golden Ratio" indices in fragment-based drug discovery. *Drug Disc. Today* 14(5–6): 321–328.

Orry, A. J. W., R. A. Abagyan, and C. N. Cavasotto. 2006. Structure-based development of target-specific compound libraries. *Drug Disc. Today* 11(5–6): 261–266.

Overington, J. P., B. Al-Lazikani, and A. L. Hopkins. 2006. How many drug targets are there? *Nat. Rev. Drug Discov.* 5(12): 993–996.

Pascual, R., J. I. Borrell, and J. Teixidó. 2003. Analysis of selection methodologies for combinatorial library design. *Mol. Divers.* 6(2): 121–133.

Patel, H., M. J. Bodkin, B. Chen et al. 2009. Knowledge-based approach to *de Novo* design using reaction vectors. *J. Chem. Inf. Model.* 49(5): 1163–1184.

Pearce, B. C., M. J. Sofia, A. C. Good et al. 2006. An empirical process for the design of high-throughput screening deck filters. *J. Chem. Inf. Model.* 46(3): 1060–1068.

Pirok, G., N. Maté, J. Varga et al. 2006. Making "Real" molecules in virtual space. *J. Chem. Inf. Model.* 46(2): 563–568.

Rajan, K. 2008. Combinatorial materials sciences: Experimental strategies for accelerated knowledge discovery. *Ann. Rev. Mater. Res.* 38(1): 299–322.

Reymond, J. L. and M. Awale. 2012. Exploring chemical space for drug discovery using the chemical universe database. *ACS Chem. Neurosci.* 3(9): 649–657.

Rishton, G. M. 2008. Molecular diversity in the context of leadlikeness: Compound properties that enable effective biochemical screening. *Curr. Opin. Chem. Biol.* 12(3): 340–351.

Rogers, D. and M. Hahn. 2010. Extended-connectivity fingerprints. *J. Chem. Inf. Model.* 50(5): 742–754.

Rognan, D. 2012. Fragment-based approaches and computer-aided drug discovery. In: *Fragment-Based Drug Discovery and X-Ray Crystallography SE–182*, Thomas

G. Davies and Marko Hyvönen, (eds.), vol. 317, pp. 201–222. Topics in Current Chemistry. Springer, Berlin Heidelberg.

Saxena, A. K. and P. Prathipati. 2006. Collection and preparation of molecular databases for virtual screening. *SAR QSAR Environ. Res.* 17(4): 371–392.

Schnur, D. M. 2008. Recent trends in library design: "Rational Design" revisited. *Curr. Opin. Drug Discov. Develop.* 11(3): 375–380.

Schuffenhauer, A., S. Ruedisser, A. L. Marzinzik et al. Library design for fragment based screening. *Curr. Top. Med. Chem.* 5(2005): 751–762.

Singh, N., H. Sun, S. Chaudhury et al. 2012. A physicochemical descriptor-based scoring scheme for effective and rapid filtering of kinase-like chemical space. *J. Cheminf.* 4(1): 4.

Tang, G. W. and R. B. Altman. 2014. Knowledge-based fragment binding prediction. Edited by Yanay Ofran. *PLoS Computational Biology* 10(4): e1003589.

Veber, D. F., S. R. Johnson, H. Y. Cheng et al. 2002. Molecular properties that influence the oral bioavailability of drug candidates. *J. Med. Chem.* 45(12): 2615–2623.

Vieth, M., M. G. Siegel, R. E. Higgs et al. 2004. Characteristic physical properties and structural fragments of marketed oral drugs. *J. Med. Chem.* 47(1): 224–232.

Villar, H. O. and M. R. Hansen. 2009. Design of chemical libraries for screening. *Exp. Opin. Drug Discov.* 4(12): 1215–1220.

Villar, H. O., M. R. Hansen, and R. Kho. 2007. Substructural analysis in drug discovery. *Curr. Comput. Aided Drug Des.* 3(1): 59–67.

Villar, H. O. and R. T. Koehler 2000. Comments on the design of chemical libraries for screening. *Mol. Divers.* 5(1): 13–24.

Wilde, F. and A. Link. 2013. Advances in the design of a multipurpose fragment screening library. *Exp. Opin. Drug Discov.* 8(5): 597–606.

Willett, P. 2006. Similarity-based virtual screening using 2D fingerprints. *Drug Disc. Today* 11(23–24): 1046–1053.

Yang, W., R. V. Fucini, B. T. Fahr et al. 2009. Fragment-based discovery of nonpeptidic BACE-1 inhibitors using tethering. *Biochemistry* 48(21): 4488–4496.

Yongye, A. B., J. Waddell, and J. L. Medina-Franco. 2012. Molecular scaffold analysis of natural products databases in the public domain. *Chem. Biol. Drug Des.* 80(5): 717–724.

4

Ligand-Based Drug Discovery and Design

Álvaro Cortés-Cabrera, Pedro A. Sánchez Murcia,
Antonio Morreale, and Federico Gago

CONTENTS

4.1 Introduction

Among the computational methods fostering the enticing drug discovery enterprise, those based on ligand structure alone have become very popular nowadays because they are fast and require only a limited amount of information for evaluation. The key concept underlying the majority of ligand-based protocols is the similarity principle, which basically states that similar molecules should have similar biological properties (Maggiora and Shanmugasundaram 2011, 2014). This means that at least one molecule or a group of molecules that bind with some affinity to the intended biomolecular target must be known beforehand. The major focus then lies on three related issues: (i) devise methods for molecular representation, alignment, and feature matching (Maggiora and Shanmugasundaram, 2011), (ii) measure molecular similarity fast and accurately, and (iii) explore the structure–activity relationship (SAR) space using the chemical information contained in the ligands. The ultimate aim is to facilitate the virtual screening (VS) of chemical libraries, that is, the *in silico* version of the high-throughput screening (HTS) campaigns that test huge amounts of existing chemicals for their ability to bind to a given target or exert a particular effect in a biochemical, biophysical, or cellular assay (Macarron et al., 2011). One obvious advantage of VS is that the compounds need not be physically available, so that extant repositories can be expanded to include molecules that have not been synthesized yet. The downside is that the real accessibility and/or synthetic feasibility of the proposed compound(s) should be ensured in advance to avoid false expectations.

The collection of molecules currently catalogued, together with a number of properties/descriptors associated with them, make up chemical space (Reymond et al. 2010), in which structurally related compounds form clusters. The discovery of new lead scaffolds can then be guided "geographically" by carrying out similarity searches in this particular region of a vast and unevenly explored "chemical universe." If relevant biological information (e.g., activity or binding energy) is incorporated as a descriptor, a new chemicobiological space (CBS) is defined that can be represented as an atlas and charted using some tailor-made navigation tool (Cortés-Cabrera et al., 2012). Without the advantages afforded by computational algorithms, medicinal chemists are compelled to explore the CBS in an iterative and blinded manner. In any case, constant feedback is required to guide the synthetic efforts toward the most prolific chemical space region(s). After several rounds of synthesis and evaluation, some structural information on the binding site of the macromolecular target can be inferred from the complementary chemical features present in the ensemble of true ligands. However, the new knowledge gained is informative regarding the binding determinants and the allowed size and character of different substituents but is too schematic and compares poorly to the full binding site description provided by the ligand–receptor complexes that can be solved using X-ray crystallography (Shoichet and Kobilka, 2012) or nuclear magnetic resonance (NMR) spectroscopy (Wirmer-Bartoschek and Bartoschek, 2012).

Nonetheless, drug discovery practitioners face many different challenges and a good piece of advice is to try to use every piece of information and tool available that can be of help in a given project. Thus, ligand-based VS (LBVS) protocols can be employed not only on their own, when structural data for the target is lacking, but also in conjunction with other methods that rely on atomic detailed knowledge of the target site. An example is their established role as cost-effective filters in target-based VS (TBVS) campaigns, with the aim of tapering the number of molecules that will be subjected to the more CPU-demanding tasks of docking and scoring. This usual order can also be reversed so that a docking protocol is first employed for selection of hits displaying good steric and electrostatic complementarity with the binding site and the resulting molecules are then used as queries to search for similar putative ligands in a database (Cortes-Cabrera et al., 2012). Another, possibly less optimal alternative is to classify molecules in a database according to their calculated probability of being active against a certain target, a result that is obtained by making a comparison between each candidate molecule and some known true ligand(s), as discussed at the end of this review. In the separate sections of this chapter, we will include a succinct theoretical description of the most popular methods, a brief discussion of their relative limitations and advantages, and recent examples in the fields of LBVS and polypharmacology.

4.1.1 Ligand-Based SAR Methods

A plethora of SAR methodologies have been developed over the years to try and correlate the observed differences in biological activities within a set of molecules with a combination of some calculated or experimentally determined physicochemical properties. To aid in this endeavor, SAR space classification indices have been introduced. Probably the best known are the structure–activity landscape index (SALI) (Guha and Van Drie, 2008) and the SAR index (SARI) (Peltason et al., 2009), which attempt to classify and quantify the different SAR spaces with the goal of highlighting the "activity cliffs" (Maggiora, 2006) that are so appealing to medicinal chemists. These discontinuities in the topography of "activity landscapes" pinpoint regions that are characterized by rather large changes in activity brought about by the introduction of a specific structural feature (e.g., a hydrogen bond donor or a metal chelating moiety). In addition, when an extensive knowledge of the SAR space is available for a series of ligands in the absence of 3D information of their target(s), some more classical approaches can be used to generate a pharmacophoric hypothesis, as discussed below, or to derive a quantitative SAR (QSAR) model that relies on molecular interaction fields, as performed in comparative molecular field analysis (CoMFA) (Cramer et al., 1988).

To represent activity landscapes, both 2D and 3D depictions are employed (Wassermann et al., 2010). In the former, pairs of compounds are represented on a plane by plotting their activity similarity against their structural or chemical similarity. In doing so, the space is usually divided into two different parts that hold interesting properties: (i) pairs presenting high activity similarity but low structural similarity delimit a "scaffold hopping" (Schneider et al., 1999) area where it is possible to find alternative, chemically diverse structures while retaining the activity; (ii) pairs displaying low activity similarity and high structural similarity represent the activity cliffs (Guha and Van Drie, 2008) in this 2D space. For 3D plots, x and y coordinates can be used to represent the projection of the chemical space onto a plane while the z-coordinate is used for the potency. These representations provide a very intuitive categorization of SAR into (i) continuous, where small structural changes bring about small changes in activity; (ii) discontinuous, where large differences in activity appear as a result of small structural changes, that is, where activity cliffs are more likely to be found; and (iii) heterogeneous, where both regions coexist.

These approaches, together with the numerical frameworks that SALI and SARI provide, have been successfully used to explain the different SARs of many targets including cyclooxygenase-2 and blood coagulation factor Xa (Bajorath et al., 2009).

4.1.2 Pharmacophore Modeling

It was the noted German physician and Nobel Prize winner, Paul Ehrlich, who at the beginning of the twentieth century referred to "a molecular framework that carries (*phoros*) the essential features responsible for a drug's (*pharmakon*) biological activity" (Ehrlich, 1909). About 90 years later, the International Union of Pure and Applied Chemistry (IUPAC) defined a pharmacophore as "an ensemble of steric and electronic features that is necessary to ensure the optimal supramolecular interactions with a specific biological target and to trigger (or block) its biological response" (Wermuth et al., 1998). Over the years, a pharmacophore has been usually described as the relative spatial orientation (in terms of distances, angles, planes, and centroids) of structural and stereoelectronic elements derived from a group of molecules that are responsible for binding to a common target (Figure 4.1). The chemical features that are most commonly taken into account are hydrogen bond acceptors and donors, positively and negatively charged groups, aromatic rings, and aliphatic or aromatic moieties (Leach and Gillet, 2007). Sometimes exclusion volume spheres (Toba et al., 2006) are also included to provide information about disallowed regions in the vicinity of the site, particularly in cases where the 3D structure of the target is known in atomic detail.

Ligand-based pharmacophore modeling requires two main steps: (a) exploration of the ligands' conformational space and (b) determination of the common essential chemical features that are responsible for the binding

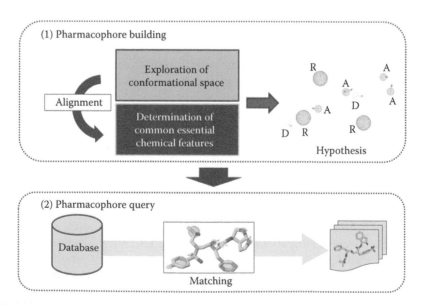

FIGURE 4.1
(**See color insert.**) Schematic showing how a 3D pharmacophore hypothesis is built and then used as a query for database searching. A: hydrogen bond acceptor; D: hydrogen bond donor; R: aromatic.

interactions. Consequently, the nature and completeness of the conformational analysis will directly determine the probability of finding the hypothetical bioactive conformation of the most flexible ligands. Thus, program Catalyst (Sprague and Hoffmann, 1997), for example, typically generates up to 250 possible conformers for a molecule within an energy cut-off value above the global minimum. However, this sort of limited enumeration, which was introduced at the time to increase the computational efficiency, may result in missing the bioactive conformation if the molecule has many degrees of freedom. If CPU time is not an issue, the conformationally sampled pharmacophore (CSP) approach (Acharya et al., 2011) addresses this problem by exhaustively sampling conformational space using replica-exchange molecular dynamics simulations (or other methods). Analysis of the trajectories first provides 1D and 2D probability distributions of various pharmacophoric feature points. Overlap coefficients of the conformational distributions are then combined with the physicochemical properties of the ligands to obtain a set of molecular descriptors that are subjected to single-variable and multivariable linear regression analysis against the biological activity of interest, with the aim of identifying the combination that best explains the variability of the response.

Before determining the essential pharmacophoric elements, most methods require a previous alignment of the generated conformers. Several procedures have been used for efficient pharmacophore mapping, including constrained systematic search, clique detection, maximum likelihood and genetic algorithms (Leach and Gillet, 2007). On the contrary, some programs merge the flexibility analysis and the alignment into one single step. GASP (Jones et al., 2000), for example, employs a genetic algorithm to generate conformational diversity during the alignment process, thus avoiding the need to pre-explore the phase space available to the ligands. PharmaGist, a free tool with an intuitive web interface (Schneidman-Duhovny et al., 2008), explores the flexibility of the ligands *in situ* using pairwise alignments and then multiple alignments. Program GALAHAD (Genetic Algorithm with Linear Assignment for Hypermolecule Alignment of Datasets) handles the components of molecular configuration, namely conformation versus rotation and translation in 3D space, separately (Richmond et al., 2006). A multiobjective genetic algorithm is first used to minimize strain while maximizing steric and pharmacophoric concordance and then optimal overlays in Cartesian space are obtained by applying a 3D hypermolecule construction method that identifies optimal feature correspondences between ligands by means of linear assignment.

Successful examples of this approach include the pharmacophore-supported combinatorial design of selective purinergic A_{2A} receptor antagonists (Schneider and Nettekoven, 2003), the retrospective retrieval from virtual libraries of known neurotransmitter receptor blockers (Evers et al., 2005), and the discovery of allosteric activators of rhodopsin with a manually designed pharmacophore (Taylor et al., 2010). Among reported applications in projects focusing on protein–protein interfaces potentially relevant to anticancer therapy are the discovery of c-Myc/Max heterodimer disruptors using a GALAHAD pharmacophore model (Mustata et al., 2009) and the identification of selective and dual hits against MDM4/p53 interactions using a pharmacophore-assisted knowledge-based approach (Jacoby et al., 2009).

Because of their inherent simplicity, 3D pharmacophores have become common components of manifold drug discovery workflows (Braga and Andrade, 2013; Cabrera et al., 2011). Their usefulness as queries to identify candidate molecules present in virtual libraries can be increased by employing them as filters in target-based methodologies to process the output of VS protocols (Singh et al., 2011) or to reduce the false-positive rate before or after ligand docking (Muthusamy et al., 2013). In this regard, the ZINCPharmer web server (Koes and Camacho, 2012) may be particularly beneficial to extract a pharmacophore from the structure of either a free ligand or a ligand–receptor complex and then search for matches in the huge and publicly available ZINC database (Irwin and Shoichet, 2005). *De novo* design is also possible because novel candidate structures can be stochastically built up from fragments that conform to the requirements of a given 3D pharmacophore (Lippert et al., 2011).

4.1.3 Molecular Similarity Analysis (MSA)

The number of features that can be compared between any two molecules is quite large (e.g., size, shape, charge distribution, conformational states, etc.) and some may contain redundant information. Apart from that, a variety of descriptors and algorithms are used to capture the essential characteristics of these features and quantitate the matching. For these reasons, it must be borne in mind that different representations and their corresponding similarity measures can lead to significantly different results.

4.1.3.1 Shape Methods

This category encompasses a group of methodologies (Table 4.1) whose leitmotiv is the basic assumption that the binding of a ligand to a given pocket in a macromolecular target requires shape and size complementarity. Shape methods, therefore, implicitly demand 3D models and consideration of a diverse set of conformers for inherently flexible molecules.

4.1.3.1.1 Approximate Shape Methods

Methods of this kind do not explicitly account for the volume or the shape themselves. Ultra-shape recognition (USR) is possibly the most popular and was conceived (Ballester et al., 2009) under the premise that the shape of a molecule can be uniquely determined by a selected set of distances measured from every atom to four distinct locations, namely the molecular centroid (*ctd*), the closest atom to *ctd* (*cst*), the farthest atom from *ctd* (*fct*), and the farthest atom from *fct* (*ftf*). Each molecular conformation is thus described

TABLE 4.1

Summary of Approximate Shape-Based Methods

Method	Number of Variables	Advantages	Limitations	Reference
USR	3	Fast comparison; Descriptors generation	Chirality not recognized; Chemical incompatibilities	Ballester et al. (2009)
CSR	3	Chirality recognition	Chemical incompatibilities	Armstrong et al. (2009)
ElectroShape	4 (charge) or 5 (charge and ClogP)	Chirality recognition; Charge/lipophilic compatibility	Dependence on charge and ClogP calculations	Armstrong et al. (2010)
UFSRAT	3 and pharmacophoric sets	Pharmacophoric compatibility	Centroids' dependence on atom types	Hsin et al. (2011)
USRCAT	3 and pharmacophoric sets	Pharmacophoric compatibility with aromaticity; Real-time screening		Schreyer and Blundell (2012)

by four distributions of atomic distances, the number of the latter being proportional to the number of atoms. To circumvent the difficulty inherent in comparing molecules with different numbers of atoms, three rotationally invariant moments are defined for each 1D distribution. The first (average distance), second (square root of the variance), and third (cube root of the skewness) moments of these four distributions make up a vector of 12 shape descriptors that uniquely encodes molecular shape and size (Figure 4.2).

These vectors can be easily compared by means of different distance metrics to establish the degree of shape similarity between any two molecules. If, for example, the Manhattan distance (Black 2006) is used, the dissimilarity is monotonically inverted so as to define a normalized similarity score that is close to 1 in cases of great shape similarity. USR vectors can be stored with minimum space requirements and employed in different projects to determine which molecules in a database have a shape most similar to that of a given query molecule. The pregeneration of the descriptors and the simplicity of the comparison, which typically requires summation of squares and a final square root calculation, yield a very fast method capable of screening millions of molecules in just a few seconds.

However, the initial USR implementation had several drawbacks that were addressed in subsequent upgrades of the algorithm. Foremost among them was the finding that the original centroids were not able to distinguish between enantiomers due to a flaw in the selection of these points. This problem was fixed with the introduction of a different calculation procedure known as chiral shape recognition (CSR) (Armstrong et al., 2009). Another important

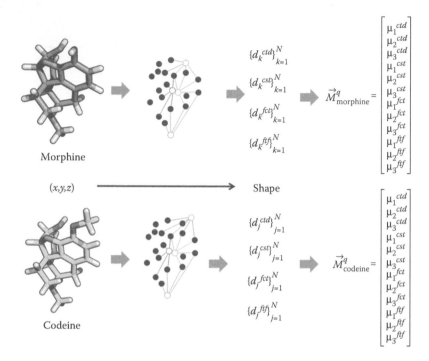

FIGURE 4.2

(See color insert.) Ultra-shape recognition. An example of how the shapes and sizes of two molecules, morphine and codeine, can be encoded as two sets of 12 distance descriptors (μ) that make up the vectors $\overrightarrow{M}{}^q_{\text{morphine}}$ and $\overrightarrow{M}{}^q_{\text{codeine}}$, which can be used in a similarity calculation. The locations of *ctd*, *cst*, *fct*, and *ftf* are depicted by hollow circles and, for simplicity, only some distances are shown (see text for details).

issue was the realization that two molecules could share an identical shape and still not be able to bind to the same pocket due to polar incompatibilities, mostly due to charge–charge repulsions and/or large desolvation costs. For this reason, a fourth (partial atomic charge) and a fifth (cLogP) variable were later introduced, giving birth to the ElectroShape method (Armstrong et al., 2010). These new variables were suitably scaled using an optimization procedure trained with common VS test sets. Besides, the USR concept was extended at the University of Edinburgh (Hsin et al., 2011), where the ultra-fast shape recognition with atom types (UFSRAT) method was developed by adding three more distributions for user-definable hydrophobic and hydrogen bond acceptor/donor atoms. A more recent variant is USR with CREDO atom types (USRCAT) (Schreyer and Blundell, 2012), which defines subsets of hydrophobic, aromatic, hydrogen bond donor and hydrogen bond acceptor atoms with the help of SMARTS substructural patterns that are used for atom typing in CREDO (Cummings et al., 2005), a database of protein–ligand interactions present in the Protein Data Bank (Braga and Andrade, 2013). USRCAT is reported to preserve the ability of the original method to retrieve hits with very low structural similarity and to improve the VS performance significantly because of a better discrimination between compounds with similar shape but distinct pharmacophoric features.

Despite the efforts expended in fixing the design problems introduced in the first version of the USR method, the result of a comparison is a 1D metric (a single coefficient), which cannot be visually inspected. This shortcoming makes this approach unsuitable for many modeling applications including optimal molecular superimpositions and QSAR studies, although it is perfectly functional for LBVS campaigns. Moreover, it is difficult to assess its validity and real performance due to the scarcity of information on its success/failure ratio, a problem that is common to other ligand-based methods. One possible solution would be to develop specific test sets (Irwin, 2008; Mysinger et al., 2012) even though this choice entails the risk of a general overestimation of its success rate (von Korff et al., 2009), particularly in comparison with other target-based ligand-docking methods (Cabrera et al., 2011). Nevertheless, and due to their simplicity, approximate shape-based methods are widely used in VS (Ballester et al., 2010; Schreyer and Blundell, 2012; Taylor et al., 2008), network analysis in polypharmacology (Cortés-Cabrera et al., 2013), and conformational sampling studies (Klett et al., 2014).

4.1.3.1.2 Gaussian Shape Methods

In 1995, Grant and Pickup pioneered the concept of replacing the collection of intersecting hard spheres of differing radii conventionally used to represent a molecule with a set of overlapping atom-centered Gaussian functions (Grant and Pickup, 1995). This way of describing molecular shape was soon used for comparing two molecules by analytically optimizing their volume intersection and applied to the prediction of the relative orientation of series of ligands binding to several protein targets (Grant et al., 1996).

Gaussian-based methods (Table 4.2) represent each atomic site in a molecule with a spherically symmetric Gaussian function and measure the integral volume over all Gaussians. The volume overlap between any two given molecules is calculated very efficiently on the computer and can be used as an estimation of their shape similarity.

Nonetheless, the overlap between two molecules depends on their relative position in 3D space and the comparison procedure must obtain, in the first place, the best possible superimposition through an optimization or fitting procedure (Grant et al., 1996). Besides, it must be borne in mind that optimization procedures are very sensitive to the initial position and orientation of the molecules that are compared, which means that in some cases the correct answer might not be found. Positional dependency can be easily avoided by translating both molecules to a common origin. However, the orientation problem is a more difficult task. Usually, different starting orientations are given as input to an optimization algorithm such as SIMPLEX (Nelder and Mead, 1965), Broyden–Fletcher–Goldfarb–Shanno (BFGS) (Liu and Nocedal, 1989), or Monte-Carlo simulated annealing (Grant et al., 1996), all of which

TABLE 4.2

Summary of Gaussian- and Shape-Based Methods

Implementation	Description	Reference
ROCS (Rapid Overlay Chemical Structures)	Traditional implementation	Rush et al. (2005)
PAPER	GPU accelerated	Haque and Pande (2010)
SHAFTS (SHApe-FeaTure Similarity)	Pharmacophore-shape hybrid method	Liu et al. (2011)
ShaEP (Shape and Electrostatic Potential)	Field and volume overlap hybrid method	Vainio et al. (2009)
MolShaCS	Charge overlap instead of feature coloring	Vaz de Lima and Nascimento (2013)
SABRE (Shape Approach-Based Routines Enhanced)	Consensus molecular shape patterns	Hamza and Wei (2014)
Weighted Gaussian algorithm (WEGA)	Shape description improved over that of traditional implementation	Yan et al. (2013)
Phase shape	Fast pharmacophore-shape hybrid method	Sastry et al. (2011)

have been proved to be successful for molecular alignment in VS (Haque and Pande, 2010). This optimization step can be speeded up by precalculating the potential overlap of certain atom types onto the reference molecule. Compared to USR-like methods, two deficiencies are apparent: (i) they are much slower, even though the computation time has been greatly reduced upon implementation of the algorithm on graphics processing units (GPU) (Haque and Pande, 2010) and (ii) the results cannot be stored and reutilized. However, a clear advantage is that their applicability extends to other modeling techniques beyond VS because results can be visually checked (Ballester et al., 2009).

The metric typically used to calculate the overlap between two molecules, as originally implemented in program rapid overlay of chemical structures (ROCS) (Rush et al., 2005), is the Tanimoto coefficient (T_c), which is defined as

$$T_c = \frac{overlap_{ab}}{overlap_{ab} - overlap_{aa} - overlap_{bb}}$$

where $overlap_{ab}$, $overlap_{aa}$, and $overlap_{bb}$ are the volume overlaps of molecule *a* with molecule *b*, of molecule *a* with itself, and of molecule *b* with itself, respectively. Values for T_c range from 0 (no similarity) to 1 (a perfect match).

These matches rely just on the volume overlap of optimally aligned molecules so that they are practically independent of the atom types and bonding patterns present in both query and search molecules. The goal of this approach, when used in a VS context, is therefore to identify molecules in the chemical library that can adopt shapes highly similar to that of the target-bound ligand and, in so doing, to increase the chances of scaffold hopping (Canela et al., 2014; Schneider et al., 1999).

An improvement recently described in a commercial ROCS implementation (OpenEye, 2013) incorporates the propensity of each group to form a hydrogen bond (Mills and Dean, 1996) so that some form of chemical complementarity can also be measured and used to refine the shape-based superpositions.

ShaEP (Shape and Electrostatic Potential) was developed with the aim of capturing the strengths of both field-based and volumetric approaches (Vainio et al., 2009). For the initial alignment of the two molecules, it uses a matching algorithm on graphs that coarsely represent their electrostatic potential and local shape at points close to the molecular surfaces. This superimposition is then optimized by maximizing the overlap of their molecular volumes, which are computed using atom-centered Gaussian functions, thus avoiding the need to start from several different orientations. On the one hand, the volume method treats all parts of space equally and is especially well suited for comparing similarly sized molecules, but this alone could miss good partial superimpositions. On the other hand, the field alignment is able to recognize those partial matches but is not as fast as the volume overlap method and is generally impractical from the computational point of view.

SHAFTS (SHApe FeaTure Similarity) (Liu et al., 2011) and Phase Shape (Sastry et al., 2011) resemble ShaEP in that they use a hybrid approach. First, they detect the pharmacophoric points on reference and target molecules and then index all possible triplets of points. Second, the algorithm superimposes all these triplets using a least squares fitting routine. Third, these initial superimpositions are used to calculate a shape score (the molecular volume overlap), which is optimized by means of a SIMPLEX (Nelder and Mead, 1965) routine. Finally, the sum of the pharmacophoric best fit and the volume overlap provides the overall score.

The representation of the shape density of a molecule as the plain sum of all individual atomic shapes can lead, in some cases (e.g., amantadine), to significant overestimations using the hard-sphere model as the reference. This error can be corrected upon introduction, for every atom, of a weight factor that reflects how crowded this atom is in relation to its neighbors, as performed by the weighted Gaussian algorithm (WEGA) (Yan et al., 2013). The representation of molecular shape density as a linear combination of weighted atomic Gaussian functions improves the accuracy of molecular volumes and reduces the error of shape similarity calculations.

However, disregarding dissimilar structures in LBVS experiments that use a single reference molecule per query can lead to high false-negative rates. For this reason, if a set of chemically diverse ligands bound to the same target site is available, it can be advantageous for filtering purposes to generate a consensus recognition pattern by means of a linear combination of weighted Gaussian functions of the pharmacophoric groups present in the set (Hamza and Wei, 2014) derived by means of data fusion techniques (Hert et al., 2006).

Generally speaking, and despite their limitations, Gaussian shape-based algorithms have provided some successful examples in VS. The first publication of a tool based on these methods described the discovery of several compounds that were able to interfere with FtsZ-ZipA interaction at micromolar concentrations (Rush et al., 2005). Likewise, use of SHAFTS (Lu et al., 2011) led to the finding of active molecules with new scaffolds targeting the p90 ribosomal S6 protein kinase 2 (RSK2). More recently, several DNA G-quadruplex binders were discovered (Alcaro et al., 2013) using multiple selection protocols including Gaussian shape similarity with ROCS.

4.1.3.1.3 *Local Surface Methods*

These tools use a morphological similarity (Jain, 2000) function based on molecular surfaces, as implemented in the Surflex-sim methodology (Jain, 2004). In a first step, a set of points is defined around the molecule. These "observation points" are then used to measure several types of distances to the molecular surface (Figure 4.3) that enable the capture of local surface features that can be compared later for alignment and similarity evaluation purposes.

Local surface methods have been used in molecular superimposition for QSAR studies (Jain et al., 1994), VS (Jain, 2004), and off-target predictions (Yera et al., 2011). In VS, both ligand-based and target-based strategies have been described, the former for comparing molecules to a reference (Ruppert et al., 1997) and the latter for extracting the complementary features from a binding site and compare them with those of the putative ligands (Jain, 2007).

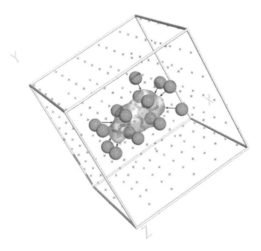

FIGURE 4.3
(See color insert.) Representation of a set of observation points (green) around the surface enveloping the adrenaline molecule (sticks). The shortest distances are shown as arrows from some selected points within a cutoff radius of 5 Å.

TABLE 4.3

Different Fingerprints Discussed in the Text

Type	Examples	Reference
Structural keys	MDL MACCS	Durant et al. (2002)
Extended	ECFP, FCFP	Rogers and Hahn (2010)
Atom distances	TAD (typed atom distances)/TGT (typed graph triangles)	Bender et al. (2009)
Path-based	Daylight	Bender et al. (2009)
Pharmacophoric	CATS (2D), piDAPH3 (pharmacophore atom triangle)	Schneider et al. (1999)

4.1.3.2 Fingerprints and Structural Keys

This category groups together a number of methods (Table 4.3) that have in common the encoding of molecular information. Most of them rely on a reduced 2D molecular representation, that is, a graph, but they are also applicable to 3D molecular structures.

4.1.3.2.1 Traditional Fingerprints

The original idea of a "molecular fingerprint" dates back to the 1980s when it was necessary to develop fast algorithms to compare and find similarities between molecules. The rationale is that the structural properties of a molecule can be represented by a more or less broad dictionary of relevant entities such as atoms, bonds, and fragments that are classified into different types (Figure 4.4). Accordingly, the structure is encoded as a series of binary flags indicating the presence (1) or absence (0) of these particular units (Taylor et al., 2008). 0s and 1s are then stored in strings (a.k.a. bitstrings) commonly

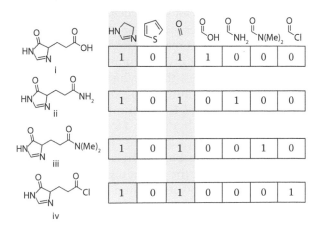

FIGURE 4.4

An example of structural key encoding into fingerprints for molecule *i* and three closely similar analogs.

referred to as "structural keys." Bitstrings are extremely fast to compare computationally due to their binary nature. Besides, their storage requirements are also minimal since the typical string size does not exceed one or two thousand positions (Cabrera et al., 2011).

However, arbitrary building of dictionaries and lack of generality (as not all possible fragments can be included within a dictionary) are the two main drawbacks (Eckert and Bajorath et al. 2007). To overcome these problems, other methods have been developed. Hashing fingerprints such as those from Daylight (Butina 1999) or Unilever Centre (Bender et al., 2004b) extract the chemical information from a graph and then encode each chemical pattern using a hashing method at the expense of a larger bit space as compared to traditional fingerprints. The size of this space will determine the likelihood of a collision, that is, an event that occurs when two or more chemical patterns activate the same bit, giving rise to some loss of information. Most common fingerprints include general chemical patterns or fragments such as multiple bonded atoms (typically up to 7), branches and cycles, pairwise topological distances (i.e., distances measured as the number of bonds between two selected points in the graph), and so on, each of which is assigned an integer value.

4.1.3.2.2 Extended Connectivity Fingerprints

The fingerprints described above were mainly designed to be efficient for similarity searches and substructure comparisons. However, extended connectivity fingerprints (ECFP) (Rogers and Hahn, 2010) were developed to encode molecular features useful in SAR modeling. These methods are based, to some extent, on a modified version of the original Morgan algorithm that unambiguously labels atoms in molecules (Landrum, 2013). These labels form the basis of the fingerprint and they are generated iteratively on the basis of atoms' connectivities and neighbors until all atoms in the molecule have a unique identifier (as in the original Morgan algorithm), a maximum number of iterations is reached (as in ECFP), or another stop criterion is met. Depending on the initial atomic labels, there are two types of fingerprints: (i) ECFP, which use the Daylight invariants, namely, six values that do not depend on the numbering order (atomic number, atomic mass, partial atomic charge, connectivity, number of bonds to non-hydrogen atoms, and number of attached hydrogen atoms), and (ii) functional class fingerprints (FCFP), which attempt to be less specific regarding atom types so as to be more generally applicable. In this case, the six initial values are set either *on* or *off* depending on the following atom types: hydrogen bond acceptor, hydrogen bond donor, positively and negatively charged, aromatic, and halogen.

ECFP and FCFP have been successfully employed in a wide variety of ligand-based applications such as quantification of relationships among drug classes (Hert et al., 2008), prospective VS studies (Kellenberger et al.,

2007; Pan et al., 2011), and chemogenomic analysis (Cortés-Cabrera et al., 2013). These fingerprints have also been massively used in the comparison and benchmarking of many types of 2D and 3D methods (Bender et al., 2009). It appears that ECFP and FCFP slightly outperform other types of fingerprints in recent comparisons, while their performance is comparable to that of other 3D methods such as volume overlap (Hu et al., 2012). However, it should be remarked, once again, that this type of evaluation is not a trivial task and that a method's potential use is commonly overestimated due to the little resemblance of the test scenarios in which they are employed to those of real VS campaigns.

4.1.3.2.3 Pharmacophoric Fingerprints

Although pharmacophores were reviewed in Section 4.1.2, the case of pharmacophoric encoding and its relation to fingerprint bitstrings deserves a separate brief discussion. The distances between distinct pharmacophore points in a molecule, whether calculated in Cartesian space or measured as topological distances in a molecular graph, can be sorted into bins of a certain size. Given that the number of possible ranges is discrete, reduction to distance ranges allows the encoding of this information as bits (1, if the distance is met, or 0, otherwise) and enables the so-called chemically advanced template search (CATS) (Reutlinger et al., 2013), in which distances are measured as the number of intermediate bonds needed to reach one pharmacophoric point from another. For CATS, five chemotypes (hydrogen bond acceptors and donors, positive and negative charges, and hydrophobic/lipophilic moieties) are defined and 10 bins for distances (number of bonds between any two chemotypes). This amounts to a total of 150 bits per fingerprint if only pairs are stored. For 3D pharmacophoric fingerprints, three, four, or even five points are taken into account at the expense of increasing the storage needs. Sometimes, at the bins' boundaries, both bins can be activated (with half the value, for example) to try to increase the coverage of the fingerprint and to avoid the effects of distance discretization (Bonachéra et al., 2006).

4.1.3.3 Alternative Methods

The methods described so far basically study the similarity of one molecule with respect to a reference structure that displays some activity. Other methods in ligand-based drug discovery address the task of identifying new active molecules as if it were a classification problem. Therefore, they classify members of a chemical library as active or inactive depending on some properties that are extracted from training datasets composed of either only active compounds or a mixture of active/inactive molecules. In what follows, an overview will be provided of support vector machines (SVMs), Bayesian methods, and decision trees.

4.1.3.3.1 Support Vector Machines

The methods that make use of SVMs require the availability of binding information on positive ("active") and negative ("low activity" or "inactive") molecules (Hasegawa and Funatsu, 2010). In the first stage, the dataset is divided into training and test sets and a series of descriptors are calculated that properly represent the most physically meaningful properties responsible for binding to the target of interest. These descriptors define a space where the molecules are represented as points. Then, it is possible to build a set of hyperplanes that differentiate the points of the active molecules from the points of the inactive molecules and to select the hyperplane that maximizes this difference.

Originally, an SVM implementation could deal only with linearly separable cases. However, to deal with more complicated situations, that is, nonlinear problems, kernel functions were introduced (e.g., Gaussian kernels) to map the original finite-dimensional space onto a higher-dimensional space where compounds are easily separated (Boser et al., 1992). Once the hyperplane is defined, test compounds are used to validate the binary classifier. The hyperplane is highly dependent on the nature (chemical composition and descriptors used) of the active and inactive molecules, the kernel and its parameters. Besides, it has been found that the source of negative cases can induce a high variability on the SVM results (Heikamp and Bajorath, 2013), a tendency that has already been mentioned regarding the overestimation in SVM performance when certain test sets from common sources are utilized (Hähnke et al., 2013; Irwin and Shoichet, 2005).

SVM models were recently shown to identify 10 butyrylcholinesterase micromolar inhibitors within an in-house dataset of 3601 compounds, three of which displayed novel scaffolds (Fang et al., 2013). 2P2I Hunter is a web-based server (Basse et al., 2013) that has been built using a combination of SVM and general profiles ("rule-of-4") of inhibitors of protein–protein interactions (PPI) with the aim of filtering general chemical libraries and defining more focused collections of compounds with a greater potential of being PPI disruptors.

4.1.3.3.2 Bayesian Methods

Methods based on Bayes' theorem, widely used in probability theory and statistics, aim to quantify a given compound's likelihood of being active against a selected target. The estimation relies on the probability distributions of the fingerprints or the descriptors used to define the compounds. Naïve Bayesian classifiers are popular methods based on the use of datasets of molecules with calculated descriptors (vectors) and an associated known class (Bender et al., 2004a). The classifier predicts the probability of a molecule belonging to a given class as

$$P(\text{class}_n \mid V) = \frac{P(V \mid \text{class}_n)P(\text{class}_n)}{P(V)}$$

where $P(\text{class}_n)$ is the probability of class$_n$, $P(V)$ is the vector probability, and $P(V|\text{class}_n)$ is the probability of the vector in class$_n$, which in this case is equal to $\Pi P(v_i|\text{class}_n)$, where v_i is the ith element in the vector.

4.1.3.3.3 Decision Trees

These algorithms start from a group of descriptors (parameters) calculated from active and inactive datasets, and use a recursive partitioning scheme in which each parameter is applied to split the data. The classifier has a tree structure where the data are propagated along the branches. At each decision node of the tree, a group of molecules is placed either on one branch or the other. To classify an unknown compound, a path is traced through the tree, taking into account the values for the calculated parameters or descriptors, until a leaf (terminal node) is reached.

There are only a few recent examples illustrating the use of a decision tree in the drug discovery field, mostly in VS of natural products (Ehrman et al., 2007) and QSAR studies (Zhou et al., 2009). This is most likely due to the fact that this technique compares unfavorably to SVM or Bayesian methods because of its higher noise and tendency to overfit the data.

4.2 Concluding Remarks

In this chapter we have briefly outlined the methods most commonly used in ligand-based drug discovery and design. Our tentative division has been into traditional methods that have evolved within the computer-aided drug design field, such as those based on molecular shape, pharmacophores, SAR and molecular fingerprints, and alternative methods that apply "machine learning" techniques from other disciplines to the process of drug identification, such as SVMs (from classification and regression analysis), Bayesian models (from probability theory and statistics), and decision trees (from decision analysis). Both groups have their own advantages and drawbacks, and the same can be said about individual methods within each group. Being aware of the limitations of each particular technique is essential to its successful application and inexperienced users must be advised on what can and cannot be achieved. A critical analysis of the outcome is of foremost importance and one must always bear in mind that only a fraction of the factors that actually govern the binding affinity and account for the differences in activity can be embodied in a simplified molecular representation.

Combining ligand-based knowledge with target-based 3D information would appear as the most robust means of (i) understanding SAR, (ii) paving the way to the identification of ligand candidates from chemical libraries, and (iii) designing new chemical entities with a given pharmacological profile.

References

Acharya, C., A. Coop, J.E. Polli, and A.D. MacKerell Jr. 2011. Recent advances in ligand-based drug design: Relevance and utility of the conformationally sampled pharmacophore approach. *Curr. Comput. Aided Drug Des.* 7(1): 10–22.

Alcaro, S., C. Musetti, S. Distinto et al. 2013. Identification and characterization of new DNA G-quadruplex binders selected by a combination of ligand and structure-based virtual screening approaches. *J. Med. Chem.* 56(3): 843–855.

Armstrong, M.S., G.M. Morris, P.W. Finn et al. 2010. ElectroShape: Fast molecular similarity calculations incorporating shape, chirality and electrostatics. *J. Comput. Aided Mol. Des.* 24(9): 789–801.

Armstrong, M.S., G.M. Morris, P.W. Finn, R. Sharma, and W.G. Richards. 2009. Molecular similarity including chirality. *J. Mol. Graph. Modell.* 28(4): 368–370.

Bajorath, J., L. Peltason, M. Wawer et al. 2009. Navigating structure–activity landscapes. *Drug Discov. Today* 14(13): 698–705.

Ballester, P.J., I. Westwood, N. Laurieri, E. Sim, and W.G. Richards. 2010. Prospective virtual screening with ultrafast shape recognition: The identification of novel inhibitors of arylamine N-acetyltransferases. *J. R. Soc. Interface* 7(43): 335–342.

Ballester, P.J., P.W. Finn, and W.G. Richards. 2009. Ultrafast shape recognition: Evaluating a new ligand-based virtual screening technology. *J. Mol. Graph. Modell.* 27(7): 836–845.

Basse, M.J., S. Betzi, R. Bourgeas et al. 2013. 2P2Idb: A structural database dedicated to orthosteric modulation of protein-protein interactions. *Nucl. Acids Res.* 41(Database issue): D824–D827.

Bender, A., H.Y. Mussa, R.C. Glen, and S. Reiling. 2004a. Molecular similarity searching using atom environments, information-based feature selection, and a naive Bayesian classifier. *J. Chem. Inf. Comput. Sci.* 44(1): 170–178.

Bender, A., H.Y. Mussa, R.C. Glen, and S. Reiling. 2004b. Similarity searching of chemical databases using atom environment descriptors (MOLPRINT 2D): Evaluation of performance. *J. Chem. Inf. Comput. Sci.* 44(5): 1708–1718.

Bender, A., J.L. Jenkins, J. Scheiber et al. 2009. How similar are similarity searching methods? A principal component analysis of molecular descriptor space. *J. Chem. Inf. Model.* 49(1): 108–119.

Black, P.E. 2006. Manhattan distance. V. Pieterse and P. E. Black (eds.). http://www.nist.gov/dads/HTML/manhattanDistance.html.

Bonachéra, F., B. Parent, F. Barbosa, N. Froloff, and D. Horvath. 2006. Fuzzy tricentric pharmacophore fingerprints. 1. Topological fuzzy pharmacophore triplets and adapted molecular similarity scoring schemes. *J. Chem. Inf. Model.* 46(6): 2457–2477.

Boser, B.E., I.M. Guyon, and V.N. Vapnik. 1992. A training algorithm for optimal margin classifiers. Paper read at COLT '92 *Proceedings of the Fifth Annual Workshop on Computational Learning Theory*, Pittsburgh, PA, USA, pp. 144–152.

Braga, R.C. and C.H. Andrade. 2013. Assessing the performance of 3D pharmacophore models in virtual screening: How good are they? *Curr. Top. Med. Chem.* 13(9): 1127–1138.

Butina, D. 1999. Unsupervised database clustering based on daylight's fingerprint and Tanimoto similarity: A fast and automated way to cluster small and large data sets. *J. Chem. Inf. Comput. Sci.* 39(4): 747–750.

Cabrera, Á.C., R. Gil-Redondo, A. Perona, F. Gago, and A. Morreale. 2011. VSDMIP 1.5: An automated structure-and ligand-based virtual screening platform with a PyMOL graphical user interface. *J. Comput. Aided Mol. Des.* 25(9): 813–824.

Canela, M.D., M.J. Perez-Perez, S. Noppen et al. 2014. Novel colchicine-site binders with a cyclohexanedione scaffold identified through a ligand-based virtual screening approach. *J. Med. Chem.* 57(10): 3924–3938.

Cortés-Cabrera, Á., A. Morreale, F. Gago, and C. Abad-Zapatero. 2012. AtlasCBS: A web server to map and explore chemico-biological space. *J. Comput. Aided Mol. Des.* 26(9): 995–1003.

Cortes-Cabrera, A., F. Gago, and A. Morreale. 2012. A reverse combination of structure-based and ligand-based strategies for virtual screening. *J. Comput. Aided Mol. Des.* 26(3): 319–327.

Cortés-Cabrera, A., G.M. Morris, P.W. Finn, A. Morreale, and F. Gago. 2013. Comparison of ultra-fast 2D and 3D ligand and target descriptors for side effect prediction and network analysis in polypharmacology. *Br. J. Pharmacol.* 170(3): 557–567.

Cramer, R.D., D.E. Patterson, and J.D. Bunce. 1988. Comparative molecular field analysis (CoMFA). 1. Effect of shape on binding of steroids to carrier proteins. *J. Am. Chem. Soc.* 110(18): 5959–5967.

Cummings, M.D., R.L. DesJarlais, A.C. Gibbs, V. Mohan, and E.P. Jaeger. 2005. Comparison of automated docking programs as virtual screening tools. *J. Med. Chem.* 48(4): 962–976.

Durant, J.L., B.A. Leland, D.R. Henry, and J.G. Nourse. 2002. Reoptimization of MDL keys for use in drug discovery. *J. Chem. Inf. Comput. Sci.* 42(6): 1273–1280.

Eckert, H. and J. Bajorath. 2007. Molecular similarity analysis in virtual screening: foundations, limitations and novel approaches. *Drug Discov. Today* 12(5): 225–233.

Ehrlich, P. 1909. Present status of chemotherapy. *Ber. Dtsch. Chem. Ges.* 42: 17–47.

Ehrman, T.M., D.J. Barlow, and P.J. Hylands. 2007. Virtual screening of Chinese herbs with random forest. *J. Chem. Inf. Model.* 47(2): 264–278.

Evers, A., G. Hessler, H. Matter, and T. Klabunde. 2005. Virtual screening of biogenic amine-binding G-protein coupled receptors: Comparative evaluation of protein-and ligand-based virtual screening protocols. *J. Med. Chem.* 48(17): 5448–5465.

Fang, J., R. Yang, L. Gao et al. 2013. Predictions of BuChE inhibitors using support vector machine and naive Bayesian classification techniques in drug discovery. *J. Chem. Inf. Model.* 53(11): 3009–3020.

Grant, J.A. and B. Pickup. 1995. A Gaussian description of molecular shape. *J. Phys. Chem.* 99(11): 3503–3510.

Grant, J.A., M. Gallardo, and B.T. Pickup. 1996. A fast method of molecular shape comparison: A simple application of a Gaussian description of molecular shape. *J. Comput. Chem.* 17(14): 1653–1666.

Guha, R. and J.H. Van Drie. 2008. Structure–activity landscape index: Identifying and quantifying activity cliffs. *J. Chem. Inf. Model.* 48(3): 646–658.

Hähnke, V., E.E. Bolton, and S.H. Bryant. 2013. PubChem: Atom environments for molecule standardization. *J. Cheminform.* 5(Suppl 1): P38.

Hamza, A. and N.-n. Wei. 2014. SABRE: Ligand/structure-based virtual screening approach using consensus molecular-shape pattern recognition. *J. Chem. Inf. Model.* 54: 338–346. doi: 10.1021/ci4005496.

Haque, I.S. and V.S. Pande. 2010. PAPER—Accelerating parallel evaluations of ROCS. *J. Comput. Chem.* 31(1): 117–132.

Hasegawa, K. and K. Funatsu. 2010. Non-linear modeling and chemical interpretation with aid of support vector machine and regression. *Curr. Comput. Aided Drug Des.* 6(1): 24–36.

Heikamp, K. and J. Bajorath. 2013. Comparison of confirmed inactive and randomly selected compounds as negative training examples in support vector machine-based virtual screening. *J. Chem. Inf. Model.* 53(7): 1595–1601.

Hert, J., M.J. Keiser, J.J. Irwin, T.I. Oprea, and B.K. Shoichet. 2008. Quantifying the relationships among drug classes. *J. Chem. Inf. Model.* 48(4): 755–765.

Hert, J., P. Willett, D.J. Wilton et al. 2006. New methods for ligand-based virtual screening: use of data fusion and machine learning to enhance the effectiveness of similarity searching. *J. Chem. Inf. Model.* 46(2): 462–470.

Hsin, K.Y., H.P. Morgan, S.R. Shave et al. 2011. EDULISS: A small-molecule database with data-mining and pharmacophore searching capabilities. *Nucl. Acids Res.* 39(Database issue): D1042–D1048.

Hu, G., G. Kuang, W. Xiao et al. 2012. Performance evaluation of 2D fingerprint and 3D shape similarity methods in virtual screening. *J. Chem. Inf. Model.* 52(5): 1103–1113.

Irwin, J.J. 2008. Community benchmarks for virtual screening. *J. Comput. Aided Mol. Des.* 22(3–4): 193–199.

Irwin, J.J. and B.K. Shoichet. 2005. ZINC—A free database of commercially available compounds for virtual screening. *J. Chem. Inf. Model.* 45(1): 177–182.

Jacoby, E., A. Boettcher, L.M. Mayr et al. 2009. Knowledge-based virtual screening: Application to the MDM4/p53 protein–protein interaction. *Methods Mol. Biol.* 575: 173–194.

Jain, A.N. 2000. Morphological similarity: A 3D molecular similarity method correlated with protein–ligand recognition. *J. Comput. Aided Mol. Des.* 14(2): 199–213.

Jain, A.N. 2004. Ligand-based structural hypotheses for virtual screening. *J. Med. Chem.* 47(4): 947–961.

Jain, A.N. 2007. Surflex-Dock 2.1: Robust performance from ligand energetic modeling, ring flexibility, and knowledge-based search. *J. Comput. Aided Mol. Des.* 21(5): 281–306.

Jain, A.N., T.G. Dietterich, R.H. Lathrop et al. 1994. Compass: A shape-based machine learning tool for drug design. *J. Comput. Aided Mol. Des.* 8(6): 635–652.

Jones, G., P. Willett, and R.C. Glen. 2000. GASP: Genetic algorithm superimposition program. In: *Pharmacophore Perception, Development, and Use in Drug Design*, O. F. Güner (ed.). International University Line, La Jolla, CA, USA.

Kellenberger, E., J.-Y. Springael, M. Parmentier et al. 2007. Identification of nonpeptide CCR5 receptor agonists by structure-based virtual screening. *J. Med. Chem.* 50(6): 1294–1303.

Klett, J., A. Cortés-Cabrera, R. Gil-Redondo, F. Gago, and A. Morreale. 2014. ALFA: Automatic ligand flexibility assignment. *J. Chem. Inf. Model.* 54(1): 314–323.

Koes, D.R. and C.J. Camacho. 2012. ZINCPharmer: Pharmacophore search of the ZINC database. *Nucleic Acids Res.* 40(W1): W409–W414.

Landrum, G. 2013. *Rdkit: Open-Source Cheminformatics*. Available at http://www.rdkit.org/.

Leach, A.R. and V.J. Gillet. 2007. *An Introduction to Chemoinformatics*. Springer, Netherlands.

Lippert, T., T. Schulz-Gasch, O. Roche, W. Guba, and M. Rarey. 2011. *De novo* design by pharmacophore-based searches in fragment spaces. *J. Comput. Aided Mol. Des.* 25(10): 931–945.

Liu, D.C. and J. Nocedal. 1989. On the limited memory BFGS method for large scale optimization. *Math. Program.* 45(1–3): 503–528.

Liu, X., H. Jiang, and H. Li. 2011. SHAFTS: A hybrid approach for 3D molecular similarity calculation. 1. Method and assessment of virtual screening. *J. Chem. Inf. Model.* 51(9): 2372–2385.

Lu, W., X. Liu, X. Cao et al. 2011. SHAFTS: A hybrid approach for 3D molecular similarity calculation. 2. Prospective case study in the discovery of diverse p90 ribosomal S6 protein kinase 2 inhibitors to suppress cell migration. *J. Med. Chem.* 54(10): 3564–3574.

Macarron, R., M.N. Banks, D. Bojanic et al. 2011. Impact of high-throughput screening in biomedical research. *Nat. Rev. Drug Discov.* 10(3): 188–195.

Maggiora, G., M. Vogt, D. Stumpfe, and J. Bajorath. 2014. Molecular similarity in medicinal chemistry. *J. Med. Chem.* 57(8): 3186–3204.

Maggiora, G.M. 2006. On outliers and activity cliffs—Why QSAR often disappoints. *J. Chem. Inf. Model.* 46(4): 1535.

Maggiora, G.M. and V. Shanmugasundaram. 2011. Molecular similarity measures. *Methods Mol. Biol.* 672: 39–100.

Mills, J.E. and P.M. Dean. 1996. Three-dimensional hydrogen-bond geometry and probability information from a crystal survey. *J. Comput. Aided Mol. Des.* 10(6): 607–622.

Mustata, G., A.V. Follis, D.I. Hammoudeh et al. 2009. Discovery of novel Myc–Max heterodimer disruptors with a three-dimensional pharmacophore model. *J. Med. Chem.* 52(5): 1247–1250.

Muthusamy, K., K.D. Singh, S. Chinnasamy et al. 2013. High throughput virtual screening and E-pharmacophore filtering in the discovery of new BACE-1 inhibitors. *Interdiscip. Sci. Comput. Life Sci.* 5(2): 119–126.

Mysinger, M.M., M. Carchia, J.J. Irwin, and B.K. Shoichet. 2012. Directory of useful decoys, enhanced (DUD-E): Better ligands and decoys for better benchmarking. *J. Med. Chem.* 55(14): 6582–6594.

Nelder, J.A. and R. Mead. 1965. A simplex method for function minimization. *Comput. J.* 7(4): 308–313.

OpenEye. 2013. *ROCS (Shape Similarity for Virtual Screening & Lead Hopping)*. Available at http://www.eyesopen.com/docs/rocs/current/html/index.html.

Pan, Y., L. Li, G. Kim et al. 2011. Identification and validation of novel human pregnane X receptor activators among prescribed drugs via ligand-based virtual screening. *Drug Metab. Dispos.* 39(2):337–344.

Peltason, L., Y. Hu, and J. Bajorath. 2009. From structure–activity to structure–selectivity relationships: Quantitative assessment, selectivity cliffs, and key compounds. *Chem. Med. Chem.* 4(11): 1864–1873.

Reutlinger, M., C.P. Koch, D. Reker et al. 2013. Chemically Advanced Template Search (CATS) for scaffold-hopping and prospective target prediction for "Orphan" molecules. *Mol. Inf.* 32(2): 133–138.

Reymond, J.-L., R. van Deursen, L.C. Blum, and L. Ruddigkeit. 2010. Chemical space as a source for new drugs. *Med. Chem. Commun.* 1(1): 30–38.

Richmond, N.J., C.A. Abrams, P.R. Wolohan et al. 2006. GALAHAD: 1. Pharmacophore identification by hypermolecular alignment of ligands in 3D. *J. Comput. Aided Mol. Des.* 20(9): 567–587.

Rogers, D. and M. Hahn. 2010. Extended-connectivity fingerprints. *J. Chem. Inf. Model.* 50(5): 742–754.

Ruppert, J., W. Welch, and A.N. Jain. 1997. Automatic identification and representation of protein binding sites for molecular docking. *Protein Sci.* 6(3): 524–533.

Rush, T.S., J.A. Grant, L. Mosyak, and A. Nicholls. 2005. A shape-based 3-D scaffold hopping method and its application to a bacterial protein–protein interaction. *J. Med. Chem.* 48(5): 1489–1495.

Sastry, G.M., S.L. Dixon, and W. Sherman. 2011. Rapid shape-based ligand alignment and virtual screening method based on atom/feature-pair similarities and volume overlap scoring. *J. Chem. Inf. Model.* 51(10): 2455–2466.

Schneider, G. and M. Nettekoven. 2003. Ligand-based combinatorial design of selective purinergic receptor (A_{2A}) antagonists using self-organizing maps. *J. Comb. Chem.* 5(3): 233–237.

Schneider, G., W. Neidhart, T. Giller, and G. Schmid. 1999. "Scaffold-Hopping" by topological pharmacophore search: A contribution to virtual screening. *Angew. Chem. Int. Ed. Engl.* 38(19): 2894–2896.

Schneidman-Duhovny, D., O. Dror, Y. Inbar, R. Nussinov, and H.J. Wolfson. 2008. PharmaGist: A webserver for ligand-based pharmacophore detection. *Nucl. Acids Res.* 36 (Suppl 2): W223–W228.

Schreyer, A.M. and T. Blundell. 2012. USRCAT: Real-time ultrafast shape recognition with pharmacophoric constraints. *J. Cheminf.* 4(1): 1–12.

Shoichet, B.K. and B.K. Kobilka. 2012. Structure-based drug screening for G-protein-coupled receptors. *Trends Pharmacol. Sci.* 33(5): 268–272.

Singh, K.D., M. Karthikeyan, P. Kirubakaran, and S. Nagamani. 2011. Pharmacophore filtering and 3D-QSAR in the discovery of new JAK2 inhibitors. *J. Mol. Graph. Modell.* 30: 186–197.

Sprague, P.W. and R. Hoffmann. 1997. CATALYST pharmacophore models and their utility as queries for searching 3D databases. In: *Computer-Assisted Lead Finding and Optimization: Current Tools for Medicinal Chemistry*, H. v. d. Waterbeemd, B. Testa, and G. Folkers (eds.). Wiley.

Taylor, C.M., N.B. Rockweiler, C. Liu et al. 2010. Using ligand-based virtual screening to allosterically stabilize the activated state of a GPCR. *Chem. Biol. Drug Des.* 75(3): 325–332.

Taylor, P., E. Blackburn, Y.G. Sheng et al. 2008. Ligand discovery and virtual screening using the program LIDAEUS. *Br. J. Pharmacol.* 153(Suppl 1): S55–S67.

Toba, S., J. Srinivasan, A.J. Maynard, and J. Sutter. 2006. Using pharmacophore models to gain insight into structural binding and virtual screening: An application study with CDK2 and human DHFR. *J. Chem. Inf. Model.* 46(2): 728–735.

Vainio, M.J., J.S. Puranen, and M.S. Johnson. 2009. ShaEP: Molecular overlay based on shape and electrostatic potential. *J. Chem. Inf. Model.* 49(2): 492–502.

Vaz de Lima, L.A.C., and A.S. Nascimento. 2013. MolShaCS: A free and open source tool for ligand similarity identification based on Gaussian descriptors. *Eur. J. Med. Chem.* 59: 296–303.

von Korff, M., J. Freyss, and T. Sander. 2009. Comparison of ligand- and structure-based virtual screening on the DUD data set. *J. Chem. Inf. Model.* 49(2): 209–231.

Wassermann, A.M., M. Wawer, and J. Bajorath. 2010. Activity landscape representations for structure–activity relationship analysis. *J. Med. Chem.* 53(23): 8209–8223.

Wermuth, C.-G., C.R. Ganellin, P. Lindberg, and L.A. Mitscher. 1998. Glossary of terms used in medicinal chemistry (IUPAC Recommendations 1998). *Pure Appl. Chem.* 70(5): 1129–1143.

Wirmer-Bartoschek, J. and S. Bartoschek. 2012. NMR in drug discovery on membrane proteins. *Future Med. Chem.* 4(7): 869–875.

Yan, X., J. Li, Z. Liu et al. 2013. Enhancing molecular shape comparison by weighted Gaussian functions. *J. Chem. Inf. Model.* 53(8): 1967–1978.

Yera, E.R., A.E. Cleves, and A.N. Jain. 2011. Chemical structural novelty: On-targets and off-targets. *J. Med. Chem.* 54(19): 6771–6785.

Zhou, Y.-P., L.-J. Tang, J. Jiao et al. 2009. Modified particle swarm optimization algorithm for adaptively configuring globally optimal classification and regression trees. *J. Chem. Inf. Model.* 49(5): 1144–1153.

5

Pharmacophore Modeling and Pharmacophore-Based Virtual Screening

Muhammad Akram, Teresa Kaserer, and Daniela Schuster

CONTENTS

5.1 Introduction

The concept of a pharmacophore originated from Paul Ehrlich's understanding of toxophores (chemical groups responsible for toxic effects) and haptophores (chemical groups responsible for binding) for explaining the interaction between a drug and its receptor. Paul Ehrlich hypothesized that specific chemical groups are responsible for the activity of a certain drug molecule (Ehrlich, 1909). The first modern definition of a pharmacophore was proposed by Schueler in the 1960s. He proposed that "abstract features" are responsible for biological activity rather than "chemical groups" (Schueler, 1961). The first pharmacophore model was reported by Beckett in 1963 for muscarinic receptors (Beckett et al., 1963). In 1967, the first computed model of muscarinic receptor ligands was introduced by Kier (Kier, 1967). The modern definition of a 3D pharmacophore by the International Union of Pure and Applied Chemistry (IUPAC) is based on the definition of Schueler as "an ensemble of steric and electronic features that is necessary to ensure the optimal supramolecular interactions with a specific biological target and to trigger (or block) its biological response" (Wermuth et al., 1998). A comprehensive review on the development of the pharmacophore concept has been recently published by Güner and Bowen (2014). The core idea of the pharmacophore concept is the molecular recognition of a biological target by a group of compounds having some common features that interact with compatible sites of the biological target (Leach et al., 2010). A pharmacophore model, therefore, represents the spatial arrangement and the electrochemical properties that are required for a compound to interact with a macromolecular biomolecule (a protein or DNA/RNA). It supposedly reflects the binding mode for a specific binding site.

A pharmacophore model is composed of physicochemical features, which represent these molecular interactions. Such a feature is not entitled to be a specific functional group such as carbonic acid or amine, but merges the electrochemical properties that a whole set of functionalities share. Therefore, different functional groups can be represented by the same feature (Leach et al., 2010). This allows also for the identification of novel compound classes (novel scaffolds) that possess the required electrochemical properties to interact with a target, a concept that is called scaffold-hopping (Hessler and Baringhaus, 2010; Perez-Pineiro et al., 2009).

Although the exact definition and the underlying algorithms for the recognition of chemical functionalities differ in the various pharmacophore modeling programs, all of them include pharmacophore features describing hydrogen bond donor (HBD) and hydrogen bond acceptor (HBA) groups, hydrophobic regions, aromatic rings, positively or negatively charged/ionizable groups, and metal–ion interactions.

Hydrogen bonding is a weak type of electrostatic interaction that can be formed between a hydrogen atom covalently bound to a heavy atom, the

HBD, and a lone pair of electrons of an electronegative atom (e.g., nitrogen, oxygen, or fluorine) of another molecule or the same molecule (intramolecular hydrogen bonding), which serve as HBAs. In general, hydrogen bonding partners have a distance of less than 2.5 Å and a donor-hydrogen-acceptor angle between 90° and 180° (Hubbard and Kamran, 2010). However, due to the resolution and flexibility limitation of protein–ligand x-ray crystal structures, pharmacophore modeling software may vary these limitations to retrieve better screening results (Table 5.1). Technically, Catalyst (Sprague, 1995) and LigandScout (Wolber and Langer, 2005) model HBD and HBA positions for the heavy atom and a projection point in the environment (the protein site), where a vector indicates the direction of the hydrogen bond. Phase uses SMART patterns for defining the hydrogen bonding in one out of three ways, that is, point, vector, or group (Dixon et al., 2006). Molecular operating environment (MOE) models the HBD/HBA features with multiple feature definitions including vectored and unvectored ones (MOE, 2011). The default HBD and HBA feature in MOE is an unvectored feature, for example, a HBA without a projected point (Figure 5.1).

TABLE 5.1

Summary of Chemical Feature Settings in Common Pharmacophore Modeling Programs

Features	DS Catalyst	LigandScout	MOE	Phase
Hydrogen bond acceptor	$d_{O,N...D} = 1.9$ Å $d_{D-X} = 1.0$ Å	$d = 2.2–3.8$ Å	$d = 2.8$ Å	$d \leq 2.5$ Å $\angle_{Y-H...X\,min} = 120°$
Hydrogen bond donor	$d_{H...A} = 1.9$ Å $d_{A-Y} = 1.23$ Å	$d = 2.2–3.8$ Å	$d = 2.8$ Å	$d \leq 2.5$ Å $\angle_{Y-H...X\,min} = 120°$
Hydrophobic	$d = 4$ Å	$d = 1.0–5.9$ Å	$d \leq 4.5$ Å	$d \leq 4.0$ Å
Aromatic	$d = 4$ Å or 6 Å (above and below the aromatic ring plane)[a]	$d = 2.8–4.5$ Å for parallel and orthogonal ring interactions or 3.5–5.5 Å for cation-π interactions	$d = 2.1$ Å for π normal projection	$d \leq 4.0$ Å also applies for aromatic–hydrophobic interactions
Ionic		$d = 1.5–5.5$ Å (1.0–10.0 Å for cation- π interactions)		$d \leq 5.0$ Å
Metal-binding		depending on the metal between 1.0 and 4.0 Å		

Sources: DS Catalyst (Böhm, H. J. 1992. *J. Comput. Aided Mol. Des.* 6(1): 61–78); LigandScout (Wolber, G. and T. Langer. 2005. *J. Chem. Inf. Model.* 45(1): 160–169); MOE (MOE help and documentation, MOE version 2011.10, Chemical Computing Group Inc., Montreal, Canada); and Phase (Dixon, S. L. et al. 2006. *J. Comput. Aided Mol. Des.* 20(10–11): 647–671.)

Note: O... oxygen; N... nitrogen; D... donor; X... accepting atom on the protein side; H... hydrogen; Y... donating atom on the protein side; C... carbon; L... ligand; A... acceptor.

[a] Special rules apply for amide and sulfur-containing aromatic interactions.

(a)   (b)

(c)   (d)

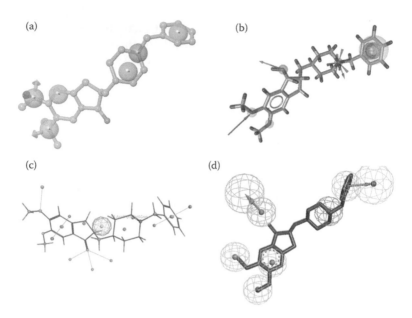

FIGURE 5.1
(See color insert.) Pharmacophore models generated by four different software packages using the crystal structure of the aricept–acetylcholinesterase complex (PDB entry 1EVE). (From Kryger, G., I. Silman, and J. L. Sussman. *Structure* 7(3): 297–307.) (a) Pharmacophore hypothesis generated by Phase. (From Dixon, S. L. et al. 2006. *J. Comput. Aided Mol. Des.* 20(10–11): 647–671.) Red sphere = hydrogen bond acceptor, blue sphere = positively ionizable group, and green sphere = hydrophobic group. (b) Pharmacophore query from LigandScout. (From Wolber, G. and T. Langer. 2005. *J. Chem. Inf. Model.* 45(1): 160–169.) Green arrow = hydrogen bond donor, red arrow = hydrogen bond acceptor, yellow sphere = hydrophobic contact, blue star = positively ionizable group, and blue rings = aromatic interaction. (c) Pharmacophore model developed by MOE. (From MOE version 2010.10. Chemical Computing Group Inc., Montreal, Canada.) Yellow sphere = hydrophobic interaction, cyan line = hydrogen bond acceptor, orange line = aromatic ring, green dots = hydrophobic feature. (d) Pharmacophore query generated by Discovery Studio. (From Sprague, P. W. 1995. *Perspect. Drug Discov. Des.* 3(1): 1–20.) Cyan sphere = hydrophobic group, orange sphere = aromatic ring, green sphere = hydrogen bond acceptor, and red sphere = positively ionizable group.

Hydrophobic areas are represented by tolerance spheres on lipophilic centers, chains, or groups, like, for example, alkanes (Greene et al., 1994). As the size and shape of lipophilic areas in a molecule are not geometrically restricted (as is the case for hydrogen bonds), the actual form of the lipophilic ligand part may only poorly be represented by a ball-shaped sphere. Enlarging the default sphere size or placing several hydrophobic features onto the lipophilic area can help to represent the molecule's lipophilicity more accurately.

Aromatic interactions can be defined with or without geometric constraints. An aromatic ring plane is included when geometric constraints are allowed, and the direction of the interaction is included. In general, interacting aromatic rings preferentially orient themselves in an off-centered, parallel orientation. Alternatively, they may adapt a T-shaped arrangement (90°) toward each other (Li et al., 2013). MOE (MOE, 2011) represents the aromatic interaction without geometric constraints, while Catalyst (Sprague, 1995), Phase (Dixon et al., 2006), and LigandScout (Wolber and Langer, 2005) model these interactions with geometric constraints (Figure 5.1). More details on the aromatic feature settings of the programs are provided in Table 5.1.

Charge-transfer interactions are produced by positively or negatively ioniz-able areas of a single atom or groups of atoms. Also, atoms and groups of atoms that already have a positive or negative charge are covered by this kind of features (ionic interactions). These interactions are dependent on the protonation state of the affected atoms. Since the protonation state of a group of atoms is depending on its environment (pH, surrounding amino acids), it may be challenging to accurately define the protonation state for each ligand when generating a screening database. Therefore, in some programs pharmacophore features are available that allow a group to be "ionizable." For example, a negatively ionizable feature will recognize protonated and deprotonated carboxylic groups alike. In contrast, a negative charge feature will only allow for deprotonated acids to be counted as a mapping structure. While Catalyst offers ionizable and charge features separately, LigandScout only includes ionizable features. Phase handles charge-transfer interac-tions with the so-called positively or negatively charged features. However, these features also recognize non-ionized groups such as carboxylic acids. LigandScout (Wolber and Langer, 2005), Catalyst (Sprague, 1995), and Phase (Dixon et al., 2006) by default use input structures without adaption to the pH. However, assigning protonation states during conformational analysis is an optional feature available in Catalyst and Phase. Assigning the compre-hensive charges and definition of charge-transfer interactions in MOE (MOE, 2011) is done during the preparation of the molecules. The positively or nega-tively charged areas, which are recognized by MOE, are limited to single atoms. Table 5.1 describes the program settings for chemical features in the different described software packages.

Exclusion volumes represent areas in the 3D pharmacophore model, into which ligands are forbidden to intrude. They mimic the size and shape of the binding pocket and, therefore, a ligand's extension into these areas is expected to cause steric clashes with surrounding amino acids. In structure-based pharmacophore modeling, exclusion volumes are defined by the pro-tein side-chains forming the ligand-binding site, while an exclusion volume coat surrounding aligned ligands can be created in ligand-based modeling. Exclusion volumes help to make pharmacophore models more restrictive by limiting the mapping compounds to only those who can fit into the binding pocket and excluding compounds that are too large for binding. This results in an improvement of model selectivity, decrease in false-positive (FP) hits, and can increase enrichment rates in virtual screening experiments (Toba et al., 2006). Although all discussed pharmacophore modeling tools offer exclusion volumes for modeling, they handle them quite differently in the screening of databases (Spitzer et al., 2010). In Phase and Catalyst, the area occupied by the exclusion volume sphere is forbidden for the mapping ligand. In detail, the van der Waals radii of ligand heavy atoms are not allowed to clash with the exclusion volumes. In Catalyst, a modest receptor flexibility can be mimicked by adjusting the so-called "ExcludedVolumeXFactor" parameter. This setting makes the spheres "soft," allowing a ligand to protrude into the exclusion volume to a certain extent. In Phase, also the radii of the hydrogen atoms can be considered. MOE only counts a steric clash with an exclusion volume when a ligand heavy atom center lies within (Spitzer et al., 2010). LigandScout represents the exclusion volumes spheres as single spheres (Wolber and Langer, 2005).

In some cases, the default pharmacophore feature definitions will not meet the needs of the modeler, and a *customization of the features* is required. Simple adaptations of the features comprise modifications of the feature size and feature weight. For more sophisticated changes, almost all software programs allow for the creation of customized features, where the functional groups or substructures covered by the feature can be individually defined, for example, substructures suitable to act as Michael acceptors (Steindl et al., 2005).

In general, LigandScout (Wolber and Langer, 2005) and Phase (Dixon et al., 2006) have the ability to set more than one feature on a heavy atom, while Catalyst (Sprague, 1995) only allows for one feature definition for every heavy atom at one time. MOE can include several properties into one feature. So technically, it is one feature that can describe several chemical functionalities at the same molecule location.

In addition to the above described four most commonly used algorithms, there are a number of algorithms available, that can be used for pharmacophore modeling and virtual screening (Table 5.2).

5.2 Pharmacophore Model Generation

Nowadays, the most widely used programs for pharmacophore modeling are Catalyst implemented in Discovery Studio, Genetic Algorithm with Linear Assignment for Hypermolecular Alignment of Datasets (GALAHAD) (Richmond et al., 2006), Genetic Algorithm Similarity Program (GASP) (Jones et al., 2000), LigandScout (Wolber and Langer, 2005), Phase (Dixon et al., 2006), and pharmacophore module of MOE (MOE, 2011). Two types of approaches are used for pharmacophore model generation, depending on the available data concerning the 3D structure of the target, for example protein or DNA and RNA, and known bioactive molecules.

TABLE 5.2

An Overview of Available Pharmacophore Modeling and Screening Algorithms

Name	Short Description	References
DS Catalyst	Commercially available algorithm for pharmacophore modeling, generation of 3D databases, virtual screening, shape-based screening, and ligand conformer generation. It is available as a part of Discovery Studio	http://accelrys.com/ products/discovery-studio/ pharmacophore.html BioVia, Sprague (1995)
FLAP	Commercially available software package for pharmacophore modeling and virtual screening	http://www.moldiscovery. com/soft_flap.php Cross et al. (2012)
FORECASTER Suite	Commercially available tool for performing docking, pdb superposition, protein setup, ligand setup, converting 2D to 3D, pharmacophore search, clustering, filtering, and asymmetric catalysis	http://fitted.ca/suite.html
GASP	Ligand-based pharmacophore modeling tool using genetic algorithm, distributed by Tripos	http://www.certara.com/ products/molmod/ sybyl-x/simpharm/ (Tripos International) Jones et al. (2000)
LigandScout	Commercial structure- and ligand-based pharmacophore modeling and virtual screening software suite	http://www.inteligand.com/ ligandscout, Wolber and Langer (2005)
MOE	Commercial drug discovery software package for pharmacophore modeling and screening, but also for docking, fragment-based design, cheminformatics, molecular simulations, and more	http://www.chemcomp. com/MOE-Molecular_ Operating_Environment. htm MOE (2011)
PharmaGist	Open source online algorithm for pharmacophore modeling; the desktop version also has the ability to perform virtual screening	http://bioinfo3d.cs.tau.ac.il/ pharma/about.html Schneidman-Duhovny et al. (2008), Dror et al. (2009)
Pharmer	An open source pharmacophore modeling and screening software	http://smoothdock.ccbb.pitt. edu/pharmer/ Koes and Camacho (2011)
PharmMapper	Open source online tool for target fishing using pharmacophore mapping	http://59.78.96.61/ pharmmapper/ Liu et al. (2010)
Phase	Pharmacophore modeling, virtual screening, database calculation and docking, and more	http://www.schrodinger. com/Phase/ Dixon et al. (2006)
QUASI	It creates pharmacophore models and performs virtual screening. It is distributed by *De Novo* Pharmaceuticals	http://www.denovopharma. com/page2. asp?PageID=485, Todorov et al. (2007)

(Continued)

TABLE 5.2 (*Continued*)

An Overview of Available Pharmacophore Modeling and Screening Algorithms

Name	Short Description	References
Silicos it	Open source command line toolkit for performing various functions such as filtering unwanted molecules, pharmacophore modeling, and for extracting molecular scaffolds according to predefined rules	http://silicos-it.be
ZINCPharmer	Open source online tool for screening ZINC database by using pharmacophore models of LigandScout and MOE	http://zincpharmer.csb.pitt.edu/ Koes and Carlos (2012)

5.2.1 Structure-Based Pharmacophore Models

Structure-based pharmacophore models can be generated for targets, where a known 3D structure is available. These can be experimentally determined x-ray crystal structures, NMR structures, or *in silico* calculated homology models. The most important source for publicly available target x-ray crystal structures is the Protein Data Bank (PDB) (Berman et al., 2000). Structure-based pharmacophore modeling follows a simple key and lock principle for protein–ligand complexes. It combines all the data of interactions from the ligand and the binding site along with shape and volume information (Horvath, 2011). The principle of structure-based pharmacophore modeling is based on the analysis of complementary chemical features of the active site and the ligand. Structure-based pharmacophore modeling can be divided into two types, protein–ligand complex-based and protein-based, depending on the availability of a ligand. The protein–ligand-based technique extracts the key interactions between ligand and protein and offers a lot of information about the mode of action. Several software programs such as LigandScout (Wolber and Langer, 2005), Pocket v.2 (Chen and Lai, 2006), grid-based pharmacophore modeling (Ortuso et al., 2006), Discovery Studio Catalyst (BioVia), and MOE (MOE, 2011) can automatically generate pharmacophore models from protein–ligand complexes. When a protein–ligand complex is not available, protein-based pharmacophore modeling can be applied. The LUDI tool implemented in Discovery Studio (BioVia), for example, is able to convert the properties of the protein-binding site directly into pharmacophore features (Böhm, 1992).

5.2.2 Ligand-Based Pharmacophore Models

The ligand-based pharmacophore modeling approach is considered as key computational strategy in today's drug discovery, when no 3D structure of the target protein is available. Ligand-based pharmacophore models consist of features that a group of known active ligands share, the so-called common features. The generation of ligand-based pharmacophore models differs in the various tools.

LigandScout generates the common feature pharmacophore models from a set of at least two training set molecules. If not previously available, LigandScout calculates conformers of the training set molecules. In the next step, all dataset molecules are ranked according to their flexibility, starting with the least-flexible compound, and pharmacophore features (e.g., hydrogen bonds, aromatic features, etc.) are assigned to all conformers. The features of all conformers of the two top-ranked training set molecules are aligned to generate common feature intermediate pharmacophore models. These intermediate pharmacophore models are then ranked by using the chemical feature overlap, the steric overlap scoring function, or both. The top-ranked intermediate pharmacophore model is then aligned with all conformations of the third-ranked molecule in the training set. This process is repeated until all training set molecules have been processed or no further conformation from a training set molecule does match with the intermediate pharmacophore model. For a successful pharmacophore model generation, the final model must consist of at least three features (LigandScout 3.1 User manual, Inte:Ligand).

Phase (Dixon et al., 2006) also generates preliminary pharmacophore models for every conformation of the active ligand set (those potential models are called variants). Every variant is then categorized using a binary decision tree that progressively splits the variants based on inter-feature distances. Such a description of an intermediate pharmacophore model is named as a box. A final common pharmacophore feature model is defined if at least one conformation of the minimum number of active compounds required is classified into the same box. Since the investigation of all theoretically possible models is computationally expensive, the Phase program filters all variants according to predefined parameters, which can be manually adapted. Those include the number of matching ligands, the minimum and maximum number of features, and the minimum and maximum occurrence number of a specific feature (Dixon et al., 2006).

MOE generates common feature pharmacophore models based on the annotation points of aligned ligand conformations in the active compounds dataset. Annotation points within a defined distance from each other, the so-called neighbors, are only kept, if they are above the minimum consensus score. This score is based on the number of conformations represented by the annotation point. In the next step, the consensus score is calculated for a cluster of annotation points (also called components), and components below the minimum consensus score are eliminated. In the end, pharmacophore features are defined for every component, and all suggested features are listed according to their consensus score (MOE, 2011).

Discovery Studio Catalyst HipHop creates common feature pharmaco-phore models from training set molecules, which are evaluated against the test-set molecules. HipHop starts by recognizing the common pharmaco-phore configurations automatically in the training set molecules. This search starts from a small set of features and is extended to larger common phar-macophore configurations, discarding no common pharmacophore configu-rations in the training set molecules. The matching of a test set molecule with pharmacophore configurations is only possible, if it has the structural features and at least one conformation that can be placed within specific tol-erances of the corresponding ideal locations. The pharmacophore configu-rations are then scored on the basis of the fitting of training set molecules (Barnum et al., 1996). The HipHop algorithm provides a qualitative hypoth-esis to distinguish between active and inactive molecules. The final result of a HipHop run is a user-defined number of hypotheses ranked from highest to lowest score.

In Catalyst, it is also possible to include information from inactive com-pounds already in the model building process. If inactive molecules are present in the training set, then the pharmacophore models are refined by adding space restrictions with the HipHopRefine algorithm (Sutter et al., 2011). Exclusion volumes are added to the hypothesis at sites that are solely occupied by inactive compounds from the training set.

Besides HipHop, Discovery Studio Catalyst provides the HypoGen algo-rithm (Kurogi and Güner, 2004; Li et al., 2000) that generates quantitative pharmacophore models by identifying chemical features that are common in the 3D training set. For a reliable model, at least 16 compounds in the training set are required along with their activity data. The activities (IC_{50}, EC_{50}, K_I) of the training set molecules should be spread over at least 4 orders of magnitude. The weight of each feature of the resulting pharmacophore model is depending on its relative contribution to the compounds activities. HypoGen generates the pharmacophore hypothesis, which is common in all active compounds of the training set molecules, but not in the inactive ones. It creates pharmacophore models in three phases: the constructive phase, the subtractive phase, and the optimization phase. The constructive phase is similar to HipHop and creates common feature pharmacophore models of the two most active compounds from the training set molecules. The sub-tractive phase removes the pharmacophore models that map inactive mol-ecules in the dataset. In the optimization phase, remaining hypotheses are improved by making small perturbations. Finally, the resulting 10 pharma-cophore models with the highest score and lowest cost are reported to the user (Kurogi and Güner, 2004).

Catalyst HypoRefine is an extension of the HypoGen algorithm. The con-structive phase of HypoRefine is similar to the HypoGen; however, there is no subtractive phase in the HypoRefine algorithm. For further improvement of the pharmacophore hypothesis, exclusion volumes are added in the opti-mization phase (BioVia).

5.3 Design of Datasets

The quality of the underlying dataset for modeling determines the quality of the calculated pharmacophore models. In general, the data used to model a specific protein–ligand interaction should come from direct binding assays, not from functional (e.g., cell-based) assays. From the *in vitro* data, it must be evident that the compound used for modeling is indeed directly binding to the pharmacological target. In the past, molecular modelers had to dig through hundreds of papers to assemble datasets for model generation and validation. In recent years, however, with the release of publicly available compound–activity databases (PubChem, ChEMBL and Open PHACTS), the situation has improved a lot. PubChem (Wang et al., 2010) (http://pubchem. ncbi.nlm.nih.gov/) and ChEMBL (Gaulton et al., 2012) (https://www.ebi. ac.uk/chembl/) allow searching for binding data sorted by compound or by bioassay. While ChEMBL derives its data directly from over 47 international, peer-reviewed journals, PubChem provides full activity data from high-throughput screening (HTS), many of which are not published anywhere else. Both the ChEMBL and PubChem have each other's data linked, so a search in the ChEMBL will also report compounds from PubChem Bioassay screenings and the PubChem search will show activities from the literature as well. Open PHACTS is a freely available database that has been created to increase the speed of the drug discovery process. It has been developed by a collaboration of academia, industry, and small business enterprises. Currently, 29 organizations take part in Open PHACTS and provide pharmacological data. Open PHACTS also has a platform for the validation and standardization of chemical structures (Williams et al., 2012). ChEMBL, PubChem, and Open PHACTS are by no means the only database sources for small molecule activities; however, they are publicly available and are the most important ones due to their large number of entries (Bolton et al., 2008; Gaulton et al., 2012).

Several kinds of datasets can be employed for both the generation and theoretical validation of pharmacophore models. The training set usually comprises a collection of known active ligands, which serve as templates for the generation of the models. Additional active compounds are to be included in the test set, which allows for the investigation of whether the model also maps other active compounds besides the ones from the training set. Active compounds have to be selected on the basis of identical binding sites at the target protein, because one pharmacophore model can only represent one specific binding mode. However, a pharmacophore model should not only be able to identify active molecules, but also filter out inactive molecules. Therefore, known inactive compounds can be combined in a so-called inactive dataset, which should not be found by the model.

When screening a large number of compounds against a biological activity, usually the majority of tested compounds will be inactive. The chances to randomly find an active compound for a specific target using HTS have been reported to be 0.02% for protein tyrosine phosphatase inhibitors (Doman et al., 2002), 0.07% for cruzain inhibitors (Ferreira et al., 2010), 0.55% for glycogen synthase kinase-3β inhibitors (Polgar et al., 2005), and 0.1% for formyl-peptide receptor ligands (Young et al., 2005).

A virtual screening validation should mimic such a scenario by assembling the validation database from a high number of inactive and a small number of active compounds. It is suggested that a representative ratio of number of active:number of inactive compounds is about 1:40 (Huang et al., 2006). However, inactive compounds are rarely published, which hampers this endeavor. With the release of the PubChem (Wang et al., 2010), ChEMBL (Gaulton et al., 2012), OpenPHACTS (Williams et al., 2012), and Drugmatrix (Ganter et al., 2006) datasets, the situation has improved a lot; however, a large number of experimentally verified inactive compounds may still be hard to find.

If insufficient data on inactive molecules is available, a decoy dataset may be used to substitute the large number of inactive compounds needed for model validation. Decoys are compounds with unknown biological activity, but assumed to be inactive (because the probability for a random compound to be active is really low, see above). According to the number of hits retrieved by screening the decoy dataset, it can be estimated how restrictive a pharmacophore model is. The generation of a high-quality decoy dataset is achieved by the selection of molecules with similar physiochemical properties compared to the active compounds dataset (Kirchmair et al., 2008). For this purpose, Verdonk et al. suggested to use several physicochemical properties, including the number of HBDs, the number of HBAs, and the number of nonpolar atoms. However, these compounds should possess a diverse topology from each other and from the active compounds to exclude potentially active molecules from the dataset (Verdonk et al., 2004). Table 5.3 lists the commonly used databases that provide data for model building and validation.

5.4 Theoretical Validation Metrics for Assessing the Performance of Pharmacophore Models

To verify the reliability of a pharmacophore model, the active and inactive compounds that were not used for model generation can be used for theoretical validation. The validation of a pharmacophore model with active compounds indicates the reliability of the model to identify active molecules from a dataset of both active and inactive entries. In contrast, the validation of a pharmacophore model with inactive compounds analyzes its capability to distinguish active from inactive molecules (Vuorinen et al., 2014).

The result from screening a validation database with N entries will lead to a hit-list comprising n compounds fitting the model. Active compounds

TABLE 5.3

List of Commonly Used Databases for Model Building and Validation

Database	Data Provided	Reference
BindingDB	Binding data for 6795 protein targets and 442,444 small molecules (June 2014)	http://www.bindingdb.org/ bind/index.jsp Chen et al. (2001), Liu et al. (2007)
ChEMBL	>1.3 million distinct compounds with annotated biological data (version 18)	https://www.ebi.ac.uk/chembl/ Gaulton et al. (2012)
Directory of Useful Decoys (DUD)	2950 actives compounds and 106,200 decoys for model generation and validation (version 2.0)	http://dud.docking.org Huang et al. (2006)
DrugBank	7685 drug molecules (version 4.1)	http://www.drugbank.ca/ Law et al. (2014)
MDL Drug Data Report	>150,000 compounds	http://lib.stanford.edu/ mdl-drug-data-report (MDDR)
Open PHACTS	29 organizations from academia, pharmaceutical companies, and other enterprises created an "open pharmacological space" network	http://www.openphacts.org/ index.php Williams et al. (2012)
Protein Data Bank (PDB)	>100,000 experimentally derived target structures	http://www.rcsb.org/ Berman et al. (2000)
PubChem	>50 million nonunique compounds with annotated biological data	http://pubchem.ncbi.nlm.nih.gov/ Bolton et al. (2008)
STITCH	Over 300,000 chemical–protein interactions	http://stitch.embl.de/ Kuhn et al. (2008, 2010, 2012, 2014)
WOMBAT	270,918 unique compounds and 1996 targets (version 2013.1)	http://www.sunsetmolecular. com/index.php Olah et al. (2005, 2008), Olah and Oprea (2007)

that were correctly found by the model are true-positive (TP) hits. Inactive compounds mapping the models are FP hits. An active compound that is not found by the model is a false-negative (FN) molecule. Correctly classified, inactive compounds are termed true-negative (TN) compounds (Figure 5.2).

The following metrics are most commonly used to determine the quality of the pharmacophore models.

5.4.1 Sensitivity (Se)

The Sensitivity (Se) determines the ability of a pharmacophore model to retrieve TP compounds in a virtual screening experiment. It is defined as the ratio of TP compounds to all active compounds in the validation dataset (Equation 5.1) (Triballeau et al., 2005). Its value ranges from zero to one, where zero indicates that the pharmacophore model did not find any of the

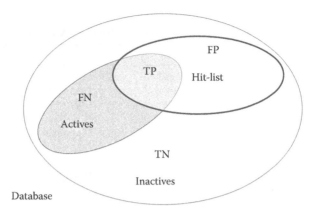

FIGURE 5.2

In a typical virtual screening experiment, a database containing a small number of active molecules embedded in a large number of inactive molecules is searched with a model. The resulting hit-list comprises correctly recognized active molecules (TP) and inactive compounds wrongly assessed as active (FP). Active molecules not recognized by the model are FN, while correctly classified inactive compounds are TN.

TP molecules in a selected dataset during a virtual screening process, and one indicates that it found all of them

$$Se = \frac{TP}{(TP + FN)} \tag{5.1}$$

5.4.2 Specificity (Sp)

Specificity (Sp) is the ability of a pharmacophore model to reject inactive compounds in a virtual screening experiment. It is calculated as the ratio of the rejected TN compounds to all the compounds present in the dataset, (Equation 5.2) (Triballeau et al., 2005). Similar to the sensitivity, its values range from zero to one. Zero indicates that all inactive compounds map the model, while one represents the correct rejection of all inactive compounds during a virtual screening process.

$$Sp = \frac{TN}{(TN + FP)} \tag{5.2}$$

5.4.3 Accuracy (Acc)

Accuracy is the ratio of TP and TN to the active (P) and inactive (N) compounds in the dataset (Equation 5.3) (Gao et al., 1999; Jacobsson et al., 2003). It determines the number of correctly classified compounds.

$$\text{Acc} = \frac{(\text{TP} + \text{TN})}{(\text{P} + \text{N})} \tag{5.3}$$

5.4.4 Yield of Actives (Ya)

The yield of actives (Ya) is defined as the ratio of the TP compounds retrieved in a virtual screening process to the total number of hits (n) or the size of the hit-list (Equation 5.4). It therefore determines the fraction of TP hits in the hit-list (Güner and Henry, 2000; Jacobsson et al., 2003).

$$\text{Ya} = \frac{\text{TP}}{\text{n}} \tag{5.4}$$

5.4.5 Goodness of Hit-List (GH)

The goodness of hit-list (GH) combines the Se, Sp, and Ya (Equation 5.5). It has more capability to evaluate the discriminatory power of a pharmacophore model than Se, Sp, or Ya alone. It accounts for both the TP and TN ratio (Güner et al., 2004). Its value ranges from zero to one. A value of one indicates that the pharmacophore model is very good and is providing a perfect hit-list containing only actives (Güner and Henry, 2000).

$$\text{GH} = \left(\frac{3}{4} \text{Ya} + \frac{1}{4} \text{Se} \right) \times (\text{Sp}) \tag{5.5}$$

5.4.6 Enrichment Factor (EF)

The enrichment factor (EF) is defined as the ratio of TP hits in a hit-list and the active compounds in the entire database (Equation 5.6) (Güner and henry, 2000). It is calculated as follows:

$$\text{EF} = \frac{\text{TP}/\text{n}}{n_{\text{act}}/\text{N}} \tag{5.6}$$

n_{act} = number of active molecules in the whole database.

The EF, therefore, measures the enrichment of active compounds in the hit-list compared to pure random selection. This metric relates the retrieval of active compounds to the composition of the validation database. However, the EF has two major drawbacks. First, it is strongly depending on the size and ratio of the datasets used in the experiments. The larger the inactive dataset is in comparison to the active dataset, the higher the maximum EF can be. However, datasets with approximately the same size of active and inactive compounds can always reach only relatively small EFs. The second drawback concerns the ranking of active compounds within a hit-list. The EF does not give any information about the ordering of active and inactive hits, so it is not known whether active molecules are among the top-ranked hits. To overcome the first issue, a relative EF (calculated EF divided through the maximum EF for the used dataset) can be calculated. Regarding the latter issue, the next described metric offers a solution.

5.4.7 Receiver Operating Characteristics (ROC) Curve

The ROC curve is a widely applied quality metric to overcome the limitations mentioned above. While the pharmacophore evaluating metrics explained above give one-digit answers to determine the quality of the pharmacophore model, the ROC curve is a 2D graph, in which the number of active compounds is plotted against the number of inactive compounds (also referred to as 1-specificity) according to their ranking in the hit-list (Triballeau et al., 2005) (Figure 5.3). It therefore describes the TP from a database of N entries as a function of (1–FP rate) (Zweig and Campbell, 1993). The ROC curve is independent of the composition of the datasets and can help to determine the efficiency of a single candidate pharmacophore model as well as compare the differences in the results of various virtual screening experiments.

In the ideal ROC curve, all active molecules are ranked before the inactive molecules, and there is no overlap between them. This curve proceeds from the origin to the upper left corner and ends at the upper right corner (Figure

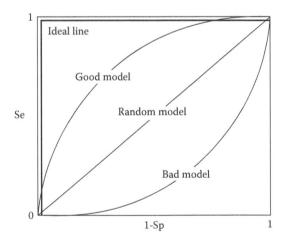

FIGURE 5.3
Exemplary depiction of ROC curves indicating models of different quality. The diagonal shows a random selection of hits, while all curves above and below this line represent models with an enrichment of active and inactive molecules in the hit-list, respectively. The ideal ROC curve is shown as a bold line. Se = selectivity, 1-Sp = 1-specificity.

5.3). Randomly selected compounds would lead to a curve that directly connects the lower left and the upper right corner (diagonale). Curves lower than this one indicate models that are worse than random and lead to an actual enrichment of inactive molecules in the hit-list (Figure 5.3). The area under the curve (AUC) of the ROC curve is another useful evaluation metric for determining the discriminatory power of virtual screening methods. Similar to the ROC curve, the AUC does not depend on the ratio of the active and inactive molecules in a database. The ideal ROC curve would lead to an AUC of 1, while a random distribution of active and inactive compounds results in an AUC of 0.5. Everything below an AUC of 0.5, again, indicates a worse than random performance of the investigated model (Triballeau et al., 2005).

5.4.8 Advanced Enrichment Descriptors

Classical enrichment descriptors such as AUC and EF do not differentiate between a virtual screening algorithm, which ranks one-half of actives at the start and the other half at the end of an ordered list, and a virtual screening protocol that ranks active hits only at the start of list. This issue of early recognition can be overcome by the use of advanced enrichment descriptors as recently reviewed by Braga and Andrade. Some of the advanced evaluation descriptors such as robust initial enhancement (RIE), Boltzmann-enhanced discrimination of ROC (BED-ROC), normalized partial AUC (pAUC), and hit rate (HR) are currently available (Braga and Andrade, 2013).

5.5 Pharmacophore Model Refinement

Due to the rapid knowledge gain in the field of medicinal chemistry, there is need to improve the quality of pharmacophore models on a regular basis. This will help to improve the quality of pharmacophore models. There are two steps of pharmacophore model refinement (Figure 5.4). The first one is the optimization of a model by using a dataset of both active and inactive compounds. In this step, the pharmacophore features are optimized by adjusting their size and volume, and exclusion volumes are added or deleted. In the second step, the pharmacophore model is used in a prospective screening and virtual hits are tested experimentally. The results of the biological examination can then be used again to refine the model. A recent study conducted by Vuorinen et al. is an excellent example of pharmacophore model refinement. They systematically refined 11β-hydroxysteroid dehydrogenase (HSD) inhibitor pharmacophore models. The refined pharmacophore models of 11β-HSD inhibitors covered more active scaffolds compared to the initial models (Schuster et al., 2006; Vuorinen et al., 2014).

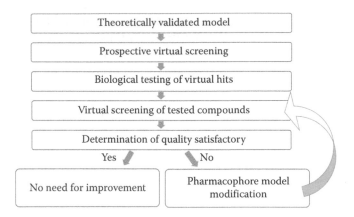

FIGURE 5.4
Flowchart of pharmacophore model refinement.

5.6 Pharmacophore-Based Virtual Screening

The first step in a virtual screening run is the selection and preparation of a 3D database. This includes the calculation of low energy conformers and the addition of physicochemical descriptors for each participating molecule. Different algorithms are available to filter out compounds with a high likelihood to be bioactive using 3D pharmacophore models. Catalyst's FAST search is an example for a rigid pharmacophore fitting algorithm, which screens a database of precalculated conformations. Catalyst's BEST algorithm in contrast allows for a limited conformational flexibility of the ligands in the database. During the screening, the mapping of a compound to the model is followed by a minimization step. Several studies proved that the BEST algorithm was superior to the FAST (Kirchmair et al., 2006), however, this advantage is at the cost of screening time. OMEGA from OpenEye (Hawkins et al., 2010; Hawkins and Nicholls, 2012; OMEGA) is implemented in LigandScout for calculating conformers and generation of screening databases. In LigandScout, the mapping of compounds is based on pharmacophore feature overlay (Wolber et al., 2006), whereas in MOE the annotation points of the molecule are mapped to the features of the model (MOE, 2011). Pharmacophore mapping in Phase is conducted in two steps: First, the database is screened to identify compounds with the required spatial arrangements of the desired features, for example, appropriate inter-feature distance and correct feature type, and in the second step the conformers are aligned to the model (Dixon et al., 2006).

Another option for pharmacophore-based screening is partial mapping, in which features can be marked as optional or a maximum number of omitted features can be defined (Cottrell et al., 2006; Schuster and Wolber, 2010). This is especially advantageous if it is still unknown, whose features are crucial for the ligand–target interaction.

5.7 Strategies for Selecting Compounds for Biological Testing from Hit-Lists

The ultimate purpose of the refinement is to improve the efficiency of the hits in terms of lead-likeness and, in case of very large hit-lists, to reduce the original hit-list to a reasonable size. Further processing of hit-lists can include the following steps.

5.7.1 Lipsinki Filter

The Lipsinki filter is a well-known criterion for selecting compounds in the hit-list using their predicted oral bioavailability (Lipinski et al., 2001). Lipinski et al. observed that 90% of the orally active drugs, which entered into phase II of clinical trials, and therefore are more likely to become an approved drug, shared several properties. These parameters, which he called the "rule of 5" (RO5) according to the determined properties, are molecular weight ≤ 500, clogP value ≤ 5, HBDs ≤ 5, and HBAs (sum of O and N atoms) ≤ 10 (Lipinski et al., 2001; Lipinski, 2004). However, this rule is restricted to those drugs that are administered orally and are absorbed via passive mechanisms. The drug candidates that do not satisfy Lipinski's RO5, therefore, could have poor absorption or permeation properties. For selecting putative lead compounds from virtual screening hits, a molecular weight range of 200–350 and less lipophilic regions will provide the possibility for further optimization of a lead compound (Oprea et al., 2001). Lipsinki filters can be applied, for example, with BioVia's Pipeline Pilot tool (BioVia).

5.7.2 Molecular Similarity Evaluation

Another important strategy for the selection of lead and/or drug-likeness of compounds is by molecular similarity evaluation. If the chemical structure of a hit is closely related to already-known active drug molecules, then it may have a high likelihood to also be active. Another aspect concerns the size of the hit-list. If the modeler retrieves lots and lots of similar hits, the application of a clustering tool based on 2D similarity can help to focus experimental testing on structurally diverse compounds. However, most clustering methods are not 100% reliable. They often group chemicals from the same scaffold into different clusters. In addition, the clustering algorithm is always asking for the number of clusters to be calculated. If the user calculates only a few clusters in a big hit-list, many scaffolds will be lost. *Vice versa*, computing many clusters for small hit-lists will result in very similar cluster centers, often containing the same chemical scaffold (Reddy et al., 2007). Hit clustering is challenging and there are still novel approaches to this important step (Ertl, 2014).

Two-dimensional fingerprinting methods can also be used for the refinement of hit-lists, in which a specific characteristic appears to be beneficial or unwanted for the biological activity. These fingerprints can be defined and the hit-lists are filtered according to the pre-defined parameters. For example, Markt et al. used pharmacophore modeling, 3D shape, and electrostatic similarity screening as a combination for virtual screening to find novel scaffolds for peroxisome proliferator-activated receptor (PPAR) ligands. It was observed that 5 out of 10 virtual screening hits showed PPAR activity (Markt et al., 2008). Again, the PipelinePilot tool of BioVia software package is an excellent example for this purpose. So, similarity-based filtering and 2D fingerprinting can be used in both ways for filtering specific hits or for removing compounds with undesired properties from the hit-list.

5.7.3 Consensus Hits

To increase the likelihood of selecting active compounds for biological testing or to reduce the number of compounds from the hit-list, the so-called consensus approaches are more and more applied. Thereby, compounds are screened against two or more models for the same target and only compounds that fulfill the criteria of several or all of them are subjected to the experimental investigation. The applied models can either be generated using the same or different programs. However, it has also be shown that pharmacophore models can produce complementary hit-lists with low overlap and in each hit-list unique active compounds can be found (Spitzer et al., 2010).

Additionally, pharmacophore models are also often combined with different approaches like shape-based screening (Temml et al., 2014) or docking (Wang et al., 2014). In a recent study, Wang et al. applied a pharmacophore-based and a docking-based virtual screening workflow either alone or in combination for the identification of novel inhibitors for R-like endoplasmic reticulum kinase. Their results highlight the advantage of the consensus approach in terms of improved ranking of active molecules in the hit-list and enrichment rates (Wang et al., 2014).

5.7.4 Visual Inspection

Besides the use of algorithms, the eye of an experienced computational chemist is often more powerful than any software package. So, visual inspection of the hit-list is highly recommended for the selection of compounds for testing.

5.8 Parallel Screening (PS) and Bioactivity Profiling

In conventional pharmacophore-based virtual screening, large datasets of compounds are screened against high-quality pharmacophore models to identify novel bioactive compounds for a specific target (Schuster et al., 2010). However, in parallel screening (PS), a single chemical entity is screened against a collection of high-quality pharmacophore models in order to generate an *in silico* bioactivity profile (Steindl et al., 2006). Therefore, PS focuses rather on the ligand than on a single-receptor protein. In general, activity profiling involves the following steps: (a) selection of the compound of interest, (b) selection of a set of pharmacophore models, ready to be screened against the molecule, (c) virtual screening, (d) analysis of the hit-list that represents the *in silico* pharmacologic profile of the compound, and (e) selection of promising targets for the biological testing (Steindl et al., 2006). This kind of screening can be used for various purposes, for example, to identify promising targets for the selected compound in the course of target fishing (Schuster and Wolber, 2010), to investigate the potential toxicity of a compound, or to identify additional application fields for an already approved drug (Schuster, 2010).

5.9 Toxicity Predictions and Structure–Activity Relationship (SAR) Studies

Computer-aided drug development techniques are widely used to save time and costs in the drug development process (Duffy et al., 2012; Ooms, 2000). Although originally intended for the identification of novel lead structures, pharmacophore-based virtual screening can also aid in the prediction of toxic side effects that could lead to the termination of a drug development project. Every drug–protein interaction in addition to the pharmacologically desired target can lead to potential unwanted side effects. These interactions can be predicted for a specific protein of interest (in this case called anti-target as the interaction is disadvantageous) or for a whole set of potential interaction partners investigated in the course of a parallel screening. For example, Nashev et al. reported an example of successful toxicity prediction involving endocrine disruptors in sun cream. 17β-hydroxysteroid dehydrogenase 3 (17β-HSD3) is an enzyme responsible for the catalysis of the last step in testosterone synthesis in human testes. Any chemical inhibiting 17β-HSD3 can lead to a decrease in the plasma concentration of testosterone, which would result in imperfect development of the male reproductive system. The obtained hit-list from virtual screening for 17β-HSD3 inhibitors was analyzed and several UV-filter chemicals were experimentally tested against

17β-HSD3 inhibition. Subsequent SAR studies were performed to analyze the differences in the toxicity of the tested compounds (Nashev et al., 2010). This led to the identification of a specific unwanted moiety shared by all active compounds, which all inactive compounds from the same compound class lack. Pharmacophore modeling is therefore, cannot only be used to predict unwanted side effects, but can also help to avoid them.

5.10 Drug Repurposing

Drug repositioning or repurposing is a recent development in drug discovery in which new application fields for already established drugs are discovered (drug-centric) or already established drugs are studied to be used for the treatment of neglected diseases (disease-centric) (Ekins et al., 2011). Neglected diseases occur in only small populations; hence pharmaceutical companies lack the interest to develop drugs for their treatment (Liu et al., 2013). Since a lot of data are already available for approved drugs, especially with regard to pharmacokinetic properties and toxicity, drug repurposing enables fast access to treatment of these diseases with low costs. For instance, astemizole was withdrawn as antihistaminic drug from the market because of its potential to cause arrhythmias at higher doses. Recently, it was repositioned as an anticancer drug with an IC_{50} value of 1.62 ± 0.75 μM against the voltage-gated potassium channel EAG1 that inhibits the proliferation of tumor cells (García-Quiroz et al., 2012; Garcia-Quiroz and Camacho, 2011). Astemizole was also repositioned as an antimalarial agent with IC_{50} values of 227, 457, and 734 nM against the 3D7, Dd2, and ItG stains of *Plasmodium falciparum*, respectively (Chong et al., 2006).

5.11 Target Fishing

A parallel screening approach can also be applied for the prediction of potential interaction partners for a certain compound (also referred to as target-fishing). In a normal screening process ligands are screened against a specific pharmacophore model, while in pharmacophore-based parallel screening and target fishing, the virtual screening is performed with one compound against several pharmacophore models. This type of technique is especially advantageous for newly isolated natural products or newly developed synthetic compounds. For example, Rollinger et al. extracted 16 secondary metabolites from the medicinal plant *Ruta graveolens* and performed a parallel screening against 2208 pharmacophore models generated for over 280 different targets. Selected hits were biologically evaluated and the activity of several compounds could be confirmed: Arborinine, the highest scoring virtual hit for acetylcholinesterase (AchE), showed an inhibitory activity in the biological testing with an IC_{50} value of 34.7 μM. The antiviral activity of arborinine and 6,7,8-trimethoxycoumarin with IC_{50} values of 3.19 and 11.98 μM, respectively, was confirmed. Finally, the only compound that was virtually predicted for the cannabinoid-2 receptor, rutamarin, showed selective activity with a K_i value of 7.4 μM (Rollinger et al., 2009).

5.12 General Remarks on Success Rates

In silico methods, in general, are nowadays well integrated in the drug development process (Tanrikulu et al., 2013). Although originally considered as independent approaches, experimental HTS and virtual screening perfectly complement each other. The two approaches represent opposing strategies: one is experimental while the other is theoretical, offering the opportunity to increase the output of the drug discovery process (Bajorath, 2002).

Drug development projects can benefit from the advantages of both methods. As a matter of fact, no drug can reach the market without extensive experimental testing. However, *in silico* techniques can provide a rationale for selecting compounds with a preferable pharmacological profile to proceed in the drug development pipeline. Also, original screening libraries can be limited to the most promising candidates using *in silico* approaches (Babaoglu et al., 2008). A study conducted by Schuster et al. specifically investigated the success rate of pharmacophore modeling in comparison to random selection of test compounds. Within the course of identifying novel acetylcholine inhibitors, hits derived from a pharmacophore-based virtual screening and randomly selected compounds were experimentally tested. The group observed a distinct enrichment of active compounds in the virtual hit-list compared to the randomly composed screening library. While 57.1% of all compounds from the pharmacophore-based screening were at least weakly active, this was only the case for 14% of the molecules derived from the random selection (Schuster et al., 2010). These results illustrate the impact pharmacophore modeling can have on a drug development project, and the contributions it can account for.

5.13 Limitations and Caveats of Pharmacophore-Based Screening

One of the main limitations of all *in silico* methods including pharmacophore modeling concerns the quantity and quality of the data used for the dataset generation. As already mentioned in the "theoretical validation metrics" section, most of these theoretical quality determinants are largely depending on the size and composition of the datasets. Representation of only one chemical scaffold in the dataset makes the identification of diverse molecules in the hit-list rather unlikely, and lets the quality metrics of the model appear more successful than it actually was. Similar to that, also the decoy set has to be of high quality and diversity. If one uses a decoy set that is composed of compounds that have nothing in common with the true active compounds, it will not be challenging to generate a model that can discriminate between these two populations. However, in the prospective screening, the model will retrieve a high number of FP hits, because it was not trained to distinguish between active and inactive compounds from the same chemical space. It has been recently shown that using experimentally confirmed inactive compounds for model building instead of decoys systematically improves the quality of the generated models. Although this study did not use pharmacophore models as screening tools, this finding can be expected to be true also for other virtual screening approaches such as pharmacophore models (Heikamp and Bajorath, 2013). Also, the quality of the data included in the dataset has to be examined. One can carefully optimize and refine a model, it will not lead to improvements if no high-quality data were used. Therefore, the initial steps of dataset generation comprise the careful selection of the biological test system used for the generation of the experimental data, the determination of a reasonable activity cut-off for the compounds included in the dataset, and the manual inspection of the original reference for checking the values and 2D structures. In general, binding assay data are preferred over functional assay data, because it confirms the interaction with the intended target. Functional assays describe the biological effect, but give no further information about the underlying mode of action.

In most cases when ligand-based pharmacophore modeling is applied, no experimental data concerning the orientation of a bioactive ligand in the binding site is available. One big challenge, therefore, is to cover the conformational space of a molecule, and accordingly select a conformation similar to the bioactive one. This often appears to be challenging, because the bioactive conformation might not be the one close to the energy minimum (Schwab, 2010). These issues are of subordinate relevance in the extraction of ligand–target interactions applied in structure-based modeling, however, the conformer generation concerns both approaches when it comes to model refinement, theoretical validation, and prospective screening. Also, in the preparation of the database selected for screening, the whole conformational space should be explored. Otherwise, the risk rises to miss a compound that actually was active, but not identified in the course of the screening because the appropriated conformer was not included in the database (Steindl et al., 2006).

The main limitation in structure-based pharmacophore modeling, obviously, is the availability of a 3D structure. Without structural data about the target, independently from the source (x-ray crystallography, NMR, or homology modeling), no structure-based approach can be conducted. Still, these structures, if accessible, are snapshots of a specific state and neglect the flexibility of a protein. However, with the constant progress and increase of computer performance and power, molecular dynamics simulations will be examined on a more regular basis and can help to address this issue (Durrant and McCammon, 2011).

Improvement could also lie in the refinement of pharmacophore features. Halogens, for example, were long considered as solely hydrophobic residues. However, halogen bonding can considerably contribute to ligand–target interactions (Wilcken et al., 2013), but may still be neglected in the definition of the default pharmacophore features of most commonly used pharmacophore modeling programs.

There is still room for improvement in the field of pharmacophore-based modeling and virtual screening. However, being aware of the current limitations already allows to avoid certain caveats, and to correctly interpret the obtained data. Both of them are important steps that guarantee optimum results.

Most of the available pharmacophore model generation algorithms have very good performance (Dixon et al., 2006; MOE, 2011; Sprague, 1995; Wolber and Langer, 2005), and some of them are even available free of charge (Table 5.2) (Dixon et al., 2006; Koes and Camacho, 2011). Pharmacophore modeling in combination with other methods is currently used extensively in drug research and development. Also in the future, it will be an essential tool for finding the new bioactive compounds.

Acknowledgments

We are grateful to the Austrian Science Fund (P26782) and Young Talent Grants from the University of Innsbruck for supporting this work. Teresa Kaserer is supported by the "Verein zur Förderung der wissenschaftlichen Ausbildung und Tätigkeit von Südtirolern an der Landesuniversität Innsbruck." Daniela Schuster is financed by Erika Cremer Habilitation Program of the University of Innsbruck.

References

Babaoglu, K., A. Simeonov, J. J. Irwin et al. 2008. Comprehensive mechanistic analysis of hits from high-throughput and docking screens against beta-lactamase. *J. Med. Chem.* 51(8): 2502–2511.

Bajorath, J. 2002. Integration of virtual and high-throughput screening. *Nat. Rev. Drug. Discov.* 1(11): 882–894.

Barnum, D., J. Greene, A. Smellie, and P. Sprague. 1996. Identification of common functional configurations among molecules. *J. Chem. Inf. Comput. Sci.* 36(3): 563–571.

Beckett, A. H., N. J. Harper, and J. W. Clitherow. 1963. The importance of stereoisomerism in muscarinic activity. *J. Pharm. Pharmacol.* 15(1): 362–371.

Berman, H. M., J. Westbrook, Z. Feng et al. 2000. The protein data bank. *Nucl. Acids Res.* 28(1): 235–242.

Böhm, H. J. 1992. The computer program LUDI: A new method for the *de novo* design of enzyme inhibitors. *J. Comput. Aided Mol. Des.* 6(1): 61–78.

Bolton, E. E., Y. Wang, P. A. Thiessen, and S. H. Bryant. 2008. PubChem: Integrated platform of small molecules and biological activities. In: *Annual Reports in Computational Chemistry*, A. W. Ralph and C. S. David (eds.), Oxford, UK; Amsterdam, The Netherlands: Elsevier, pp. 217–241.

Braga, R. C. and C. H. Andrade. 2013. Assessing the performance of 3D pharmacophore models in virtual screening: How good are they. *Curr. Top. Med. Chem.* 13(9): 1127–1138.

Chen, J. and L. Lai. 2006. Pocket v.2: Further developments on receptor-based pharmacophore modeling. *J. Chem. Inf. Model.* 46(6): 2684–2691.

Chen, X., Y. Lin, and M. K. Gilson. 2001. The binding database: Overview and user's guide. *Biopolymers* 61(2): 127–141.

Chong, C. R., X. Chen, L. Shi, J. O. Liu, and D. J. Sullivan, Jr. 2006. A clinical drug library screen identifies astemizole as an antimalarial agent. *Nat. Chem. Biol.* 2(8): 415–416.

Cottrell, S. J., V. J. Gillet, and R. Taylor. 2006. Incorporating partial matches within multiobjective pharmacophore identification. *J. Comput. Aided Mol. Des.* 20: 735–749.

Cross, S., M. Baroni, L. Goracci, and G. Cruciani. 2012. GRID-based three-dimensional pharmacophores I: FLAPpharm, a novel approach for pharmacophore elucidation. *J. Chem. Inf. Model.* 52(10): 2587–2598.

Dixon, S. L., A. M. Smondyrev, E. H. Knoll, S. N. Rao, D. E. Shaw, and R. A. Friesner. 2006. PHASE: A new engine for pharmacophore perception, 3D QSAR model development, and 3D database screening: 1. Methodology and preliminary results. *J. Comput. Aided Mol. Des.* 20(10–11): 647–671.

Doman, T. N., S. L. McGovern, B. J. Witherbee et al. 2002. Molecular docking and high-throughput screening for novel inhibitors of protein tyrosine phosphatase-1B. *J. Med. Chem.* 45(11): 2213–2221.

Dror, O., D. Schneidman-Duhovny, Y. Inbar, R. Nussinov, and H. J. Wolfson. 2009. Novel approach for efficient pharmacophore-based virtual screening: Method and applications. *J. Chem. Inf. Model.* 49(10): 2333–2343.

Duffy, B. C., L. Zhu, H. Decornez, and D. B. Kitchen. 2012. Early phase drug discovery: Cheminformatics and computational techniques in identifying lead series. *Bioorg. Med. Chem.* 20(18): 5324–5342.

Durrant, J. D. and J. A. McCammon. 2011. Molecular dynamics simulations and drug discovery. *BMC Biol.* 9: 71–80.

Ehrlich, P. 1909. Über den jetzigen Stand der Chemotherapie. *Ber. Dtsch. Chem. Ges.* 42(1): 17–47.

Ekins, S., A. J. Williams, M. D. Krasowski, and J. S. Freundlich. 2011. *In silico* repositioning of approved drugs for rare and neglected diseases. *Drug Discov. Today* 16(7–8): 298–310.

Ertl, P. 2014. Intuitive ordering of scaffolds and scaffold similarity searching using scaffold keys. *J. Chem. Inf. Model.* 54(6): 1617–1622.

Ferreira, R. S., A. Simeonov, A. Jadhav et al. 2010. Complementarity between a docking and a high-throughput screen in discovering new cruzain inhibitors. *J. Med. Chem.* 53(13): 4891–4905.

Ganter, B., R. D. Snyder, D. N. Halbert, and M. D. Lee. 2006. Toxicogenomics in drug discovery and development: Mechanistic analysis of compound/class-dependent effects using the DrugMatrix® database. *Pharmacogenomics* 7(7):1025–1044.

Gao, H., C. Williams, P. Labute, and J. Bajorath. 1999. Binary quantitative structure–activity relationship (QSAR) analysis of estrogen receptor ligands. *J. Chem. Inf. Comput. Sci.* 39(1): 164–168.

Garcia-Quiroz, J. and J. Camacho. 2011. Astemizole: An old anti-histamine as a new promising anti-cancer drug. *Anticancer Agents Med. Chem.* 11(3): 307–314.

García-Quiroz, J., R. García-Becerra, D. Barrera et al. 2012. Astemizole synergizes calcitriol antiproliferative activity by inhibiting CYP24A1 and upregulating VDR: A novel approach for breast cancer therapy. *PLoS ONE* 7(9): e45063.

Gaulton, A., L. J. Bellis, A. P. Bento et al. 2012. ChEMBL: A large-scale bioactivity database for drug discovery. *Nucleic Acids Res.* 40(Database issue): D1100– D1107.

Greene, J., S. Kahn, H. Savoj, P. Sprague, and S. Teig. 1994. Chemical function queries for 3D database search. *J. Chem. Inf. Comput. Sci.* 34(6): 1297–1308.

Güner, F. and R. Henry. 2000. Metric for analyzing hit-lists and pharmacophores. In: *Pharmacophore Perception, Development, and Use in Drug Design*, F. G. Osman (ed.), La Jolla, CA: International University Line, pp. 193–12.

Güner, O., O. Clement, and Y. Kurogi. 2004. Pharmacophore modeling and three dimensional database searching for drug design using catalyst: Recent advances. *Curr. Med. Chem.* 11(22): 2991–3005.

Güner, O. F. and J. P. Bowen. 2014. Setting the record straight: The origin of the pharmacophore concept. *J. Chem. Inf. Model.* 54(5): 1269–1283.

Hawkins, P. C. and A. Nicholls. 2012. Conformer generation with OMEGA: Learning from the data set and the analysis of failures. *J. Chem. Inf. Model.* 52(11): 2919–2936.

Hawkins, P. C. D., A. G. Skillman, G. L. Warren, B. A. Ellingson, and M. T. Stahl. 2010. Conformer generation with OMEGA: Algorithm and validation using high quality structures from the protein databank and Cambridge structural database. *J. Chem. Inf. Model.* 50(4): 572–584.

Heikamp, K. and J. Bajorath. 2013. Comparison of confirmed inactive and randomly selected compounds as negative training examples in support vector machine-based virtual screening. *J. Chem. Inf. Model.* 53(7): 1595–1601.

Hessler, G. and K. H. Baringhaus. 2010. The scaffold hopping potential of pharmacophores. *Drug Discov. Today Technol.* 7(4): e263–e269.

Horvath, D. 2011. Pharmacophore-based virtual screening. In: *Chemoinformatics and Computational Chemical Biology*, J. Bajorath (ed.), New York, NY: Humana Press, pp. 261–298.

Huang, N., B. K. Shoichet, and J. J. Irwin. 2006. Benchmarking sets for molecular docking. *J. Med. Chem.* 49(23): 6789–6801.

Hubbard, R. E. and H. M. Kamran. 2010. Hydrogen bonds in proteins: Role and strength. In: *eLS*, J. M. Valpuesta (ed.), Chichester: John Wiley & Sons, Ltd. DOI: 10.1002/9780470015902.a0003011.pub2.

Jacobsson, M., P. Liden, E. Stjernschantz, H. Bostrom, and U. Norinder. 2003. Improving structure-based virtual screening by multivariate analysis of scoring data. *J. Med. Chem.* 46(26): 5781–5789.

Jones, G., P. Willett and R. C. Glen. 2000. GASP: Genetic Algorithm Superimposition Program. In: *Pharmacophore Perception, Development, and Use in Drug Design*, O. F. Güner (ed.), La Jolla, CA: International University Line, pp. 85–106.

Kier, L. B. 1967. Molecular orbital calculation of preferred conformations of acetylcholine, muscarine, and muscarone. *Mol. Pharmacol.* 3(5): 487–494.

Kirchmair, J., G. Wolber, C. Laggner, and T. Langer. 2006. Comparative performance assessment of the conformational model generators omega and catalyst: A large-scale survey on the retrieval of protein-bound ligand conformations. *J. Chem. Inf. Model.* 46(4): 1848–1861.

Kirchmair, J., P. Markt, S. Distinto, G. Wolber, and T. Langer. 2008. Evaluation of the performance of 3D virtual screening protocols: RMSD comparisons, enrichment assessments, and decoy selection—What can we learn from earlier mistakes? *J. Comput. Aided Mol. Des.* 22(3–4): 213–228.

Koes, D. R. and C. J. Camacho. 2011. Pharmer: Efficient and exact pharmacophore search. *J. Chem. Inf. Model.* 51(6): 1307–1314.

Koes, D. R. and J. C. Carlos. 2012. ZINCPharmer: Pharmacophore search of the ZINC database. *Nucleic Acids Res.* 40(Web Server issue): W409–W414.

Kryger, G., I. Silman and J. L. Sussman. 1999. Structure of acetylcholinesterase complexed with E2020 (Aricept): Implications for the design of new anti-Alzheimer drugs. *Structure* 7(3): 297–307.

Kuhn, M., C. Von-Mering, M. Campillos, L. J. Jensen, and P. Bork. 2008. STITCH: Interaction networks of chemicals and proteins. *Nucleic Acids Res.* 36(Database issue): D684–D688.

Kuhn, M., D. Szklarczyk, A. Franceschini et al. 2010. STITCH 2: An interaction network database for small molecules and proteins. *Nucleic Acids Res.* 38(Database issue): D552–D556.

Kuhn, M., D. Szklarczyk, A. Franceschini, C. Von-Mering, L. J. Jensen, and P. Bork. 2012. STITCH 3: Zooming in on protein–chemical interactions. *Nucleic Acids Res.* 40(Database issue): D876–D880.

Kuhn, M., D. Szklarczyk, S. Pletscher-Frankild et al. 2014. STITCH 4: Integration of protein–chemical interactions with user data. *Nucleic Acids Res.* 42(Database issue): D401–D407.

Kurogi, Y. and O. F. Güner. 2004. Pharmacophore modeling and three-dimensional database searching for drug design using catalyst. *Curr. Med. Chem.* 8(9): 1035–1055.

Law, V., C. Knox, Y. Djoumbou et al. 2014. DrugBank 4.0: Shedding new light on drug metabolism. *Nucleic Acids Res.* 42(Database issue): D1091–D1097.

Leach, A. R., V. J. Gillet, R. A. Lewis, and R. Taylor. 2010. Three-dimensional pharmacophore methods in drug discovery. *J. Med. Chem.* 53(2): 539–558.

Li, H., J. Sutter, and R. Hoffman. 2000. HypoGen: An automated system for generating 3D predictive pharmacophore models. In: *Pharmacophore Perception, Development and Use in Drug Design*, O. F. Güner (ed.), La Jolla, CA: International University Line, pp. 171–190.

Li, S., Y. Xu, Q. Shen et al. 2013. Non-covalent interactions with aromatic rings: Current understanding and implications for rational drug design. *Curr. Pharm. Des.* 19(36): 6522–6533.

LigandScout 3.1 User Manual, Inte:Ligand GmbH, Vienna, Austria, 1999–2015, www.inteligand.com.

Lipinski, C. A. 2004. Lead- and drug-like compounds: The rule-of-five revolution. *Drug Discov. Today Technol.* 1(4): 337–341.

Lipinski, C. A., F. Lombardo, B. W. Dominy, and P. J. Feeney. 2001. Experimental and computational approaches to estimate solubility and permeability in drug discovery and development settings. *Adv. Drug. Deliv. Rev.* 46(1–3): 3–26.

Liu, T., Y. Lin, X. Wen, R. N. Jorissen, and M. K. Gilson. 2007. BindingDB: A web-accessible database of experimentally determined protein–ligand binding affinities. *Nucleic Acids Res.* 35(Database issue): D198–D201.

Liu, X., S. Ouyang, B. Yu et al. 2010. PharmMapper server: A web server for potential drug target identification using pharmacophore mapping approach. *Nucleic Acids Res.* 38(Web Server issue): W609–W614.

Liu, Z., H. Fang, K. Reagan et al. 2013. *In silico* drug repositioning—What we need to know. *Drug Discov. Today* 18(3–4): 110–115.

Markt, P., R. K. Petersen, E. N. Flindt et al. 2008. Discovery of novel PPAR ligands by a virtual screening approach based on pharmacophore modeling, 3D shape, and electrostatic similarity screening. *J. Med. Chem.* 51(20): 6303–6317.

MDDR licensed by Molecular Design, Ltd., San Leandro, CA. www.mdli.com.

Molecular Operating Environment (MOE), 2011.10; Chemical Computing Group Inc., 1010 Sherbooke St. West, Suite #910, Montreal, QC, Canada, H3A 2R7, 2011.

Nashev, L. G., D. Schuster, C. Laggner et al. 2010. The UV-filter benzophenone-1 inhibits 17β-hydroxysteroid dehydrogenase type 3: Virtual screening as a strategy to identify potential endocrine disrupting chemicals. *Biochem. Pharmacol.* 79(8): 1189–1199.

Olah, M., M. Mracec, L. Ostopovici et al. 2005. WOMBAT: World of molecular bioactivity. In: *Chemoinformatics in Drug Discovery*, B. Jürgen (ed.), Weinheim, Germany: Wiley-VCH Verlag GmbH & Co. KGaA, pp. 221–239.

Olah, M., R. Rad, L. Ostopovici et al. 2008. WOMBAT and WOMBAT-PK: Bioactivity databases for lead and drug discovery. In: *Chemical Biology*, L. S. Stuart, M. K. Tarun, and W. Günther (eds.), Weinheim, Germany: Wiley-VCH Verlag GmbH, pp. 760–786.

Olah, M. and T. I. Oprea. 2007. 3.14–Bioactivity databases. In: *Comprehensive Medicinal Chemistry II*, J. B. Taylor, and D. J. Triggle. (eds.), Oxford: Elsevier, pp. 293–313.

OMEGA 2.5.1.4: OpenEye Scientific Software, Santa Fe, NM. http://www.eyesopen.com. Hawkins, P.C.D.; Skillman, A.G.; Warren, G.L.; Ellingson, B.A.; Stahl, M.T.

Ooms, F. 2000. Molecular modeling and computer aided drug design. Examples of their applications in medicinal chemistry. *Curr. Med. Chem.* 7(2): 141–158.

Oprea, T. I., A. M. Davis, S. J. Teague, and P. D. Leeson. 2001. Is there a difference between leads and drugs? A historical perspective. *J. Chem. Inf. Comput. Sci.* 41(5): 1308–1315.

Ortuso, F., T. Langer, and S. Alcaro. 2006. GBPM: GRID-based pharmacophore model: Concept and application studies to protein-protein recognition. *Bioinformatics* 22(12): 1449–1455.

Perez-Pineiro, R., A. Burgos, D. C. Jones et al. 2009. Development of a novel virtual screening cascade protocol to identify potential trypanothione reductase inhibitors. *J. Med. Chem.* 52(6): 1670–1680.

Polgar, T., A. Baki, G. I. Szendrei, and G. M. Keseru. 2005. Comparative virtual and experimental high-throughput screening for glycogen synthase kinase-3beta inhibitors. *J. Med. Chem.* 48(25): 7946–7959.

Reddy, A. S., S. P. Pati, P. P. Kumar, H. N. Pradeep, and G. N. Sastry. 2007. Virtual screening in drug discovery—A computational perspective. *Curr. Protein Pept. Sci.* 8(4): 329–351.

Richmond, N. J., C. A. Abrams, P. R. Wolohan, E. Abrahamian, P. Willett, and R. D. Clark. 2006. GALAHAD: 1. pharmacophore identification by hypermolecular alignment of ligands in 3D. *J. Comput. Aided Mol. Des.* 20(9): 567–587.

Rollinger, J. M., D. Schuster, B. Danzl et al. 2009. *In silico* target fishing for rationalized ligand discovery exemplified on constituents of Ruta graveolens. *Planta Med.* 75(3): 195–204.

Schneidman-Duhovny, D., O. Dror, Y. Inbar, R. Nussinov, and H. J. Wolfson. 2008. PharmaGist: A webserver for ligand-based pharmacophore detection. *Nucleic Acids Res.* 36(Web Server issue): W223–W228.

Schueler, F.W. 1961. Chemobiodynamics and drug design. *J. Pharm. Sci.* 50(1): 92–92.

Schuster, D. 2010. 3D pharmacophores as tools for activity profiling. *Drug Discov. Today Technol.* 7(4): e205–e211.

Schuster, D., E. M. Maurer, C. Laggner et al. 2006. The discovery of new 11β-Hydroxysteroid dehydrogenase type 1 inhibitors by common-feature pharmacophore modeling and virtual screening. *J. Med. Chem.* 49(12): 3454–3466.

Schuster, D. and G. Wolber. 2010. Identification of bioactive natural products by pharmacophore-based virtual screening. *Curr. Pharm. Des.* 16(15): 1666–1681.

Schuster, D., M. Spetea, M. Music et al. 2010. Morphinans and isoquinolines: Acetylcholinesterase inhibition, pharmacophore modeling, and interaction with opioid receptors. *Bioorg. Med. Chem.* 18(14): 5071–5080.

Schwab, C. H. 2010. Conformations and 3D pharmacophore searching. *Drug Discov. Today Technol.* 7(4): e245–e253.

Spitzer, G. M., M. Heiss, M. Mangold et al. 2010. One concept, three implementations of 3D pharmacophore-based virtual screening: Distinct coverage of chemical search space. *J. Chem. Inf. Model.* 50(7): 1241–1247.

Sprague, P. W. 1995. Automated chemical hypothesis generation and database searching with Catalyst®. *Perspect. Drug Discov. Des.* 3(1): 1–20.

Steindl, T., C. Laggner, and T. Langer. 2005. Human rhinovirus 3C protease: Generation of pharmacophore models for peptidic and nonpeptidic inhibitors and their application in virtual screening. *J. Chem. Inf. Model.* 45(3): 716–724.

Steindl, T. M., D. Schuster, C. Laggner, and T. Langer. 2006. Parallel screening: A novel concept in pharmacophore modeling and virtual screening. *J. Chem. Inf. Model.* 46(5): 2146–2157.

Sutter, J., J. Li, A. J. Maynard, A. Goupil, T. Luu, and K. Nadassy. 2011. New features that improve the pharmacophore tools from Accelrys. *Curr. Comput. Aided Drug Des.* 7(3): 173–180.

Tanrikulu, Y., B. Krüger, and E. Proschak. 2013. The holistic integration of virtual screening in drug discovery. *Drug Discov. Today* 18(7–8): 358–364.

Temml, V., C. V. Voss, V. M. Dirsch, and D. Schuster. 2014. Discovery of new liver X receptor agonists by pharmacophore modeling and shape-based virtual screening. *J. Chem. Inf. Model.* 54(2): 367–371.

Toba, S., J. Srinivasan, A. J. Maynard, and J. Sutter. 2006. Using pharmacophore models to gain insight into structural binding and virtual screening: An application study with CDK2 and human DHFR. *J. Chem. Inf. Model.* 46(2): 728–735.

Todorov, N. P., I. L. Alberts, I. J. P. De-Esch, and P. M. Dean. 2007. QUASI: A novel method for simultaneous superposition of multiple flexible ligands and virtual screening using partial similarity. *J. Chem. Inf. Model.* 47(3): 1007–1020.

Triballeau, N., F. Acher, I. Brabet, J. P. Pin, and H. O. Bertrand. 2005. Virtual screening workflow development guided by the "eceiver operating characteristic" curve approach. Application to high-throughput docking on metabotropic glutamate receptor subtype 4. *J. Med. Chem.* 48(7): 2534–2547.

Tripos International, SYBYL 8.0, 1699 South Hanley Rd., St. Louis, Missouri, 63144, USA.

Verdonk, M. L., V. Berdini, M. J. Hartshorn et al. 2004. Virtual screening using protein–ligand docking: Avoiding artificial enrichment. *J. Chem. Inf. Comput. Sci.* 44(3): 793–806.

Vuorinen, A., L. G. Nashev, A. Odermatt, J. M. Rollinger, and D. Schuster. 2014. Pharmacophore model refinement for 11β-Hydroxysteroid dehydrogenase inhibitors: Search for modulators of intracellular glucocorticoid concentrations. *Mol. Inf.* 33(1): 15–25.

Wang, Q., J. Park, A. K. Devkota, E. J. Cho, K. N. Dalby, and P. Ren. 2014. Identification and validation of novel PERK inhibitors. *J. Chem. Inf. Model.* 54(5): 1467–1475.

Wang, Y., E. Bolton, S. Dracheva et al. 2010. An overview of the PubChem BioAssay resource. *Nucleic Acids Res.* 38(Database issue): D255–D266.

Wermuth, C. G., C. R. Ganellin, P. Lindberg, and L. A. Mitscher. 1998. Glossary of terms used in medicinal chemistry (IUPAC reccomendations 1998). *Pure Appl. Chem.* 70(5): 1129–1143.

Wilcken, R., M. O. Zimmermann, A. Lange, A. C. Joerger, and F. M. Boeckler. 2013. Principles and applications of halogen bonding in medicinal chemistry and chemical biology. *J. Med. Chem.* 56(4): 1363–1388.

Williams, A. J., L. Harland, P. Groth et al. 2012. Open PHACTS: Semantic interoperability for drug discovery. *Drug Discov. Today* 17(21–22): 1188–1198.

Wolber, G., A. Dornhofer, and T. Langer. 2006. Efficient overlay of small organic molecules using 3D pharmacophores. *J. Comput. Aided Mol. Des.* 20(12): 773–788.

Wolber, G. and T. Langer. 2005. LigandScout: 3-D pharmacophores derived from protein-bound ligands and their use as virtual screening filters. *J. Chem. Inf. Model.* 45(1): 160–169.

Young, S. M., C. Bologa, E. R. Prossnitz, T. I. Oprea, L. A. Sklar, and B. S. Edwards. 2005. High-throughput screening with HyperCyt flow cytometry to detect small molecule formylpeptide receptor ligands. *J. Biomol. Screen.* 10(4): 374–382.

Zweig, M. H. and G. Campbell. 1993. Receiver-operating characteristic (ROC) plots: A fundamental evaluation tool in clinical medicine. *Clin. Chem.* 39(4): 561–577.

6

Protein–Ligand Docking: From Basic Principles to Advanced Applications

Christoph A. Sotriffer

CONTENTS

6.1 The Docking Problem

Given the three-dimensional (3D) structure of a protein and the molecular constitution of a ligand, what is the binding mode of the ligand, that is, its position, orientation, and conformation when bound to the protein? This is the fundamental question of the "docking problem" (Sotriffer et al. 2003b). Although at first sight it reminds of a 3D jigsaw puzzle, where two complementary shapes have to be matched, the complexity of the docking problem goes far beyond. In fact, the binding partners are not rigid bodies, but flexible molecules surrounded by water and governed in their energetics not simply by hard-sphere potentials, but rather by complex enthalpic and entropic contributions (Bissantz et al. 2010; Sotriffer et al. 2003a,b). Moreover, to deal with the problem a workflow for appropriate setup and handling of the underlying molecular structures is required (Cole et al. 2011; ten Brink and Exner

2009). Accordingly, the constitutive elements of any docking approach are (1) a suitable representation of the interacting molecular structures; (2) a search algorithm to generate meaningful binding poses of the ligand at the protein's binding site; and (3) a scoring method to evaluate the generated configurations and identify the best one, ideally corresponding to the true, experimentally verifiable binding mode. These three components are tightly related to each other, as not every type of molecular representation or scoring function can be combined with every possible search algorithm. In the following, commonly used approaches for "representing," "searching," and "scoring" in the context of docking are briefly outlined (cf. Figure 6.1), without attempting to fully cover the large variety of methods grown over the past years. As docking is a well and frequently reviewed subject in the literature, the interested reader is referred to more extensive reviews for further details and additional approaches (Brooijmans and Kuntz 2003; Halperin et al. 2002; Moitessier et al. 2008; Muegge and Rarey 2001; Sotriffer 2011; Sotriffer et al. 2003a,b; Sousa et al. 2006, 2013; Yuriev and Ramsland 2013; Yuriev et al. 2011). For links to the distributor websites of docking programs, the "Click2Drug" Directory of

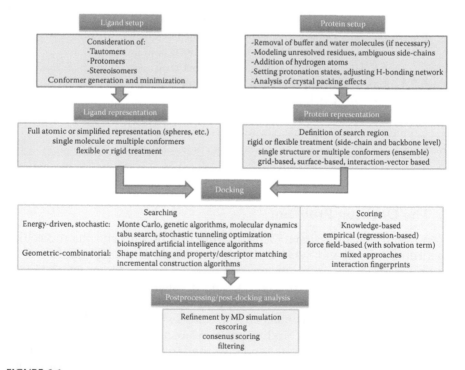

FIGURE 6.1
(See color insert.) Simplified overview of the docking workflow, illustrating the major components, the required steps in ligand and protein setup, and the available approaches for solving the docking problem with respect to "representing molecular structures," "searching," and "scoring." The individual items are explained in Section 6.2.

computer-aided Drug Design of the Swiss Institute of Bioinformatics should be consulted (http://www.click2drug.org/index.html#Docking).

6.2 Components of Docking

6.2.1 Molecular Representations

Every docking method needs a suitable way of handling the molecular structures involved in the docking process. The choice of the molecular representation is related to the applied search algorithm and scoring method. As far as the *protein* is concerned, it is often not the entire structure with all its coordinates that is used in the docking process, but rather a simplified or reduced representation prepared from the original structure. This is generally required to make the optimization problem computationally tractable and to render the search more efficient. On the one hand, the search region is often confined to the area of the binding site, which in most of the practically relevant cases is at least approximately known. Otherwise, "blind docking" to the entire protein surface has to be carried out, which is more challenging but not necessarily hopeless (cf. below). On the other hand, simplified representations of the 3D structure are used. This includes the application of surface or sphere representations of the binding site (as used by DOCK [Kuntz et al. 1982; Oshiro and Kuntz 1998]), the definition of interaction vectors and interaction spheres to be matched by complementary interaction groups of the ligand (as used by FlexX [Rarey et al. 1996a,b]), or the generation of grid representations (as used by AutoDock [Goodsell and Olson 1990; Morris et al. 1998] or Glide [Friesner et al. 2004]). Especially the grid approach has found widespread application, as it provides a straightforward surrogate representation of the protein search space in terms of the chosen interaction potentials. All these approaches were originally developed for rigid protein representations and are not equally well amenable to the consideration of protein flexibility (Sotriffer 2011).

Regardless of the actual representation used, the preparation always starts with a protein coordinate file, most commonly obtained from structure determination by X-ray crystallography and provided in the PDB format (Berman et al. 2000). It is important to be aware of the fact that the outcome of a docking calculation critically depends on the quality and the further setup of this structure file (Cole et al. 2011). Crystal structures and the underlying experimental methods have their own limitations, which must be considered. Accordingly, the protein structure needs to be checked for residues with missing density, low occupancy, and alternative conformations. Ambiguous side chain orientations (of asparagine, glutamine, and histidine residues) may have to be fixed based on a hydrogen-bonding network analysis (Hooft et al. 1996). Crystal packing close to the binding site can severely affect the relevance of the structure (Bergner et al. 2001; Sotriffer et al. 2000). Buffer molecules should be recognized and removed, cofactors have to be adequately treated, and choices regarding the inclusion of water molecules have to be made (cf. below). Furthermore, the addition of hydrogen atoms (normally not visible in protein crystal structures) and the definition of the protonation state (in particular for histidine residues) deserve special attention (Bietz et al. 2014).

With respect to the *ligand*, a full atomic treatment is much more common. Depending on the docking approach, it may be necessary to transform the ligand into a representation complementary to that used for the protein, such as a set of spheres or interaction vectors. In grid-based methods, the atomic coordinates are used directly for evaluating the position-dependent interaction energies based on the precalculated grid values by interpolation between the grid points and summation over all ligand atoms. With other methods, the handling depends on the treatment of ligand flexibility and requires multiple pregenerated conformers, an incremental construction procedure, or an explicit search in torison-angle space. The ligand setup for docking must also carefully consider the possible stereoisomers, tautomers, and protonation states. The influence of these factors and the related setup steps on the final docking result has gained increasing attention over the past years, and any practitioner in the docking field is strongly encouraged to consult the corresponding studies (e.g., ten Brink and Exner 2009, 2010).

6.2.2 Search Algorithms

Docking is essentially an optimization problem. Given the individual structures of the two binding partners, the goal is to identify the structure of the binary complex with optimal binding free energy. If this free energy of binding was readily amenable to computation, the docking problem could be reduced to a pure minimization problem. However, as outlined in the scoring section below, the binding free energy as ideal target variable is not easily accessible, making approximate and simplified scoring schemes necessary. Correspondingly, the search for the optimal binding mode is based either on energy-driven (often stochastic) methods or on geometric-combinatorial search procedures.

The energy-driven methods aim for optimizing the ligand position, orientation, and conformation based on a suitable target function. This function has to model the protein–ligand binding energy as a function of the interaction geometry of the binding partners. If only translation and rotation is considered, a systematic search (possibly combined with some heuristics for computational speed-up) is actually feasible and frequently used in the context of protein–protein docking (Gabb et al. 1997; Katchalski-Katzir et al. 1992; May and Zacharias 2008). The additional consideration of torsional degrees of freedom of the ligand, however, makes a systematic search normally impractical due to the higher dimensionality of the problem and the resulting combinatorial explosion. Nevertheless, attempts have been published to overcome this problem and allow for an exhaustive search, such as GLIDE (Friesner et al. 2004), which relies on an exhaustive systematic search within a prescreened and drastically reduced region of phase space, or the SKATE program (Feng and Marshall 2010), which decouples systematic sampling from scoring.

Docking requires optimization procedures that can cope well with the high dimensionality and the very rugged interaction energy landscape. Most commonly, stochastic global optimization techniques are used for this purpose. Monte-Carlo-based methods are one such class (Leach 2001). Starting from an arbitrary configuration of the ligand within the search area, new configurations are randomly generated within certain thresholds for maximal changes in translational, rotational, and torsional degrees of freedom. The acceptance of a new configuration is governed by the Metropolis algorithm (Metropolis et al. 1953), which ensures that more favorable configurations (configurations lower in energy) are always accepted, while configurations higher in energy are only probabilistically accepted (based on the comparison of a random number between 0 and 1 with a Boltzmann factor calculated from the energy difference between the current and the previously accepted configuration). Accordingly, the search can also proceed "uphill" on the energy landscape and may cross barriers for reaching deeper minima. Examples of docking programs using Monte Carlo techniques (either in the form of simulated annealing or as "Monte Carlo minimization") include AutoDock (Goodsell and Olson 1990; Morris et al. 1996), ICM (Abagyan et al. 1994; Totrov and Abagyan 1997), MCDOCK (Liu and Wang 1999), ProDock (Trosset and Scheraga 1998, 1999), QXP (McMartin and Bohacek 1997), and RosettaLigand (Davis and Baker 2009).

A further prominent class of stochastic optimization techniques is given by genetic algorithms (GAs), which are inspired by the principles of evolution (Clark and Westhead 1996). In the context of docking, an initial population of ligand poses is randomly generated, where the position, orientation, and conformation of each pose is encoded in a chromosome of genes for translation, rotation, and torsion variables. A set of genetic operators (crossover, mutation) is then applied to this population to generate a new generation, whereby individuals with higher fitness (i.e., better docking score) have a higher chance of reproduction into the next generation. This process continues until a termination criterion is reached, such as a constant optimal fitness, a minimal root-mean-square deviation (RMSD) of the fittest individual, or simply a maximum number of generations. Many different variants of GA-based docking algorithms exist, with GOLD (Jones et al. 1995, 1997) and AutoDock (Morris et al. 1998) as the most widely used examples. While GOLD uses a direct encoding of hydrogen-bonding motifs in the chromosome, a special feature of AutoDock is the Lamarckian GA, which combines a standard GA with a local search method to perform energy minimization of a certain fraction of the population in phenotypic space to increase the overall search efficiency. An example of a more recent addition to the class of GA-based docking programs is the program FITTED (Flexibility Induced Through Targeted Evolutionary Description), developed to account also for water molecules as well as protein flexibility at the side-chain and backbone level in the docking process (Corbeil et al. 2007, 2008; Corbeil and Moitessier 2009).

As a technique to sample configuration space, molecular dynamics (MD) simulations provide another approach to energy-driven search methods. Based on a suitable force field and Newton's equation of motion, MD simulations allow to analyze the dynamic properties of biomolecular systems in solution (Karplus 2002; Rognan 1998; Tuckerman and Martyna 2000; van Gunsteren and Berendsen 1990). In principle, this could also include the association of a ligand with a protein, corresponding to the simulation of the actual docking process. In practice, however, the access to a computationally straightforward docking approach is precluded by the low efficiency of standard MD simulations in crossing energy barriers and exploring multiple minima. Accordingly, in the context of docking, MD simulations have mainly been used for preprocessing or for postdocking refinement, primarily to better account for the flexibility of the protein and the presence of water molecules. As far as preprocessing is concerned, an example is given by ensemble-based docking methods, where docking is carried out to multiple protein conformations generated by MD simulations (if not obtained with other methods) (Totrov and Abagyan 2008). Similarly, in the "relaxed complex scheme" the consideration of protein flexibility via MD simulations is decoupled from the actual ligand placement in the docking process (Amaro et al. 2008; Lin et al. 2002); originally, all snapshots saved at regular time intervals of the MD trajectory were used for this purpose, whereas later applications investigated the effect of various selection methods for multiple MD-generated protein conformations (Nichols et al. 2011) (ensemble-docking based on multiple crystal structures and the related ensemble selection methods have also been analyzed in detail [Craig et al. 2010; Korb et al. 2012]). With respect to *post-docking refinement*, the goal is often to analyze and refine already docked complexes in order to overcome the limitations of a rigid-protein docking procedure and/or to validate the obtained binding modes and discriminate between native and nonnative binding positions. Many examples of such combined docking and MD studies are available (Alonso et al. 2006; Kranjc et al. 2009; Wang et al. 1999).

Despite the more common use of MD before or after the actual docking process, various attempts to make direct use of MD simulations in docking have also been presented. Supported by the continuous increase in computing power, the approaches are becoming more and more attractive for solving the docking problem under most realistic conditions (i.e., full inclusion of protein flexibility and solvation). As an early example, the MD docking (MDD) algorithm may be mentioned (Di Nola et al. 1994; Mangoni et al. 1999), which separates the ligand's center-of-mass motion from its internal motions to obtain enhanced sampling. A more recent and increasingly attractive method is given by the metadynamics approach, which allows to explore different binding poses by providing the free energy profile of the docking and undocking mechanism, hence also leading to mechanistic insights into the docking path (cf. Barducci et al. [2011] for a review on metadynamics and Branduardi et al. [2005]; Gervasio et al. [2005]; and Masetti et al. [2009] for metadynamics-based applications in the context of docking).

Besides the MC-, GA-, and MD-based docking approaches, a large variety of other energy-driven search strategies has found application in the context of docking. This includes Tabu Search methods (Baxter et al. 1998, 2000; Westhead et al. 1997), Stochastic Tunneling Optimization (Fischer et al. 2007), and bioinspired artificial intelligence algorithms such as Ant Colony Optimization and Particle Swarm Optimization (Chen et al. 2007; Namasivayam and Gunther 2007). Moreover, docking programs are often not only based on a single optimization method, but rather on a workflow of different methods applied at different stages of the entire docking process. A prominent example is the widely used Glide program (Friesner et al. 2004). Glide follows a docking hierarchy where a series of filters is applied to search for possible ligand poses. It starts with ligand conformer generation and initial rough, but systematic positioning and scoring in different stages. This is followed by force field-based, torsionally flexible energy minimization of the best (typically some hundred) candidate poses from the previous step. Finally, the three to six best poses are sent to a Monte Carlo sampling procedure, which examines nearby torsional minima to obtain optimal pose conformations. Taken together, this corresponds to a funnel-like docking procedure, where a large number of potential ligand poses is progressively reduced and optimized with different methods (Friesner et al. 2004).

Besides the energy-driven/stochastic approaches, the group of geometric/combinatorial search procedures represents the second major class of search algorithms. These are generally built on concepts of shape complementarity or matching of compatible recognition motifs of molecules represented by structural (geometrical) and/or physicochemical descriptors with the help of alignment procedures. Once suitable alignments or appropriate matches of protein and ligand interaction features are generated, the solutions are ranked based on appropriate scoring schemes. As one of the first docking methods published, the pioneering program DOCK used a negative sphere image of the binding pocket onto which the ligand was superimposed with a distance-matching algorithm followed by least-squares fitting (DesJarlais et al. 1988; Kuntz et al. 1982). Other programs represent the binding site by interaction points onto which the ligand atoms have to be matched. Normally, these points do not only represent shape information, but also the physicochemical type of the interaction possible at this position. The program SLIDE uses such an approach and carries out the search by exhaustively mapping all triangles of appropriate atoms in the ligand onto triangles of interactions points with compatible properties (Schnecke and Kuhn 2000). Based on the resulting initial placements of the molecule, a series of further steps is used to refine the initial position. The matching of hydrogen-bond patterns, as used, for example, in ADAM (Mizutani et al. 1994) or H-Dock (Luo et al. 2010), is encountered as a further variant. Other algorithms focus more on shape complementarity, by making use of alpha spheres (ASEdock [Goto et al. 2008]), the beta-complex theory and Voronoi diagrams (BetaDock [Kim et al. 2011]), or the so-called quadratic shape descriptors (QSDOCK [Goldman and Wipke 2000]). The interested reader is referred to the corresponding references for details on these shape-matching methods.

Application of the concept of shape complementarity and descriptor matching in docking is always faced with the problem of ligand flexibility, as the bioactive conformation of the molecule is normally not known in advance. Accordingly, one needs to perform rigid docking with a set of pregenerated conformers, as done, for example, by the programs EUDOC (Pang et al. 2001), FLOG (Miller et al. 1994), or FRED (McGann 2011). The challenge here is shifted to the conformer generation program, in particular for larger molecules with many rotatable bonds: on the one hand, it has to ensure that the bioactive conformation is included in the set, while on the other the number of conformers has to remain handable by the docking algorithm within a reasonable time frame to avoid combinatorial explosion (Bostrom 2001; Kirchmair et al. 2006). An alternative to the rigid docking of pregenerated conformers is given by incremental construction methods. Here, the ligand is dissected into smaller fragments, typically by cutting at all single bonds which are not part of a cyclic system. After selection of a base fragment and its placement at suitable positions in the binding site, the molecule is incrementally reconstructed from the base fragment within the binding pocket by step-wise addition of the next fragments. The placement of these fragments is based on the matching algorithm of the docking method (e.g., superposition of triples or pairs of interaction centers) in combination with rules regarding the torsional preferences. An incremental construction algorithm lies at the heart of the widely used docking program FlexX (Kramer et al. 1999; Rarey et al. 1996a,b). Also the anchor-and-grow method implemented in DOCK is an example of an incremental construction technique (Ewing et al. 2001).

As mentioned previously, however, docking programs are often not based on a single method only, but rather on a workflow or combination of different approaches. In DOCK, for example, the originally purely geometric descriptor matching has been augmented with various additional features over time, such as the "sphere coloring" to better account for physicochemical complementarity (DesJarlais and Dixon 1994; Shoichet and Kuntz 1993) or the energy minimization routines to optimize the positions obtained by initial descriptor matching (Gschwend and Kuntz 1996; Meng et al. 1993).

6.2.3 Scoring Methods

Every ligand pose generated in the docking process must somehow be evaluated. Simple matching criteria may initially suffice for geometric/descriptor-based search methods, but ultimately more sophisticated surrogates of the actual binding free energy are required as scoring functions. Scoring functions are generally applied for binding-mode prediction, relative affinity ranking, and/or estimation of absolute binding free energy. The possibility to rapidly and accurately calculate the actual affinity would solve all three tasks simultaneously. The available methods, however, are either computationally too expensive or not accurate enough to be of practical value in this context; in fact, correct affinity prediction remains a major challenge (Sotriffer and Matter 2011). Accordingly, current scoring functions are rather expected to reveal the correct binding pose in docking and/or to provide a meaningful ranking of ligands in a docking-based virtual screening than to predict the absolute affinity. In the following, the focus will be on pose prediction.

As rigorous calculation methods based on simulations and principles of statistical thermodynamics can hardly be applied in the context of routine docking tasks, current scoring functions are generally based on assumptions and simplifications. Most importantly, scoring functions normally attempt to estimate the quality of a protein–ligand complex based on a single configuration of the complex without considering ensemble averages and/or the unbound state of the binding partners. Furthermore, the energy functions are in most of the cases based on the assumption of additivity of pairwise molecular interactions, without considering cooperative effects. Keeping these general simplifications in mind, three different approaches of scoring functions can be distinguished: the knowledge-based scoring functions, the force field-based methods, and the empirical scoring functions. Although transitions and combinations among these approaches exist, it is still useful to present them as individual classes.

6.2.3.1 Knowledge-Based Scoring Functions

Structural databases of protein–ligand complexes contain a wealth of information beyond the value of the individual structure. Knowledge-based scoring functions make use of this structural information. Starting from a statistical analysis of the propensity of contacts between protein and ligand atom types within predefined distance ranges in an ensemble of experimental structures, atom-type- and distance-dependent pseudopotentials are derived. This makes use of the inverse Boltzmann law and the assumption that interactions between certain atom types at a particular distance observed more frequently than seen in a reference distribution of unspecific protein–ligand contacts (irrespective of atom type) are energetically favorable. Accordingly, these potentials can then be used to score the quality of a docking pose in a protein–ligand complex.

Importantly, the knowledge-based scoring functions are exclusively derived from structural data, without the use of experimental affinity values. This also explains why their major strength lies in the assessment of the binding mode quality, as shown in large-scale comparative test studies (Cheng et al. 2009). Typical examples include the DrugScore functions (Gohlke et al. 2000; Neudert and Klebe 2011; Velec et al. 2005), PMF (Muegge 2000, 2006), and BLEEP (Mitchell et al. 1999a,b).

The quality of the functions critically depends on the structural data basis (quality and number, i.e., statistically significant observations of contacts between a particular pair of atom types). Most commonly, subsets of the PDB (Berman et al. 2000) selected by certain quality criteria are used, but also the Cambridge Structural Database (CSD) (Allen 2002; Allen et al. 1991) has been mined to derive potentials from the intermolecular crystal packing contacts in a huge number of crystal structures of small organic molecules (Velec et al. 2005). Further differences among the scoring functions arise from the definition of the atom types, the considered distance ranges, the reference state, and the addition of other terms, such as surface-dependent interaction potentials (Gohlke et al. 2000), terms accounting for solvation effects and/or the configurational entropy of the ligand (Huang and Zou 2010).

6.2.3.2 Force Field-Based Scoring Functions

The application of a molecular mechanics (MM) force field provides another possibility to score protein–ligand interactions and drive the docking process toward a binding mode with optimal van der Waals and electrostatic interaction energies. The Lennard-Jones and Coulomb potentials commonly used as nonbonded interaction terms in force fields are well suited to sensitively monitor the geometric quality of a binding mode. Force fields are, in fact, normally derived to accurately model/describe the structure and conformational energies of a molecule. As they depend on empirical parameterization, care must be taken to use a force field adequately parameterized for the molecules to be investigated. In the context of docking, biomolecular force fields such as AMBER (Cornell et al. 1995; Weiner et al. 1986), CHARMM (Brooks et al. 1983), and OPLS (Kaminski et al. 2001) and their derivatives (such as GAFF [Wang et al. 2004]) are most commonly used.

Various docking programs make use of force field terms to score the generated configurations and/or optimize the docking pose, with AutoDock (Goodsell and Olson 1990; Morris et al. 1998) and Glide (Friesner et al. 2004) as two prominent examples. For ranking of different ligands and affinity estimation, however, pure force field terms are not sufficient, as they do not account for important solvation and entropic effects. Accordingly, for this purpose, at least a desolvation term needs to be added. A popular example of this is the MM-PBSA (Kollman et al. 2000; Kuhn et al. 2005; Thompson et al. 2008; Weis et al. 2006) or MM-GBSA (Guimaraes and Cardozo 2008; Lyne et al. 2006; Zhang et al. 2009) approach, where a solvent-accessible surface area (SA) term is added for nonpolar solvation and a continuum solvent Poisson–Boltzmann (PB) (Baker 2005) or generalized Born (GB) (Ghosh et al. 1998) term for polar solvation. These approaches (MM-PBSA/GBSA) are typically used for rescoring, rather than in the docking process itself. In combination with the program DOCK, different variants of desolvation terms have been investigated (Mysinger and Shoichet 2010; Wei et al. 2002), some of which can be precomputed on a grid to make their calculation fast enough for docking applications.

6.2.3.3 Empirical Scoring Functions

Regression analysis between structural descriptors and affinity data of protein–ligand complexes provides another approach to scoring functions. Because of their reliance on experimental data for both structures and affinities, the resulting functions are typically termed "empirical scoring functions." The descriptors are chosen to encode the geometric features of interaction terms thought to make important contributions to the overall affinity, such as hydrogen bonds, buried lipophilic surface area, or the number of rotatable bonds immobilized upon complex formation. For a large number of complexes of known structure and affinity (training set), these descriptors are calculated and then correlated to the experimental affinity by assigning weights in a classical regression analysis or related statistical methods, such as machine learning techniques (e.g., Random Forest, Support Vector Machines), which are becoming increasingly popular for deriving empirical scoring functions (Ballester and Mitchell 2010; Das et al. 2010; Zilian and Sotriffer 2013). The resulting function is then used to score protein–ligand complexes and obtain affinity estimates. The quality of empirical scoring functions critically depends on the size, composition, and quality of the training set, with respect to both structure and affinity data (Kalliokoski et al. 2013; Kramer et al. 2012). Typical examples of empirical scoring functions include the functions of Boehm (SCORE1 [Boehm 1994] and SCORE2 [Boehm 1998]), ChemScore (Eldridge et al. 1997), GlideScore (Friesner et al. 2006), SFCscore (Sotriffer et al. 2008), and X-Score (Wang et al. 2002). The reader is referred to other reviews for more comprehensive lists and more detailed discussions of (empirical) scoring functions (Boehm and Stahl 1999, 2002; Sotriffer and Matter 2011; Sotriffer 2012).

Empirical scoring functions are used by or included in many popular docking programs, ranging from AutoDock (Morris et al. 1998, 2009) and FlexX (Rarey et al. 1996a,b) to GOLD (Jones et al. 1997) and Glide (Friesner et al. 2004, 2006). As another, more recent example, the PLANTS$_{\text{CHEMPLP/PLP}}$ scoring function was designed explicitly for the docking algorithm PLANTS and was trained with particular emphasis on pose prediction (Korb et al. 2009).

6.2.3.4 Further Approaches to Scoring

Instead of applying only one of the mentioned scoring functions for pose prediction in docking, the combined application of multiple different scoring functions may allow to overcome deficiencies of the individual functions. This concept has been termed "consensus scoring" and was shown to lead to improvements in the overall docking performance (Charifson et al. 1999; Clark et al. 2002). However, while often decreasing the number of false positives, the approach is also prone to miss true positives, which are favorably scored by only one function. Accordingly, success is not guaranteed, and it is worthwhile to test and compare the performance of various combination schemes and workflows of consensus scoring for the target of interest (Feher 2006; Oda et al. 2006).

Instead of applying one or more of the classical scoring functions mentioned above, tailored filtering methods may also be used to eliminate decoy poses and more reliably identify near-native poses among the generated docking results. One example is given by the residue-based structural interaction fingerprints (SIFt) method (Deng et al. 2004). It extracts information about the molecular interaction between a pose and the residues in the active site and converts it to a binary fingerprint, which may then be used for similarity searching or filtering. Various applications and extensions of this approach have been described (Brewerton 2008; Kelly and Mancera 2004; Marcou and Rognan 2007; Nandigam et al. 2009). MotifScore is another example of a non-energy-based scoring function for docking (Xie and Hwang 2010). It is based on recurring network substructures ("motifs") derived from protein–ligand interactions; these motifs then serve as probability-ranked interaction templates to score docking solutions.

6.2.4 Docking Under Special "Scenarios"

Although the approaches presented above can be applied to a wide range of docking problems, the general underlying assumption in the presentation was that the target is a crystallographically determined protein with a well-defined binding site and that the ligand is a small organic molecule interacting noncovalently with the target. If this is not the case, the general principles of docking still hold true, but further particular aspects may have to be considered. The following examples very briefly provide an impression of the most important scenarios encountered.

- *Covalent docking*: Ligands interacting covalently with the protein require special treatment, as covalent bond formation (and, hence, electronic degrees of freedom) cannot be handled by the classical potentials used in docking. Most commonly, covalent docking is carried out by defining a link or geometric constraint to keep the appropriate ligand atom in proximity (or already connected) to the protein atom forming the covalent bond. The docking search for suitable ligand positions is then carried out under this constraint. Obviously, the energetics of the covalent bond formation are neglected by this approach. Further details and examples can be found in the literature (Ouyang et al. 2013; Schroeder et al. 2013). A protocol for the design of covalently interacting inhibitors with the combined, stepwise application of docking and quantum mechanical calculations has recently been presented (Schmidt et al. 2014).

- *Blind docking*: Although the active site or the approximate binding region is often known in advance, this is not always the case. Instead of relying on ligand-independent surface-mapping and binding-site prediction tools (Sotriffer and Klebe 2002), docking to the entire protein surface is a straightforward approach to localize the putative binding site of a given ligand. This approach is termed "blind docking," and validation studies have shown that respectable results can be obtained despite the much larger search area (Grosdidier et al. 2009; Zoete et al. 2010). The approach can also be helpful for identifying potential alternative binding sites, but experimental validation is mandatory, as the rate of false-positive results is expected to be high.

- *Docking to homology models*: If no experimental receptor structure is available, homology models can provide useful alternatives for structure-based investigations and docking studies (Kiss and Keserü 2011). However, even though the fold of the homology model might be correct, the side-chain orientations and conformations may deviate significantly and possibly prevent the identification of near-native ligand binding modes. Accordingly, special care is required with respect to side-chain optimization and side-chain flexibility (Cavasotto et al. 2008; Evers et al. 2003; Schafferhans and Klebe 2001). Nevertheless, valuable results can be obtained, as illustrated in particular in the GPCR field, where for a long time docking could only be carried out with homology models. With the availability of more and more crystal structures for pharmaceutically important GPCRs, the results obtained with homology models can now be compared to those obtained with crystal structures (Costanzi 2008; Mobarec et al. 2009; Tang et al. 2012).

- *Special types of ligands and/or receptors*: Particular challenges can arise for certain classes of ligands or receptors. Carbohydrates, for example, with their flexible ring systems and the many rotatable hydroxyl groups are often not well handled by standard docking programs due to their complicated binding energetics. Accordingly, validation studies for selecting the best-suited approach (Agostino et al. 2009) or methods particularly adapted to carbohydrates (Kerzmann et al. 2008) are required. As another example, docking to metalloproteins can critically depend on the model quality for the metal–ligand interaction (Rohrig et al. 2009). Detailed studies have been carried out to analyze the typical interaction motifs and apply this information in docking (Seebeck et al. 2008). If the receptor is not a protein at all, but rather a nucleic acid (RNA or DNA), electrostatics and polar interactions play a major role. Standard docking programs need careful validation or particular adaptation prior to application to RNA or DNA targets (Daldrop et al. 2011; Lang et al. 2009; Li et al. 2010), and docking methods developed specifically for nucleic acids are also available (Guilbert and James 2008; Morley and Afshar 2004). Finally, if the ligand is actually a protein as well, protein–protein docking has to be carried out, which is not further discussed here, but amply reviewed in the literature (Camacho and Vajda 2002; Cherfils et al. 1991; Ehrlich and Wade 2001; Huang 2014; Janin 2010; Smith and Sternberg 2002; Sternberg et al. 1998; Zacharias 2010).

6.3 Challenges for Docking Methods

In an extensive review on docking and scoring prepared for the 6th edition of *Burgers Handbook of Medicinal Chemistry* (Sotriffer et al. 2003a), the opinion of the authors regarding the major challenges in the further development of docking procedures was summarized as follows (the challenges related more directly to scoring and affinity prediction are omitted here):

1. The fact that protein–ligand interactions occur in aqueous solution is generally appreciated, but not yet adequately accounted for. Especially, the simultaneous placement of explicit water molecules upon docking, accurate estimates of the water versus ligand interaction-energy balance, and the fast prediction of protonation states in binding pockets await a fully satisfactory solution.
2. The consideration of a sufficient degree of protein flexibility needs to become part of standard docking approaches. This requires faster algorithms. In addition, with respect to scoring, an often overlooked aspect is that as soon as receptor flexibility is allowed, protein conformational energy changes need to be accounted for appropriately.
3. Although flexible-ligand docking has already become standard, the error rate in predictions of interaction geometries is still significant for more flexible ligands. Again, more efficient algorithms would be required to sample the conformation space more thoroughly (Sotriffer et al. 2003a).

These statements appeared more than 10 years ago, and it is worthwhile asking which progress has been made since then with respect to these challenges. As far as the *water* problem is concerned, explicit water molecules can now routinely be considered in various widely distributed docking programs, such as FlexX (Rarey et al. 1999), GOLD (Verdonk et al. 2005), and FITTED (Corbeil and Moitessier 2009). This normally relies on predefined water positions, derived either from crystal structure analysis or from computational methods to predict water sites (cf. below). Water molecules located at these positions can then be toggled "on" or "off" by the docking program, depending on an appropriate score. In some cases, orientational sampling is carried out (without modifying the position) to optimize the hydrogen-bonding network of the water molecules. However, correctly capturing the interaction energy balance with water molecules is still very challenging with the fast-scoring procedures required for docking (Cappel et al. 2011; Kirchmair et al. 2011).

With respect to protonation states, the awareness has certainly grown that protonation states in the binding pocket and the ligand may change upon complex formation (Czodrowski et al. 2006, 2007) and that setting the correct protonation state critically influences the quality of the docking results (ten Brink and Exner 2009, 2010). Computational methods for the prediction of protonation changes in protein–ligand complexes have become available (Bas et al. 2008; Czodrowski et al. 2006; Sondergaard et al. 2011). Although they were not directly designed to work "on-the-fly" with docking or virtual screening, the fast PROPKA method (Bas et al. 2008; Sondergaard et al. 2011) appears amenable to routine analysis of protein–ligand complexes obtained from docking calculations.

Consideration of various degrees of *protein flexibility* is nowadays in much more widespread use than 10 years ago. In a previous review (Sotriffer 2011), which summarized flexible-protein docking approaches up to the end of 2009, the conclusion was that "full induced-fit docking approaches for cases of moderate plasticity are becoming available and are already getting close to a range of computing time which is no longer prohibitive for routine application in docking projects (…)" (Sotriffer 2011). While side-chain modeling was judged to be in a relatively advanced state, the handling of backbone motions was far from being routine. Methods for full, simultaneous consideration of protein flexibilty upon ligand binding started to appear, which, however, did not mean that the reliable prediction of even small localized changes was routinely possible for any system of interest. Rather, the complicated energetics and the even more severe scoring problem in flexible-protein docking still present major hurdles for a true breakthrough.

With respect to *ligand flexibility*, enhanced sampling is certainly possible nowadays, but caution is still warranted with larger ligands (Mukherjee et al. 2010). As noted by Coleman et al. (2013), ligand size and flexibility is not only a sampling problem, but also a scoring issue. Of course, "conformational space grows exponentially with ligand size, and sampling this space remains challenging" (Coleman et al. 2013). Problems occur in particular with the electrostatics of very large, peptide-like and drug-like ligands, whereas no problems are encountered with ligands in the lead-like or fragment-like range (Coleman et al. 2013). Interestingly, however, in the analysis of the CSAR 2011–2012 competition results no correlation between the pose prediction metrics and chemical properties or size of the ligand was found (Damm-Ganamet et al. 2013). Apparently, major problems arise only for very large ligands, which are not typically in the focus of docking or virtual screening studies.

One may ask at this point whether progress made over the past years is also apparent in higher success rates in large-scale comparative assessments. For this purpose, the results of Warren et al.'s extensive analysis from 2006 (Warren et al. 2006) can be confronted with the observations made in the latest CSAR challenge published in 2013 (Damm-Ganamet et al. 2013). In the following, this is done with respect to the overall results as well as the results obtained for the kinase CHK1, a target addressed by both studies.

Warren et al. (2006) evaluated 10 docking programs and 37 scoring functions against ligand series of 8 proteins of 7 target types for binding mode prediction (and—not further discussed here—for lead identification and rank-ordering by affinity). In total, 136 crystal structures were used. The overall conclusion was that "all of the docking programs were able to generate ligand conformations similar to crystallographically determined protein/ligand complex structures for at least one of the targets. However, scoring functions were less successful at distinguishing the crystallographic conformation from the set of docked poses" (Warren et al. 2006). More in detail, for five of the seven targets, at least one program docked ≥50% of the ligands within 2 Å of the crystal conformation, and for several protein targets, 90% of the ligands could be docked in the correct orientation. Clearly, docking algorithms were able to explore conformational space sufficiently well to generate correctly docked poses. The top-pose statistics, however, were not as good, but nevertheless, "for five of the seven target types, at least one docking program/scoring function pair was able to identify poses within 2 Å of the crystallographic conformation for ≥40% of the compounds" (Warren et al. 2006). A large system dependency was observed, as no approach performed well across all protein targets. Protein flexibility was not found to be a major issue for the tested cases.

With respect to the target CHK1, the authors observed a comparatively good performance across many docking protocols and related this to the fact that the investigated compounds are bound to a relatively small, well-defined binding site and make a small number of key orienting interactions with protein atoms. In detail, however, the results differed quite drastically among the 10 docking programs. For the 15 crystal structures of CHK1-ligand complexes, the percentage of well-docked poses (≤2 Å RMSD) irrespective of their rank ranged between 0% and ~85%, with five programs reaching values above 60%. With respect to the top pose, values from 0% to ~65% were obtained, and only three programs reached more than 50% (percentage of top-ranked poses within ≤2 Å RMSD from the crystal structure).

A more recent, large-scale docking evaluation was organized by the CSAR benchmark exercise 2011–2012 (Damm-Ganamet et al. 2013). It included four targets with blinded, high-quality experimental data. For each target, one PDB file was suggested to be used, but the actual crystal structures (34 in total) of the ligand complexes to be investigated were released only after submission of the predictions. Twenty research groups participated, with 18 different docking programs and 38 different protocols/submissions analyzed in the final article (Damm-Ganamet et al. 2013). The challenge had multiple tasks, but the focus here is on pose prediction. The authors concluded that pose prediction "proved to be the most straightforward task, and most methods were able to successfully reproduce binding poses when the crystal structure employed was cocrystallized with a ligand of the same chemical series" (Damm-Ganamet et al. 2013). Up to three poses per ligand were submitted for each protocol. The median RMSD of the best poses (i.e., the poses with the minimum RMSD) across all group methods and targets was 3.00 Å, ranging from 1.14 Å for LpxC to 5.03 Å for ERK2. In 50.6% of the cases, the best pose was also the top pose. Of all *top poses* submitted, 33.9% had an RMSD up to 2 Å and 41.5% of more than 5 Å. Again, the results were highly system-dependent, both with respect to the target and the chemical series: good results were obtained for LpxC (top poses: 73.6% ≤2 Å, 8%> 5 Å), rather poor results for ligand series 2 of CHK1 (top poses: 5.4%≤ 2 Å, 57.8%> 5 Å). Interestingly, ligand series 1 of CHK1 led to much better results than series 2, with 61.7% of the top poses showing an RMSD ≤ 2 Å. The reason is that series 1 contained chemically similar ligands to the cocrystal structure utilized for docking. Overall, of the 477 submitted top poses for the 14 CHK1 complexes, 27.7% had an RMSD ≤ 2 Å. One of the major problems with this series observed in our own work (Zilian and Sotriffer 2013) was the occurrence of flipped binding modes leading to large RMSD values although the overall binding location was correct. Apparently, the fine-balance in the interaction terms is not sufficiently well captured by the applied scoring functions, with the consequence that the native pose is either not even generated or not correctly discriminated from other poses upon rescoring (cf. Figure 6.2).

Despite many advances and successes in the docking field, these examples may serve as an alert that the precise prediction of the binding mode is still prone to fail in individual cases, even though at first sight the binding pocket and/or the ligand type may not appear to be exceptionally complicated. Further developments are required, in particular with respect to scoring functions, to improve the reliability of the top-ranked binding-pose predictions.

6.4 Recent Advances and Selected New Approaches

To illustrate a little more in detail recent advances in the docking field, a few selected examples are presented below. They refer to the consideration of

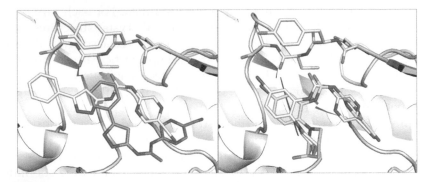

FIGURE 6.2
(See color insert.) Illustration of CHK1 docking results for closely related urea derivatives (CHK1_34 und CHK1_36) of the CSAR challenge (Damm-Ganamet et al. 2013; Zilian and Sotriffer 2013). Even though the ligands are very similar, docking with Glide led to top-ranked poses of very different quality. In the case of CHK1_36 (right figure), the top-ranked docking result (shown with green carbon atoms) differs only 1.1 Å from the crystal structure (shown with light gray carbon atoms); moreover, all 10 generated poses were found to be very similarly placed and equally well acceptable. In contrast, for CHK1_34 (left figure) the 10 generated docking poses show very different binding modes, but never the crystallographically observed one; rather, an RMSD of 5.2 Å is measured for the top-ranked pose (light blue carbon atoms) with respect to the crystal structure.The figures were generated with Pymol (The PyMOL Molecular Graphics System, Version 1.3, Schrödinger, LLC).

explicit water molecules and full protein flexibility as the two major challenges for current docking techniques.

As far as the water problem is concerned, most of the presently available approaches rely on predefined water positions. These are either derived from the analysis of high-resolution crystal structures of the investigated target (ideally one apo structure plus multiple complex structures) (Roberts and Mancera 2008; Thilagavathi and Mancera 2010) or obtained from computational water placement methods, such as GRID (Goodford 1985; Wade et al. 1993), SZMAP (Kumar and Zhang 2013), WaterMap (Beuming et al. 2012), or JAWS (Michel et al. 2009). Based on these water positions, the user may choose which water molecules to include in the docking of a particular ligand. Alternatively, the decision is left to the docking algorithm based on an empirical score, as mentioned above. In contrast to these methods, the placement of water molecules independent of predetermined positions and simultaneous with the docking process is much less common. Forli and Olson (2012) have recently presented such an approach which does not require prior knowledge of the apo or holo protein hydration state. For AutoDock4 as underlying docking methodology, they calibrated a specific hydration force field to account for enthalpic and entropic contributions of discrete water molecules to ligand binding. This modified AutoDock energy function was then used in the docking search with explicit displaceable water molecules. The central idea, however, is that the water molecules are not preplaced at specific positions in the protein-binding site, but rather attached to the ligand before docking. Water molecules (in the form of monoatomic pseudoatoms) are attached to all polar ligand sites capable of hydrogen bonding. Upon docking, these water molecules remain attached to the ligand in the defined geometry, but their presence is continuously evaluated during the search. This means that if the mediation through a water molecule stabilizes the protein–ligand interaction, it is kept, whereas otherwise it is displaced. This has the advantage that the water arrangement is not predefined or fixed in the binding site, but may vary depending on the specific hydration properties of the ligand. Moreover, novel ligands may also interact through water molecules not present in the apo or known holo structures. Extensive testing and validation of the approach showed that the method not only finds experimentally determined water molecules, but has also the ability to predict structurally conserved and ligand-stabilized water molecules that are not present in the apo structure. Significant improvements in docking accuracy for various data sets could also be shown. Finally, it is worthwhile noting that the approach can handle quite a large number of water molecules (up to 35 were used in the study) at moderate computational efforts.

Interestingly, a conceptually very similar approach with ligand-attached water molecules was published slightly earlier by Lie et al. (2011) and implemented as AWM (attached water model) into the docking program MolDock/ Molegro Virtual Docker (Thomsen and Christensen 2006). However, in contrast to the approach of Forli, which was evaluated on a total of 1649 protein–ligand complexes, it was calibrated and tested only on two small datasets of 12 complexes each.

An approach for truly simultaneous and independent placement of water molecules during ligand docking has been presented by Hoffer and Horvath with their S4MPLE conformational sampling tool (Hoffer and Horvath 2013). S4MPLE is a conformational sampling tool based on a hybrid genetic algorithm and allows simultaneous docking of multiple entities. The energy calculations are based on the AMBER (Cornell et al. 1995) and GAFF (Wang et al. 2004) force fields with an additional continuum solvation term and a term rewarding favorable interactions such as hydrogen bonds and hydrophobic enclosure. Explicit water molecules are treated as additional ligands competing for binding to the active site. In contrast to the previous approach, this introduces a significant increase in the required sampling efforts. A protocol involving the refinement of all water molecules around each of the poses kept for the ligand was found to be most successful on a test set of 16 complexes (from the Astex Diverse Set [Hartshorn et al. 2007]) in which water-mediated contacts play a key role. Taking all saved poses into account, the correct water positions (within 2 Å RMSD) were obtained in 76% of the cases. Correct ranking, however, was more problematic, as the accuracy of the top-ranked pose concerning water molecules was only 41%. However, as correctly noted by the authors, water localization is an extremely delicate issue in terms of weighing of electrostatic and desolvation terms, even more so as the targeted configurations are not necessarily the energetically most rewarding ones, because the mobile explicit water may well be trapped into site subpockets binding crystallographic waters even tighter (Hoffer and Horvath 2013). Nevertheless, the results are encouraging, given the possibility of truly simultaneous sampling of water and ligand positions with affordable computational resources.

Besides the adequate treatment of water molecules, full consideration of protein flexibility is the second major issue in current docking developments, with many reviews dedicated to this topic (Ahmed et al. 2007; B-Rao et al. 2009; Cavasotto 2011; Cavasotto and Singh 2008; Henzler and Rarey 2011; May et al. 2008; Sotriffer 2011; Totrov and Abagyan 2008). As mentioned above, one of the biggest challenges for flexible protein docking is the efficient inclusion of backbone flexibility.

One of the most recent variants for considering backbone flexibility in docking is the Backbone Perturbation-DOCK (BP-Dock) approach (Bolia et al. 2014). It is reported as a multiscale approach able to cover both backbone and side-chain conformational changes upon ligand binding. Essentially, it is a procedure for generating an ensemble of bound-like conformations of the protein by means of "perturbation response scanning" followed by clustering and all-atom energy minimization of the obtained perturbed protein conformation. Perturbation response scanning (Atilgan et al. 2010; Gerek and Ozkan 2011) is a method combining the elastic network model and linear response theory, whereby—basically—the residues of the protein are perturbed (one at a time) with a small Brownian kick (random external unit force on a single alpha-carbon atom) and the resulting relative displacements of all residues are recorded using linear response theory. Docking itself is carried out in an ensemble-docking fashion with RosettaLigand (Davis and Baker 2009; Meiler and Baker 2006) in such a way that ligands are docked to all individual conformations of the generated ensemble. The final docking result is obtained as the "lowest free energy pose" given by the lowest Rosetta energy score among all docked poses. For affinity estimation, rescoring with the X-Score scoring function (Wang et al. 2002) is carried out.

In evaluating this approach, the authors focused on the correlation of the computed scores with experimental binding affinities for five test sets (5 targets with a total of 68 complexes), finding that BP-Dock provides better correlations than rigid docking to unbound structures. The significance of this finding is somewhat difficult to judge, as the RMSD values of the binding poses obtained from docking to the rigid apo protein structure was already well below 2 Å for all but one of the 68 complexes (Table S2 of the SI [Bolia et al. 2014]), and only minor improvements (if any) in the RMSD of the binding poses were seen with the BP-DOCK protocol. It would be interesting to know whether BP-Dock can actually provide improved binding mode predictions in cases where rigid docking fails. Further tests are needed to more fully judge on the potential of the method.

MedusaDock (Ding et al. 2010) has recently been extended to cover backbone flexibility (Ding and Dokholyan 2013). Originally, MedusaDock was designed as a method to simultaneously sample conformations of the ligand and of the protein side chains by means of rotamer libraries (stochastically generated "on the fly" for the ligand, whereas for the protein side chains a predefined rotamer set is used). After generating representative ligand conformations, each of these is first docked rigidly to the binding pocket with the van der Waals repulsion between ligand and side chains turned off. This is followed by iterative minimization (with van der Waals repulsion included) and repacking of the ligand rotamers and protein side chains. The force field-based MedusaScore (Yin et al. 2008) is used as scoring function in this docking process. Backbone flexibility is then incorporated by constructing a small ensemble of representative protein backbone conformations from known experimental structures. For each of these structures with different backbone conformations, independent docking runs with MedusaDock are carried out (100 in case of the presented study), followed by clustering of a chosen number of top poses obtained for each of the backbone structures. The clusters are then ranked either by the average MedusaScore or by an effective free energy computed for each cluster from the MedusaScore.

In comparison to other submissions, MedusaDock performed very well in pose prediction in the last CSAR benchmark. Nevertheless, for the CHK1 data set the results were not yet ideal, and for the even more problematic ERK2 data set, only in 1 out of the 12 cases with a crystal structure reference a top pose with RMSD below 2 Å was obtained. Accordingly, further improvements appear to be required, most likely related to the scoring approach, as near-native poses were more often generated than recognized as top-ranked solution.

Both BP-DOCK and MedusaDock once more show that flexible protein docking is rather a workflow than a single program (Henzler and Rarey 2011). In contrast to these two methods, however, Flick et al. (2012) present an approach for explicit sampling of backbone conformational degrees of freedom during the docking process. It is built on their stochastic tunneling docking program FlexScreen, which already allowed side chain conformational sampling and was shown to improve docking and virtual screening results (Kokh and Wenzel 2008; Merlitz and Wenzel 2002, 2004; Merlitz et al. 2003). To extend this approach the authors have added a routine for sampling flexibility of a selected backbone region (such as a flexible loop) based on a loop reconstruction algorithm (Flick et al. 2012). In the applied scheme, backbone dihedral angles are randomly changed at an adjustable frequency during the simulation. After such a backbone change, a loop closure search is carried out to close the loop, and subsequently the resulting conformation is locally minimized. The probability for a backbone reconstruction move can be set by the user and altered for the different stages of the docking cascade in the stochastic tunneling algorithm. As correctly recognized by the authors, scoring provides a challenge for such flexible backbone sampling docking approaches, as the backbone–backbone and backbone–ligand inter-action energies have to be adequately balanced. The authors often found large energy differences for rather small backbone movements, probably caused by an overestimation of the internal receptor contribution. A more accurate solvent treatment could help in this context. Nevertheless, for the investigated test cases of three different kinases where rigid docking neces-sarily fails, docking to the apo structure with flexibility of the critical loop backbone and selected side chains could reproduce the experimental bind-ing mode, although not always as best-scored solution due to the scoring problem mentioned above.

6.5 Conclusion

Over the past 30 years, computational docking has grown to a firmly estab-lished and widely utilized technique. A large variety of docking programs is nowadays available, and thousands of reported docking applications can be found in the scientific literature (Sousa et al. 2013). Significant progress has been made for handling water molecules and protein flexibility in docking, but the related scoring problems are not yet satisfactorily solved. Even though binding mode prediction is generally reported to work very well, success is not yet guaranteed, and entire ligand series may fail to dock correctly even to well-known targets. As long as the situation persists that no single docking program performs equally well across all test cases and targets and as long as the most reliable program for a particular docking problem is hardly known in advance, thorough validation of the available docking approaches for the target of interest is mandatory. As noted by Yuriev and Ramsland (2013), "the docking field needs a breakthrough. And that is more likely to come from better scientific understanding of protein–ligand interplay translated into better scoring." Indeed, major advances in scoring are required to fully unleash the great potential of current docking algorithms and techniques.

References

Abagyan, R., M. Totrov, and D. Kuznetsov. 1994. ICM—A new method for protein modeling and design: Applications to docking and structure prediction from the distorted native conformation. *J. Comput. Chem.* 15: 488–506.
Agostino, M., C. Jene, T. Boyle, P. A. Ramsland, and E. Yuriev. 2009. Molecular dock-ing of carbohydrate ligands to antibodies: Structural validation against crystal structures. *J. Chem. Inf. Model.* 49(12): 2749–2760.

Ahmed, A., S. Kazemi, and H. Gohlke. 2007. Protein flexibility and mobility in structure-based drug design. *Front. Drug Des. Discov.* 3: 455–476.

Allen, F. H. 2002. The Cambridge Structural Database: A quarter of a million crystal structures and rising. *Acta cryst. B* 58 (Part 3 Part 1): 380–388.

Allen, F. H., J. E. Davies, J. J. Galloy et al. 1991. The development of version-3 and version-4 of the Cambridge Structural Database system. *J. Chem. Inf. Comput. Sci.* 31: 187–204.

Alonso, H., A. A. Bliznyuk, and J. E. Gready. 2006. Combining docking and molecular dynamic simulations in drug design. *Med. Res. Rev.* 26(5): 531–568.

Amaro, R. E., R. Baron, and J. A. McCammon. 2008. An improved relaxed complex scheme for receptor flexibility in computer-aided drug design. *J. Comput. Aided Mol. Des.* 22(9): 693–705.

Atilgan, C., Z. N. Gerek, S. B. Ozkan, and A. R. Atilgan. 2010. Manipulation of conformational change in proteins by single-residue perturbations. *Biophys. J.* 99(3): 933–943.

B-Rao, C., J. Subramanian, and S. D. Sharma. 2009. Managing protein flexibility in docking and its applications. *Drug Discov. Today* 14(7–8): 394–400.

Baker, N. A. 2005. Biomolecular applications of Poisson-Boltzmann methods. In: *Reviews in Computational Chemistry*, K. B. Lipkowitz, R. Larter, T. R. Cundari, and D. B. Boyd (Eds.), pp. 349–379, New York: Wiley-VCH.

Ballester, P. J. and J. B. Mitchell. 2010. A machine learning approach to predicting protein-ligand binding affinity with applications to molecular docking. *Bioinformatics* 26(9): 1169–1175.

Barducci, A., M. Bonomi, and M. Parrinello. 2011. Metadynamics. *Wires Comput. Mol. Sci.* 1(5): 826–843.

Bas, D. C., D. M. Rogers, and J. H. Jensen. 2008. Very fast prediction and rationalization of pKa values for protein-ligand complexes. *Proteins* 73(3): 765–783.

Baxter, C. A., C. W. Murray, D. E. Clark, D. R. Westhead, and M. D. Eldridge. 1998. Flexible docking using Tabu search and an empirical estimate of binding affinity. *Proteins* 33(3): 367–382.

Baxter, C. A., C. W. Murray, B. Waszkowycz et al. 2000. New approach to molecular docking and its application to virtual screening of chemical databases. *J. Chem. Inf. Comput. Sci.* 40(2): 254–262.

Bergner, A., J. Günther, M. Hendlich, G. Klebe, and M. Verdonk. 2001. Use of Relibase for retrieving complex three-dimensional interaction patterns including crystallographic packing effects. *Biopolymers* 61(2): 99–110.

Berman, H. M., J. Westbrook, Z. Feng et al. 2000. The protein data bank. *Nucleic Acids Res.* 28(1): 235–242.

Beuming, T., Y. Che, R. Abel, B. Kim, V. Shanmugasundaram, and W. Sherman. 2012. Thermodynamic analysis of water molecules at the surface of proteins and applications to binding site prediction and characterization. *Proteins* 80(3): 871–883.

Bietz, S., S. Urbaczek, B. Schulz, and M. Rarey. 2014. Protoss: A holistic approach to predict tautomers and protonation states in protein-ligand complexes. *J. Cheminform.* 6: 12.

Bissantz, C., B. Kuhn, and M. Stahl. 2010. A medicinal chemist's guide to molecular interactions. *J. Med. Chem.* 53(14): 5061–5084.

Boehm, H. J. 1994. The development of a simple empirical scoring function to estimate the binding constant for a protein-ligand complex of known three-dimensional structure. *J. Comput. Aided Mol. Des.* 8(3): 243–256.

Boehm, H. J. 1998. Prediction of binding constants of protein ligands: A fast method for the prioritization of hits obtained from *de novo* design or 3D database search programs. *J. Comput. Aided Mol. Des.* 12(4): 309–323.

Boehm, H. J. and M. Stahl. 1999. Rapid empirical scoring functions in virtual screening applications. *Med. Chem. Res.* 9: 445–462.

Boehm, H. J. and M. Stahl. 2002. The use of scoring functions in drug discovery applications. In: *Reviews in Computational Chemistry*, K. B. Lipkowitz and D. B. Boyd (Eds.), pp. 41–88, New York: Wiley-VCH.

Bolia, A., Z. N. Gerek, and S. B. Ozkan. 2014. BP-Dock: A flexible docking scheme for exploring protein-ligand interactions based on unbound structures. *J. Chem. Inf. Model.* 54(3): 913–925.

Bostrom, J. 2001. Reproducing the conformations of protein-bound ligands: A critical evaluation of several popular conformational searching tools. *J. Comput. Aided Mol. Des.* 15(12): 1137–1152.

Branduardi, D., F. L. Gervasio, A. Cavalli, M. Recanatini, and M. Parrinello. 2005. The role of the peripheral anionic site and cation-pi interactions in the ligand penetration of the human AChE gorge. *J. Am. Chem. Soc.* 127(25): 9147–9155.

Brewerton, S. C. 2008. The use of protein-ligand interaction fingerprints in docking. *Curr. Opin. Drug. Discov. Devel.* 11(3): 356–364.

Brooijmans, N. and I. D. Kuntz. 2003. Molecular recognition and docking algorithms. *Annu. Rev. Biophys. Biomol. Struct.* 32: 335–373.

Brooks, B. R., R. E. Bruccoleri, B. D. Olafson, D. J. States, S. Swaminathan, and M. Karplus. 1983. CHARMM: A program for macromolecular energy, minimization, and dynamics calculations. *J. Comput. Chem.* 4: 187–217.

Camacho, C. J. and S. Vajda. 2002. Protein-protein association kinetics and protein docking. *Curr. Opin. Struct. Biol.* 12(1): 36–40.

Cappel, D., R. Wahlstrom, R. Brenk, and C. A. Sotriffer. 2011. Probing the dynamic nature of water molecules and their influences on ligand binding in a model binding site. *J. Chem. Inf. Model.* 51(10): 2581–2594.

Cavasotto, C. N. 2011. Handling protein flexibility in docking and high-throughput docking: from algorithms to applications. In: *Virtual Screening. Principles, Challenges, and Practical Guidelines*, C. Sotriffer (Ed.), pp. 245–262, Weinheim: Wiley-VCH.

Cavasotto, C. N., A. J. Orry, N. J. Murgolo et al. 2008. Discovery of novel chemotypes to a G-protein-coupled receptor through ligand-steered homology modeling and structure-based virtual screening. *J. Med. Chem.* 51(3): 581–588.

Cavasotto, C. N. and N. Singh. 2008. Docking and high throughput docking: Successes and the challenge of protein flexibility. *Curr. Comput. Aid. Drug Des.* 4(3): 221–234.

Charifson, P. S., J. J. Corkery, M. A. Murcko, and W. P. Walters. 1999. Consensus scoring: A method for obtaining improved hit rates from docking databases of three-dimensional structures into proteins. *J. Med. Chem.* 42(25): 5100–5109.

Chen, H. M., B. F. Liu, H. L. Huang, S. F. Hwang, and S. Y. Ho. 2007. SODOCK: Swarm optimization for highly flexible protein-ligand docking. *J. Comput. Chem.* 28(2): 612–623.

Cheng, T., X. Li, Y. Li, Z. Liu, and R. Wang. 2009. Comparative assessment of scoring functions on a diverse test set. *J. Chem. Inf. Model.* 49(4): 1079–1093.

Cherfils, J., S. Duquerroy, and J. Janin. 1991. Protein-protein recognition analyzed by docking simulation. *Proteins* 11: 271–280.

Clark, R. D., A. Strizhev, J. M. Leonard, J. F. Blake, and J. B. Matthew. 2002. Consensus scoring for ligand/protein interactions. *Journal of Molecular Graphics & Modelling* 20(4): 281–295.

Clark, D. E. and D. R. Westhead. 1996. Evolutionary algorithms in computer-aided molecular design. *J. Comput. Aided Mol. Des.* 10: 337–358.

Cole, J. C., O. Korb, T. S. G. Olsson, and J. Liebeschuetz. 2011. The basis for target-based virtual screening: Protein structures. In: *Virtual Screening. Principles, Challenges, and Practical Guidelines*, C. Sotriffer (Ed.), pp. 87–114, Weinheim: Wiley-VCH.

Coleman, R. G., M. Carchia, T. Sterling, J. J. Irwin, and B. K. Shoichet. 2013. Ligand pose and orientational sampling in molecular docking. *PLoS One* 8(10): e75992.

Corbeil, C. R., P. Englebienne, and N. Moitessier. 2007. Docking ligands into flexible and solvated macromolecules. 1. Development and validation of FITTED 1.0. *J. Chem. Inf. Model.* 47(2): 435–449.

Corbeil, C. R., P. Englebienne, C. G. Yannopoulos et al. 2008. Docking ligands into flexible and solvated macromolecules. 2. Development and application of fitted 1.5 to the virtual screening of potential HCV polymerase inhibitors. *J. Chem. Inf. Model.* 48(4): 902–909.

Corbeil, C. R. and N. Moitessier. 2009. Docking ligands into flexible and solvated macromolecules. 3. Impact of input ligand conformation, protein flexibility, and water molecules on the accuracy of docking programs. *J. Chem. Inf. Model.* 49(4): 997–1009.

Cornell, W. D., P. Cieplak, C. I. Bayly et al. 1995. A second generation force field for the simulation of proteins, nucleic acids, and organic molecules. *J. Am. Chem. Soc.* 117: 5179–5197.

Costanzi, S. 2008. On the applicability of GPCR homology models to computer-aided drug discovery: A comparison between *in silico* and crystal structures of the beta2-adrenergic receptor. *J. Med. Chem.* 51(10): 2907–2914.

Craig, I. R., J. W. Essex, and K. Spiegel. 2010. Ensemble docking into multiple crystallographically derived protein structures: An evaluation based on the statistical analysis of enrichments. *J. Chem. Inf. Model.* 50(4): 511–524.

Czodrowski, P., I. Dramburg, C. A. Sotriffer, and G. Klebe. 2006. Development, validation, and application of adapted PEOE charges to estimate pKa values of functional groups in protein-ligand complexes. *Proteins* 65(2): 424–437.

Czodrowski, P., C. A. Sotriffer, and G. Klebe. 2007. Protonation changes upon ligand binding to trypsin and thrombin: Structural interpretation based on pK(a) calculations and ITC experiments. *J. Mol. Biol.* 367(5): 1347–1356.

Daldrop, P., F. E. Reyes, D. A. Robinson et al. 2011. Novel ligands for a purine riboswitch discovered by RNA-ligand docking. *Chem. Biol.* 18(3): 324–335.

Damm-Ganamet, K. L., R. D. Smith, J. B. Dunbar, Jr., J. A. Stuckey, and H. A. Carlson. 2013. CSAR benchmark exercise 2011–2012: Evaluation of results from docking and relative ranking of blinded congeneric series. *J. Chem. Inf. Model.* 53(8): 1853–1870.

Das, S., M. P. Krein, and C. M. Breneman. 2010. Binding affinity prediction with property-encoded shape distribution signatures. *J. Chem. Inf. Model.* 50(2): 298–308.

Davis, I. W. and D. Baker. 2009. RosettaLigand docking with full ligand and receptor flexibility. *J. Mol. Biol.* 385(2): 381–392.

Deng, Z., C. Chuaqui, and J. Singh. 2004. Structural interaction fingerprint (SIFt): A novel method for analyzing three-dimensional protein-ligand binding interactions. *J. Med. Chem.* 47(2): 337–344.

DesJarlais, R. L. and J. S. Dixon. 1994. A shape- and chemistry-based docking method and its use in the design of HIV-1 protease inhibitors. *J. Comput. Aided Mol. Des.* 8(3): 231–242.

DesJarlais, R. L., R. P. Sheridan, G. L. Seibel, J. S. Dixon, I. D. Kuntz, and R. Venkataraghavan. 1988. Using shape complementarity as an initial screen in designing ligands for a receptor binding site of known three-dimensional structure. *J. Med. Chem.* 31(4): 722–729.

Di Nola, A., D. Roccatano, and H. J. Berendsen. 1994. Molecular dynamics simulation of the docking of substrates to proteins. *Proteins* 19(3): 174–182.

Ding, F. and N. V. Dokholyan. 2013. Incorporating backbone flexibility in MedusaDock improves ligand-binding pose prediction in the CSAR2011 docking benchmark. *J. Chem. Inf. Model.* 53(8): 1871–1879.

Ding, F., S. Yin, and N. V. Dokholyan. 2010. Rapid flexible docking using a stochastic rotamer library of ligands. *J. Chem. Inf. Model.* 50(9): 1623–1632.

Ehrlich, L. P. and R. C. Wade. 2001. Protein-protein docking. In: *Reviews in Computational Chemistry*, K. B. Lipkowitz, and D. B. Boyd (Eds.), pp. 61–97, New York: Wiley-VCH.

Eldridge, M. D., C. W. Murray, T. R. Auton, G. V. Paolini, and R. P. Mee. 1997. Empirical scoring functions: I. The development of a fast empirical scoring function to estimate the binding affinity of ligands in receptor complexes. *J. Comput. Aided Mol. Des.* 11(5): 425–445.

Evers, A., H. Gohlke, and G. Klebe. 2003. Ligand-supported homology modelling of protein binding-sites using knowledge-based potentials. *J. Mol. Biol.* 334(2): 327–345.

Ewing, T. J., S. Makino, A. G. Skillman, and I. D. Kuntz. 2001. DOCK 4.0: Search strategies for automated molecular docking of flexible molecule databases. *J. Comput. Aided Mol. Des.* 15(5): 411–428.

Feher, M. 2006. Consensus scoring for protein-ligand interactions. *Drug Discov. Today* 11(9–10): 421–428.

Feng, J. A. and G. R. Marshall. 2010. SKATE: A docking program that decouples systematic sampling from scoring. *J. Comput. Chem.* 31(14): 2540–2554.

Fischer, B., S. Basili, H. Merlitz, and W. Wenzel. 2007. Accuracy of binding mode prediction with a cascadic stochastic tunneling method. *Proteins* 68(1): 195–204.

Flick, J., F. Tristram, and W. Wenzel. 2012. Modeling loop backbone flexibility in receptor-ligand docking simulations. *J. Comput. Chem.* 33(31): 2504–2515.

Forli, S. and A. J. Olson. 2012. A force field with discrete displaceable waters and desolvation entropy for hydrated ligand docking. *J. Med. Chem.* 55(2): 623–638.

Friesner, R. A., J. L. Banks, R. B. Murphy et al. 2004. Glide: A new approach for rapid, accurate docking and scoring. 1. Method and assessment of docking accuracy. *J. Med. Chem.* 47(7): 1739–1749.

Friesner, R. A., R. B. Murphy, M. P. Repasky et al. 2006. Extra precision Glide: Docking and scoring incorporating a model of hydrophobic enclosure for protein-ligand complexes. *J. Med. Chem.* 49(21): 6177–6196.

Gabb, H. A., R. M. Jackson, and M. J. Sternberg. 1997. Modelling protein docking using shape complementarity, electrostatics and biochemical information. *J. Mol. Biol.* 272(1): 106–120.

Gerek, Z. N. and S. B. Ozkan. 2011. Change in allosteric network affects binding affinities of PDZ domains: Analysis through perturbation response scanning. *PLoS Comput. Biol.* 7(10): e1002154.

Gervasio, F. L., A. Laio, and M. Parrinello. 2005. Flexible docking in solution using metadynamics. *J. Am. Chem. Soc.* 127(8): 2600–2607.

Ghosh, A., C. S. Rapp, and R. A. Friesner. 1998. Generalized born model based on a surface integral formulation. *J. Phys. Chem. B* 102(52): 10983–10990.

Gohlke, H., M. Hendlich, and G. Klebe. 2000. Knowledge-based scoring function to predict protein-ligand interactions. *J. Mol. Biol.* 295(2): 337–356.

Goldman, B. B. and W. T. Wipke. 2000. QSD Quadratic shape descriptors. 2. Molecular docking using quadratic shape descriptors (QSDock). *Proteins* 38: 79–94.

Goodford, P. J. 1985. A computational procedure for determining energetically favorable binding sites on biologically important macromolecules. *J. Med. Chem.* 28(7): 849–857.

Goodsell, D. S. and A. J. Olson. 1990. Automated docking of substrates to proteins by simulated annealing. *Proteins* 8(3): 195–202.

Goto, J., R. Kataoka, H. Muta, and N. Hirayama. 2008. ASEDock-docking based on alpha spheres and excluded volumes. *J. Chem. Inf. Model.* 48(3): 583–590.

Grosdidier, A., V. Zoete, and O. Michielin. 2009. Blind docking of 260 protein-ligand complexes with EADock 2.0. *J. Comput. Chem.* 30(13): 2021–2030.

Gschwend, D. A. and I. D. Kuntz. 1996. Orientational sampling and rigid-body minimization in molecular docking revisited: On-the-fly optimization and degeneracy removal. *J. Comput. Aided Mol. Des.* 10(2): 123–132.

Guilbert, C. and T. L. James. 2008. Docking to RNA via root-mean-square-deviation-driven energy minimization with flexible ligands and flexible targets. *J. Chem. Inf. Model.* 48(6): 1257–1268.

Guimaraes, C. R. and M. Cardozo. 2008. MM-GB/SA rescoring of docking poses in structure-based lead optimization. *J. Chem. Inf. Model.* 48(5): 958–970.

Halperin, I., B. Ma, H. Wolfson, and R. Nussinov. 2002. Principles of docking: An overview of search algorithms and a guide to scoring functions. *Proteins* 47(4): 409–443.

Hartshorn, M. J., M. L. Verdonk, G. Chessari et al. 2007. Diverse, high-quality test set for the validation of protein-ligand docking performance. *J. Med. Chem.* 50(4): 726–741.

Henzler, A. M. and M. Rarey. 2011. Protein flexibility in structure-based virtual screening: From models to algorithms. In: *Virtual Screening. Principles, Challenges, and Practical Guidelines*, C. Sotriffer (Ed.), Weinheim: Wiley-VCH.

Hoffer, L. and D. Horvath. 2013. S4MPLE—Sampler for multiple protein-ligand entities: Simultaneous docking of several entities. *J. Chem. Inf. Model.* 53(1): 88–102.

Hooft, R. W., C. Sander, and G. Vriend. 1996. Positioning hydrogen atoms by optimizing hydrogen-bond networks in protein structures. *Proteins* 26(4): 363–376.

Huang, S. Y. 2014. Search strategies and evaluation in protein-protein docking: Principles, advances and challenges. *Drug Discov. Today* 19(8): 1081–1096.

Huang, S. Y. and X. Zou. 2010. Inclusion of solvation and entropy in the knowledge-based scoring function for protein-ligand interactions. *J. Chem. Inf. Model.* 50(2): 262–273.

Janin, J. 2010. Protein-protein docking tested in blind predictions: The CAPRI experiment. *Mol. Biosyst.* 6(12): 2351–2362.

Jones, G., P. Willett, and R. C. Glen. 1995. Molecular recognition of receptor sites using a genetic algorithm with a description of desolvation. *J. Mol. Biol.* 245(1): 43–53.

Jones, G., P. Willett, R. C. Glen, A. R. Leach, and R. Taylor. 1997. Development and validation of a genetic algorithm for flexible docking. *J. Mol. Biol.* 267(3): 727–748.

Kalliokoski, T., C. Kramer, A. Vulpetti, and P. Gedeck. 2013. Comparability of mixed IC50 data—A statistical analysis. *PLoS One* 8(4): e61007.

Kaminski, G. A., R. A. Friesner, J. Tirado-Rives, and W. L. Jorgensen. 2001. Evaluation and reparametrization of the OPLS-AA force field for proteins via comparison with accurate quantum chemical calculations on peptides. *J. Phys. Chem. B* 105(28): 6474–6487.

Karplus, M. 2002. Molecular dynamics simulations of biomolecules (Editorial). *Acc. Chem. Res.* 35: 321–323.

Katchalski-Katzir, E., I. Shariv, M. Eisenstein, A. A. Friesem, C. Aflalo, and I. A. Vakser. 1992. Molecular surface recognition: Determination of geometric fit between proteins and their ligands by correlation techniques. *Proc. Natl. Acad. Sci. USA* 89(6): 2195–2199.

Kelly, M. D. and R. L. Mancera. 2004. Expanded interaction fingerprint method for analyzing ligand binding modes in docking and structure-based drug design. *J. Chem. Inf. Comput. Sci.* 44(6): 1942–1951.

Kerzmann, A., J. Fuhrmann, O. Kohlbacher, and D. Neumann. 2008. BALLDock/ SLICK: A new method for protein-carbohydrate docking. *J. Chem. Inf. Model.* 48(8): 1616–1625.

Kim, D. S., C. M. Kim, C. I. Won et al. 2011. BetaDock: Shape-priority docking method based on beta-complex. *J. Biomol. Struct. Dyn.* 29(1): 219–242.

Kirchmair, J., G. M. Spitzer, and K. R. Liedl. 2011. Consideration of water and solvation effects in virtual screening. In: *Virtual Screening. Principles, Challenges, and Practical Guidelines*, C. Sotriffer (Ed.), pp. 263–289, Weinheim: Wiley-VCH.

Kirchmair, J., G. Wolber, C. Laggner, and T. Langer. 2006. Comparative performance assessment of the conformational model generators omega and catalyst: A large-scale survey on the retrieval of protein-bound ligand conformations. *J. Chem. Inf. Model.* 46(4): 1848–1861.

Kiss, R. and G. M. Keserü. 2011. Virtual screening on homology models. In: *Virtual Screening. Principles, Challenges, and Practical Guidelines*, C. Sotriffer (Ed.), pp. 381–410, Weinheim: Wiley-VCH.

Kokh, D. B. and W. Wenzel. 2008. Flexible side chain models improve enrichment rates in *in silico* screening. *J. Med. Chem.* 51(19): 5919–5931.

Kollman, P. A., I. Massova, C. Reyes et al. 2000. Calculating structures and free energies of complex molecules: Combining molecular mechanics and continuum models. *Acc. Chem. Res.* 33(12): 889–897.

Korb, O., T. S. Olsson, S. J. Bowden et al. 2012. Potential and limitations of ensemble docking. *J. Chem. Inf. Model.* 52(5): 1262–1274.

Korb, O., T. Stutzle, and T. E. Exner. 2009. Empirical scoring functions for advanced protein-ligand docking with PLANTS. *J. Chem. Inf. Model.* 49(1): 84–96.

Kramer, C., T. Kalliokoski, P. Gedeck, and A. Vulpetti. 2012. The experimental uncertainty of heterogeneous public K(i) data. *J. Med. Chem.* 55(11): 5165–5173.

Kramer, B., M. Rarey, and T. Lengauer. 1999. Evaluation of the FLEXX incremental construction algorithm for protein-ligand docking. *Proteins* 37(2): 228–241.

Kranjc, A., S. Bongarzone, G. Rossetti et al. 2009. Docking ligands on protein surfaces: The case study of prion protein. *J. Chem. Theory Comput.* 5(9): 2565–2573.

Kuhn, B., P. Gerber, T. Schulz-Gasch, and M. Stahl. 2005. Validation and use of the MM-PBSA approach for drug discovery. *J. Med. Chem.* 48(12): 4040–4048.

Kumar, A. and K. Y. Zhang. 2013. Investigation on the effect of key water molecules on docking performance in CSARdock exercise. *J. Chem. Inf. Model.* 53(8): 1880–1892.

Kuntz, I. D., J. M. Blaney, S. J. Oatley, R. Langridge, and T. E. Ferrin. 1982. A geometric approach to macromolecule-ligand interactions. *J. Mol. Biol.* 161(2): 269–288.

Lang, P. T., S. R. Brozell, S. Mukherjee et al. 2009. DOCK 6: Combining techniques to model RNA-small molecule complexes. *RNA* 15(6): 1219–1230.

Leach, A. R. 2001. Monte Carlo simulation methods. In: *Molecular Modelling: Principles and Applications*. Essex: Pearson Education Limited.

Li, Y., J. Shen, X. Sun, W. Li, G. Liu, and Y. Tang. 2010. Accuracy assessment of protein-based docking programs against RNA targets. *J. Chem. Inf. Model.* 50(6): 1134–1146.

Lie, M. A., R. Thomsen, C. N. Pedersen, B. Schiott, and M. H. Christensen. 2011. Molecular docking with ligand attached water molecules. *J. Chem. Inf. Model.* 51(4): 909–917.

Lin, J. H., A. L. Perryman, J. R. Schames, and J. A. McCammon. 2002. Computational drug design accommodating receptor flexibility: The relaxed complex scheme. *J. Am. Chem. Soc.* 124(20): 5632–5633.

Liu, M. and S. Wang. 1999. MCDOCK: A Monte Carlo simulation approach to the molecular docking problem. *J. Comput. Aided Mol. Des.* 13: 435–451.

Luo, W., J. Pei, and Y. Zhu. 2010. A fast protein-ligand docking algorithm based on hydrogen bond matching and surface shape complementarity. *J. Mol. Model.* 16(5): 903–913.

Lyne, P. D., M. L. Lamb, and J. C. Saeh. 2006. Accurate prediction of the relative potencies of members of a series of kinase inhibitors using molecular docking and MM-GBSA scoring. *J. Med. Chem.* 49(16): 4805–4808.

Mangoni, M., D. Roccatano, and A. Di Nola. 1999. Docking of flexible ligands to flexible receptors in solution by molecular dynamics simulation. *Proteins* 35(2): 153–162.

Marcou, G. and D. Rognan. 2007. Optimizing fragment and scaffold docking by use of molecular interaction fingerprints. *J. Chem. Inf. Model.* 47(1): 195–207.

Maselli, M., A. Cavalli, M. Recanatini, and F. L. Gervasio. 2009. Exploring complex protein-ligand recognition mechanisms with coarse metadynamics. *J. Phys. Chem. B* 113(14): 4807–4816.

May, A., F. Sieker, and M. Zacharias. 2008. How to efficiently include receptor flexibility during computational docking. *Curr. Comput. Aided Drug Des.* 4: 143–153.

May, A. and M. Zacharias. 2008. Energy minimization in low-frequency normal modes to efficiently allow for global flexibility during systematic protein-protein docking. *Proteins* 70(3): 794–809.

McGann, M. 2011. FRED pose prediction and virtual screening accuracy. *J. Chem. Inf. Model.* 51(3): 578–596.

McMartin, C. and R. S. Bohacek. 1997. QXP: Powerful, rapid computer algorithms for structure-based drug design. *J. Comput. Aided Mol. Des.* 11(4): 333–344.

Meiler, J. and D. Baker. 2006. ROSETTALIGAND: Protein-small molecule docking with full side-chain flexibility. *Proteins* 65(3): 538–548.

Meng, E. C., D. A. Gschwend, J. M. Blaney, and I. D. Kuntz. 1993. Orientational sampling and rigid-body minimization in molecular docking. *Proteins* 17(3): 266–278.

Merlitz, H., B. Burghardt, and W. Wenzel. 2003. Application of the stochastic tunneling method to high throughput database screening. *J. Chem. Phys. Lett.* 370: 68–73.

Merlitz, H. and W. Wenzel. 2002. Comparison of stochastic optimization methods from receptor-ligand docking. *J. Chem. Phys. Lett.* 362: 271–277.

Merlitz, H. and W. Wenzel. 2004. Impact of receptor conformation on *in silico* screening performance. *J. Chem. Phys. Lett.* 390: 500–505.

Metropolis, N., A. W. Rosenbluth, M. N. Rosenbluth, A. H. Teller, and E. Teller. 1953. Equation of state calculations by fast computing machines. *J. Chem. Phys.* 21(6): 1087–1092.

Michel, J., J. Tirado-Rives, and W. L. Jorgensen. 2009. Prediction of the water content in protein binding sites. *J. Phys. Chem. B* 113(40): 13337–13346.

Miller, M. D., S. K. Kearsley, D. J. Underwood, and R. P. Sheridan. 1994. FLOG: A system to select "quasi-flexible" ligands complementary to a receptor of known three-dimensional structure. *J. Comput. Aided Mol. Des.* 8(2): 153–174.

Mitchell, J. B. O., R. A. Laskowski, A. Alex, and J. M. Thornton. 1999a. BLEEP—A potential of mean force describing protein-ligand interactions: I. Generating the potential. *J. Comput. Chem.* 20: 1165–1176.

Mitchell, J. B. O., R. A. Laskowski, A. Alex, M. J. Forster, and J. M. Thornton. 1999b. BLEEP—A potential of mean force describing protein-ligand interactions: II. Calculation of binding energies and comparison with experimental data. *J. Comput. Chem.* 20: 1177–1185.

Mizutani, M. Y., N. Tomioka, and A. Itai. 1994. Rational automatic search method for stable docking models of protein and ligand. *J. Mol. Biol.* 243(2): 310–326.

Mobarec, J. C., R. Sanchez, and M. Filizola. 2009. Modern homology modeling of G-protein coupled receptors: Which structural template to use? *J. Med. Chem.* 52(16): 5207–5216.

Moitessier, N., P. Englebienne, D. Lee, J. Lawandi, and C. R. Corbeil. 2008. Towards the development of universal, fast and highly accurate docking/scoring methods: A long way to go. *Br. J. Pharmacol.* 153(Suppl. 1): S7–S26.

Morley, S. D. and M. Afshar. 2004. Validation of an empirical RNA-ligand scoring function for fast flexible docking using Ribodock. *J. Comput. Aided Mol. Des.* 18(3): 189–208.

Morris, G. M., D. S. Goodsell, R. S. Halliday et al. 1998. Automated docking using a Lamarckian genetic algorithm and an empirical binding free energy function. *J. Comput. Chem.* 19(14): 1639–1662.

Morris, G. M., D. S. Goodsell, R. Huey, and A. J. Olson. 1996. Distributed automated docking of flexible ligands to proteins: Parallel applications of AutoDock 2.4. *J. Comput. Aided Mol. Des.* 10(4): 293–304.

Morris, G. M., R. Huey, W. Lindstrom et al. 2009. AutoDock4 and AutoDockTools4: Automated docking with selective receptor flexibility. *J. Comput. Chem.* 30(16): 2785–2791.

Muegge, I. 2000. A knowledge-based scoring function for protein-ligand interactions: Probing the reference state. *Persp. Drug Discov. Design* 20: 99–114.

Muegge, I. 2006. PMF scoring revisited. *J. Med. Chem.* 49(20): 5895–5902.

Muegge, I. and M. Rarey. 2001. Small molecule docking and scoring. In: *Reviews in Computational Chemistry*, K. B. Lipkowitz, and D. B. Boyd (Eds.), pp. 1–60, New York: Wiley-VCH.

Mukherjee, S., T. E. Balius, and R. C. Rizzo. 2010. Docking validation resources: Protein family and ligand flexibility experiments. *J. Chem. Inf. Model.* 50(11): 1986–2000.

Mysinger, M. M. and B. K. Shoichet. 2010. Rapid context-dependent ligand desolvation in molecular docking. *J. Chem. Inf. Model.* 50(9): 1561–1573.

Namasivayam, V. and R. Gunther. 2007. pso@autodock: A fast flexible molecular docking program based on Swarm intelligence. *Chem. Biol. Drug Des.* 70(6): 475–484.

Nandigam, R. K., S. Kim, J. Singh, and C. Chuaqui. 2009. Position specific interaction dependent scoring technique for virtual screening based on weighted protein-ligand interaction fingerprint profiles. *J. Chem. Inf. Model.* 49(5): 1185–1192.

Neudert, G. and G. Klebe. 2011. DSX: A knowledge-based scoring function for the assessment of protein-ligand complexes. *J. Chem. Inf. Model.* 51(10): 2731–2745.

Nichols, S. E., R. Baron, A. Ivetac, and J. A. McCammon. 2011. Predictive power of molecular dynamics receptor structures in virtual screening. *J. Chem. Inf. Model.* 51(6): 1439–1446.

Oda, A., K. Tsuchida, T. Takakura, N. Yamaotsu, and S. Hirono. 2006. Comparison of consensus scoring strategies for evaluating computational models of protein-ligand complexes. *J. Chem. Inf. Model.* 46(1): 380–391.

Oshiro, C. M. and I. D. Kuntz. 1998. Characterization of receptors with a new negative image: Use in molecular docking and lead optimization. *Proteins* 30(3): 321–336.

Ouyang, X., S. Zhou, C. T. Su, Z. Ge, R. Li, and C. K. Kwoh. 2013. Covalent Dock: Automated covalent docking with parameterized covalent linkage energy estimation and molecular geometry constraints. *J. Comput. Chem.* 34(4): 326–336.

Pang, Y. P., E. Perola, K. Xu, and F. G. Prendergast. 2001. EUDOC: A computer program for identification of drug interaction sites in macromolecules and drug leads from chemical databases. *J. Comput. Chem.* 22: 1750–1771.

Rarey, M., B. Kramer, and T. Lengauer. 1999. The particle concept: Placing discrete water molecules during protein-ligand docking predictions. *Proteins* 34(1): 17–28.

Rarey, M., B. Kramer, T. Lengauer, and G. Klebe. 1996a. A fast flexible docking method using an incremental construction algorithm. *J. Mol. Biol.* 261(3): 470–489.

Rarey, M., S. Wefing, and T. Lengauer. 1996b. Placement of medium-sized molecular fragments into active sites of proteins. *J. Comput. Aided Mol. Des.* 10(1): 41–54.

Roberts, B. C. and R. L. Mancera. 2008. Ligand-protein docking with water molecules. *J. Chem. Inf. Model.* 48(2): 397–408.

Rognan, D. 1998. Molecular dynamics simulations: A tool for drug design. *Persp. Drug Discov. Design* 9/10/11: 181–209.

Rohrig, U. F., A. Grosdidier, V. Zoete, and O. Michielin. 2009. Docking to heme proteins. *J. Comput. Chem.* 30(14): 2305–2315.

Schafferhans, A. and G. Klebe. 2001. Docking ligands onto binding site representations derived from proteins built by homology modelling. *J. Mol. Biol.* 307(1): 407–427.

Schmidt, T. C., A. Welker, M. Rieger et al. 2014. Protocol for rational design of covalently interacting inhibitors. *ChemPhysChem* 15(15): 3226–3235.

Schnecke, V. and L. A. Kuhn. 2000. Virtual screening with solvation and ligand-induced complementarity. *Persp. Drug Discov. Design* 20: 171–190.

Schroeder, J., A. Klinger, F. Oellien, R. J. Marhoefer, M. Duszenko, and P. M. Selzer. 2013. Docking-based virtual screening of covalently binding ligands: An orthogonal lead discovery approach. *J. Med. Chem.* 56(4): 1478–1490.

Seebeck, B., I. Reulecke, A. Kamper, and M. Rarey. 2008. Modeling of metal interaction geometries for protein-ligand docking. *Proteins* 71(3): 1237–1254.

Shoichet, B. K. and I. D. Kuntz. 1993. Matching chemistry and shape in molecular docking. *Protein Eng.* 6(7): 723–732.

Smith, G. R. and M. J. Sternberg. 2002. Prediction of protein-protein interactions by docking methods. *Curr. Opin. Struct. Biol.* 12(1): 28–35.

Sondergaard, C. R., M. H. M. Olsson, M. Rostkowski, and J. H. Jensen. 2011. Improved treatment of ligands and coupling effects in empirical calculation and rationalization of pK(a) values. *J. Chem. Theory Comput.* 7(7): 2284–2295.

Sotriffer, C. 2012. Scoring functions for protein-ligand interactions. In: *Protein-Ligand Interactions*, H. Gohlke (Ed.), pp. 237–263, Weinheim: Wiley-VCH.

Sotriffer, C. and G. Klebe. 2002. Identification and mapping of small-molecule binding sites in proteins: Computational tools for structure-based drug design. *Farmaco* 57(3): 243–251.

Sotriffer, C. and H. Matter. 2011. The challenge of affinity prediction: Scoring functions for structure-based virtual screening. In: *Virtual Screening. Principles, Challenges, and Practical Guidelines*, C. Sotriffer (Ed.), pp. 177–221, Weinheim: Wiley-VCH.

Sotriffer, C. A. 2011. Accounting for induced-fit effects in docking: What is possible and what is not? *Curr. Top. Med. Chem.* 11(2): 179–191.

Sotriffer, C. A., H. H. Ni, and J. A. McCammon. 2000. HIV-1 integrase inhibitor interactions at the active site: Prediction of binding modes unaffected by crystal packing. *J. Am. Chem. Soc.* 122(25): 6136–6137.

Sotriffer, C. A., M. Stahl, H. J. Boehm, and G. Klebe. 2003a. Docking and scoring functions/virtual screening. In: *Burger's Medicinal Chemistry and Drug Discovery*, 6th edition, D. J. Abraham (Ed.), pp. 281–333, New York: Wiley.

Sotriffer, C., M. Stahl, and G. Klebe. 2003b. The docking problem. In: *Handbook of Chemoinformatics*, J. Gasteiger (Ed.), pp. 1732–1768, Weinheim: Wiley-VCH.

Sotriffer, C. A., P. Sanschagrin, H. Matter, and G. Klebe. 2008. SFCscore: Scoring functions for affinity prediction of protein-ligand complexes. *Proteins* 73(2): 395–419.

Sousa, S. F., P. A. Fernandes, and M. J. Ramos. 2006. Protein-ligand docking: Current status and future challenges. *Proteins* 65(1): 15–26.

Sousa, S. F., A. J. Ribeiro, J. T. Coimbra et al. 2013. Protein-ligand docking in the new millennium—A retrospective of 10 years in the field. *Curr. Med. Chem.* 20(18): 2296–2314.

Sternberg, M. J., H. A. Gabb, and R. M. Jackson. 1998. Predictive docking of protein-protein and protein-DNA complexes. *Curr. Opin. Struct. Biol.* 8(2): 250–256.

Tang, H., X. S. Wang, J. H. Hsieh, and A. Tropsha. 2012. Do crystal structures obviate the need for theoretical models of GPCRs for structure-based virtual screening? *Proteins* 80(6): 1503–1521.

ten Brink, T. and T. E. Exner. 2009. Influence of protonation, tautomeric, and stereoisomeric states on protein-ligand docking results. *J. Chem. Inf. Model.* 49(6): 1535–1546.

ten Brink, T. and T. E. Exner. 2010. pK(a) based protonation states and microspecies for protein-ligand docking. *J. Comput. Aided Mol. Des.* 24(11): 935–942.

Thilagavathi, R. and R. L. Mancera. 2010. Ligand-protein cross-docking with water molecules. *J. Chem. Inf. Model.* 50(3): 415–421.

Thompson, D. C., C. Humblet, and D. Joseph-McCarthy. 2008. Investigation of MM-PBSA rescoring of docking poses. *J. Chem. Inf. Model.* 48(5): 1081–1091.

Thomsen, R. and M. H. Christensen. 2006. MolDock: A new technique for high-accuracy molecular docking. *J. Med. Chem.* 49(11): 3315–3321.

Totrov, M. and R. Abagyan. 1997. Flexible protein-ligand docking by global energy optimization in internal coordinates. *Proteins* 29(Suppl. 1): 215–220.

Totrov, M. and R. Abagyan. 2008. Flexible ligand docking to multiple receptor conformations: A practical alternative. *Curr. Opin. Struct. Biol.* 18(2): 178–184.

Trosset, J. Y. and H. A. Scheraga. 1998. Reaching the global minimum in docking simulations: A Monte Carlo energy minimization approach using Bezier splines. *Proc. Natl. Acad. Sci. USA* 95(14): 8011–8015.

Trosset, J. Y. and H. A. Scheraga. 1999. PRODOCK: Software package for protein modeling and docking. *J. Comput. Chem.* 20: 412–427.

Tuckerman, M. E. and G. J. Martyna. 2000. Understanding modern molecular dynamics: Techniques and applications. *J. Phys. Chem. B* 104: 159–178.

van Gunsteren, W. F. and H. J. C. Berendsen. 1990. Computer simulation of molecular dynamics: Methodology, applications, and perspectives in chemistry. *Angew. Chem. Int. Ed. Engl.* 29: 992–1023.

Velec, H. F., H. Gohlke, and G. Klebe. 2005. DrugScore(CSD)-knowledge-based scoring function derived from small molecule crystal data with superior recognition rate of near-native ligand poses and better affinity prediction. *J. Med. Chem.* 48(20): 6296–6303.

Verdonk, M. L., G. Chessari, J. C. Cole et al. 2005. Modeling water molecules in protein-ligand docking using GOLD. *J. Med. Chem.* 48(20): 6504–6515.

Wade, R. C., K. J. Clark, and P. J. Goodford. 1993. Further development of hydrogen bond functions for use in determining energetically favorable binding sites on molecules of known structure. 1. Ligand probe groups with the ability to form two hydrogen bonds. *J. Med. Chem.* 36(1): 140–147.

Wang, J., P. A. Kollman, and I. D. Kuntz. 1999. Flexible ligand docking: A multistep strategy approach. *Proteins* 36(1): 1–19.

Wang, J. M., R. M. Wolf, J. W. Caldwell, P. A. Kollman, and D. A. Case. 2004. Development and testing of a general amber force field. *J. Comput. Chem.* 25(9): 1157–1174.

Wang, R., L. Lai, and S. Wang. 2002. Further development and validation of empirical scoring functions for structure-based binding affinity prediction. *J. Comput. Aided Mol. Des.* 16(1): 11–26.

Warren, G. L., C. W. Andrews, A. M. Capelli et al. 2006. A critical assessment of docking programs and scoring functions. *J. Med. Chem.* 49(20): 5912–5931.

Wei, B. Q., W. A. Baase, L. H. Weaver, B. W. Matthews, and B. K. Shoichet. 2002. A model binding site for testing scoring functions in molecular docking. *J. Mol. Biol.* 322(2): 339–355.

Weiner, S. J., P. A. Kollman, D. T. Nguyen, and D. A. Case. 1986. An all atom force field for simulations of proteins and nucleic acids. *J. Comput. Chem.* 7: 230–252.

Weis, A., K. Katebzadeh, P. Soderhjelm, I. Nilsson, and U. Ryde. 2006. Ligand affinities predicted with the MM/PBSA method: Dependence on the simulation method and the force field. *J. Med. Chem.* 49(22): 6596–6606.

Westhead, D. R., D. E. Clark, and C. W. Murray. 1997. A comparison of heuristic search algorithms for molecular docking. *J. Comput. Aided Mol. Des.* 11(3): 209–228.

Xie, Z. R. and M. J. Hwang. 2010. An interaction-motif-based scoring function for protein-ligand docking. *BMC Bioinformatics* 11: 298.

Yin, S., L. Biedermannova, J. Vondrasek, and N. V. Dokholyan. 2008. MedusaScore: An accurate force field-based scoring function for virtual drug screening. *J. Chem. Inf. Model.* 48(8): 1656–1662.

Yuriev, E., M. Agostino, and P. A. Ramsland. 2011. Challenges and advances in computational docking: 2009 in review. *J. Mol. Recognit.* 24(2): 149–164.

Yuriev, E. and P. A. Ramsland. 2013. Latest developments in molecular docking: 2010–2011 in review. *J. Mol. Recognit.* 26(5): 215–239.

Zacharias, M. 2010. Accounting for conformational changes during protein-protein docking. *Curr. Opin. Struct. Biol.* 20(2): 180–186.

Zhang, X., X. Li, and R. Wang. 2009. Interpretation of the binding affinities of PTP1B inhibitors with the MM-GB/SA method and the X-score scoring function. *J. Chem. Inf. Model.* 49(4): 1033–1048.

Zilian, D. and C. A. Sotriffer. 2013. SFCscore(RF): A random forest-based scoring function for improved affinity prediction of protein-ligand complexes. *J. Chem. Inf. Model.* 53(8): 1923–1933.

Zoete, V., A. Grosdidier, M. Cuendet, and O. Michielin. 2010. Use of the FACTS solvation model for protein-ligand docking calculations. Application to EADock. *J. Mol. Recognit.* 23(5): 457–461.

7

Protein–Ligand Docking: Virtual Screening and Applications to Drug Discovery

Antonella Ciancetta and Stefano Moro

CONTENTS

7.1 Background

The term virtual screening (VS) was first reported in literature in 1997 (Horvath 1997), and refers to computational techniques aimed at stream-lining the drug discovery process through *in silico* identification of novel hits from large chemical libraries. In the early 1990s, the drug discovery paradigm was overturned by the introduction of high-throughput screen-ing (HTS) (Bleicher et al. 2003) and combinatorial chemistry (Geysen et al. 2003). These techniques promised to accelerate the drug discovery process by enabling the synthesis of large libraries of chemical compounds and the assay of their biological activity against several targets in a short period of time. However, the revolutionary approach soon proved to be expen-sive and not productive as expected, as many of the identified hits failed the lead optimization stage due to unsuitable pharmacokinetic properties. The development of alternative strategies to select appropriate compounds, while removing unsuitable structures, aimed at significantly reducing costs and required resources therefore became necessary. In the late 1990s, thanks to the advances in hardware and algorithms (Kitchen et al. 2004), the use of computational methodologies to identify *in silico* potential drug candidates became feasible and timely. Within this context, VS emerged as a strategy to reduce the time and cost of chemical synthesis and *in vitro* testing and currently represents an integral part of the drug discovery pipeline, both in the pharmaceutical industry and in academia. Depending on the amount of information available about the system of interest, VS is historically classified into two categories (Wilton et al. 2003): ligand-based virtual screening (LBVS) and structure-based virtual screening (SBVS). SBVS exploits knowledge about the three-dimensional (3D) structure of the target—gathered either experimentally by x-ray crystallography or nuclear magnetic resonance (NMR) spectroscopy, or computationally through homology modeling—and performs docking calculations to rank candi-dates on the basis of estimated binding affinity or complementarity to the binding site.

7.1.1 Designing an SBVS Study

A typical workflow of an SBVS protocol is depicted in Figure 7.1. The basic inputs are a target structure—achieved either experimentally or computa-tionally—and a library (Shoichet 2004) of compounds either physically avail-able (screening library) or synthetically feasible (virtual library). After the preparation of the input structures, each compound in the library is docked into the target-binding site. The fitness of the generated poses is then evalu-ated by a scoring function. This stage is often followed by a postprocessing phase, in which the compounds are ranked and selected on the basis of pre-defined criteria. Finally, a small subset of top-ranked compounds is chosen

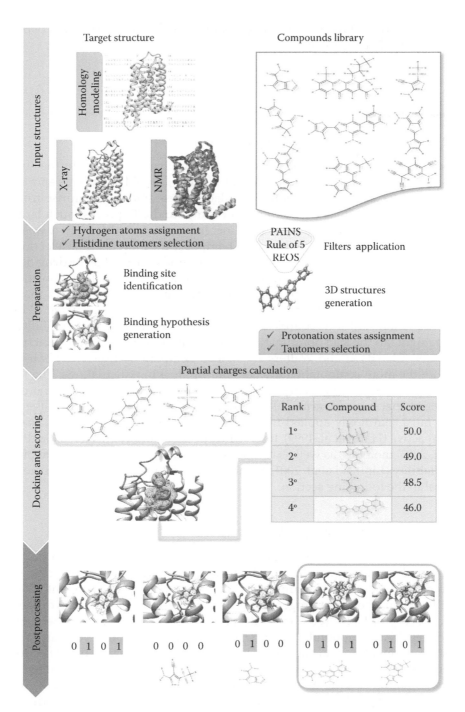

FIGURE 7.1
(**See color insert.**) General workflow of a VS experiment.

for the experimental assays. Each step of the workflow is explained in detail in Sections 7.2 through 7.6.

7.2 Compounds Library Preparation

The choice of the compounds library to screen is a key factor to the success of an SBVS project (Cummings et al. 2007). In Table 7.1, we report a list of chemical databases publicly available: these libraries comprise from tens of thousands to several millions of compounds. To process such large amount of compounds in a VS pipeline, however, would lead to a waste of time and computer resources and hamper a meaningful hits selection. Moreover, those libraries often enclose compounds unsuitable for drug discovery purposes, such as molecules containing reactive or toxic moieties (toxicophores), scaffolds that might interfere with biological assays (pan-assay interference compounds [PAINS]) giving rise to "false positives" (FP), or simply molecules with undesirable physical properties (poor solubility) that might fail the lead optimization phase. Therefore, it is common practice to filter (Charifson and Walters 2000) such compounds from the libraries before the more computationally demanding docking calculations. The filters usually rely on molecular connectivity and do not require 3D coordinates, so that large libraries (10^5–10^6 compounds) can be rapidly processed. The most commonly applied filtering strategies discard compounds bearing reactive (Hann et al. 1999), toxic (Muegge 2003), or promiscuous (Seidler et al. 2003) moieties, as well as compounds predicted to have poor oral bioavailability (Lipinski et al. 2001). Some of these filters are described in more detail in the following section.

7.2.1 Property Filters: Lipinski Rule of Five

The Lipinski "rule of five" (Lipinski et al. 2001) was derived from a statistical analysis of known drugs, which revealed that a high percentage of compounds possessed common features, such as molecular weight ≤ 500, $\log P \leq 5$, number of hydrogen bond donors ≤ 5, and number of hydrogen bond acceptors ≤ 10 (see Table 7.2). From this analysis, it was therefore deduced that compounds violating this rule might exhibit poor absorption or permeation and therefore cannot represent suitable candidates for oral bioavailable drugs. Exceptions to this generalization are encountered for compounds acting as substrates for transporters. This is the case for many natural products such as antibiotics, cardiac glycosides, and antifungal agents.

TABLE 7.1

List of Libraries of Compounds Publicly Available Online

Database Name	Webpage	Cpds #	Ref.
BindingDB	http://www. bindingdb.org/	453,657	Liu et al. (2007)
ChemDB	http://cdb.ics.uci. edu/	~5 millions	Chen et al. (2007)
Chem ID	http://chem.sis.nlm. nih.gov/ chemidplus/	404,318	ChemIDplus Advanced-Chemical Information with Searchable Synonyms, Structures, and Formulas (2014)
ChemBank	http://chembank. broadinstitute.org	1,204,720	Seiler et al. (2007)
ChEMBL	https://www.ebi. ac.uk/chembl/	1,411,786	Gaulton et al. (2012)
Chemical Entities of Biological Interest (ChEBI)	http://www.ebi. ac.uk/chebi/init.do	41,036	Hastings et al. (2013)
Chemical Structure Lookup Service	http://cactus.nci. nih.gov/cgi-bin/ lookup/search	46 millions	Chemical Structure Lookup Service (2014)
ChemMine	http://chemminedb. ucr.edu/	>6,200,000	Girke (2005)
ChemSpider	http://www. chemspider.com/	32 millions	ChemSpider	Search and Share Chemistry (2014)
Commercial Compound Collection (CoCoCo)	http://cococo.unibo. it/	~7 millions	Del Rio et al. (2010)
Developmental Therapeutics Program (DTP)	http://cactus.nci. nih.gov/ncidb2.2/	250,250	Developmental Therapeutics Program NCI/NIH (2014)
DrugBank	http://www. drugbank.ca/	7,740	Wishart et al. (2007)
Edinburgh University Ligand Selection System (EDULISS)	http://eduliss.bch. ed.ac.uk/	5 millions	Hsin et al. (2011)
Ligand.Info	http://ligand.info/	1,159,274	von Grotthuss et al. (2003)
MMsINC	http://mms.dsfarm. unipd.it/MMsINC/ search	4 millions	Masciocchi et al. (2009)
Mother of All Databases (MOAD)	http://www. bindingmoad.org/	11,173	Hu et al. (2005)
PubChem	https://pubchem. ncbi.nlm.nih.gov/	55,093,940	Bolton et al. (2008)
Therapeutic Target Database	http://bidd.nus.edu. sg/group/cjttd/	17,816	Zhu et al. (2012)
Traditional Chinese Medicine Database (TCM)	http://tcm.cmu.edu. tw/	37,170	Chen (2011)
ZINC	http://zinc.docking. org/	35 millions	Irwin et al. (2012)

TABLE 7.2

Lipinski Rule of Five Criteria

Property	Threshold Value
Molecular weight	500
log P	5
Number of hydrogen bond donor (OH, NH groups)	5
Number of hydrogen bond acceptor (O, N atoms)	10

7.2.2 Functional Group Filters: REOS

The Rapid Elimination of Swill (REOS) (Walters and Namchuk 2003) method discards problematic molecules (swills) from compounds libraries through the combination of functional group filters and counting schemes. Initial filtering is based on properties such as molecular weight, log P, number of hydrogen bond donors, number of hydrogen bond acceptors, formal charge, number of rotatable bonds, and number of heavy atoms. In a subsequent step, the compounds are filtered on the basis of about 200 rules detecting the presence of problematic substructures. The rules are in the form of SMARTS strings and were collected from literature data reporting functional groups acting as promiscuous ligands and/or frequent hitters. The default values for the property filters are listed in Table 7.3 and examples of detected functional groups are presented in Figure 7.2. Both rules and filters can be customized to the specific needs of the screening procedure.

7.2.3 Substructure Filters: PAINS

PAINS (Baell and Holloway 2010) are the major source of FP in VS campaigns (Thorne et al. 2010). The interference mechanism can be either direct on the assay signaling (Inglese et al. 2007; Shapiro et al. 2009) as is the case of strongly colored or fluorescent molecules, or indirect on components (proteins or reagents) of the assay system (Thorne et al. 2010). In the latter case, PAINS

TABLE 7.3

Default Values for REOS Property Filters

Property Min Max	Min	Max
Molecular weight	200	500
log P	−5	5
HB donors	0	5
HB acceptors	0	10
Formal charge	−2	2
Number of rotatable bonds	0	8
Number of heavy atoms	15	50

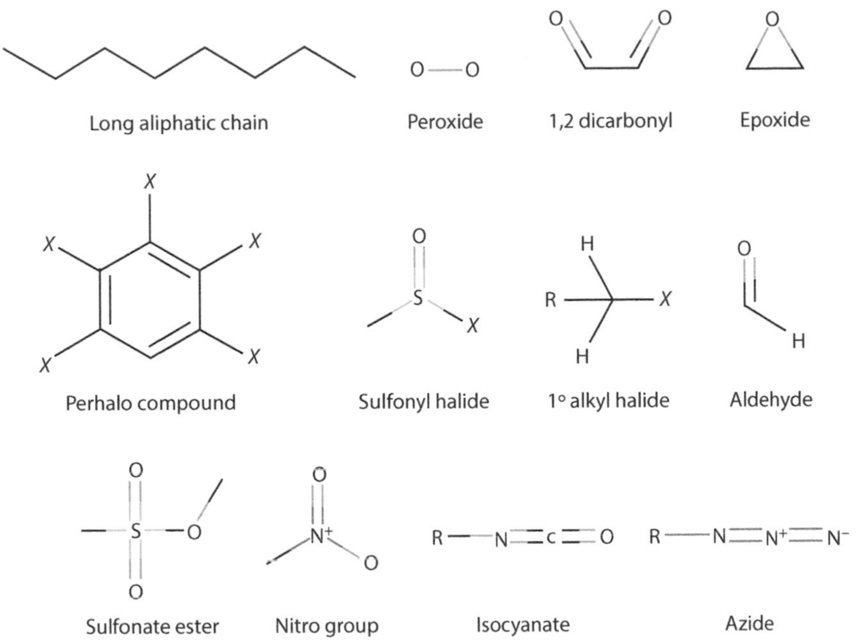

FIGURE 7.2
Examples of functional groups detected by the REOS filtering approach.

can undergo redox cycling (thus producing hydrogen peroxide) (Baell 2011), covalent binding to proteins (Rishton 2003), or metal ion chelation (Rishton 1997). Recently, a collection of 480 PAINS substructures have been reported in literature. Moreover, substructure filters that encode for such compounds have been developed and released. The structures have been grouped into 30 main (broad) classes, although the majority of the compounds enclose only 16 substructures, listed in Table 7.4 along with representative SMARTS strings. An overview of the most commonly encountered PAINS substructures is given in Figure 7.3.

7.2.4 Target-Based Filters: Pharmacophores

Another strategy to be avoided in order to process undesirable structure is to design so-called "focused" or "targeted" libraries. By contrast to "general" libraries—that are of broad interest for VS against any target-focused libraries are aimed at a family of related targets, whereas targeted libraries are aimed at a single therapeutic target. These libraries may be derived from general libraries by applying pharmacophore-based filters, which encode specific geometric and physicochemical features required to achieve binding, as deduced from observed ligand–target complexes.

TABLE 7.4

List of Main Structural Classes Recognized as PAINS

Structural Class	Example of SMART String Representation
Rhodanines	[#7]-1-[#6](= [#16])-[#16]-[#6](= [#6])-[#6]-1 = [#8]
Phenolic mannich bases	[#7]-[#6;X4]-c:1:c:c:c:c:c:1-[#8]-[#1]
Hydroxyphenylhydrazones	c:1:c:c(:c(:c:c:1)-[#6] = [#7]-[#7])-[#8]-[#1]
Alkylidene barbiturates	[#6]-1(-[#6](~[!#6&!#1] ~ [#6]-[!#6&!#1]-[#6]-1 = [!#6&!#1]) ~ [!#6&!#1]) = [#6;!R]-[#1]
Alkylidenes of 5-membered heterocycles	[#6]-1(= [#6])-[#6] = [#7]-[!#6&!#1]-[#6]-1 = [#8]
Fused tetrahydroquinolines	c:1:c:c-2:c(:c:c:1)-[#6]-3-[#6](-[#6]-[#7]-2)-[#6]-[#6] = [#6]-3
Pyrroles	n2(-[#6]:1:[!#1]:[#6]:[#6]:[#6]:[#6]:1)c(cc(c2-[#6;X4])-[#1])-[#6;X4]
Benzofurazans	[#7](-c:1:c:c:c:c:c:1)-[#16](=[#8])(=[#8])-[#6]:2:[#6]:[#6]:[#6]:[#6]:3: [#7]:[$([#8]),$([#16])]:[#7]:[#6]:2:3
2-Amino-3-carbonyl-thiophenes	[#7](-[#1])(-[#1])-c:1:c(:c(:c(:s:1)-[!#1])-[!#1])-[#6] = [#8]
Catechols	c:1:c:c(:c(:c:c:1)-[#8]-[#1])-[#8]-[#1]
Quinones	[!#6&!#1] = [#6]-1-[#6] =,:[#6]-[#6](= [!#6&!#1])-[#6] =,:[#6]-1
Azo compounds	[#7;!R] = [#7]
Cyanopyridones	[#6]-1(= [!#1]-[!#1] = [!#1]-[#7](-[#6]-1 = [#16])-[#1])-[#6]#[#7]
Divinylketones	[#6] = !@[#6](-[!#1])-@[#6](= !@[!#6&!#1])-@[#6](= !@[#6])-[!#1]
Indoles	n:1(c(c(c:2:c:1:c:c:c:c:2-[#1])-[#6;X4]-[#1])-[$([#6](-[#1])-[#1]),$([#6] = ,:[!#6&!#1]),$([#6](-[#1])-[#7]),$([#6](-[#1])(-[#6](-[#1])-[#1])-[#6](-[#1])(-[#1])-[#7](-[#1])-[#6](-[#1])-[#1])])-[$([#1]),$([#6](-[#1])-[#1])]
Tertiary anilines	[#6](-[#1])(-[#1])-[#7](-[#6](-[#1])-[#1])-c:1:c:c(:c(:c:c:1)-[$([#1]),$([#6](-[#1])-[#1]),$([#8]-[#6](-[#1])(-[#1])-[#6](-[#1])-[#1])])-[#7])-[#1]

7.2.5 Generating Compounds 3D Coordinates

Typically, information about the compounds to be screened is stored in the libraries in 2D formats, mainly line notations as SMILES (Weininger 1988), InChi (Heller et al. 2013), or SLN (Ash et al. 1997). However, the majority of docking programs requires 3D conformations as input structures. It is therefore necessary to expand the 2D representation of the compounds into 3D coordinates. This is usually performed with specialized tools such as CORINA (Sadowski and Gasteiger 1993), OMEGA (Hawkins et al. 2010), or CONCORD (Pearlman 1987). The generation of proper compounds tautomeric, stereoisomeric, and protonation states (Rapp et al. 2009; ten Brink and Exner 2010) is also fundamental for the successful outcome of the subsequent docking calculation. Special attention has to be paid to the assigned atom and bond types and to the geometry of undefined chiral centers: improperly assigned chirality and wrong atom types might strongly affect the conformational search and the resulting docking pose. Moreover, depending on

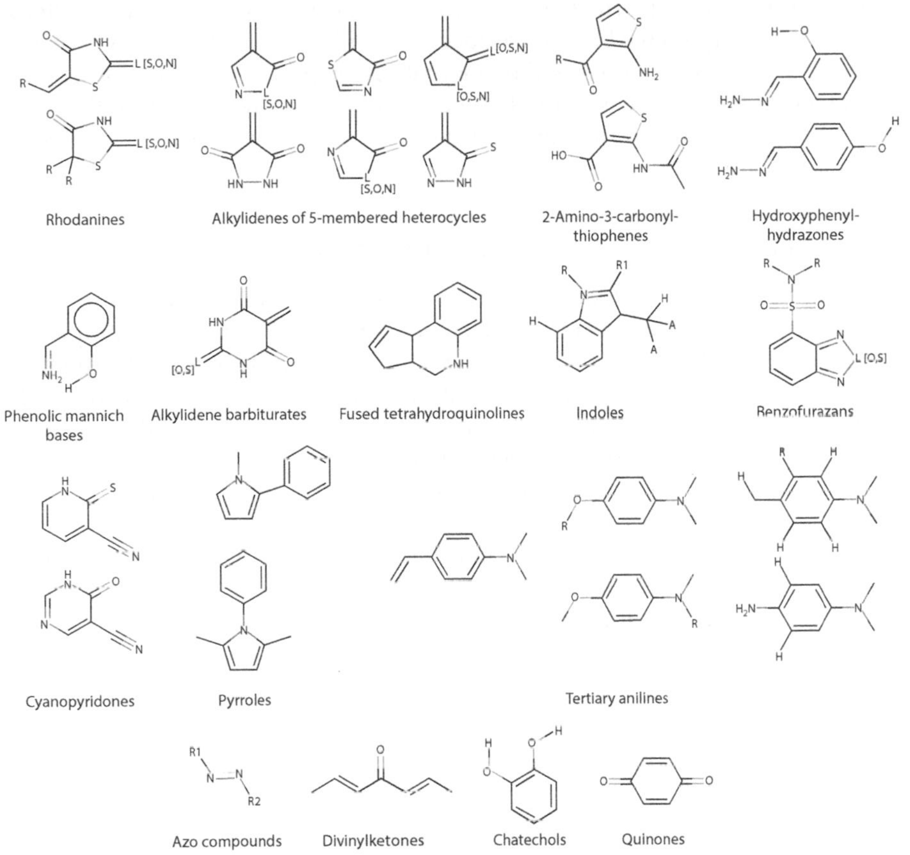

Rhodanines   Alkylidenes of 5-membered heterocycles   2-Amino-3-carbonyl-thiophenes   Hydroxyphenyl-hydrazones

Phenolic mannich bases   Alkylidene barbiturates   Fused tetrahydroquinolines   Indoles   Benzofurazans

Cyanopyridones   Pyrroles   Tertiary anilines

Azo compounds   Divinylketones   Chatechols   Quinones

FIGURE 7.3
Representation of most commonly encountered PAINS substructures.

the specific docking engine that will be used in the screen, it might also be necessary to assign atomic partial charges to the compounds.

7.3 Protein Preparation

The preparation of the protein structure is also a crucial step in SBVS. At medium resolution, hydrogen atoms are usually not solved in x-ray structures. To perform docking calculation, it is therefore necessary to add hydrogen atoms to the target structure. This is, however, not a trivial task, as it implies the assignment of appropriate protonation states to ionizable residues in the active site and the selection of correct tautomeric states for histidine residues. After hydrogen atoms have been added to the structure, it is also customary to perform an energy minimization to release eventual steric clashes that might have been introduced. Also for the protein structure, the preparation phase comprises the calculation of partial atomic charges. At this stage, the structure is ready to be carefully inspected to define the location and size of the binding site and derive at least one binding hypothesis that will guide hits selection.

7.3.1 Binding Site Identification and Inspection

In case experimental structures are available, the selection of the binding site is usually guided by the placement of the ligand in the complexes. Otherwise, the definition of binding cavity can be performed with the help of either available experimental data (mutagenesis) or specific software packages (Brylinski and Skolnick 2008; Capra et al. 2009; Roy et al. 2012). In either case, the size of the binding site needs to be carefully chosen, as it can affect the efficiency and outcome of the VS procedure: if a too small binding site is defined, potential ligands not fitting into it will be discarded; however, if a too large binding site is set much computational time will be spent in exploring regions that are not interesting. From the analysis of the binding site, a binding hypothesis is usually formulated: one or more key interactions, that all compounds should satisfy to be selected, are identified.

7.4 Docking

The docking of each compound of the library into the binding site is the most computationally demanding step of the VS procedure. As the docking methodology has been already discussed in Chapter 6, we will only discuss the following two aspects that influence the outcome of VS studies: the flexibility of the target structure and the role of water molecules.

7.4.1 Target Flexibility

A basic assumption when performing docking calculations, in general, and in the VS scenario, in particular, is that the target structure is held fixed in its initial conformation. Proteins, however, are dynamic entities and the binding site often adapts upon ligand binding through conformational changes that might involve small side-chain flips as well as the motion of larger protein portions. Although several studies have highlighted that proper consideration of target flexibility can improve the results (Rueda et al. 2009) of VS campaigns, it is still challenging to incorporate this aspect in modern docking algorithms (Cavasotto and Singh 2008). An attempt to take protein flexibility into account in SBVS is the use of a structural ensemble, obtained either from several experimental snapshots or generated by molecular dynamics (MD) simulations. However, the ensemble docking strategy requires that for each considered conformation of the target an individual docking run is performed. This practice is still computationally expensive in the VS context, therefore the choice of the pool of alternative conformations is usually limited to a few units.

7.4.2 Water Molecules

It is widely recognized that water molecules play an important role in ligand recognition. The contribution of water molecules in protein–ligand binding can either be of enthalpic or entropic nature, although the best-investigated role is the mediation of ligand–target interactions through hydrogen bonds networks (Lu et al. 2007). Although it has been demonstrated that including water molecules in docking calculations can improve VS performances (Thilagavathi and Mancera 2010), taking this aspect into account in docking calculations is still a challenging task. This methodological shortcoming arises from the difficulty to correctly predict the number and placement of water molecules into the binding site. To address this issue, sophisticated MD-based methods have been developed (Young et al. 2007; Abel et al. 2008; Michel et al. 2009; Sabbadin et al. 2014). However, these approaches are too computationally demanding to be applied for VS purposes. On the contrary, several strategies have also been proposed to account for water molecules orientation during docking calculations and this setting is currently available with several software packages. This approach, however, suffers from treating water molecules as fixed part of the protein, thus not taking into account that water arrangements depend on the size, shape, and physicochemical properties of the ligands. A solution to this issue has been proposed by a novel approach that attaches water molecules to the ligands during docking simulations (Lie et al. 2011). The proposed method, however, introduces additional degrees of freedom to the ligands and requires a modification of the scoring function to add an entropy penalty term, which accounts for water loss of rotational and translational degrees of freedom. Both features make the application of this new approach still unfeasible in the VS context.

7.5 Scoring

Once a conformation has been generated for each compound in the library, a scoring function evaluates the quality of the pose with respect to other poses of the same compound, and finally ranks the pose selected for each compound with respect to other molecules in the database. In the VS context, the scoring function is asked to handle several thousand of compounds rapidly. This implies that, despite the wide choice of scoring functions available, only the fastest ones are used in practice. To date, scoring functions represent the Achilles' heel of the docking methodology. Their inadequacy at correctly predicting binding affinities is widely recognized (Warren et al. 2006). As a consequence, if hits selection were based on the rank ordering as resulted from the docking calculations, a high number of FP would be retrieved. A popular strategy to address this issue is the use of consensus scoring as described in the following section.

7.5.1 Consensus Scoring

A common practice to reduce the number of FP in VS is to combine the results of several different scoring functions, a method usually referred to as "consensus scoring" (Charifson et al. 1999). According to this approach, multiple scoring functions are used to score the top-ranked poses and the poses common to each scoring function are selected. Several studies in literature have reported that this method enables a better accuracy with respect to the use of a single scoring function (Huang et al. 2006; Cheng et al. 2009; Chang et al. 2010; Kukol 2011). However, it has to be pointed out that the performance of individual scoring functions should be assessed prior to applying consensus scoring in order to choose the most appropriate combination for the system of interest.

7.6 Hit Selection and Confirmation

The VS of a compound library against a target yields a large amount of data comprising the predicted binding pose for each compound along with the estimated binding affinity. Of these compounds only a small subset will be tested for biological assays. Hits selection is, therefore, a crucial step in SBVS. Although in principle the selection could be made on the basis of the rank ordering or, as described in the previous paragraph, on the basis of the consensus score, it is strongly recommended to apply additional postprocessing strategies in order to minimize the number of FP. Among the devised postprocessing approaches, several automated methods (Deng et al. 2004; Kroemer et al. 2004; Marcou and Rognan 2007; Bouvier et al. 2010; Radifar et al. 2013; Ciancetta et al. 2014; Da and Kireev 2014) have been developed that focus on verifying that a previously defined binding hypothesis is satisfied. According to these strategies, only the docking poses that establish key interactions or exhibit a certain degree of surface complementarity with the binding pocket are selected. We describe in more detail a couple of these approaches in the following section. As in the case of the application of consensus scoring, it is advisable, before applying the above-mentioned methods, to calibrate them, whenever possible, with a set of ligands for which binding modes and affinities are known. Furthermore, visual inspection of the poses of selected hits is usually performed to ensure that both the ligand–protein interactions and the ligand conformation are reasonable.

7.6.1 Postprocessing Strategies

The underlying idea of *interaction fingerprints* is to encode, either explicitly (Marcou and Rognan 2007; Radifar et al. 2013) or implicitly (Da and Kireev 2014), the 3D information of ligand–protein key interactions into a binary string that can be easily managed and enables fast comparison of large amount of docking poses. A common filtering metrics used is the similarity of the strings derived from all the generated docking poses to a chosen reference compound. Notably, very recently a Python-based open source tool (Radifar et al. 2013) to compute interaction fingerprints has been developed and released. The program relies on OpenBabel (O'Boyle et al. 2011) chemical library, which is freely available at http://code.google.com/p/pyplif, and can be further developed or modified according to the specific needs.

An alternative approach to postprocess docking poses is represented by the Automatic analysis of Poses using *Self-Organizing Map* (AuPosSOM) method (Bouvier et al. 2010). This strategy ranks and clusters docking poses according to ligand–protein interactions encoded into mathematical vectors. The results of the clustering analyses are reported in a hierarchical tree, where compounds with similar binding modes belong to the same leave. Interestingly, this approach exploits information of all poses of the docked compound simultaneously. Therefore, each compound mean vectors are calculated that bear information about all the poses, their cluster size, and conformation frequencies. The tool is freely available at https://www.bio-medicale.univ-paris5.fr/aupossom.

7.6.2 Hit Selection Criteria

Once careful selection and inspection of docking poses have been performed, the next step is the synthesis or purchase of selected hits for experimental assays. The number of compounds left at this stage usually depends upon the resources available. Moreover, to reduce costs, usually additional criteria are applied to narrow the hits list. Method such as structure clustering is usually applied to favor chemical diversity in the selection, whereas ADME/Tox (Wang 2009; Gleeson et al. 2011; Huggins et al. 2011) prediction tools or drug-likeness (Walters and Murcko 2002) filters are used to aid the selection of scaffolds amenable for pharmaceutical purposes. Another widely applied yet controversial metrics for hit selection is ligand efficiency (LE) (Kuntz et al. 1999; Hopkins et al. 2004). LE is the estimated binding free energy of a ligand normalized by its molecular size, expressed in terms of heavy atom count (HAC, Equation 7.1).

$$LE = \frac{(-2.303RT)}{HAC} \times \log K_D \qquad (7.1)$$

At standard conditions (300 K, 1 M concentrations, and neutral pH), the −2.303RT term approximates to −1.37 kcal/mol. As recently pointed out, LE suffers from several deficiencies (Shultz 2014) and alternative more sophisticated metrics have been proposed (Leeson and Springthorpe 2007; Reynolds et al. 2008; Nissink 2009). In particular, it has been highlighted that LE varies for different targets (Hopkins et al. 2014) and all heavy atoms are counted the same, irrespective of the nature of the functional group they belong to. Nevertheless, judicious application of LE in conjunction with other property descriptors that counterbalance its weaknesses can be a valid help in the final selection of the chemical entities to test.

The final step of a VS campaign is to confirm the predicted activity of the selected hits with specific *in vitro* assays. This stage is of paramount importance for the successful outcome of the VS campaign, as well as for subsequent hit-to-lead and lead optimization steps. Screening assay results and potential artifacts should be carefully analyzed. The activity of the hits should be confirmed, whenever possible, by secondary assays, such as direct biophysical binding assays, orthogonal assays, or structural biology studies (Inglese et al. 2007). Moreover, pharmacological promiscuity should also be prevented by counterscreens to confirm the selectivity, especially for hits targeting kinases and G protein-coupled receptor (GPCRs).

7.7 Metrics to Evaluate the Performances of VS Protocols

A standard practice before conducting VS campaigns is to perform retrospective or benchmark studies to evaluate the performances of different methods in retrieving active compounds from inactive ones. Generally, the studies are more reliable if experimentally verified inactive compounds are available. In practice, this piece of information is difficult to achieve. Therefore, it is a common practice (Verdonk et al. 2004) to resort to the so-called "decoys" sets. Decoys are molecules putatively inactive against the target of interest, sharing similar physicochemical properties with the active compounds. Decoys are usually commercially available compounds that might be eventually purchased and tested to confirm inactivity. However, for prospective screening, decoys need to be synthetically feasible but not necessarily real

(Wallach and Lilien 2011). The largest database of decoys available to public is the Directory of Useful Decoys (DUD) (Huang et al. 2006), a collection of 36 decoys for each of the 2950 active molecules collected for 40 different targets. The DUD is a subset of the ZINC database and is available at http://dud.docking.org/. Very recently, a decoys library specific for GPCRs with 39 decoy molecules selected for each ligand has been released (Gatica and Cavasotto 2012).

Several metrics have been proposed to assess the success of retrospective SBVS studies (Kirchmair et al. 2008). They are usually divided into classic and advanced metrics: classic metrics evaluate the ability of the VS protocol to discriminate actives from decoys, whereas advanced metrics take into account the so-called "early recognition problem" by introducing a weighting factor that favors protocols ranking active molecules at the top of the list (Truchon and Bayly 2007). After discussing some fundamental definition, we will describe in the following only the most commonly used measures, such as the enrichment factor (EF), the receiver operating characteristic (ROC) curve, and the area under the receiver operating characteristic curve (AUC).

7.7.1 Evaluation Metrics: Fundamental Definitions

The result of a VS campaign is the selection of n molecules from a library of N compounds (Figure 7.4). The selected hits might enclose active molecules or "true positives" (TP) and decoys or "false positives" (FP). Active molecules that are not in the selected hits are defined "false negatives" (FN), whereas the unselected decoys represent "true negatives" (TN).

The *sensitivity* (Se, Equation 7.2) or TP rate describes the ratio of the number of active molecules retrieved by the VS protocol with respect to the number of all active compounds in the library.

$$Se = \frac{\text{selected actives}}{\text{total actives}} = \frac{TP}{TP + FN} \qquad (7.2)$$

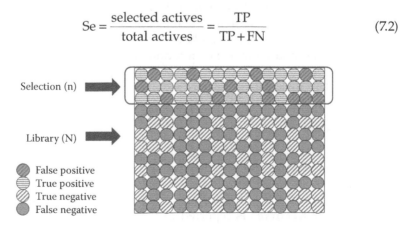

FIGURE 7.4
(See color insert.) Selection of n compounds from a library of N entries.

Se can vary between 0 (all active compounds missed) and 1 (all active compounds selected) and provide insights on the FN: the closer to 1 is the value, the lower is their number and the better is the protocol in retrieving active compounds.

The *specificity* (Sp, Equation 7.3) or FP rate represents the ratio of the number of inactive compounds that were not selected by the VS protocol with respect to the number of all inactive molecules in the library.

$$Sp = \frac{discarded\ inactives}{total\ inactives} = \frac{TN}{TN + FP} \qquad (7.3)$$

Sp can vary between 0 (all inactive compounds selected) and 1 (all inactive compounds discarded), and provide insights on the FP: the closer to 1 is the value, the lower is their number and the better is the VS protocol in discarding inactive compounds.

7.7.2 Enrichment Factor

The enrichment factor (EF, Equation 7.4) describes the improvement of the hit rate as compared to a random selection. It is usually referred to the percentage of the ranked list screened and is expressed as the ratio of active compounds in the selected subset divided by the number of active compounds in a randomly chosen subset of equal size.

$$EF_\% = \frac{TP/n}{A/N} = \frac{TP}{(TP + FN)} \times \frac{N}{n} \qquad (7.4)$$

where A is the total number of active compounds in the library of N compounds. A VS protocol with EF equals to 1 is equally good as random selection. As frequently highlighted (Triballeau et al. 2005; Kirchmair et al. 2008), the EF metrics suffers from several deficiencies: it depends upon the ratio of active molecules and all active compounds contribute equally to the value, as no distinction is made between those at the top and the ones at the end of the rank-ordered list.

7.7.3 ROC Curves

The ROC curve represents the TP rate as a function of the FP rate. The curve is obtained by plotting the "activity signal" (TP rate, Se) versus the "detected noise" (FP rate, $1 - Sp$) at various activity thresholds. This implies that quantitative activity measures are required to perform such analysis. A theoretical depiction of ROC curves is reported in Figure 7.5: A VS protocol that performs random distribution causes the ROC curve to tend to the $Se = 1 - Sp$ line (a diagonal rising from the origin to the upper right corner), whereas

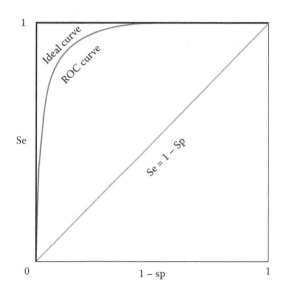

FIGURE 7.5
Examples of ROC curves.

a VS protocol able to detect the correct signal would have an ROC plot that curves above that diagonal. For ideal distributions, the curve rises vertically to the upper-left corner and then runs horizontally to the upper-right corner. Therefore, the more an ROC curve bends toward the upper-left corner, the better the VS protocols perform at separating active from inactive compounds.

7.7.4 AUC Plots

A different way to interpret the results of ROC plots is to derive the area under the ROC curve (AUC). The AUC is a metrics useful to assess the probability that the screening method assigns higher ranks to randomly chosen active compounds than to inactive compounds. The AUC at a specific percentage of the ranked library is calculated as the sum of all rectangles formed by the Se and $1 - Sp$ values for the different thresholds Equation 7.5.

$$\text{AUC} = \sum_{i}^{n} \left[(Se_{i+1})(Sp_{i+1} - Sp_i) \right] \qquad (7.5)$$

The AUC value is 1 for an ideal distribution, whereas a random distribution yields an AUC value of 0.5. VS protocols that perform better than random return AUC values between 0.5 and 1, whereas VS protocols that assign better scores to inactive compounds yield AUC values lower than 0.5.

7.8 Some Recent Successful Stories

Over the past two decades, SBVS has been successfully applied to identify new lead compounds. We briefly describe below a couple of exemplar VS studies on two widely investigated target families, Kinases and GPCRs, of paramount pharmaceutical interest.

7.8.1 Case Study on Kinases

Kinases are one of the largest families of enzymes. These multidomain proteins play an important role in several biological processes, especially in the signaling pathways that control cell proliferation and differentiation. Downregulation of such cellular events is implicated in many disorders, including inflammatory diseases and cancer (Catapano and Manji 2008; Zhang et al. 2009). Nowadays, protein kinases represent about 25% of putative drug targets.

A VS campaign on fibroblast growth factors receptor 1 (FGFR1) kinase has led to the discovery of new scaffold for inhibitors development (Ravindranathan et al. 2010). The two most potent identified hits showed potencies falling into the low micromolar range ($IC_{50} = 23$ and $50\,\mu M$), whereas subsequent lead optimization led to a compound with significantly enhanced potency ($IC_{50} = 1.9\,\mu M$).

Two alternative enzyme conformations taken from the same crystallographic snapshot (PDB ID: 3JS2) were used for the prospective VS study. The ZINC database consisting of 2.2 million small molecules was selected as compounds library. Multiple protonation and tautomeric states were generated for the molecules and 41 known FGFR1 inhibitors were included in the collection to assess the ability of the VS protocol to place them in the top-ranked list. A binding hypothesis to filter docking poses was also defined: poses not reporting at least one hydrogen bond with either Glu562 or Ala564 were discarded.

A first docking run with a fast-scoring function was performed. The resulting top 40,000 poses were then docked with a more accurate scoring function. The top 1000 compounds for both conformations from this second docking run were also docked into five additional kinase structures, to select compounds that could selectively inhibit FGFR1. Only compounds that were ranked in the top 100 for FGFR1 but not in the top 100 for any of the other five kinases were further processed. Finally, after careful visual inspection of the selected protein–ligand complexes and the check of ligand conformational strain in the pose, 23 compounds were purchased and tested *in vitro* for inhibition of FGFR1 kinase. Two of the 23 compounds resulted active. Subsequently, Monte Carlo/free-energy perturbation calculations were applied to compute relative free energies of binding in order to guide initial modifications of active compounds, leading to the final structure.

7.8.2 Case Study on GPCRs

GPCRs are the largest family of surface receptor. The human genome encodes for more than 800 members of this superfamily. Owing to their participation in several physiopathologic processes, about 350 member of this superfamily represent potential drug targets for the treatment of, among other diseases, cardiovascular and mental disorders (Moreno et al. 2013), cancer (O'Hayre et al. 2014), and viral infections (Sodhi et al. 2004). Currently, about 50% of marketed drugs act by interfering with a GPCR-mediated signaling pathway.

A VS campaign on dopamine D3 receptor (D3R) led to the discovery of 22 novel ligands being either D3R antagonists or negative allosteric modulators (Lane et al. 2013). The highest achieved binding affinity and antagonism potency were both in the nanomolar range ($K_i = 77$ nM and $IC_{50} = 57$ nM).

Retrospective VS studies were performed to assess the ability of the selected screening protocol to retrieve known ligands from decoys. For the benchmark study, the human D3R crystallographic structure in complex with etoclopride (PDB ID: 3PBL) was used as target structure. The selected compounds library consisted of 28 known selective antagonists with affinities values in the low nanomolar range collected from the ChEMBL database (Gaulton et al. 2012) and 300 randomly chosen decoys compiled from the Chemdiv library of commercially available drug-like compounds.

Two different receptor models (based on the 3PBL template) were used for the prospective VS studies: a model with the empty binding site representing the receptor in the apo state and a model with the binding site occupied by dopamine representing the receptor in the agonist-bound state. The models were constructed with the aim to search for ligands targeting either the orthosteric binding site (apo state) and putative allosteric sites on the extracellular side (dopamine bound state).

For each receptor model, an independent VS campaign was performed. A screening library of 4.1 million compounds was prepared from the Molsoft ScreenPub library of drug-like compounds available from chemical vendors by filtering compounds with reactive groups and molecular weight exceeding 500 Da. The top 300 compounds in each model hit list as ranked by the docking scores were selected and clustered by chemical similarity. Finally, up to 25 compounds for each model were selected for ligand binding and functional assays on the basis of predicted LE values, chemical properties, and onshelf availability from vendors.

7.9 Challenges and Perspectives

SBVS is a drug discovery strategy routinely applied both in pharmaceutical companies and in academic groups. Being a computational methodology based on molecular docking, SBVS faces all its challenges: to tackle target flexibility, to account for the role of water molecules in ligand binding, and to accurately estimate entropic contributions in a computationally feasible and timely fashion. As briefly discussed in this chapter, the main issue that hampers the progress of the field concerns the quality of the scoring functions employed. Although in principle for VS purposes, scoring functions do not necessarily need for ranking true hits correctly, but they should simply be able to discern true hits from decoys, the numbers of FP remains high.

We are confident that the progress in the development of computational methodologies and algorithms will solve or at least efficiently address these issues in the next decade. Moreover, much effort is currently devoted to streamlining the entire computational procedure through the development of user-friendly tools that fully automatize VS protocols. However, as hopefully as we have been able to show, VS is much more than just a docking exercise. The difference for a successful outcome of a VS campaign can be made by the attention paid in the preparation of the input structures and in the analysis of the output docking poses. The wise application of filtering and postprocessing strategies and after all their judicious application after careful calibration can help in minimizing the risk of wasting money and resources with nonpromising drug candidates.

After all, as Louis Pasteur said, "chance favors only the prepared mind."

References

Abel, R., T. Young, R. Farid, B. J. Berne, and R. A. Friesner. 2008. Role of the active-site solvent in the thermodynamics of factor Xa ligand binding. *J. Am. Chem. Soc.* 130(9): 2817–2831.

Ash, S., M. A. Cline, R. W. Homer, T. Hurst, and G. B. Smith. 1997. SYBYL Line Notation (SLN): A versatile language for chemical structure representation. *J. Chem. Inf. Model.* 37(1): 71–79.

Baell, J. B. 2011. Redox-active nuisance screening compounds and their classification. *Drug Discov. Today* 16(17–18): 840–841.

Baell, J. B. and G. A. Holloway. 2010. New substructure filters for removal of Pan Assay Interference Compounds (PAINS) from screening libraries and for their exclusion in bioassays. *J. Med. Chem.* 53(7): 2719–2740.

Bleicher, K. H., H.-J. Böhm, K. Müller, and A. I. Alanine. 2003. A guide to drug discovery: Hit and lead generation: Beyond high-throughput screening. *Nat. Rev. Drug Discov.* 2(5): 369–378.

Bolton, E. E., Y. Wang, P. A. Thiessen, and S. H. Bryant. 2008. PubChem: Integrated platform of small molecules and biological activities. *Annu. Rep. Comput. Chem.*, 4: 217–241.

Bouvier, G., N. Evrard-Todeschi, J.-P. Girault, and G. Bertho. 2010. Automatic clustering of docking poses in virtual screening process using self-organizing map. *Bioinformatics* 26(1): 53–60.

Brylinski, M. and J. Skolnick. 2008. A threading-based method (FINDSITE) for ligand-binding site prediction and functional annotation. *Proc. Natl. Acad. Sci. USA* 105(1): 129–134.

Capra, J. A., R. A. Laskowski, J. M. Thornton, M. Singh, and T. A. Funkhouser. 2009. Predicting protein ligand binding sites by combining evolutionary sequence conservation and 3D structure. *PLoS Comput. Biol.* 5(12): e1000585.

Catapano, L. A. and H. K. Manji. 2008. Kinases as drug targets in the treatment of bipolar disorder. *Drug Discov. Today* 13(7–8): 295–302.

Cavasotto, C. and N. Singh. 2008. Docking and high throughput docking: Successes and the challenge of protein flexibility. *Curr. Comput. Aided Drug Des.* 4(3): 221–234.

Chang, M. W., C. Ayeni, S. Breuer, and B. E. Torbett. 2010. Virtual screening for HIV protease inhibitors: A comparison of AutoDock 4 and Vina. *PloS One* 5(8): e11955.

Charifson, P.l S., J. J. Corkery, M. A. Murcko, and W. P. Walters. 1999. Consensus scoring: A method for obtaining improved hit rates from docking databases of three-dimensional structures into proteins. *J. Med. Chem.* 42(25): 5100–5109.

Charifson, P. S. and W. P. Walters. 2000. Filtering databases and chemical libraries. *Mol. Divers.* 5(4): 185–197.

Chemical Structure Lookup Service. 2014. Accessed November 18. http://cactus.nci.nih.gov/cgi-bin/lookup/search.

ChemIDplus Advanced–Chemical Information with Searchable Synonyms, Structures, and Formulas. 2014. Accessed November 18. http://chem.sis.nlm.nih.gov/chemidplus/.

ChemSpider | Search and Share Chemistry. 2014. Accessed November 18. http://www.chemspider.com/.

Chen, C. Y.-C. 2011. TCM Database: The world's largest traditional Chinese medicine database for drug screening *in silico*. Edited by Andreas Hofmann. *PLoS ONE* 6(1): e15939. doi:10.1371/journal.pone.0015939.

Chen, J. H., E. Linstead, S. J. Swamidass, D. Wang, and P. Baldi. 2007. ChemDB update full-text search and virtual chemical space. *Bioinformatics* 23(17): 2348–2351.

Cheng, T., X. Li, Y. Li, Z. Liu, and R. Wang. 2009. Comparative assessment of scoring functions on a diverse test set. *J. Chem. Inf. Model.* 49(4): 1079–1093.

Ciancetta, A., A. Cuzzolin, and S. Moro. 2014. Alternative quality assessment strategy to compare performances of GPCR-ligand docking protocols: The human adenosine A $_{2A}$ receptor as a case study. *J. Chem. Inf. Model.* 54(8): 2243–2254.

Cummings, M. D., A. C. Maxwell, and R. L. DesJarlais. 2007. Processing of small molecule databases for automated docking. *Med. Chem.* 3(1): 107–113.

Da, C. and D. Kireev. 2014. Structural Protein–Ligand Interaction Fingerprints (SPLIF) for structure-based virtual screening: Method and benchmark study. *J. Chem. Inf. Model.* 54(9): 2555–2561.

Del Rio, A., A. J. Moura Barbosa, F. Caporuscio, and G. F. Mangiatordi. 2010. CoCoCo: A free suite of multiconformational chemical databases for high-throughput virtual screening purposes. *Mol. BioSyst.* 6(11): 2122.

Deng, Z., C. Chuaqui, and J. Singh. 2004. Structural Interaction Fingerprint (SIFt): A novel method for analyzing three-dimensional protein-ligand binding interactions. *J. Med. Chem.* 47(2): 337–344.

Developmental Therapeutics Program NCI/NIH. 2014. Accessed November 18. http://dtp.nci.nih.gov/.

Gatica, E. A. and C. N. Cavasotto. 2012. Ligand and decoy sets for docking to G protein-coupled receptors. *J. Chem. Inf. Model.* 52(1): 1–6.

Gaulton, A., L. J. Bellis, A. P. Bento, J. Chambers, M. Davies, A. Hersey, Y. Light et al. 2012. ChEMBL: A large-scale bioactivity database for drug discovery. *Nucleic Acids Res.* 40(D1): D1100–D1107.

Geysen, M. H., F. Schoenen, D. Wagner, and R. Wagner. 2003. A guide to drug discovery: Combinatorial compound libraries for drug discovery: An ongoing challenge. *Nat. Rev. Drug Discov.* 2(3): 222–230.

Girke, T. 2005. ChemMine. A compound mining database for chemical genomics. *Plant Physiol.* 138(2): 573–577.

Gleeson, M. P., A. Hersey, D. Montanari, and J. Overington. 2011. Probing the links between *in vitro* potency, ADMET and physicochemical parameters. *Nat. Rev. Drug Discov.* 10(3): 197–208.

Hann, M., B. Hudson, X. Lewell, R. Lifely, L. Miller, and N. Ramsden. 1999. Strategic pooling of compounds for high-throughput screening. *J. Chem. Inf. Model.* 39(5): 897–902.

Hastings, J., P. de Matos, A. Dekker, M. Ennis, B. Harsha, N. Kale, V. Muthukrishnan et al. 2013. The ChEBI reference database and ontology for biologically relevant chemistry: Enhancements for 2013. *Nucleic Acids Res.* 41(D1): D456–D463.

Hawkins, P. C. D., A. G. Skillman, G. L. Warren, B. A. Ellingson, and M. T. Stahl. 2010. Conformer generation with OMEGA: Algorithm and validation using high quality structures from the protein databank and Cambridge structural database. *J. Chem. Inf. Model.* 50(4): 572–584.

Heller, S., A. McNaught, S. Stein, D. Tchekhovskoi, and I. Pletnev. 2013. InChI–the worldwide chemical structure identifier standard. *J. Cheminform.* 5(1): 7.

Hopkins, A. L., C. R. Groom, and A. Alex. 2004. Ligand efficiency: A useful metric for lead selection. *Drug Discov. Today* 9(10): 430–431.

Hopkins, A. L., G. M. Keserü, P. D. Leeson, D. C. Rees, and C. H. Reynolds. 2014. The role of ligand efficiency metrics in drug discovery. *Nat. Rev. Drug Discov.* 13(2): 105–121.

Horvath, D. 1997. A virtual screening approach applied to the search for trypanothione reductase inhibitors. *J. Med. Chem.* 40(15): 2412–2423.

Hsin, K.-Y., H. P. Morgan, S. R. Shave, A. C. Hinton, P. Taylor, and M. D. Walkinshaw. 2011. EDULISS: A small-molecule database with data-mining and pharmacophore searching capabilities. *Nucleic Acids Res.* 39(Database issue): D1042–D1048.

Huang, N., B. K. Shoichet, and J. J. Irwin. 2006. Benchmarking sets for molecular docking. *J. Med. Chem.* 49(23): 6789–6801.

Huggins, D. J., A. R. Venkitaraman, and D. R. Spring. 2011. Rational methods for the selection of diverse screening compounds. *ACS Chem. Biol.* 6(3): 208–217.

Hu, L., M. L. Benson, R. D. Smith, M. G. Lerner, and H. A. Carlson. 2005. Binding MOAD (Mother Of All Databases). *Proteins* 60(3): 333–340.

Inglese, J., R. L. Johnson, A. Simeonov, M. Xia, W. Zheng, C. P. Austin, and D. S. Auld. 2007. High-throughput screening assays for the identification of chemical probes. *Nat. Chem. Biol.* 3(8): 466–479.

Irwin, J. J., T. Sterling, M. M. Mysinger, E. S. Bolstad, and R. G. Coleman. 2012. ZINC: A free tool to discover chemistry for biology. *J. Chem. Inf. Model.* 52(7): 1757–1768.

Kirchmair, J., P. Markt, S. Distinto, G. Wolber, and T. Langer. 2008. Evaluation of the performance of 3D virtual screening protocols: RMSD comparisons, enrichment assessments, and decoy selection—What can we learn from earlier mistakes? *J. Comput. Aided Mol. Des.* 22(3–4): 213–228.

Kitchen, D. B., H. Decornez, J. R. Furr, and J. Bajorath. 2004. Docking and scoring in virtual screening for drug discovery: Methods and applications. *Nat. Rev. Drug Discov.* 3(11): 935–949.

Kroemer, R. T., A. Vulpetti, J. J. McDonald, D. C. Rohrer, J.-Y. Trosset, F. Giordanetto, S. Cotesta, C. McMartin, M. Kihlén, and P. F. W. Stouten. 2004. Assessment of docking poses: Interactions-Based Accuracy Classification (IBAC) versus crystal structure deviations. *J. Chem. Inf. Comput. Sci.* 44(3): 871–881.

Kukol, A. 2011. Consensus virtual screening approaches to predict protein ligands. *Eur. J. Med. Chem.* 46(9): 4661–4664.

Kuntz, I. D., K. Chen, K. A. Sharp, and P. A. Kollman. 1999. The maximal affinity of ligands. *Proc. Natl. Acad. Sci. USA* 96(18): 9997–10002.

Lane, J. R., P. Chubukov, W. Liu, M. Canals, V. Cherezov, R. Abagyan, R. C. Stevens, and V. Katrich. 2013. Structure-based ligand discovery targeting orthosteric and allosteric pockets of dopamine receptors. *Mol. Pharmacol.* 84(6): 794–807.

Leeson, P. D. and B. Springthorpe. 2007. The influence of drug-like concepts on decision-making in medicinal chemistry. *Nat. Rev. Drug Discov.* 6(11): 881–890.

Lie, M. A., R. Thomsen, C. N. S. Pedersen, B. Schiøtt, and M. H. Christensen. 2011. Molecular docking with ligand attached water molecules. *J. Chem. Inf. Model.* 51(4): 909–917.

Lipinski, C. A., F. Lombardo, B. W. Dominy, and P. J. Feeney. 2001. Experimental and computational approaches to estimate solubility and permeability in drug discovery and development settings. *Adv. Drug Deliv. Rev.* 46(1–3): 3–26.

Liu, T., Y. Lin, X. Wen, R. N. Jorissen, and M. K. Gilson. 2007. BindingDB: A web-accessible database of experimentally determined protein-ligand binding affinities. *Nucleic Acids Res.* 35(Database issue): D198–D201.

Lu, Y., R. Wang, C.-Y. Yang, and S. Wang. 2007. Analysis of ligand-bound water molecules in high-resolution crystal structures of protein-ligand complexes. *J. Chem. Inf. Model.* 47(2): 668–675.

Marcou, G. and D. Rognan. 2007. Optimizing fragment and scaffold docking by use of molecular interaction fingerprints. *J. Chem. Inf. Model.* 47(1): 195–207.

Masciocchi, J., G. Frau, M. Fanton, M. Sturlese, M. Floris, L. Pireddu, P. Palla, F. Cedrati, P. Rodriguez-Tomé, and S. Moro. 2009. MMsINC: A large-scale chemoinformatics database. *Nucleic Acids Res.* 37(Database issue): D284–D290.

Michel, J., J. Tirado-Rives, and W. L. Jorgensen. 2009. Prediction of the water content in protein binding sites. *J. Phys. Chem. B* 113(40): 13337–13346.

Moreno, J. L., T. Holloway, and J. González-Maeso. 2013. G protein-coupled receptor heterocomplexes in neuropsychiatric disorders. *Prog. Mol. Biol. Transl. Sci.* 117: 187–205.

Muegge, I. 2003. Selection criteria for drug-like compounds. *Med. Res. Rev.* 23(3): 302–321.

Nissink, J. W. M. 2009. Simple size-independent measure of ligand efficiency. *J. Chem. Inf. Model.* 49(6): 1617–1622.

O'Boyle, N. M., M. Banck, C. A. James, C. Morley, T. Vandermeersch, and G. R. Hutchison. 2011. Open babel: An open chemical toolbox. *J. Cheminf.* 3(1): 33.

O'Hayre, M., M. S. Degese, and J. S. Gutkind. 2014. Novel insights into G protein and G protein-coupled receptor signaling in cancer. *Curr. Opin. Cell Biol.* 27: 126–135.

Pearlman, R. S. 1987. Rapid generation of high quality approximate 3D molecular structures. *Chem. Des. Auto. News* 2: 1–7.

Radifar, M., N. Yuniarti, and E. P. Istyastono. 2013. PyPLIF: Python-based protein-ligand interaction fingerprinting. *Bioinformation* 9(6): 325–328.

Rapp, C. S., C. Schonbrun, M. P. Jacobson, C. Kalyanaraman, and N. Huang. 2009. Automated site preparation in physics-based rescoring of receptor ligand complexes. *Proteins* 77(1): 52–61.

Ravindranathan, K. P., V. Mandiyan, A. R. Ekkati, J. H. Bae, J. Schlessinger, and W. L. Jorgensen. 2010. Discovery of novel fibroblast growth factor receptor 1 kinase inhibitors by structure-based virtual screening. *J. Med. Chem.* 53(4): 1662–1672.

Reynolds, C. H., B. A. Tounge, and S. D. Bembenek. 2008. Ligand binding efficiency: Trends, physical basis, and implications. *J. Med. Chem.* 51(8): 2432–2438.

Rishton, G. M. 1997. Reactive compounds and *in vitro* false positives in HTS. *Drug Discov. Today* 2(9): 382–384.

Rishton, G. M. 2003. Nonleadlikeness and leadlikeness in biochemical screening. *Drug Discov. Today* 8(2): 86–96.

Roy, A., J. Yang, and Y. Zhang. 2012. COFACTOR: An accurate comparative algorithm for structure-based protein function annotation. *Nucleic Acids Res.* 40(W1): W471–W477.

Rueda, M., G. Bottegoni, and R. Abagyan. 2009. Consistent improvement of cross-docking results using binding site ensembles generated with elastic network normal modes. *J. Chem. Inf. Model.* 49(3): 716–725.

Sabbadin, D., A. Ciancetta, and S. Moro. 2014. Perturbation of fluid dynamics properties of water molecules during G protein-coupled receptor–ligand recognition: The human A $_{2A}$ adenosine receptor as a key study. *J. Chem. Inf. Model.* 54(10): 2846–2855.

Sadowski, J. and J. Gasteiger. 1993. From atoms and bonds to three-dimensional atomic coordinates: Automatic model builders. *Chem. Rev.* 93(7): 2567–2581.

Seidler, J., S. L. McGovern, T. N. Doman, and B. K. Shoichet. 2003. Identification and prediction of promiscuous aggregating inhibitors among known drugs. *J. Med. Chem.* 46(21): 4477–4486.

Seiler, K. P., G. A. George, M. P. Happ, N. E. Bodycombe, H. A. Carrinski, S. Norton, S. Brudz et al. 2007. ChemBank: A small-molecule screening and cheminformatics resource database. *Nucleic Acids Res.* 36(Database issue): D351–D359.

Shapiro, A. B., G. K. Walkup, and T. A. Keating. 2009. Correction for interference by test samples in high-throughput assays. *J. Biomol. Screen.* 14(8): 1008–1016.

Shoichet, B. K. 2004. Virtual screening of chemical libraries. *Nature* 432(7019): 862–865.

Shultz, M. D. 2014. Improving the plausibility of success with inefficient metrics. *ACS Med. Chem. Letters* 5(1): 2–5.

Sodhi, A., S. Montaner, and J. S. Gutkind. 2004. Viral hijacking of G-protein-coupled-receptor signalling networks. *Nat. Rev. Mol. Cell Biol.* 5(12): 998–1012.

ten Brink, T. and T. E. Exner. 2010. pKa based protonation states and microspecies for protein–ligand docking. *J. Comput. Aided Mol. Des.* 24(11): 935–942.

Thilagavathi, R. and R. L. Mancera. 2010. Ligand–Protein cross-docking with water molecules. *J. Chem. Inf. Model.* 50(3): 415–421.

Thorne, N., D. S. Auld, and J. Inglese. 2010. Apparent activity in high-throughput screening: Origins of compound-dependent assay interference. *Curr. Opin. Chem. Biol.* 14(3): 315–324.

Triballeau, N., F. Acher, I. Brabet, J.-P. Pin, and H.-O. Bertrand. 2005. Virtual screening workflow development guided by the "Receiver Operating Characteristic" curve approach. Application to high-throughput docking on metabotropic glutamate receptor subtype 4. *J. Med. Chem.* 48(7): 2534–2547.

Truchon, J.-F. and C. I. Bayly. 2007. Evaluating virtual screening methods: Good and bad metrics for the "Early Recognition" problem. *J. Chem. Inf. Model.* 47(2): 488–508.

Verdonk, M. L., V. Berdini, M. J. Hartshorn, W. T. M. Mooij, C. W. Murray, R. D. Taylor, and P. Watson. 2004. Virtual screening using protein-ligand docking: Avoiding artificial enrichment. *J. Chem. Inf. Model.* 44(3): 793–806.

von Grotthuss, M., J. Pas, and L. Rychlewski. 2003. Ligand-info, searching for similar small compounds using index profiles. *Bioinformatics* 19(8): 1041–1042.

Wallach, I. and R. Lilien. 2011. Virtual decoy sets for molecular docking benchmarks. *J. Chem. Inf. Model.* 51(2): 196–202.

Walters, W. P. and M. A. Murcko. 2002. Prediction of "Drug-Likeness." *Adv. Drug Deliv. Rev.* 54(3): 255–271.

Walters, W. P. and M. Namchuk. 2003. A guide to drug discovery: Designing screens: How to make your hits a hit. *Nat. Rev. Drug Discov.* 2(4): 259–266.

Wang, J. 2009. Comprehensive assessment of ADMET risks in drug discovery. *Curr. Pharm. Des.* 15(19): 2195–2219.

Warren, G. L., C. W. Andrews, A.-M. Capelli, B. Clarke, J. LaLonde, M. H. Lambert, M. Lindvall et al. 2006. A critical assessment of docking programs and scoring functions. *J. Med. Chem.* 49(20): 5912–5931.

Weininger, D. 1988. SMILES, a chemical language and information system. 1. Introduction to methodology and encoding rules. *J. Chem. Inf. Model.* 28(1): 31–36.

Wilton, D., P. Willett, K. Lawson, and G. Mullier. 2003. Comparison of ranking methods for virtual screening in lead-discovery programs. *J. Chem. Inf. Model.* 43(2): 469–474.

Wishart, D. S., C. Knox, A. C. Guo, D. Cheng, S. Shrivastava, D. Tzur, B. Gautam, and M. Hassanali. 2007. DrugBank: A knowledgebase for drugs, drug actions and drug targets. *Nucleic Acids Res.* 36(Database issue): D901–D906.

Young, T., R. Abel, B. Kim, B. J. Berne, and R. A. Friesner. 2007. Motifs for molecular recognition exploiting hydrophobic enclosure in protein-ligand binding. *Proc. Natl. Acad. Sci. USA* 104(3): 808–813.

Zhang, J., P. L. Yang, and N. S. Gray. 2009. Targeting cancer with small molecule kinase inhibitors. *Nat. Rev. Cancer* 9(1): 28–39.

Zhu, F., Z. Shi, C. Qin, L. Tao, X. Liu, F. Xu, L. Zhang et al. 2012. Therapeutic target database update 2012: A resource for facilitating target-oriented drug discovery. *Nucleic Acids Res.* 40(D1): D1128–D1136.

8

Protein Structure Modeling in Drug Design

Damián Palomba and Claudio N. Cavasotto

CONTENTS

8.1 Introduction

Homology or comparative, also known as template-based modeling, is a technique aimed at predicting an unknown protein structure (target or query receptor) from a homologous protein (template) whose three-dimensional (3D) structure has been experimentally solved (Fiser 2004). The premise of this methodology lies in the assumption that homologous proteins, which share a detectable sequence similarity, have similar 3D structures, that is, the extent of structural changes is directly related to the extent of sequence changes. Thus, the expected degree of success in predicting the structure of a protein from its sequence, using structures of known homologous proteins, depends on the extent of sequence identity or similarity (Chothia and Lesk 1986). It should be noted, however, that in some protein families such as G protein-coupled receptors (GPCRs) (Cavasotto and Phatak 2009), the 3D structure is more conserved than their amino-acid sequences.

The 3D structures of proteins are often extracted from the Protein Data Bank (PDB) (Berman et al. 2000, 2002), which collects ~108,000 experimentally solved structures (May 2015). Nowadays, even though the number of experimental structures in the PDB has enormously increased during the last 10 years, a huge surge of new sequences triggered by progress in DNA sequencing technology (Activities at the Universal Protein Resource [UniProt] 2014) renders unfeasible to experimentally determine the 3D structures of all therapeutic relevant proteins, at least with current techniques (Schwede 2013). Moreover, and specifically concerning membrane proteins such as GPCRs, there are additional challenges in obtaining diffracting crystals so as to achieve x-ray structures (Congreve et al. 2014). Thus, homology modeling

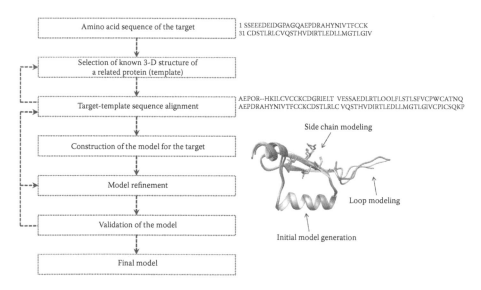

FIGURE 8.1
Simplified flowchart of the comparative modeling process. The first stage involves selecting homologous sequences to align them to the target sequence. Next, a target-template sequence alignment is carried out. If the alignment is not satisfactory, other templates can be selected. Based on the alignment, an initial model is built, which must be refined at the backbone, side chains, and loops level. The refined model is validated and, if successful, conserved. Otherwise, the process should be re-examined. In some cases, after model evaluation, the whole process should be started allover even from the alignment stage in order to adjust and rebuild the model. (Figure prepared using Chimera [https://www.cgl.ucsf.edu/chimera/]).

appears as an appealing tool that, while with limitations, has many uses in structure-based drug discovery. Depending on the accuracy of the obtained model, which in turn depends, among other things, on the sequence similarity between target and template, homology modeling can provide medium-quality models, well suited to construct site-directed mutants (Vernal et al. 2002), and high-quality models comparable to low-resolution x-ray structures or medium-resolution nuclear magnetic resonance (NMR) (Ohlendorf 1994; Sanchez and Sali 1997b).

In comparative modeling, the following sequential steps can be distinguished (Figure 8.1):

(1) Selection of one (or more) known 3D structure(s) from a sequence homologue protein, which is used as a template; (2) target-template sequence alignment; (3) construction of an initial model for the target based on the template structure and the sequence alignment; and (4) refinement of the initial model, validation and evaluation of the model. Each of these steps, which involve different technical aspects, could be iterated in order to generate a positive feedback in the entire process and, finally, to obtain an acceptable model (Marti-Renom et al. 2000).

8.2 Homology Modeling Procedure

8.2.1 Selection of Template Structures of Related Proteins

8.2.1.1 Amino Acid Sequence of the Target

To start working on homology modeling, the user must identify the sequence of the target protein. There are several databases where the protein sequences can be extracted, such as the ExPASy Proteomics Server (http://www.expasy.org) (Bioinformatics Resource Portal from the Swiss Institute of Bioinformatics, which provides access to scientific databases and software tool, e.g., UniProt Knowledgebase -UniProtKB-) (Artimo et al. 2012), and NCBI (http://www.ncbi.nlm.nih.gov/protein) (Acland et al. 2014) (Figure 8.2).

8.2.1.2 Template Selection

After retrieving the target protein sequence, the user must select a suitable template structure. To do so, there should be a detectable similarity between the template and the target protein. The template structure can be extracted from databases such as the PDB (RCSB Protein Data Bank [RCSB PDB][http://www.rcsb.org/pdb/home/home.do]) (Berman et al. 2014), SCOP (Structural Classifications of Proteins 2 [SCOP2] [http://scop2.mrc-lmb.cam.ac.uk/]) (Andreeva et al. 2014), and CATH (Protein Structure Classification Database at UCL [CATH] [http://www.cathdb.info/]) (Sillitoe et al. 2013), by using the target sequence as the query. There are several statistical measures to

>sp|P29274|AA2AR_HUMAN Adenosine receptor A2a OS=Homo sapiens GN=ADORA2A PE=1 SV=2
MPIMGSSVYITVELAIAVLAILGNVLVCWAVWLNSNLQNVTNYFVVSLAAADIAVGVLAI
PFAITISTGFCAACHGCLFIACFVLVLTQSSIFSLLAIAIDRYIAIRIPLRYNGLVTGTR
AKGIIAICWVLSFAIGLTPMLGWNNCGQPKEGKNHSQGCGEGQVACLFEDVVPMNYMVYF
NFFACVLVPLLLMLGVYLRIFLAARRQLKQMESQPLPGERARSTLQKEVHAAKSLAIIVG
LFALCWLPLHIINCFTFFCPDCSHAPLWLMYLAIVLSHTNSVVNPFIYAYRIREFRQTFR
KIIRSHVLRQQEPFKAAGTSARVLAAHGSDGEQVSLRLNGHPPGVWANGSAPHPERRPNG
YALGLVSGGSAQESQGNTGLPDVELLSHELKGVCPEPPGLDDPLAQDGAGVS

FIGURE 8.2
A sample FASTA file of the sequence for Human A_{2A} Adenosine Receptor. Each sequence line contains less than 80 characters.

quantify similarity, such as E-value and Z-score, depending on the approach adopted.

Ideally, one would search for a high identity match between the target and the template, covering the full span of the sequence. However, in many cases, this is not possible, and multiple templates covering non-overlapping regions are a way to model the target "by pieces." It has been shown that better results are obtained with several templates than with a single one, at least below 40% target-template sequence identity (Fernandez-Fuentes et al. 2007). Even the use of multiple templates covering overlapping regions and displaying a certain degree of structural conformational diversity is usually useful since it allows the use of multiple sequence alignments (MSAs), which are generally more accurate than pairwise ones.

As a general rule, the crystal structure with the highest sequence homology to the receptor is chosen, although this rule has been lately questioned (Rataj et al. 2014). However, other criteria could be taken into account in the selection of the template(s), such as a specific functional conformation (active or inactive state of the receptor), bound- or apo-structure, experimental accuracy (e.g., number of restraints per residue in NMR structures, and resolution and R-factor in x-ray structures), biological information (pH, solvent, quaternary interactions), metal ionic state in metalloproteins, and conservation of residues in the active site. Furthermore, it is worth noting that even the same template structure could lead to large differences in the resulting homology model (Rataj et al. 2014).

The degree of sequence identity or similarity between target and template, is an accepted criterion that indicates the "confidence" of the model (i.e., if target and template actually share a common fold). The threshold value of sequence identity widely accepted is 30% (Cavasotto and Phatak 2009; Lushington 2015), although Chothia and Lesk in their pioneering article (Chothia and Lesk 1986) proposed a 50% identity to find highly similar structures with less than 1 Å of root-mean-square deviation ([RMSD], distance between corresponding Cα atoms). While model quality is usually related to sequence similarity, this rule does not necessarily apply to all cases. The family of membrane proteins GPCRs displays a strong conservation of the transmembrane (TM) structure even at low sequence identity (lower than 20%) (Cavasotto and Phatak 2009; Gonzalez et al. 2014). On the contrary, an overall high-sequence identity may either mask dissimilarities in flexible regions like loops (Cavasotto and Phatak 2009) or ignore other already-stated factors such as a specific functional conformation, which can greatly influence the accuracy of a model.

There are different methods of target-template alignment, which are described in the next section.

8.2.2 Target-Template Sequence Alignment

Even though there are different classifications, in general, three main types of sequence–structure relationships can be identified:

1. Pairwise sequence alignment approaches for related protein sequences with >30% sequence similarity (Figure 8.3). These methods compare the sequences of the target with those of a template database using a substitution matrix and penalties for gap initiation and extension. Two of the most used programs are BLAST (Altschul et al. 1997) and FASTA (Lipman and Pearson 1985; Pearson 1994). The advantage of this strategy lies in its speed, as it allows comparing thousands of sequences in a short period of time. It should be mentioned that for alignments to be accurate in a structural sense, a range of 40–50% sequence identity and few or no gaps might be necessary (Venclovas 2012). The downside of these methods is low sensitivity since they are not able to identify remote homologs.

2. Sequence-profile and profile–profile alignment methods are used in the "twilight zone," which corresponds to relationships with statistically significant sequence identity (10–30% sequence similarity). The profile of a sequence stems from a MSA and determines the occurrences of each type of residue for each alignment position.

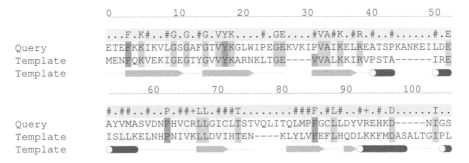

FIGURE 8.3
Example of a sequence alignment. The type of residue conservation is showed above the Query sequence. The Template secondary structure (α-helices, β-sheets, loops) is also displayed below its sequence. (Alignment and figure prepared with ICM program [http://www.molsoft.com]).

There are two main types of profiles: The position-specific scoring matrix (PSSM) (Henikoff and Henikoff 1994), and the Hidden Markov Model (HMM) (Krogh et al. 1994; Eddy 1998). In this type of method the profile of the target sequence is utilized to seek template sequences in a database. Profile-based algorithms perform much better than pairwise sequence-based methods (Sauder et al. 2000). There are several computer programs for profile-sequence alignment such as BUILD_PROFILE (part of MODELLER [Sali and Blundell 1993]), PSI-BLAST (Altschul et al. 1997), SAM (Karplus et al. 1998), HHsearch (Soding 2005), and HHBlits (Remmert et al. 2012). The profile-sequence alignment methods have paved the way for the rise of profile–profile alignment approaches, which seek proper template structures by scanning the profile of the target sequence versus a database of template profiles (instead of template sequences). These methods have outperformed profile-sequence alignment strategies (Ohlson et al. 2004; Wang and Dunbrack 2004). FFAS (Jaroszewski et al. 2005), HHsearch (Soding 2005), and SP3 (Zhou and Zhou 2005) are some examples of computer programs that use profile–profile algorithms.

3. *Threading methods*: These are employed when it is not possible to build sequence profiles (below the "twilight zone"). In this technique, the target sequence is matched against a library of 3D profiles in terms of residue-by-residue similarity. Since sequence identity is often less useful for evaluating threading templates, a consensus Z-score is employed with the aim of measuring statistical significance for the quality of a candidate template. The Z-score offers insight into the likelihood of both target and template belonging to a common protein family, sharing a common fold, or having no evident relationship. GenTHREADER (McGuffin and Jones 2003), 3D-PSSM (Kelley et al. 2000), and MUSTER (Wu and Zhang 2008) are frequently used threading programs.

Methods of MSA align a set of homologous sequences already detected by other methods. These approaches may be utilized not only to improve the quality of MSA, but also to directly align target to template, as long as both template and target are in the set of sequences to be aligned. In practice, MSA methods can usually generate good alignments using moderate computational resources. Many MSA tools utilize heuristics known as progressive alignment. ClustalW (Larkin et al. 2007) and ClustalΩ (Sievers et al. 2011) are examples of computer programs that employ this strategy. In order to address the inaccuracies of progressive alignment, an iterative refinement is sometimes performed. Two MSA methods that use this iterative refinement are MAFFT (Katoh and Standley 2013) and MUSCLE (Edgar 2004). Another method to improve progressive alignments is to employ consistency information. T-Coffee (Notredame et al. 2000) and ProbCons (Do et al. 2005) are representative methods of this approach. Broadly speaking, consistency-based approaches show higher accuracy than those based on iterative refinement, but are more computationally expensive.

8.2.3 Initial Model Generation

Once the template(s) has (have) been selected and the sequence alignment performed, the next step is the construction of an initial structural model of the target, also called crude model. There are three approaches, which take into account information from the template structure:

1. *Modeling by rigid body assembly*: In this method, a comparative model of target segments is assembled from a number of rigid bodies derived from the aligned template protein structures (Browne et al. 1969; Blundell et al. 1987; Greer 1990). This strategy relies on the natural separation of conserved core regions linked by variable flexible loops, and side chains attached to the backbone (Topham et al. 1993). The accuracy of a model can be improved when more than one template structure is used to build the framework, and also when templates are averaged into the framework using weights related to sequence similarity (Srinivasan and Blundell 1993). Computer programs such as Composer (Sutcliffe et al. 1987), SWISS-MODEL (Schwede et al. 2003), RosettaCM (Song et al. 2013), and 3D-JIGSAW (Bates et al. 2001) implement this approach.

2. *Modeling by segment matching or coordinate reconstruction*: In this approach, the comparative model is built by means of a subset of atomic positions from template structures as "guiding" positions, usually $C\alpha$ or $C\alpha$–C–N atoms. These guiding positions are used to identify and assemble short, all-atom segments that fit these positions. The identified atom segments are obtained either by scanning all known protein structures (Claessens et al. 1989; Holm and Sander 1991), or by a conformational search restricted by an energy function (Bruccoleri and Karplus 1987; van Gelder et al. 1994). Not only main-chain atoms may be constructed by this method, but also side-chain atoms (Chinea et al. 1995). The SegMod program (Levitt 1992) implements this kind of strategy.

3. *Modeling by satisfaction of spatial restraints*: The process of this method is conceptually similar to that used in the determination of protein structures from NMR-derived restraints. By using the target alignment as a guide, many restraints are generated on the structure of the target sequence. These constraints are usually complemented by stereochemical restraints obtained from a molecular mechanics force field, and combined into an objective function. Then the model is derived by optimizing the objective function in Cartesian space.

This approach is implemented in the computer program MODELLER (Sali and Blundell 1993; Fiser and Sali 2003).

8.2.4 Structural Homology Model Refinement

The initial or crude model described above usually inherits the template backbone structure. Although progress has been observed in the refinement process of the model (Jamroz and Kolinski 2011; Lin and Head-Gordon 2011), there might be cases where large-scale backbone displacements could be difficult to model with available modeling tools. In spite of this, small- and midrange displacements could be modeled through molecular dynamics (MD) (Amaro and Li 2010). Reports also show that normal mode analysis-based methods can also be used for this purpose (Cavasotto et al. 2005b; Kovacs et al. 2005; Rai et al. 2010; Sperandio et al. 2010; Cavasotto 2012). The analysis of refinement strategies is divided into loop modeling, side chains, and the use of ligand information to structurally shape and optimize the binding site.

8.2.4.1 Modeling of Loops

Loop modeling is a crucial stage in homology modeling owing to the fact that loops usually represent the most characteristic differences between the template and the target, and thus may be involved in functional differences. It is common that some loops exhibit poor sequence conservation, or are present in gapped regions of the alignment. In the range of 30–50% sequence identity, although core regions are relatively conserved and accurately aligned, loops between homologs vary. Loop modeling can be viewed as a mini protein folding problem, due to the fact that the correct conformation of a given polypeptide chain segment must be mainly predicted from the sequence of the segment itself (i.e., not through using a structural template). Yet, loops are mostly too short to furnish enough information about their local fold (Mezei 1998). Broadly speaking, gaps covering five amino acids or less entail little concern since they can be predicted in with a sensible accuracy (Levitt 1992; Kolodny et al. 2002; Fernandez-Fuentes et al. 2006). Nevertheless, it is still a challenge to model loops accurately with gap lengths longer than 10 residues (Zhu et al. 2006).

There are two main types of loop modeling: database search approaches and conformational search approaches. In addition, there are methods that blend these two strategies with the aim of exploiting the advantages of each one (van Vlijmen and Karplus 1997; Deane and Blundell 2001).

1. In the database search approach (also named as fragment-based), a database of known protein structures is scanned in order to find segments fitting anchor regions (Jones and Thirup 1986; Chothia and Lesk 1987). The efficiency of this strategy is maximal when a database of specific loops is created to tackle the modeling of loops either on the same class (e.g., β-hairpins [Sibanda et al. 1989]), or on a specific fold

(for instance, some regions in the immunoglobulin fold [Chothia et al. 1989]). Furthermore, to extend the applicability of this approach, efforts have been made to classify loop conformations into wider categories (Rufino et al. 1997). The growth of the PDB in the last 10 years paved the way for these efforts (Fernandez-Fuentes and Fiser 2006).

2. The conformational searching method (also known as *ab initio, de novo,* or optimization-based) is based on minimizing an energy-based scoring function (Moult and James 1986; Bruccoleri and Karplus 1987). The search protocol includes the minimum perturbation method (Fine et al. 1986), genetic algorithms (Ring et al. 1993), multiple-copy simultaneous search (Zheng et al. 1993), Monte Carlo and simulated annealing (Higo et al. 1992; Abagyan and Totrov 1994), self-consistent field optimization (Koehl and Delarue 1995), MD simulations (Bruccoleri and Karplus 1990; vanVlijmen and Karplus 1997), enumeration-based on graph theory (Samudrala and Moult 1998), dihedral angle search through a rotamer library (Zhu et al. 2006; Sellers et al. 2008), and robotics-inspired kinematic closure (Mandell et al. 2009). An advantage of such methods is that they can be applied both to the simultaneous modeling of several loops, and to loops that interact with ligands, unlike the database search approach (Fiser 2010).

8.2.4.2 Modeling of Side Chains

Various methods for modeling side-chain packing have been developed. In the backbone-dependent rotamer libraries (Dunbrack and Karplus 1993; Lovell et al. 2000; Dunbrack 2002; Canutescu et al. 2003; Jiang et al. 2005), the library content relates to the probability of occurrence for each amino acid rotamers, and the sum of the overall probability of the side-chain rotamers is calculated. The computer program SCWRL (Bower et al. 1997) implements this kind of modeling by using a search method based on graph theory. Besides, sampling methods such as simulated annealing (Liang and Grishin 2002), rotamer substitutions (Xiang and Honig 2001), and self-consistent mean field approaches (Koehl and Delarue 1994) are used to create stable conformations. Of note is the Monte Carlo-based global energy minimization method implemented in the Internal Coordinates Mechanics (ICM) software (Abagyan et al. 1994; Abagyan and Totrov 1994; ICM 2012), where bond lengths and bond angles are considered fixed, and sampling is carried out in the torsional angle space. This methodology was successfully used, for example, to optimize ligand and side-chain conformations in bovine rhodopsin (bRho) bound to retinal, starting from a random conformation (Cavasotto et al. 2003).

8.2.4.3 Integral Modeling Using Existing Ligand Information

Since target proteins may bind structurally diverse ligands, it is reasonable to incorporate receptor flexibility upon modeling binding sites (Cavasotto et al. 2005a; Cavasotto and Singh 2008; Cavasotto 2011a). It would be natural to incorporate, whenever possible, information about existing ligands in the process of binding site modeling. Ligand–protein restraints derived from manual or rigid-receptor docking were incorporated in MODELLER (Evers and Klebe 2004a), and models thus developed successfully used to identify antagonists for neurokinin-1 (Evers and Klebe 2004b). Moro et al. (2006) developed models with diverse side-chain orientations generated from a crude model on which small molecules were soft-docked, thus creating an ensemble of ligands poses. This was followed by a local energy minimization step of the side chains and ligand. Costanzi used combined the use of experimental knowledge of ligand binding with *in silico* modeling of induced fit effects (Sherman et al. 2006); this approach was used to obtain β_2 adrenergic structural models from bRho (Costanzi 2008). In the ligand-steered homology modeling (LSHM) method, existing ligands are used to optimize the binding site through flexible ligand-flexible receptor docking protocol, using Monte Carlo sampling of the side-chain dihedral angles, and the free torsions and six rigid coordinates of the ligand (Orry and Cavasotto 2006; Cavasotto et al. 2008). In fact, this approach is a natural extension to comparative modeling of a methodology previously developed to optimize the binding site of a target when complexed with nonnative ligands, and where target flexibility is accounted for in the process (Cavasotto and Abagyan 2004; Cavasotto et al. 2005b; Kovacs et al. 2005; Monti et al. 2007, 2009). The LSHM method was initially used to develop structural models of the melanin concentrating hormone receptor 1 (MCH-R1), an antiobesity Class-A GPCR target, taking bRho as the structural template, the only GPCR structure available by then. The quality of the models was assessed through small-scale high-throughput docking (HTD), and the top-scoring model was then used in a prospective structure-based virtual screening of ~200,000 small-molecule library. After a postscreening protocol, top-ranking compounds were evaluated and six low-micromolar inhibitors were found (Cavasotto et al. 2008). The validation of the LSHM method using cross modeling of GPCRs with available structures has been also published (Phatak et al. 2010) (see details below). The ligand-steered method was also used to rationalize SAR data of ligand binding to the cannabinoid CB2 receptor (Diaz et al. 2009a,b; Petrov et al. 2013). Following this concept, GPCR models generated using an induced fit docking approach were used to assess their performance in HTD (McRobb et al. 2010). It should be mentioned that MD has also been used for GPCR refinement (Varady et al. 2003; Kimura et al. 2008; Wolf et al. 2008).

8.3 Limitations and Errors

Generally speaking, sequence identity between the target and templates, and quality of the alignment are the major determinants of the accuracy of comparative modeling. Typically, depending on both the level of sequence similarity and the quality of the alignment, the accuracy of comparative models compared to the actual native structure can be up to approximately 1–2 Å Cα atom RMSD (Ginalski 2006; Burley et al. 2008). Sequence identity higher than 50% usually results in reliable models with errors mainly in side chains and loops. Between 30% and 50%, more errors may be obtained. And below 30% sequence similarity, homology models are even less trustworthy and serious inaccuracies might happen. Moreover, significant errors might occur in protein regions that share little sequence identity with the templates, even when the remainder of the protein may show a high sequence similarity. Needless to say these are general observations; there are cases like GPCRs, where a low target-template sequence similarity is compensated by a strong structural similarity, and the presence of strongly conserved key residues in each helix throughout the whole class A family (Cavasotto et al. 2008; Cavasotto and Phatak 2009; Phatak et al. 2010).

Typical errors in homology modeling are often grouped into five classes:

1. *Errors arising in a target region that is properly aligned with templates*: As a result of issues either related to inherent defects of the experimental determination, or to the structural determination of the template in different environments (in particular, solvent, ligand, crystal packing, etc.), sometimes there might be structural differences between the model and the actual structure of the target. This type of error can be minimized by using simultaneously multiple templates (Srinivasan and Blundell 1993; Sanchez and Sali 1997a). However, one should be cautious when using template structures with mutated residues; in this case, mutated amino acids in the crystal structure should be changed into the corresponding residues of the wild-type receptor.

2. *Errors due to misalignments*: This is one of the major problems in homology modeling. Particularly, when sequence similarity falls below 30%, this kind of error is often coupled with the difficulty of identifying appropriate templates. At this level of sequence identity, about 20% of residues are expected to be misaligned and thus their backbone atoms could have an RMSD error greater than 3 Å (Fiser 2010). Again, a MSA can reduce this type of error (Taylor et al. 1994). Additionally, a good strategy is to repeatedly adjust the alignment parts corresponding to inaccuracies in the model (John and Sali 2003). Close attention should be paid to proline target residues aligned to residues in template helices, as well as to the relative position of cysteine residues involved in disulfide bonds, and ionic residues participating in salt bridges. Manual curation may be carried out in order to mitigate such errors, with the cost of opening or extending gaps in exposed loops, provided that reasonable penalties

are used in the overall alignment score. In this regard, the mounting alignment problems identified for a determined target/template pair could be useful to prioritize template suitability with respect to other candidates.

3. *Inaccuracies in target segments that have no equivalent in templates*: Insertions and deletions are the most challenging areas in protein modeling. As already explained, gap lengths larger than 10 amino acids are difficult model (Zhu et al. 2006). Necessary conditions for the successful prediction of these areas are both proper alignment, and gap-surrounding regions precisely modeled. Special care should be taken with gaps larger than two or three residues in core regions, as well as with gaps greater than one amino acid in helices and sheets of templates, though some exceptions to this could be found in some GPCRs (Gonzalez et al. 2012).

4. *Errors arising from erroneous templates*: As noted above, this difficulty is primarily evidenced for sequence similarity below 30%. Preservation of structural or functional key residues of the target sequence is of utmost importance when selecting a template (Webb and Sali 2014).

5. *Failure to model side-chain conformation*: Errors in side chains that are involved in protein function, for example, in active and ligand binding sites. It could have a strong impact on the application of target models in structure-based drug design. This highlights the importance of accounting for ligand–protein interaction at the modeling stage, as described above.

8.4 Model Evaluation

In general, there are two types of assessment of model accuracy:

1. *"Internal" evaluation*: For the sake of achieving a consistent model, an assessment is made to guarantee that the constraints used to calculate the model are satisfied. The stereo-chemistry of a model (e.g., bond lengths, bond angles, dihedral angles, and nonbonded contacts) (cf. Figure 8.4) can be evaluated by using programs such as PROCHECK (Laskowski et al. 1993), WHATCHECK (Hooft et al. 1996), and MolProbity (Davis et al. 2007). Despite errors in stereochemistry are unusual and less instructive than errors discovered by statistical potentials, a set of stereo-chemical errors could indicate major inaccuracies in that region. It should be stressed that this is an

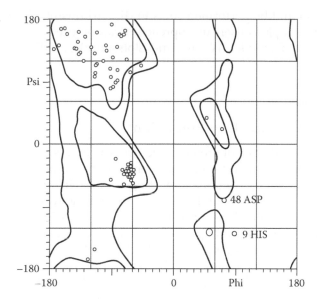

FIGURE 8.4
Ramachandran plot as a measure of model quality. Two residues (Asp 48 and His 9), which are in disallowed regions, could be noted. (Figure created using MolProbity [http://molprobity. biochem.duke.edu/].)

internal consistency check, and brings no information whatsoever regarding the accuracy of the model with respect to the actual structure of the target.

2. *"External" evaluation*: This assessment, which is based on information that was not included in the construction of the model, is made in order to test template suitability. With sequence similarity below 30%, an additional complication is that the alignment usually possesses many errors. This problem is reflected in the difficulty to differentiate between an improper template on the one hand, and a wrong alignment with a proper template, on the other. There are various approaches that use 3D profiles and statistical potential (Sippl 1990; Luthy et al. 1992; Melo et al. 2002) to evaluate the compatibility between the sequence and modeled structure. Methods such as VERIFY3D (Eisenberg et al. 1997), ANOLEA (Melo and Feytmans 1998), DFIRE (Zhou and Zhou 2002), and QMEAN (Benkert et al. 2011) may be used to assess the template viability. Furthermore, other issues may arise by using templates that contain either errors or modifications (e.g., mutations). Moreover, as stated above, other factors such as the "environment" can impact the quality of the model. Validation analyses on candidate templates prior

to use should be performed so as to discard unsuitable structures. Besides, simple consensus approaches can be used to evaluate the reliability of a model (Wallner and Elofsson 2005, 2007).

8.5 Automated Structure Prediction

At present, the prediction of protein structure is an accessible task, which was largely facilitated by increasing improvements in automated user-friendly servers. In this regard, assessment meetings of protein structure prediction methods, such as CASP and GPCR-Dock, opened the way for the development and optimization of these services (see Sections 8.7 and 8.10).

There are many servers that perform automated homology protein modeling, some of the most important are I-TASSER (http://zhanglab.ccmb.med. umich.edu/I-TASSER/) (Zhang 2008; Roy et al. 2010), RaptorX (http://raptorx. uchicago.edu/about/) (Kallberg et al. 2012), SwissModel (http://swissmodel. expasy.org/) (Biasini et al. 2014), Robetta (http://robetta.bakerlab.org/) (Kim et al. 2004), HHpred (http://toolkit.tuebingen.mpg.de/hhpred) (Biegert et al. 2006), Phyre2 (http://www.sbg.bio.ic.ac.uk/~phyre2/html/page.cgi?id=index) (Kelley and Sternberg 2009), IntFOLD (http://www.reading.ac.uk/bioinf/ IntFOLD/) (Roche et al. 2011), M4T (http://manaslu.aecom.yu.edu/M4T/) (Fernandez-Fuentes et al. 2007), and ModWeb (https://modbase.compbio. ucsf.edu/modweb/) (Pieper et al. 2014). Anyway, users should use these servers with caution, and evaluate selected templates, alignments, and refinement approaches, in order to have greater control and insight over the entire process. In addition, validation remains crucial: regardless of whether evaluation data were, or were not provided by the automated service, the user must carefully examine the final 3D structure for the intended use.

8.6 Repositories of Homology Models

There are several repositories where protein models generated by different methods can be found. Protein Model Portal (http://www.proteinmodelportal.org/) (Haas et al. 2013), SWISS-MODEL Repository (http://swissmodel. expasy.org/repository/) (Kiefer et al. 2009), and ModBase (http://modbase. compbio.ucsf.edu/modbase-cgi/index.cgi) (Pieper et al. 2014) are some examples. Also, there are repositories of 3D models of specific receptors, such as GPCRs (GPCRDB [http://www.gpcr.org/7tm/]) (Vroling et al. 2011), GPCR-HGmod (http://zhanglab.ccmb.med.umich.edu/GPCR-HGmod/), and GPCR-SSFE (http://www.ssfa-7tmr.de/ssfe/) (Worth et al. 2011), and nuclear receptors (NucleaRDB [http://www.receptors.org/nucleardb/] [Vroling et al. 2012]).

8.7 Assessments of Protein Modeling

The Critical Assessment of Techniques for Protein Structure Prediction (CASP) (Moult et al. 1995), tests methods for modeling of protein structure, including homology modeling, and has been continuously carried out biannually since 1994. In this competition, worldwide scientific groups submit 3D models of target proteins with unknown structures. The 3D structures of the targets, solved either by x-ray crystallography or by NMR methods, are available after each team presents their predicted models. Thus, modeling methods of protein structure are blindly and genuinely evaluated. Description of the experiments and full data of each CASP competition are available to the public in the protein structure prediction center website (http://predictioncenter.org/). Recent advances in protein structure prediction, and where future efforts should be aimed, were announced and discussed at the CASP 11 Meeting held in December 2014. After the meeting, progress and future directions are discussed in a special issue of *Proteins: Structure, Function and Bioinformatics*. Thus, this meeting held every two years since 1994 has undoubtedly accelerated the progress of protein prediction techniques.

The advancement that has been made in the last decade, that is, since CASP5, on protein structure prediction methods, can be synthesized as follows (Kryshtafovych et al. 2014): There is an important progress in template-based model accuracy. This fact is evidenced in the successful modeling of certain regions hardly obtained from a single template, which in turn reveals not only the intense work within the modeling community in the development of approaches that utilize multiple templates, but also the increased number of experimental structures available. On the contrary, total backbone accuracy of models shows a minor change in the last 10 years. This can be justified both by the development of larger databases (making it more difficult to select the best available templates), and by an increase in the intrinsic difficulty of CASP targets (since the experimental work has improved to larger and unusual structures). On the contrary, the accuracy of sequence alignments seems to have saturated since CASP5.

Besides CASP, the community-wide GPCR modeling and docking (GPCR Dock) assessment was created to evaluate the advancement of molecular modeling of, and ligand docking to GPCRs (Michino et al. 2009; Kufareva et al. 2011, 2014) (see below).

8.8 Applications of Homology Models

Since comparative modeling is based on the homology between target and template, three types of uses can be addressed in accordance with the level of sequence similarity: higher than 50%, between 30% and 50%, and sequence identity lower than 30%.

The mean accuracy of models based on 50% sequence identity or higher approximates that of low-resolution x-ray structures (3 Å resolution) or medium-resolution NMR structures (10 interproton distance restraints per residue [Sanchez and Sali 1997b]), which means that they are accurate enough either for refining crystallographic structures by the molecular replacement method (Schwarzenbacher et al. 2004), or for structure-based drug design (Hillisch et al. 2004). Medium quality models, which are generated by using templates with sequence identity between 30% and 50%, have roughly 85% of Cα atoms within 3.5 Å of their correct positions. They are appropriate both for evaluating target druggability and for building site-directed mutants that might test hypotheses about structure–function relationships (Hillisch et al. 2004). Models arising from sequence identity below 30% are in the "twilight zone," and are supposed to have less than 50% of Cα atoms within 3.5 Å of the native 3D structure. This kind of models could be used to check a match between remotely related proteins (Sanchez and Sali 1997a).

8.9 Use of Homology Models in Structure-Based Drug Discovery

Homology models have been applied in many settings in the context of drug discovery, including structure–function relationships (Song et al. 2007; Guimaraes et al. 2008), identification of binding sites (Soga et al. 2007), and to aid mutagenesis experiments (Gagnidze et al. 2008). Furthermore, with regard to structure-based virtual screening, the usefulness of homology models has been proven not only in retrospective analyses (Skolnick et al. 2013; Costanzi 2013), but also in prospective campaigns (Ripphausen et al. 2010; Cavasotto 2011b).

The performance of homology models in HTD is usually assessed by comparison with the performance on the corresponding crystal structures. However, it is an open question about how the quality of the model in the context of structure-based drug discovery should be measured. It should be stressed that model quality should correlate not only with high docking enrichment factors, but also with accurate docking poses of known ligands. Clearly, the performance of models in docking and HTD will also depend on many factors such as the availability of template structures, and others not directly related with the modeling process, such as the docking program of choice, the ligand and decoy databases (cfr. [Cavasotto and Phatak 2011; Gatica and Cavasotto 2012]), and small molecule preparation. Obviously, results could also be target-dependent, as in the case in docking to crystal structures (Warren et al. 2006). Furthermore, the outcome of HTD experiments could deteriorate due to the use of the rigid receptor approximation, and a single-receptor approach (Cavasotto and Abagyan 2004; Cavasotto and Singh 2008; Vilar et al. 2011), even if high-quality models are used.

Studying the performance of homology models of four protein kinases in virtual screening (Diller and Li 2003) (the epidermal growth factor receptor [EGFR], the fibroblast growth factor receptor 1 [FGFR1], the P38 mitogen-activated protein kinase [P38], and the Src protein tyrosine kinase [SRC]), it was found that models performed reasonably well (EGFR), even better than crystal structures in the case of SRC. The performance of P38 models was rather poor, in agreement with another study showing that even correctly docked ligands did not rank very well in crystal structures (Cavasotto and Abagyan 2004). In FGFR1 structures, HTD was poor using both experimental and modeled structures.

An extensive study on the performance of HTD in unbound, bound, and homology models in nine protein families (acetylcholinesterase [AchE], androgen receptor [AR], dihydrofolate reductase [DHFR], glycisamide ribonucleotide phosphorylase [GART], poly ADP-ribose polymerase [PARP], purine nucleoside phophorylase [PNP], S-adenosylhomocysteine hydrolase [SAHH], thrombin, and thymilidate synthase [TS]) (McGovern and Shoichet 2003), showed that bound structures exhibited the best performance in HTD, and while homology models also performed reasonably well.

HTD studies on models of AChE, carboxypeptidase A, CDK2, Factor Xa, and peroxisome proliferator-activated receptor α (PPARα) (Kairys et al. 2006), and on CDK2, protein tyrosine phosphatase 1B (PTP1B), renin and thrombin (Novoa et al. 2010), confirmed the suitability of homology models for docking-based high-throughput screening. A study of modeling and docking to 38 targets, using molecules from the DUD library (Huang et al. 2006) showed that the use of models in HTD usually outperform random selection (Fan et al. 2009).

A study regarding the use of homology models in docking and HTD was presented for Class A GPCRs (Phatak et al. 2010) using the LSHM method to cross model the bRho, β_2 adrenergic, and adenosine A_{2A} receptors, and then comparing the performance of HTD both on crystal structures and models. Using the LSHM method, a small ensemble of homology models of those GPCRs was generated, while incorporating protein flexibility at the modeling stage. The ligand-steered generated models showed good performance in docking when compared to experimental structures, initial homology models prior to refinement (crude models), and to random selection. However, no model outperformed its corresponding crystal structure. Interestingly, models with low ligand RMSD performed well in small-scale HTD experiments, and also in selectivity prediction, comparable to experimental structures. This study highlighted the importance of adequate model refinement, which can offset a poor target-template sequence similarity whenever structural similarity is observed, and also suggested an adequate quality control to determine which models could perform well in HTD. Furthermore, a study of the accuracy of ligand-protein docking on homology models (Bordogna et al. 2011) reached similar conclusions regarding the necessity of using accurate binding sites in docking campaigns.

For a review of recent applications of homology models in structure-based virtual screening, cfr. Cavasotto (2011b).

8.10 Case Study: Modeling of GPCRs

GPCRs are proteins expressed in the plasma membrane that trigger intercellular responses by activating key signal-transduction pathways (Pierce et al. 2002). Class I (also known as class A) GPCRs are the target for about 27% of all FDA-approved drugs (Overington et al. 2006). Due to the great challenges that entail crystallization of membrane receptors such as GPCRs (Congreve et al. 2011), the first GPCR (bRho) was not crystallized until 2000 (Palczewski et al. 2000), while the first human GPCR structure, β_2 adrenergic receptor, was not solved until 2007 (Rasmussen et al. 2007; Cherezov et al. 2007). While in the last few years there have been technological innovations in membrane protein crystallization that triggered an accelerated growth in the amount of experimentally solved structures of GPCRs, the receptors with publicly available structures so far are still only a small fraction of more than 350 nonolfactory/taste GPCRs in the human genome (Fredriksson et al. 2003; Ono et al. 2005; Lagerstrom and Schioth 2008). Hence, it is evident that there is a need for reliable GPCRs homology models, which may contribute to elucidate specificity, function, and structural details of ligand interactions of receptors that remain experimentally unsolved, besides their use in drug discovery campaigns.

Although the sequence identity of the seven transmembrane helices is generally low in GPCRs, they retain analogous secondary/tertiary structures at these segments (Gonzalez et al. 2012). In Class A GPCR proteins, there is at least one highly conserved residue in each transmembrane domain (Mirzadegan et al. 2003). This GPCR feature was utilized by Ballesteros and Weinstein (1995) to create a nomenclature system. In this scheme, GPCR residues are described by X.YY, where X indicates the number of the helix to which the residue belongs, and YY represents its position within the transmembrane domain relative to the most conserved amino acid in the helix, arbitrarily assigned as 50. Subsequently, a modification was added whereby each amino acid is first identified with its original sequence number and is then followed by the Ballesteros and Weinstein numbering scheme (van Rhee and Jacobson 1996). The knowledge of this structural conservation ratifies the usefulness of these key residues for sequence alignment, and thus for building of homology models of unsolved structures (Gonzalez et al. 2014).

Taking into account only the class A GPCR family, homology modeling of these proteins faces several challenges, such as editing the PDB file before the alignment, the sequence alignment, the choice of template, loop modeling, the Gα subunit, consideration of internal water molecules, and model refinement (Cavasotto 2011b; Costanzi 2012; Strasser and Wittmann 2013). Since a PDB file may contain multiple receptor molecules, they should be properly edited prior to sequence alignment. One of the chains should be chosen based on its B-factor, its completeness and other factors, while the remaining ones could be deleted (Costanzi 2012). After selecting the most suitable chain, the ATOM records corresponding to the TM segments of the template must be conserved. All other records among which those belonging to cofactors and ligands as well as intracellular and extracellular regions could be removed. Moreover, ATOM records correspond to a cocrystallized fragment antigen binding (Fab) and the T4-lysozyme could be eliminated.

The main strategy in sequence alignment of the target to the 7TM domains of the candidate templates is typically a multiple template approach, which comprises the division of the target into several segments, and the further selection of the most proper template for each of these segments. Sequence identity should not be the only criterion for template selection. Another important factor to consider is the detection of specific features and motifs identified in the target sequence, such as the presence of specific amino acids responsible for helical kinks (glycine and proline), and/or cysteine residues supposedly engaged in the formation of disulfide bridges, especially in the extracellular loop 2 (EL2) (Worth et al. 2009).

Since the extracellular and intracellular regions of class A GPCRs possess high-length variability, and very low-sequence identity, sequence alignment of these domains is a much more complex task than that of the seven transmembrane segments. In case of existing short loops in the target, a feasible way to build these loops could be found in *de novo* modeling. If the *de novo* modeling approach has to be avoided, then it is advisable to use template loops with a length similar to the corresponding domains of the target. Instead of using a MSA of loops, the alignment is better performed in a pairwise fashion by comparing the target to one template at the time (Costanzi 2012).

Some loops deserve a special interest in GPCRs. For instance, in certain biogenic amine receptors, the EL2 possesses a role in ligand binding to the receptor (Lim et al. 2008; Brunskole et al. 2011). For this reason, an accurate modeling of some loops may be convenient, especially of EL2. Whereas most loops are solved by crystal structures, this is usually not the case with respect to EL2 and let alone the case concerning the intracellular loop 3 (IL3). EL2 links TM4 and TM5 and, in the majority of class I GPCRs, is characterized by a highly conserved cysteine amino acid that connects to the upper part of helix 3 through a disulfide bond. Not only a great structural variability of EL2 has been observed among the several experimentally solved receptors, but also diverse arrays of disulfide bonds have been identified in their extracellular regions (Hanson and Stevens 2009). For example, from the various crystal structures that have been obtained for the human β_2 adrenergic receptor, it is observed that this receptor has two disulfide bridges in the EL2 and a part thereof displays a helical structure, while in other GPCRs there is only one disulfide bridge in EL2 connecting with the helix 3, and a helical structure is not present.

According to various studies, GPCRs in the active conformation interact in the intracellular region with the $G\alpha$ subunit (Venkatakrishnan et al. 2013). A comprehensive analysis of crystal structures reveals that the C-terminus of the $G\alpha$ subunit is deeply bound in a pocket between the transmembrane domains (Scheerer et al. 2008; Rasmussen et al. 2011). Accordingly, in MD simulations, excluding the C-terminal part of $G\alpha$ protein and its replacement by water molecules, which are obviously highly polar and exhibit different surface properties, may cause lack of receptor stability. Therefore, either the whole $G\alpha$ or at least the C-terminal part of $G\alpha$ should be included if an accurate model of that region is sought. Noteworthy, each GPCR is coupled to a different $G\alpha$ subunit (Simon et al. 1991).

On the contrary, several studies have shown that internal and highly conserved water molecules are involved in hydrogen bonding within the receptor. Therefore, it has been suggested that these water molecules are crucial either for stabilizing, or for activating the receptor (Pardo et al. 2007), and their inclusion might be considered into the comparative model. It has been shown that the presence of water molecules bridging the interaction of the ligand with the protein within the binding site of the A_{2A} adenosine receptor is important in small-molecule docking (Gatica and Cavasotto 2012).

Before concluding the modeling process, some basic controls should be carried out in order to obtain a suitable model, such as checking the existence of the disulfide bridge between the EL2 and the helix 3, and absence of clashes between residue side chains. The model can be energetically optimized in two steps. During the first minimization, the backbone of the helical bundle is subject to positional restraints. In a second stage, the receptor may be minimized without any position restraints.

According to the 2013 Modeling and Docking Assessment (Kufareva et al. 2014), some issues about specific class A GPCRs, namely $5HT_{1B}$ and $5HT_{2B}$, were discussed. These two receptors, which both were in complexes with the agonist ergotamine, were difficult to predict because ergotamine makes different and extensive contacts with the mobile extracellular loops. These interactions could only be modeled with modest accuracy. Most successful predictions were obtained by using the computer program MODELLER (Sali and Blundell 1993; Fiser and Sali 2003) and a multiple template approach. With respect to model selection, those models derived from the ability to recognize known ligands among similar inactive molecules (property-matched decoys) displayed good performance. Moreover, some of the better complexes had been refined by MD simulations. Visual inspection and semi-automatic model selection utilizing subfamily-specific amino acid contacts, ligand SAR, and mutagenesis data also proved to be useful. On the contrary, many of the submitted models did not detect the biased state of $5HT_{2B}$. The shortfall of appropriate predictions for $5HT_{2B}$ stresses the need for either experimental determination of multiple functional states of GPCRs, or for the improvement of computational methods for their prediction.

8.11 Conclusions

Currently, the PDB has ~108,000 experimentally solved deposited structures. In spite of this number, and the ongoing structural genomics efforts, it is foreseeable that in the near future, high-quality structures of important drug targets will not be available for drug discovery endeavors. Thus, homology modeling appears as a promising and cost-effective tool, offering the actual possibility of expanding by two orders of magnitude the collection of available target structures (Pieper et al. 2009). The use of comparative models in structure-based drug discovery projects is already established (Cavasotto and Orry 2007; Cavasotto and Phatak 2009; Tuccinardi 2009; Cavasotto 2011b). However, there is an actual need to develop better methods to accurately characterize binding sites, and to validate those methods in small-scale and full-scale docking and HTD experiments. This brings refinement approaches to the center of the scene, both at the backbone and side-chain levels.

During the last decade, there has been an obvious improvement in the accuracy of models obtained by homology modeling. The features and inaccuracies that arise at different stages of the construction of a comparative model have been identified and gradually reduced, respectively. These latest advances have been achieved as a result not only of better methods and practices, but also of a large number of experimentally solved protein structures. In the several steps that involve homology modeling, sequence alignment and template selection are critical. The use of several templates, rather than a single one, seems to be a better approach, and the same holds true for sequence alignment by using a MSA strategy. Modeling loops still remain a challenging task, while errors in amino acids that are involved in protein function, for instance in active binding sites, are fundamental, which highlights the importance of incorporating the knowledge about ligand binding in the modeling process (Cavasotto et al. 2008; Phatak et al. 2010). Regarding automated structure prediction services, there are multiple servers that facilitate and accelerate homology modeling, but a careful analysis should be undertaken to check the final quality of those models.

From the CASP competition, held every two years since 1994, it is observed that the accuracy of sequence alignment seems to have saturated from CASP5, and that there has been a development of successful approaches that use multiple templates, taking advantage of the increased number of experimental structures available. Conversely, overall backbone accuracy of models exhibits a small change in the last 10 years. This could be explained by the greater difficulty in selecting the best templates available, and/or an increase in the intrinsic difficulty of the CASP targets.

With respect to Class A GPCRs in the community-wide GPCR modeling and docking assessments, extracellular loops and their interactions could only be modeled with modest accuracy. Homology models obtained from the ability to recognize known ligands among property-matched decoys played out well. Visual inspection and semiautomatic model selection, by means of subfamily-specific amino acid contacts, ligand SAR, and mutagenesis data, have also proved to be successful. The lack of suitable predictions for the biased state of 5HT2B emphasizes the need for either experimental determination of multiple functional states of GPCRs, calling also for an improvement of computational methods for their prediction.

Acknowledgment

Funding from the Agencia Nacional de Promoción Científica y Tecnológica, Argentina (PICT-2011-2778) FOCEM-Mercosur (COF 03/11) is acknowledged. CNC thanks MolSoft LLC for providing an academic license for the ICM program.

References

Abagyan, R. and M. Totrov. 1994. Biased probability Monte Carlo conformational searches and electrostatic calculations for peptides and proteins. *J. Mol. Biol.* 235(3): 983–1002.

Abagyan, R., M. Totrov, and D. Kuznetsov. 1994. ICM—A new method for protein modeling and design—Applications to docking and structure prediction from the distorted native conformation. *J. Comput. Chem.* 15(5): 488–506.

Activities at the Universal Protein Resource (UniProt). 2014. *Nucleic Acids Res.* 42(Database issue): D191–D198.

Acland, A., R. Agarwala, T. Barrett et al. 2014. Database resources of the National Center for Biotechnology Information. *Nucleic Acids Res.* 42(Database issue): D7–D17.

Altschul, S. F., T. L. Madden, A. A. Schaffer et al. 1997. Gapped BLAST and PSI-BLAST: A new generation of protein database search programs. *Nucleic Acids Res.* 25(17): 3389–3402.

Amaro, R. E. and W. W. Li. 2010. Emerging methods for ensemble-based virtual screening. *Curr. Top. Med. Chem.* 10(1): 3–13.

Andreeva, A., D. Howorth, C. Chothia, E. Kulesha, and A. G. Murzin. 2014. SCOP2 prototype: A new approach to protein structure mining. *Nucleic Acids Res.* 42(Database issue): D310–D314.

Artimo, P., M. Jonnalagedda, K. Arnold et al. 2012. ExPASy: SIB bioinformatics resource portal. *Nucleic Acids Res.* 40(Web Server issue): W597–W603.

Ballesteros, J. and H. Weinstein. 1995. Integrated methods for the construction of three-dimensional models of structure-function relations in G protein-coupled receptors. *Methods Neurosci.* 25: 366–428.

Bates, P. A., L. A. Kelley, R. M. MacCallum, and M. J. Sternberg. 2001. Enhancement of protein modeling by human intervention in applying the automatic programs 3D-JIGSAW and 3D-PSSM. *Proteins* 45(Suppl 5): 39–46.

Benkert, P., M. Biasini, and T. Schwede. 2011. Toward the estimation of the absolute quality of individual protein structure models. *Bioinformatics* 27(3): 343–350.

Berman, H. M., G. J. Kleywegt, H. Nakamura, and J. L. Markley. 2014. The Protein Data Bank archive as an open data resource. *J. Comput. Aided Mol. Des.* 28(10): 1009–1014.

Berman, H. M., J. Westbrook, Z. Feng et al. 2000. The protein data bank. *Nucl. Acids Res.* 28(1): 235–242.

Berman, H. M., T. Battistuz, T. N. Bhat et al. 2002. The protein data bank. *Acta Crystallogr. D Biol. Crystallogr.* 58(Part 6 No. 1): 899–907.

Biasini, M., S. Bienert, A. Waterhouse et al. 2014. SWISS-MODEL: Modelling protein tertiary and quaternary structure using evolutionary information. *Nucleic Acids Res.* 42(Web Server issue): W252–W258.

Biegert, A., C. Mayer, M. Remmert, J. Soding, and A. N. Lupas. 2006. The MPI Bioinformatics Toolkit for protein sequence analysis. *Nucleic Acids Res.* 34(Web Server issue): W335–W339.

Blundell, T. L., B. L. Sibanda, M. J. Sternberg, and J. M. Thornton. 1987. Knowledge-based prediction of protein structures and the design of novel molecules. *Nature* 326(6111): 347–352.

Bordogna, A., A. Pandini, and L. Bonati. 2011. Predicting the accuracy of protein-ligand docking on homology models. *J. Comput. Chem.* 32(1): 81–98.

Bower, M. J., F. E. Cohen, and R. L. Dunbrack, Jr. 1997. Prediction of protein side-chain rotamers from a backbone-dependent rotamer library: A new homology modeling tool. *J. Mol. Biol.* 267(5): 1268–1282.

Browne, W. J., A. C. North, D. C. Phillips, K. Brew, T. C. Vanaman, and R. L. Hill. 1969. A possible three-dimensional structure of bovine alpha-lactalbumin based on that of hen's egg-white lysozyme. *J. Mol. Biol.* 42(1): 65–86.

Bruccoleri, R. E. and M. Karplus. 1987. Prediction of the folding of short polypeptide segments by uniform conformational sampling. *Biopolymers* 26(1): 137–168.

Bruccoleri, R. E. and M. Karplus. 1990. Conformational sampling using high-temperature molecular dynamics. *Biopolymers* 29(14): 1847–1862.

Brunskole, I., A. Strasser, R. Seifert, and A. Buschauer. 2011. Role of the second and third extracellular loops of the histamine H(4) receptor in receptor activation. *Naunyn. Schmiedebergs Arch. Pharmacol.* 384(3): 301–317.

Burley, S. K., A. Joachimiak, G. T. Montelione, and I. A. Wilson. 2008. Contributions to the NIH-NIGMS protein structure initiative from the PSI production centers. *Structure* 16(1): 5–11.

Canutescu, A. A., A. A. Shelenkov, and R. L. Dunbrack, Jr. 2003. A graph-theory algorithm for rapid protein side-chain prediction. *Protein Sci.* 12(9): 2001–2014.

Cavasotto, C. N. 2011a. Handling protein flexibility in docking and high-throughput docking. In: *Virtual Screening. Principles, Challenges and Practical Guidelines*, C. Sotriffer (ed.), Wiley-VCH, Verlag, Weinheim, Germany.

Cavasotto, C. N. 2011b. Homology models in docking and high-throughput docking. *Curr. Top. Med. Chem.* 11(12): 1528–1534.

Cavasotto, C. N. 2012. Normal mode-based approaches in receptor ensemble docking. *Methods Mol. Biol.* 819: 157–168.

Cavasotto, C. N. and A. J. Orry. 2007. Ligand docking and structure-based virtual screening in drug discovery. *Curr. Top. Med. Chem.* 7(10): 1006–1014.

Cavasotto, C. N., A. J. Orry, N. J. Murgolo et al. 2008. Discovery of novel chemotypes to a G-protein-coupled receptor through ligand-steered homology modeling and structure-based virtual screening. *J. Med. Chem.* 51(3): 581–588.

Cavasotto, C. N., A. J. Orry, and R. A. Abagyan. 2003. Structure-based identification of binding sites, native ligands and potential inhibitors for G-protein coupled receptors. *Proteins* 51(3): 423–433.

Cavasotto, C. N., A. J. W. Orry, and R. A. Abagyan. 2005a. The challenge of considering receptor flexibility in ligand docking and virtual screening. *Curr. Comput.-Aided Drug Des.* 1(4): 423–440.

Cavasotto, C. N., J. A. Kovacs, and R. A. Abagyan. 2005b. Representing receptor flexibility in ligand docking through relevant normal modes. *J. Am. Chem. Soc.* 127(26): 9632–9640.

Cavasotto, C. N. and N. Singh. 2008. Docking and high throughput docking: Successes and the challenge of protein flexibility *Curr. Comput.-Aided Drug Design* 4(3): 221–234.

Cavasotto, C. N. and R. A. Abagyan. 2004. Protein flexibility in ligand docking and virtual screening to protein kinases. *J. Mol. Biol.* 337(1): 209–225.

Cavasotto, C. N. and S. S. Phatak. 2009. Homology modeling in drug discovery: Current trends and applications. *Drug Discov. Today* 14(13–14): 676–683.

Cavasotto, C. N. and S. S. Phatak. 2011. Docking methods for structure-based library design. *Methods Mol. Biol.* 685: 155–174.

Cherezov, V., D. M. Rosenbaum, M. A. Hanson et al. 2007. High-resolution crystal structure of an engineered human beta2-adrenergic G protein-coupled receptor. *Science* 318(5854): 1258–1265.

Chinea, G., G. Padron, R. W. Hooft, C. Sander, and G. Vriend. 1995. The use of position-specific rotamers in model building by homology. *Proteins* 23(3): 415–421.

Chothia, C. and A. M. Lesk. 1986. The relation between the divergence of sequence and structure in proteins. *EMBO J.* 5(4): 823–826.

Chothia, C. and A. M. Lesk. 1987. Canonical structures for the hypervariable regions of immunoglobulins. *J. Mol. Biol.* 196(4): 901–917.

Chothia, C., A. M. Lesk, A. Tramontano et al. 1989. Conformations of immunoglobulin hypervariable regions. *Nature* 342(6252): 877–883.

Claessens, M., E. Van Cutsem, I. Lasters, and S. Wodak. 1989. Modelling the polypeptide backbone with "spare parts" from known protein structures. *Protein Eng.* 2(5): 335–345.

Congreve, M., C. Langmead, and F. H. Marshall. 2011. The use of GPCR structures in drug design. *Adv. Pharmacol.* 62: 1–36.

Congreve, M., J. M. Dias, and F. H. Marshall. 2014. Structure-based drug design for G protein-coupled receptors. *Prog. Med. Chem.* 53: 1–63.

Costanzi, S. 2008. On the applicability of GPCR homology models to computer-aided drug discovery: A comparison between *in silico* and crystal structures of the beta2-adrenergic receptor. *J. Med. Chem.* 51(10): 2907–2914.

Costanzi, S. 2012. Homology modeling of class a G protein-coupled receptors. *Methods Mol. Biol.* 857: 259–279.

Costanzi, S. 2013. Modeling G protein-coupled receptors and their interactions with ligands. *Curr. Opin. Struct. Biol.* 23(2): 185–190.

Davis, I. W., A. Leaver-Fay, V. B. Chen et al. 2007. MolProbity: All-atom contacts and structure validation for proteins and nucleic acids. *Nucleic Acids Res.* 35(Web Server issue): W375–W383.

Deane, C. M. and T. L. Blundell. 2001. CODA: A combined algorithm for predicting the structurally variable regions of protein models. *Protein Sci.* 10(3): 599–612.

Diaz, P., S. S. Phatak, J. Xu et al. 2009a. 2,3-Dihydro-1-benzofuran derivatives as a series of potent selective cannabinoid receptor 2 agonists: Design, synthesis, and binding mode prediction through ligand-steered modeling. *ChemMedChem* 4(10): 1615–1629.

Diaz, P., S. S. Phatak, J. Xu, F. Astruc-Diaz, C. N. Cavasotto, and M. Naguib. 2009b. 6-Methoxy-N-alkyl isatin acylhydrazone derivatives as a novel series of potent selective cannabinoid receptor 2 inverse agonists: Design, synthesis and binding mode prediction. *J. Med. Chem.* 52(2): 433–444.

Diller, D. J. and R. Li. 2003. Kinases, homology models, and high throughput docking. *J. Med. Chem.* 46(22): 4638–4647.

Do, C. B., M. S. Mahabhashyam, M. Brudno, and S. Batzoglou. 2005. ProbCons: Probabilistic consistency-based multiple sequence alignment. *Genome Res.* 15(2): 330–340.

Dunbrack, R. L., Jr. 2002. Rotamer libraries in the 21st century. *Curr. Opin. Struct. Biol.* 12(4): 431–440.

Dunbrack, R. L., Jr. and M. Karplus. 1993. Backbone-dependent rotamer library for proteins. Application to side-chain prediction. *J. Mol. Biol.* 230(2): 543–574.

Eddy, S. R. 1998. Profile hidden Markov models. *Bioinformatics* 14(9): 755–763.

Edgar, R. C. 2004. MUSCLE: Multiple sequence alignment with high accuracy and high throughput. *Nucleic Acids Res.* 32(5): 1792–1797.

Eisenberg, D., R. Luthy, and J. U. Bowie. 1997. VERIFY3D: Assessment of protein models with three-dimensional profiles. *Methods Enzymol.* 277: 396–404.

Evers, A. and G. Klebe. 2004a. Ligand-supported homology modeling of G-protein-coupled receptor sites: Models sufficient for successful virtual screening. *Angew. Chem. Int. Ed. Engl.* 43(2): 248–251.

Evers, A. and G. Klebe. 2004b. Successful virtual screening for a submicromolar antagonist of the neurokinin-1 receptor based on a ligand-supported homology model. *J. Med. Chem.* 47(22): 5381–5392.

Fan, H., J. J. Irwin, B. M. Webb, G. Klebe, B. K. Shoichet, and A. Sali. 2009. Molecular docking screens using comparative models of proteins. *J. Chem. Inf. Model.* 49(11): 2512–2527.

Fernandez-Fuentes, N. and A. Fiser. 2006. Saturating representation of loop conformational fragments in structure databanks. *BMC Struct. Biol.* 6: 15.

Fernandez-Fuentes, N., B. Oliva, and A. Fiser. 2006. A supersecondary structure library and search algorithm for modeling loops in protein structures. *Nucleic Acids Res.* 34(7): 2085–2097.

Fernandez-Fuentes, N., B. K. Rai, C. J. Madrid-Aliste, J. E. Fajardo, and A. Fiser. 2007. Comparative protein structure modeling by combining multiple templates and optimizing sequence-to-structure alignments. *Bioinformatics* 23(19): 2558–2565.

Fernandez-Fuentes, N., C. J. Madrid-Aliste, B. K. Rai, J. E. Fajardo, and A. Fiser. 2007. M4T: A comparative protein structure modeling server. *Nucleic Acids Res.* 35(Web Server issue): W363–W368.

Fine, R. M., H. Wang, P. S. Shenkin, D. L. Yarmush, and C. Levinthal. 1986. Predicting antibody hypervariable loop conformations. II: Minimization and molecular dynamics studies of MCPC603 from many randomly generated loop conformations. *Proteins* 1(4): 342–362.

Fiser, A. 2004. Protein structure modeling in the proteomics era. *Expert Rev. Proteomics* 1(1): 97–110.

Fiser, A. 2010. Template-based protein structure modeling. *Methods Mol. Biol.* 673: 73–94.

Fiser, A. and A. Sali. 2003. Modeller: Generation and refinement of homology-based protein structure models. *Methods Enzymol.* 374: 461–491.

Fredriksson, R., M. C. Lagerstrom, L. G. Lundin, and H. B. Schioth. 2003. The G-protein-coupled receptors in the human genome form five main families. Phylogenetic analysis, paralogon groups, and fingerprints. *Mol. Pharmacol.* 63(6): 1256–1272.

Gagnidze, K., Sachchidanand, R. Rozenfeld, M. Mezei, M. M. Zhou, and L. A. Devi. 2008. Homology modeling and site-directed mutagenesis to identify selective inhibitors of endothelin-converting enzyme-2. *J. Med. Chem.* 51(12): 3378–3387.

Gatica, E. A. and C. N. Cavasotto. 2012. Ligand and decoy sets for docking to G protein-coupled receptors. *J. Chem. Inf. Model.* 52: 1–6.

Ginalski, K. 2006. Comparative modeling for protein structure prediction. *Curr. Opin. Struct. Biol.* 16(2): 172–177.

Gonzalez, A., A. Cordomi, G. Caltabiano, and L. Pardo. 2012. Impact of helix irregularities on sequence alignment and homology modeling of G protein-coupled receptors. *ChemBioChem* 13(10): 1393–1399.

Gonzalez, A., A. Cordomi, M. Matsoukas, J. Zachmann, and L. Pardo. 2014. Modeling of G protein-coupled receptors using crystal structures: From monomers to signaling complexes. *Adv. Exp. Med. Biol.* 796: 15–33.

Greer, J. 1990. Comparative modeling methods: Application to the family of the mammalian serine proteases. *Proteins* 7(4): 317–334.

Guimaraes, A. J., A. J. Hamilton, M. Guedes H. L. de, J. D. Nosanchuk, and R. M. Zancope-Oliveira. 2008. Biological function and molecular mapping of M antigen in yeast phase of Histoplasma capsulatum. *PLoS One* 3(10): e3449.

Haas, J., S. Roth, K. Arnold et al. 2013. The protein model portal—A comprehensive resource for protein structure and model information. *Database (Oxford)* 2013: bat031.

Hanson, M. A. and R. C. Stevens. 2009. Discovery of new GPCR biology: One receptor structure at a time. *Structure* 17(1): 8–14.

Henikoff, S. and J. G. Henikoff. 1994. Position-based sequence weights. *J. Mol. Biol.* 243(4): 574–578.

Higo, J., V. Collura, and J. Garnier. 1992. Development of an extended simulated annealing method: Application to the modeling of complementary determining regions of immunoglobulins. *Biopolymers* 32(1): 33–43.

Hillisch, A., L. F. Pineda, and R. Hilgenfeld. 2004. Utility of homology models in the drug discovery process. *Drug Discov. Today* 9(15): 659–669.

Holm, L. and C. Sander. 1991. Database algorithm for generating protein backbone and side-chain co-ordinates from a C alpha trace application to model building and detection of co-ordinate errors. *J. Mol. Biol.* 218(1): 183–194.

Hooft, R. W., G. Vriend, C. Sander, and E. E. Abola. 1996. Errors in protein structures. *Nature* 381(6580): 272.

Huang, N., B. K. Shoichet, and J. J. Irwin. 2006. Benchmarking sets for molecular docking. *J. Med. Chem.* 49(23): 6789–6801.

ICM Version 3.7.2. 2012. MolSoft, LLC, La Jolla, CA.

Jamroz, M. and A. Kolinski. 2011. Modeling of loops in proteins: A multi-method approach. *BMC Struct. Biol.* 10: 5.

Jaroszewski, L., L. Rychlewski, Z. Li, W. Li, and A. Godzik. 2005. FFAS03: A server for profile—Profile sequence alignments. *Nucleic Acids Res.* 33(Web Server issue): W284–W288.

Jiang, L., B. Kuhlman, T. Kortemme, and D. Baker. 2005. A "solvated rotamer" approach to modeling water-mediated hydrogen bonds at protein-protein interfaces. *Proteins* 58(4): 893–904.

John, B. and A. Sali. 2003. Comparative protein structure modeling by iterative alignment, model building and model assessment. *Nucleic Acids Res.* 31(14): 3982–3992.

Jones, T. A. and S. Thirup. 1986. Using known substructures in protein model building and crystallography. *EMBO J.* 5(4): 819–822.

Kairys, V., M. X. Fernandes, and M. K. Gilson. 2006. Screening drug-like compounds by docking to homology models: A systematic study. *J. Chem. Inf. Model.* 46(1): 365–379.

Kallberg, M., H. Wang, S. Wang et al. 2012. Template-based protein structure modeling using the RaptorX web server. *Nat. Protoc.* 7(8): 1511–1522.

Karplus, K., C. Barrett, and R. Hughey. 1998. Hidden Markov models for detecting remote protein homologies. *Bioinformatics* 14(10): 846–856.

Katoh, K. and D. M. Standley. 2013. MAFFT multiple sequence alignment software version 7: Improvements in performance and usability. *Mol. Biol. Evol.* 30(4): 772–780.

Kelley, L. A. and M. J. Sternberg. 2009. Protein structure prediction on the Web: A case study using the Phyre server. *Nat. Protoc.* 4(3): 363–371.

Kelley, L. A., R. M. MacCallum, and M. J. Sternberg. 2000. Enhanced genome annotation using structural profiles in the program 3D-PSSM. *J. Mol. Biol.* 299(2): 499–520.

Kiefer, F., K. Arnold, M. Kunzli, L. Bordoli, and T. Schwede. 2009. The SWISS-MODEL Repository and associated resources. *Nucleic Acids Res.* 37(Database issue): D387–D392.

Kim, D. E., D. Chivian, and D. Baker. 2004. Protein structure prediction and analysis using the Robetta server. *Nucleic Acids Res.* 32(Web Server issue): W526–W531.

Kimura, S. R., A. J. Tebben, and D. R. Langley. 2008. Expanding GPCR homology model binding sites via a balloon potential: A molecular dynamics refinement approach. *Proteins* 71(4): 1919–1929.

Koehl, P. and M. Delarue. 1994. Application of a self-consistent mean field theory to predict protein side-chains conformation and estimate their conformational entropy. *J. Mol. Biol.* 239(2): 249–275.

Koehl, P. and M. Delarue. 1995. A self consistent mean field approach to simultaneous gap closure and side-chain positioning in homology modelling. *Nat. Struct. Biol.* 2(2): 163–170.

Kolodny, R., P. Koehl, L. Guibas, and M. Levitt. 2002. Small libraries of protein fragments model native protein structures accurately. *J. Mol. Biol.* 323(2): 297–307.

Kovacs, J. A., C. N. Cavasotto, and R. A. Abagyan. 2005. Conformational sampling of protein flexibility in generalized coordinates: Application to ligand docking. *J. Comp. Theor. Nanosci.* 2: 354–361.

Krogh, A., M. Brown, I. S. Mian, K. Sjolander, and D. Haussler. 1994. Hidden Markov models in computational biology. Applications to protein modeling. *J. Mol. Biol.* 235(5): 1501–1531.

Kryshtafovych, A., K. Fidelis, and J. Moult. 2014. CASP10 results compared to those of previous CASP experiments. *Proteins* 82(Suppl 2): 164–174.

Kufareva, I., M. Rueda, V. Katritch, R. C. Stevens, and R. Abagyan. 2011. Status of GPCR modeling and docking as reflected by community-wide GPCR Dock 2010 Assessment. *Structure* 19(8): 1108–1126.

Kufareva, I., V. Katritch, R. C. Stevens, and R. Abagyan. 2014. Advances in GPCR modeling evaluated by the GPCR Dock 2013 assessment: Meeting new challenges. *Structure* 22(8): 1120–1139.

Lagerstrom, M. C. and H. B. Schioth. 2008. Structural diversity of G protein-coupled receptors and significance for drug discovery. *Nat. Rev. Drug Discov.* 7(4): 339–357.

Larkin, M. A., G. Blackshields, N. P. Brown et al. 2007. Clustal W and Clustal X version 2.0. *Bioinformatics* 23(21): 2947–2948.

Laskowski, R. A., M. W. MacArthur, D. S. Moss, and J. M. Thornton. 1993. PROCHECK: A program to check the stereochemical quality of protein structures. *J. Appl. Cryst.* (26): 283–291.

Levitt, M. 1992. Accurate modeling of protein conformation by automatic segment matching. *J. Mol. Biol.* 226(2): 507–533.

Liang, S. and N. V. Grishin. 2002. Side-chain modeling with an optimized scoring function. *Protein Sci.* 11(2): 322–331.

Lim, H. D., A. Jongejan, R. A. Bakker, E. Haaksma, I. J. de Esch, and R. Leurs. 2008. Phenylalanine 169 in the second extracellular loop of the human histamine H4 receptor is responsible for the difference in agonist binding between human and mouse H4 receptors. *J. Pharmacol. Exp. Ther.* 327(1): 88–96.

Lin, M. S. and T. Head-Gordon. 2011. Reliable protein structure refinement using a physical energy function. *J. Comput. Chem.* 32(4): 709–717.

Lipman, D. J. and W. R. Pearson. 1985. Rapid and sensitive protein similarity searches. *Science* 227(4693): 1435–41.

Lovell, S. C., J. M. Word, J. S. Richardson, and D. C. Richardson. 2000. The penultimate rotamer library. *Proteins* 40(3): 389–408.

Lushington, G. H. 2015. Comparative modeling of proteins. *Methods Mol. Biol.* 1215: 309–330.

Luthy, R., J. U. Bowie, and D. Eisenberg. 1992. Assessment of protein models with three-dimensional profiles. *Nature* 356(6364): 83–85.

Mandell, D. J., E. A. Coutsias, and T. Kortemme. 2009. Sub-angstrom accuracy in protein loop reconstruction by robotics-inspired conformational sampling. *Nat. Methods* 6(8): 551–552.

Marti-Renom, M. A., A. C. Stuart, A. Fiser, R. Sanchez, F. Melo, and A. Sali. 2000. Comparative protein structure modeling of genes and genomes. *Annu. Rev. Biophys. Biomol. Struct.* 29: 291–325.

McGovern, S. L. and B. K. Shoichet. 2003. Information decay in molecular docking screens against holo, apo, and modeled conformations of enzymes. *J. Med. Chem.* 46(14): 2895–2907.

McGuffin, L. J. and D. T. Jones. 2003. Improvement of the GenTHREADER method for genomic fold recognition. *Bioinformatics* 19(7): 874–881.

McRobb, F. M., B. Capuano, I. T. Crosby, D. K. Chalmers, and E. Yuriev. 2010. Homology modeling and docking evaluation of aminergic G protein-coupled receptors. *J. Chem. Inf. Model.* 50(4): 626–637.

Melo, F. and E. Feytmans. 1998. Assessing protein structures with a non-local atomic interaction energy. *J. Mol. Biol.* 277(5): 1141–1152.

Melo, F., R. Sanchez, and A. Sali. 2002. Statistical potentials for fold assessment. *Protein Sci.* 11(2): 430–448.

Mezei, M. 1998. Chameleon sequences in the PDB. *Protein Eng.* 11(6): 411–414.

Michino, M., E. Abola, C. L. Brooks, 3rd, J. S. Dixon, J. Moult, and R. C. Stevens. 2009. Community-wide assessment of GPCR structure modelling and ligand docking: GPCR Dock 2008. *Nat. Rev. Drug Discov.* 8(6): 455–463.

Mirzadegan, T., G. Benko, S. Filipek, and K. Palczewski. 2003. Sequence analyses of G-protein coupled receptors: Similarities to rhodopsin. *Biochemistry* 42(10): 2759–2767.

Monti, M. C., A. Casapullo, C. N. Cavasotto, A. Napolitano, and R. Riccio. 2007. Scalaradial, a dialdehyde-containing marine metabolite that causes an unexpected noncovalent PLA(2) inactivation. *Chem. Bio. Chem.* 8(13): 1585–1591.

Monti, M. C., A. Casapullo, C. N. Cavasotto et al. 2009. The binding mode of petrosaspongiolide M to the human group IIA phospholipase A(2): Exploring the role of covalent and noncovalent interactions in the inhibition process. *Chem.-Eur. J.* 15(5): 1155–1163.

Moro, S., F. Deflorian, M. Bacilieri, and G. Spalluto. 2006. Ligand-based homology modeling as attractive tool to inspect GPCR structural plasticity. *Curr. Pharm. Des.* 12(17): 2175–2185.

Moult, J., J. T. Pedersen, R. Judson, and K. Fidelis. 1995. A large-scale experiment to assess protein structure prediction methods. *Proteins* 23(3): ii–v.

Moult, J. and M. N. James. 1986. An algorithm for determining the conformation of polypeptide segments in proteins by systematic search. *Proteins* 1(2): 146–163.

Notredame, C., D. G. Higgins, and J. Heringa. 2000. T-Coffee: A novel method for fast and accurate multiple sequence alignment. *J. Mol. Biol.* 302(1): 205–217.

Novoa, E. M., L. Ribas de Pouplana, X. Barril, and M. Orozco. 2010. Ensemble docking from homology models. *J. Chem. Theory Comput.* 6: 2547–2557.

Ohlendorf, D. H. 1994. Acuracy of refined protein structures. II. Comparison of four independently refined models of human interleukin 1beta. *Acta Crystallogr. D Biol. Crystallogr.* 50(Part 6): 808–812.

Ohlson, T., B. Wallner, and A. Elofsson. 2004. Profile-profile methods provide improved fold-recognition: A study of different profile-profile alignment methods. *Proteins* 57(1): 188–197.

Ono, Y., W. Fujibuchi, and M. Suwa. 2005. Automatic gene collection system for genome-scale overview of G-protein coupled receptors in eukaryotes. *Gene* 364: 63–73.

Orry, A.J.W. and C.N. Cavasotto. 2006. Ligand-docking-based homology model of the melanin-concentrating hormone 1 receptor. Paper read at 231st Meeting of the American Chemical Society, at Atlanta, GA.

Overington, J. P., B. Al-Lazikani, and A. L. Hopkins. 2006. How many drug targets are there? *Nat. Rev. Drug Discov.* 5(12): 993–996.

Palczewski, K., T. Kumasaka, T. Hori et al. 2000. Crystal structure of rhodopsin: A G protein-coupled receptor. *Science* 289(5480): 739–745.

Pardo, L., X. Deupi, N. Dolker, M. L. Lopez-Rodriguez, and M. Campillo. 2007. The role of internal water molecules in the structure and function of the rhodopsin family of G protein-coupled receptors. *Chem. Bio. Chem.* 8(1): 19–24.

Pearson, W. R. 1994. Using the FASTA program to search protein and DNA sequence databases. *Methods Mol. Biol.* 24: 307–331.

Petrov, R. R., L. Knight, S. R. Chen et al. 2013. Mastering tricyclic ring systems for desirable functional cannabinoid activity. *Eur. J. Med. Chem.* 69: 881–907.

Phatak, S. S., E. A. Gatica, and C. N. Cavasotto. 2010. Ligand-steered modeling and docking: A benchmarking study in Class A G-Protein-Coupled Receptors. *J. Chem. Inf. Model.* 50(12): 2119–2128.

Pieper, U., B. M. Webb, G. Q. Dong et al. 2014. ModBase, a database of annotated comparative protein structure models and associated resources. *Nucleic Acids Res.* 42(Database issue): D336–D346.

Pieper, U., N. Eswar, B. M. Webb et al. 2009. MODBASE, a database of annotated comparative protein structure models and associated resources. *Nucleic Acids Res.* 37(Database issue): D347–D354.

Pierce, K. L., R. T. Premont, and R. J. Lefkowitz. 2002. Seven-transmembrane receptors. *Nat. Rev. Mol. Cell Biol.* 3(9): 639–650.

Rai, B. K., G. J. Tawa, A. H. Katz, and C. Humblet. 2010. Modeling G protein-coupled receptors for structure-based drug discovery using low-frequency normal modes for refinement of homology models: Application to H3 antagonists. *Proteins* 78(2): 457–473.

Rasmussen, S. G., B. T. DeVree, Y. Zou et al. 2011. Crystal structure of the beta2 adrenergic receptor-Gs protein complex. *Nature* 477(7366): 549–555.

Rasmussen, S. G., H. J. Choi, D. M. Rosenbaum et al. 2007. Crystal structure of the human beta2 adrenergic G-protein-coupled receptor. *Nature* 450(7168): 383–387.

Rataj, K., J. Witek, S. Mordalski, T. Kosciolek, and A. J. Bojarski. 2014. Impact of template choice on homology model efficiency in virtual screening. *J. Chem. Inf. Model.* 54(6): 1661–1668.

Remmert, M., A. Biegert, A. Hauser, and J. Soding. 2012. HHblits: Lightning-fast iterative protein sequence searching by HMM-HMM alignment. *Nat. Methods* 9(2): 173–175.

Ring, C. S., E. Sun, J. H. McKerrow et al. 1993. Structure-based inhibitor design by using protein models for the development of antiparasitic agents. *Proc. Natl. Acad. Sci. USA* 90(8): 3583–3587.

Ripphausen, P., B. Nisius, L. Peltason, and J. Bajorath. 2010. Quo vadis, virtual screening? A comprehensive survey of prospective applications. *J. Med. Chem.* 53(24): 8461–8467.

Roche, D. B., M. T. Buenavista, S. J. Tetchner, and L. J. McGuffin. 2011. The IntFOLD server: An integrated web resource for protein fold recognition, 3D model quality assessment, intrinsic disorder prediction, domain prediction and ligand binding site prediction. *Nucleic Acids Res.* 39(Web Server issue): W171–W176.

Roy, A., A. Kucukural, and Y. Zhang. 2010. I-TASSER: A unified platform for automated protein structure and function prediction. *Nat. Protoc.* 5(4): 725–738.

Rufino, S. D., L. E. Donate, L. H. Canard, and T. L. Blundell. 1997. Predicting the conformational class of short and medium size loops connecting regular secondary structures: Application to comparative modelling. *J. Mol. Biol.* 267(2): 352–367.

Sali, A. and T. L. Blundell. 1993. Comparative protein modelling by satisfaction of spatial restraints. *J. Mol. Biol.* 234(3): 779–815.

Samudrala, R. and J. Moult. 1998. A graph-theoretic algorithm for comparative modeling of protein structure. *J. Mol. Biol.* 279(1): 287–302.

Sanchez, R. and A. Sali. 1997a. Advances in comparative protein-structure modelling. *Curr. Opin. Struct. Biol.* 7(2): 206–214.

Sanchez, R. and A. Sali. 1997b. Evaluation of comparative protein structure modeling by MODELLER-3. *Proteins* 29(Suppl 1): 50–58.

Sauder, J. M., J. W. Arthur, and R. L. Dunbrack, Jr. 2000. Large-scale comparison of protein sequence alignment algorithms with structure alignments. *Proteins* 40(1): 6–22.

Scheerer, P., J. H. Park, P. W. Hildebrand et al. 2008. Crystal structure of opsin in its G-protein-interacting conformation. *Nature* 455(7212): 497–502.

Schwarzenbacher, R., A. Godzik, S. K. Grzechnik, and L. Jaroszewski. 2004. The importance of alignment accuracy for molecular replacement. *Acta Crystallogr. D Biol. Crystallogr.* 60(Part 7): 1229–1236.

Schwede, T. 2013. Protein modeling: What happened to the "protein structure gap?" *Structure* 21(9): 1531–1540.

Schwede, T., J. Kopp, N. Guex, and M. C. Peitsch. 2003. SWISS-MODEL: An automated protein homology-modeling server. *Nucleic Acids Res.* 31(13): 3381–3385.

Sellers, B. D., K. Zhu, S. Zhao, R. A. Friesner, and M. P. Jacobson. 2008. Toward better refinement of comparative models: Predicting loops in inexact environments. *Proteins* 72(3): 959–971.

Sherman, W., T. Day, M. P. Jacobson, R. A. Friesner, and R. Farid. 2006. Novel procedure for modeling ligand/receptor induced fit effects. *J. Med. Chem.* 49(2): 534–553.

Sibanda, B. L., T. L. Blundell, and J. M. Thornton. 1989. Conformation of beta-hairpins in protein structures. A systematic classification with applications to modelling by homology, electron density fitting and protein engineering. *J. Mol. Biol.* 206(4): 759–777.

Sievers, F., A. Wilm, D. Dineen et al. 2011. Fast, scalable generation of high-quality protein multiple sequence alignments using Clustal Omega. *Mol. Syst. Biol.* 7: 539.

Sillitoe, I., A. L. Cuff, B. H. Dessailly et al. 2013. New functional families (FunFams) in CATH to improve the mapping of conserved functional sites to 3D structures. *Nucleic Acids Res.* 41(Database issue): D490–D498.

Simon, M. I., M. P. Strathmann, and N. Gautam. 1991. Diversity of G proteins in signal transduction. *Science* 252(5007): 802–808.

Sippl, M. J. 1990. Calculation of conformational ensembles from potentials of mean force. An approach to the knowledge-based prediction of local structures in globular proteins. *J. Mol. Biol.* 213(4): 859–883.

Skolnick, J., H. Zhou, and M. Gao. 2013. Are predicted protein structures of any value for binding site prediction and virtual ligand screening? *Curr. Opin. Struct. Biol.* 23(2): 191–197.

Soding, J. 2005. Protein homology detection by HMM-HMM comparison. *Bioinformatics* 21(7): 951–960.

Soga, S., H. Shirai, M. Kobori, and N. Hirayama. 2007. Identification of the druggable concavity in homology models using the PLB index. *J. Chem. Inf. Model.* 47(6): 2287–2292.

Song, L., C. Kalyanaraman, A. A. Fedorov et al. 2007. Prediction and assignment of function for a divergent N-succinyl amino acid racemase. *Nat. Chem. Biol.* 3(8): 486–491.

Song, Y., F. DiMaio, R. Y. Wang et al. 2013. High-resolution comparative modeling with RosettaCM. *Structure* 21(10): 1735–1742.

Sperandio, O., L. Mouawad, E. Pinto, B. O. Villoutreix, D. Perahia, and M. A. Miteva. 2010. How to choose relevant multiple receptor conformations for virtual screening: A test case of Cdk2 and normal mode analysis. *Eur. Biophys. J.* 39(9): 1365–1372.

Srinivasan, N. and T. L. Blundell. 1993. An evaluation of the performance of an automated procedure for comparative modelling of protein tertiary structure. *Protein Eng.* 6(5): 501–512.

Strasser, A. and H. J. Wittmann. 2013. Molecular modeling studies give hint for the existence of a symmetric hbeta(2)R-Galphabetagamma-homodimer. *J. Mol. Model.* 19(10): 4443–4457.

Sutcliffe, M. J., I. Haneef, D. Carney, and T. L. Blundell. 1987. Knowledge based modelling of homologous proteins, Part I: Three-dimensional frameworks derived from the simultaneous superposition of multiple structures. *Protein Eng.* 1(5): 377–384.

Taylor, W. R., T. P. Flores, and C. A. Orengo. 1994. Multiple protein structure alignment. *Protein Sci.* 3(10): 1858–1870.

Topham, C. M., A. McLeod, F. Eisenmenger, J. P. Overington, M. S. Johnson, and T. L. Blundell. 1993. Fragment ranking in modelling of protein structure. Conformationally constrained environmental amino acid substitution tables. *J. Mol. Biol.* 229(1): 194–220.

Tuccinardi, T. 2009. Docking-based virtual screening: Recent developments. *Comb. Chem. High Throughput Screen.* 12(3): 303–314.

van Gelder, C. W., F. J. Leusen, J. A. Leunissen, and J. H. Noordik. 1994. A molecular dynamics approach for the generation of complete protein structures from limited coordinate data. *Proteins* 18(2): 174–185.

van Rhee, A. M. and K. A. Jacobson. 1996. Molecular architecture of G protein-coupled receptors. *Drug Dev. Res.* 37(1): 1–38.

van Vlijmen, H. W., and M. Karplus. 1997. PDB-based protein loop prediction: Parameters for selection and methods for optimization. *J. Mol. Biol.* 267(4): 975–1001.

Varady, J., X. Wu, X. Fang et al. 2003. Molecular modeling of the three-dimensional structure of dopamine 3 (D3) subtype receptor: Discovery of novel and potent D3 ligands through a hybrid pharmacophore- and structure-based database searching approach. *J. Med. Chem.* 46(21): 4377–4392.

Venclovas, C. 2012. Methods for sequence-structure alignment. *Methods Mol. Biol.* 857: 55–82.

Venkatakrishnan, A. J., X. Deupi, G. Lebon, C. G. Tate, G. F. Schertler, and M. M. Babu. 2013. Molecular signatures of G-protein-coupled receptors. *Nature* 494(7436): 185–194.

Vernal, J., A. Fiser, A. Sali, M. Muller, J. J. Cazzulo, and C. Nowicki. 2002. Probing the specificity of a trypanosomal aromatic alpha-hydroxy acid dehydrogenase by site-directed mutagenesis. *Biochem. Biophys. Res. Commun.* 293(1): 633–639.

Vilar, S., G. Ferino, S. S. Phatak, B. Berk, C. N. Cavasotto, and S. Costanzi. 2011. Docking-based virtual screening for GPCRs ligands: Not only crystal structures but also *in silico* models. *J. Mol. Graphics Modell.* 29: 614–623.

Vroling, B., D. Thorne, P. McDermott et al. 2012. NucleaRDB: Information system for nuclear receptors. *Nucleic Acids Res.* 40(Database issue): D377–D380.

Vroling, B. M. Sanders, C. Baakman et al. 2011. GPCRDB: Information system for G protein-coupled receptors. *Nucleic Acids Res.* 39(Database issue): D309–D319.

Wallner, B. and A. Elofsson. 2005. Pcons5: Combining consensus, structural evaluation and fold recognition scores. *Bioinformatics* 21(23): 4248–4254.

Wallner, B. and A. Elofsson. 2007. Prediction of global and local model quality in CASP7 using Pcons and ProQ. *Proteins* 69(Suppl 8): 184–193.

Wang, G. and R. L. Dunbrack, Jr. 2004. Scoring profile-to-profile sequence alignments. *Protein Sci.* 13(6): 1612–1626.

Warren, G. L., C. W. Andrews, A. M. Capelli et al. 2006. A critical assessment of docking programs and scoring functions. *J. Med. Chem.* 49(20): 5912–5931.

Webb, B. and A. Sali. 2014. Comparative protein structure modeling using MODELLER. *Curr. Protoc. Bioinformatics* 47: 5.6.1–5.6.32.

Wolf, S., M. Bockmann, U. Howeler, J. Schlitter, and K. Gerwert. 2008. Simulations of a G protein-coupled receptor homology model predict dynamic features and a ligand binding site. *FEBS Lett.* 582(23–24): 3335–3342.

Worth, C. L., A. Kreuchwig, G. Kleinau, and G. Krause. 2011. GPCR-SSFE: A comprehensive database of G-protein-coupled receptor template predictions and homology models. *BMC Bioinformatics* 12: 185.

Worth, C. L., G. Kleinau, and G. Krause. 2009. Comparative sequence and structural analyses of G-protein-coupled receptor crystal structures and implications for molecular models. *PLoS One* 4(9): e7011.

Wu, S. and Y. Zhang. 2008. MUSTER: Improving protein sequence profile-profile alignments by using multiple sources of structure information. *Proteins* 72(2): 547–556.

Xiang, Z. and B. Honig. 2001. Extending the accuracy limits of prediction for side-chain conformations. *J. Mol. Biol.* 311(2): 421–430.

Zhang, Y. 2008. I-TASSER server for protein 3D structure prediction. *BMC Bioinformatics* 9: 40.

Zheng, Q., R. Rosenfeld, S. Vajda, and C. DeLisi. 1993. Determining protein loop conformation using scaling-relaxation techniques. *Protein Sci.* 2(8): 1242–1248.

Zhou, H. and Y. Zhou. 2002. Distance-scaled, finite ideal-gas reference state improves structure-derived potentials of mean force for structure selection and stability prediction. *Protein Sci.* 11(11): 2714–2726.

Zhou, H. and Y. Zhou. 2005. Fold recognition by combining sequence profiles derived from evolution and from depth-dependent structural alignment of fragments. *Proteins* 58(2): 321–328.

Zhu, K., D. L. Pincus, S. Zhao, and R. A. Friesner. 2006. Long loop prediction using the protein local optimization program. *Proteins* 65(2): 438–452.

9

Implicit Solvation Methods in the Study of Ligand–Protein Interactions

William Zamora, Josep M. Campanera, and F. Javier Luque

CONTENTS

9.1 Ligand–Receptor Interaction

The affinity between a small compound and its macromolecular target can be related to macroscopic observables through the laws of thermodynamics. Thus, the binding affinity can be expressed in terms of the equilibrium constant (K) for the formation of the ligand–receptor complex, which can be related to the difference in the standard Gibbs free energy between bound and unbound states (ΔG°; Equation 9.1).

$$\Delta G^\circ = -RT \ln K \tag{9.1}$$

where R is the gas constant and T is the temperature.

The binding affinity reflects a subtle balance between a number of separate enthalpic and entropic contributions (Gohlke and Klebe 2002; Bissantz et al. 2010). The structural and chemical complementarity between the functional groups that are present at the binding interface renders the net stabilizing energy that is required to compensate unfavorable contributions to the binding. Thus, the binding between ligand and receptor is often accompanied by conformational changes, which can encompass a range of potential scenarios such as the "induced fit" mechanism, the "conformational selection" process, or even more complex models that combine the selection of specific conformations with the induction of structural readjustments upon binding (Csermely et al. 2010; Spyrakis et al. 2011). Predicting the energy cost associated with conformational changes in the ligand has proved to be very challenging, as noted by the uncertainties associated with the choice of the level of theory used to determine the cost of selecting the bioactive conformation (Tirado-Rives and Jorgensen 2006; Butler et al. 2009).

The energy gain as a result of the seemingly favorable interactions formed in the complex must counterbalance the cost due to dehydration of the separate partners prior to their mutual interaction. For simple neutral organic compounds, the hydration-free energies are generally in a narrow range, as noted in the experimental values for the transfer from gas phase to water for compounds that mimic the side chain of noncharged amino acids, which vary from +2 to −11 kcal/mol (Table 9.1; Wolfenden et al. 1981). However, the hydration-free energy of charged compounds is much larger, as expected from the strengthening of the interactions with water molecules, leading to hydration-free energies of −77 kcal/mol for acetate anion and −71 kcal/mol for the protonated *n*-butylamine (Pliego and Riveros 2002). Hence, there must be a sizable compensation between the dehydration energy cost and binding site residues and the energy gain triggered upon burial of the ligand in the binding pocket.

Finally, the ligand–receptor interactions must also compensate for the entropy changes arising upon molecular association, such as the loss of translational and rotational degrees of freedom, the reduction in the accessible states for internal rotations of both ligand and protein, and the reorganization of water molecules upon formation of the complex. This can be illustrated by the fact that binding of amprenavir to HIV protease is accompanied by a configurational entropy loss of 26.4 kcal/mol, which primarily

TABLE 9.1

Experimental Hydration-Free Energies (ΔG_{hyd}; kcal mol^{-1}) of Organic Compounds Chosen as Analogs of the Side Chains of Neutral Amino Acids

Residue	Side Chain Analog	ΔG_{hyd}	Residue	Side Chain Analogue	ΔG_{hyd}
Ala	Methane	2.0	Leu	Isobutane	2.3
Ile	Butane	2.1	Met	Methyl ethyl sulfide	−1.5
Val	Propane	2.0	Phe	Toluene	−0.9
Phe	*p*-Cresol	−6.1	Trp	Methylindole	−5.9
His	Methylimidazole	−10.3	Ser	Methanol	−5.1
Thr	Ethanol	−5.1	Cys	Methanethiol	−1.2
Asn	Acetamide	−9.7	Gln	Propionamide	−9.4
Asp	Acetic acid	−6.7	Glu	Propionic acid	−6.5
Lys	*N*-butylamine	−4.3	Arg	*N*-propylguanidine	−10.9

arises from narrowness of the energy wells of bound amprenavir relative to free ligand (Chang et al. 2007).

The net balance between enthalpic and entropic components leads to ligand–protein binding affinities that generally fall between 10^{-2} and 10^{-12} M (Gohlke and Klebe 2002). Unfortunately, small uncertainties in determining the magnitude of the different free energy components may have a drastic impact on the accuracy of the binding affinity (Williams et al. 2004; Reynolds and Holloway 2011). Thus, an error of 1.36 kcal/mol changes the predicted binding constant (at 298 K) by one order of magnitude. Predicting with chemical accuracy the binding free energy is a formidable challenge to current computational methods due to the magnitude of the separate contributions to the binding free energy, and the compensation between enthalpic and entropic terms. However, this is a fundamental ingredient for the success of drug discovery, especially keeping in mind that the maximal free energy contribution per non-hydrogen atom in a drug-like ligand amounts to ~–1.5 kcal/mol (higher values per atom are found in the case of metals, small anions, and ligands that form covalent bonds; Kuntz et al. 1999).

The aim of this chapter is to examine the use of implicit solvation models in the calculation of the binding affinity of ligand–receptor complexes. To this end, the chapter is divided into two major sections. The first is focused on the use of implicit solvation models in the context of classical force field methods, dealing specifically with molecular mechanics Poisson–Boltmann surface area (MM-PBSA) and its Generalized Born counterpart (MM-GBSA). Attention is paid to the details of the underlying formalism and to the different strategies undertaken in order to improve the accuracy of the predicted binding affinities. In the second section, a brief overview of the application of implicit solvation methods in the framework of quantum mechanics is given in order to highlight the progressive development of novel implementations and their application in drug discovery.

9.2 Molecular Mechanics and Implicit Solvation Models

Free energy perturbation (FEP) and thermodynamic integration (TI) are the most valuable computational methods for the prediction of binding affinities of small drug-candidate compounds (Brandsdal et al. 2003; Chipot and Pohorille 2007; Jorgensen 2009). These techniques rely on the alchemical transformation of ligands (or amino acid residues in the wild-type protein and a mutated variant) in two states, which correspond to the ligand free in solution, and the ligand bound to the receptor. This transformation is performed by means of a series of simulations carried out at intermediate points along the transition path that connects the Hamiltonians of the initial and final states. As noted by Michel and Essex (2010), it seems reasonable to expect that free energy calculations cannot predict binding free energies more accurately than solvation-free energies, where the uncertainties obtained for small organic compounds are approximately 1 kcal mol^{-1} (see also Merz 2010).

These calculations can provide the missing links between the experimental binding affinities and the atomic details of the protein–ligand complexes. However, when there are substantial differences in the chemical scaffold of the ligands, which differ by large substituents, or even when drastic mutations occur between the native protein and the mutated variant (e.g., tryptophan to alanine), the reliability and chemical accuracy of these calculations can be affected by convergence problems due to numerical instabilities and the limited conformational sampling. Hence, reliable computational schemes for the systematic prediction of ligand binding and mutagenesis effects are the subject of intense research (Pitera and van Gunsteren 2002; Steinbrecher et al. 2007; Lawrenz et al. 2011; Boukharta et al. 2014).

The high computational cost of these techniques is primarily due to the large number of intermediate states that must be defined in the alchemical transformation, but also to the explicit treatment of the molecular environment. These factors can be alleviated by treating solvent effects only implicitly using continuum solvent methods, and by considering only the endpoint states in the free energy calculations. These approximations lead to the so-called endpoint, implicit solvent-free energy methods, which encompass MM-PBSA and MM-GBSA. The main advantage of these methods is the huge reduction in the computational cost, which enables the screening of large datasets of ligands against a common receptor in a reasonable time span. Thus, MM-PB(GB)SA has been widely used in solving a broad range of topics valuable in ligand–receptor interactions, and specifically in drug discovery, such as determining hot spots in ligand-binding pockets and protein–protein interfaces, rescoring of docking poses, estimating binding affinities, and evaluating the stability of macromolecular assemblies. Nevertheless, the simplified description of the molecular system can also affect the chemical accuracy in predicting both the binding pose and the binding affinity, which makes it necessary to carry out a rigorous calibration of these methods.

9.2.1 Methodological Formalism of MM-PB(GB)SA Methods

In MM-PB(GB)SA, the binding free energy between ligand and receptor (ΔG_{bin}) is determined by combining three terms (Figure 9.1): the gas-phase free energy (ΔG_{MM}), the solvation-free energy (ΔG_{sol}), and the change in the configurational entropy ($-T\Delta S$) upon binding (Equation 9.2).

$$\Delta G_{bin} = \Delta G_{MM} + \Delta G_{sol} - T\Delta S \qquad (9.2)$$

The gas-phase component is determined from the molecular mechanics energy of the molecule, including bonded and nonbonded terms as implemented in a given force field. If the configurational space of the bound state

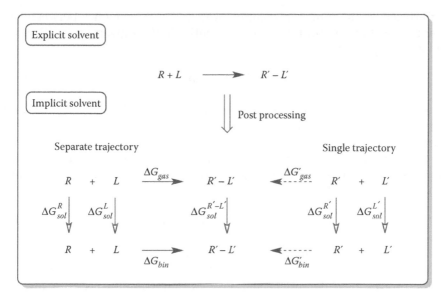

FIGURE 9.1

Thermodynamic cycle for the calculation of the binding affinity between ligand and receptor. Generally, MM-PB(GB)SA is used as a postprocessing method using representative snapshots taken from the trajectory sampled in a molecular dynamics simulation. In the single trajectory approach, ligand and receptor are taken from the snapshots sampled for the ligand-receptor complex ($R'-L'$). Other approaches use separate trajectories for receptor (R', R) and ligand (L', L). As noted in Equation 9.2, the binding affinity (ΔG_{bin}; $\Delta G'_{bin}$) combines the gas phase term (ΔG_{gas}; $\Delta G'_{gas}$), which combines the molecular mechanics (ΔG_{MM}) and entropic ($-T\Delta S$) terms, and the solvation contribution of complex ($\Delta G_{sol}^{R'-L'}$), receptor (ΔG_{sol}^{R}; $\Delta G_{sol}^{R'}$), and ligand (ΔG_{sol}^{L}; $\Delta G_{sol}^{L'}$).

is assumed to be representative of the configurations sampled by separate ligand and receptor, then the ΔG_{MM} term is merely given by the addition of Coulomb (ΔG_{elec}) and van der Waals (ΔG_{vdW}) contributions (Equation 9.3).

$$\Delta G_{MM} = \Delta G_{elec} + \Delta G_{vdW} \qquad (9.3)$$

The solvation-free energy is divided into polar (ΔG_{sol-p}) and nonpolar (ΔG_{sol-np}) components (Equation 9.4). The polar term reflects the change in free energy for the transfer from the gas phase to the aqueous solvent, typically modeled as homogeneous medium characterized with dielectric constant of 1 and 78.4, respectively. This term is calculated by resorting to numerical methods for solving the Poisson–Boltzmann equation through a finite-difference approach, or alternatively by means of the GB theory (for a review, see Orozco and Luque 2000).

$$\Delta G_{sol} = \Delta G_{sol-p} + \Delta G_{sol-np} \qquad (9.4)$$

In a continuum electrostatics model, a hydrated solute molecule is treated as a charge distribution in a low-dielectric cavity, which is embedded in a high-dielectric medium representing water. The dependence between the charge distribution and the electric potential is then given by the Poisson equation (Equation 9.5).

$$\nabla\varepsilon(r)\nabla\phi(r) = -\rho(r) \tag{9.5}$$

where $\varepsilon(r)$ denotes the dielectric constant, $\phi(r)$ is the electric potential, and $\rho(r)$ is the charge distribution.

In the presence of an ionic atmosphere, Equation 9.5 adopts the form given by the nonlinear Poisson–Boltzmann equation, which under the assumption that $\varphi(r)$ is small can be linearized (using the approximation that sinh $\varphi(r) \approx \varphi(r)$; Equation 9.6).

$$\nabla\varepsilon(r)\nabla\phi(r) - \kappa^2\phi(r) = -\rho(r) \tag{9.6}$$

where κ is the Debye–Hückel inverse screening length.

Equations 9.5 and 9.6 must be solved numerically. The finite-difference method solves the differential equations by discretizing the region of interest into grid points (typically a cubic grid). Accordingly, the solute partial charges are fractionally distributed among the nearby grid points, the dielectric constants are assigned to each grid point according to the geometry of the dielectric boundary, and the second derivatives of the potential at each grid point can be expressed in terms of the potentials at neighboring points. The coupled expressions for the potentials on the grid produce a linear system of equations that can be solved to yield the potential at each grid point. It is worth noting, however, that estimates of the electrostatic component from grid-based solvers of the Poisson equation inevitably contain numerical grid-discretization errors, and that a careful assessment of these errors must be performed (Harris et al. 2013). Other approaches, such as the finite element method or the boundary element method, are also available (for details, see Tomasi and Persico 1994).

The GB model offers a simpler, computationally less-expensive approach to the electrostatic component of the solvation-free energy (Equation 9.7; Still et al. 1990).

$$\Delta G_{sol-p} = \frac{1}{2}\left(1 - \frac{1}{\varepsilon_{out}}\right)\sum_{i,j}\frac{q_iq_j}{f_{GB}} \tag{9.7}$$

where q_i denotes the partial atomic charges of the solute, ε_{out} is the dielectric constant of the solvent environment, and f_{GB} stands for the screening function, which is generally expressed as noted in Equation 9.8 (for a review, see Bashford and Case 2000).

$$f_{GB}(r_{ij}) = \left[r_{ij}^2 + \alpha_i\alpha_j\exp\left(\frac{-r_{ij}^2}{(4\alpha_i\alpha_j)}\right)\right]^{1/2} \tag{9.8}$$

where r_{ij} is the interatomic distance between particles i and j, α_i stands for the effective Born radius of particle i.

The use of Equation 9.7 makes the calculation of the electrostatic solvation term to be the sum of pairwise interactions, thus making it suitable for implementation in molecular dynamics (MD) programs. Furthermore, the pairwise nature of the method also facilitates decomposition of free energies into individual atomic contributions (see below).

The nonpolar contribution (ΔG_{sol-np}) is generally estimated by using a linear expression with the solvent-accessible surface (SAS; Equation 9.9), which is intended to account for the contributions due to the cavity formation within the solvent and the change in nonpolar interactions between solute and solvent (Sitkoff et al. 1994).

$$\Delta G_{sol-np} = \gamma SAS + \beta \qquad (9.9)$$

Finally, the change in configurational entropy of the solute is usually estimated by means of a normal mode analysis of harmonic frequencies calculated at the MM level. This analysis can be performed for simplified structures containing the residues within a given sphere centered at the ligand, and the energy-minimized structures are obtained by using a distance-dependent dielectric, which is introduced to mimic the solvent dielectric (Kongsted and Ryde 2009; Genheden and Ryde 2011; Hou et al. 2011). However, this contribution is often neglected when the primary interest is the prediction of relative binding affinities between structurally similar ligands.

9.2.2 Computational Aspects of MM-PB(GB)SA Calculations

Calculation of the binding affinity between a ligand and its receptor can be performed using two computational approaches, which involves a single trajectory of the ligand–receptor complex or separate trajectories of the ligand–receptor complex, the receptor and the ligand (Figure 9.1; Wang et al. 2006). Although this latter approach is formally more rigorous, because it takes into account the differences in conformational flexibility of the bound and unbound states, the single trajectory strategy is usually adopted because it benefits from the cancellation of intramolecular contributions in the prediction of the binding affinity, especially in cases where no large structural differences are expected to occur upon binding.

MM-PB(GB)SA calculations are generally performed for ensembles of structures sampled along the trajectories obtained from MD simulations. Then, a set of representative structures is extracted from the trajectory, water molecules and counterions are subsequently removed, and the free energy is calculated as noted in Equation 9.2. At this point, it has been pointed out that selecting a relatively small number of representative snapshots may suffice to obtain an accurate prediction comparable to using the full MD trajectory (Lill and Thompson 2011).

Since a single MD simulation may often not provide a complete description of the conformational space available for the ligand–receptor complex (and even for the separate receptor), it is then unclear whether the binding affinity estimated from a single trajectory can be representative or not. Adler and Beroza (2013) have recently considered this issue. Thus, replicate MM-PBSA calculations were performed for four distinct ligand–receptor complexes. Separate trajectories were generated using nearly identical starting coordinates (1% randomly perturbed by 0.001 Å), and they were found to lead to significantly different calculated binding free energies. Thus, even though the binding affinity did converge in each separate run, the variation across separate runs implies that a single trajectory may inadequately sample the system. Hence, the authors recommend that combining MM-PB(GB)SA with multiple samples of the initial starting coordinates will lead to more accurate estimates of the binding affinity.

However, it is worth noting that the inclusion of specific structural water molecules has been found to be important for the accurate description of MM-PB(GB)SA energetics. For instance, it has been reported that the difference in binding affinity of nevirapine to the wild-type HIV-1 reverse transcriptase and the Y181C mutant was better discriminated upon inclusion of key water molecules as part of the protein (Treesuwan and Hannongbua 2009). Similarly, the protein–protein interaction between the T-cell receptor and its staphylococcal enterotoxin 3 (SEC3) binding partner was only effectively discriminated against two mutated SEC3 variants only when key explicit water molecules were included in the calculations (Wong et al. 2009). On the contrary, a protocol for the inclusion of water molecules that mediate ligand–protein interactions, denoted water-MM-PBSA, has been reported (Zhu et al. 2014), leading to improved correlation between the binding affinities estimated for a series of JNK3 kinase inhibitors and the experimental IC_{50} values compared to that obtained from classical MM-PBSA calculations.

The averaged contributions obtained from the whole set of snapshots enable to check the time convergence and internal consistency of the binding affinity and its free energy components (Stoica et al. 2008), while they take into account the effect due to conformational fluctuations of the molecular system. However, it has been advocated that the conformational sampling of the simulated system should be performed using simulations with explicit treatment of the solvent molecules, avoiding the use of continuum solvent simulations (Weis et al. 2006). Furthermore, the mixing of force fields for collecting the snapshots along the discrete MD simulation and for the MM-PB(GB)SA calculation is not recommended, as it may give inaccuracies (Weis et al. 2006).

Even though MM-PB(GB)SA has proven to be successful in various ligand–protein complexes, the results also demonstrate that the overall performance is highly system-dependent. For instance, a systematic analysis of 59 ligands interacting with six distinct receptors showed that MM-PBSA gives good predictions for homologous ligands and has a variable performance for ligands with diverse structures (Figure 9.2; Hou et al. 2011). Furthermore, MM-PBSA

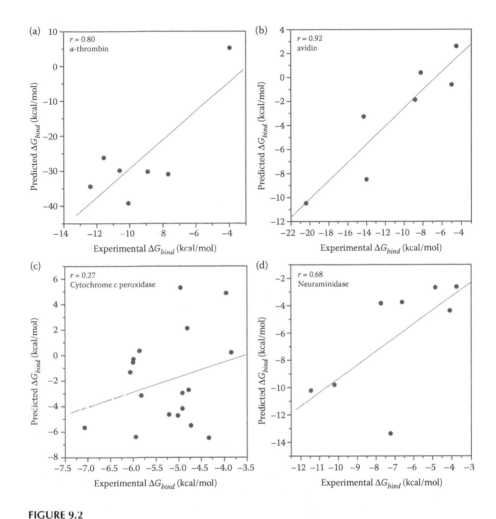

FIGURE 9.2
Correlations between the MM/PBSA binding affinities and the experimental values for (a) a-thrombin, (b) avidin, (c) cytochrome c peroxidase, (d) neuraminidase, (e) P450cam, and (f) penicillopepsin. (Reprinted with permission from Hou, T. et al. 2011. Assessing the performance of the MM/PBSA and MM/GBSA Methods. 1. The accuracy of binding free energy calculations based on molecular dynamics simulations. *J. Chem. Inf. Model.* 51(1): 69–82. Copyright 2011, American Chemical Society.) *(Continued)*

predictions were found to be very sensitive to the solute dielectric constant, which is related to the physicochemical features of the binding interface. In fact, Hou et al. (2011) reported that for highly charged binding interfaces, a higher solute dielectric constant ($\varepsilon_{in} \sim 4$) is preferred, whereas for moderately charged or hydrophobic binding interfaces values of ε_{in} equal to 2 or 1, respectively, are more adequate. At this point, the authors suggested the change in the solvent-accessible surface area (SASA) of the groups involved in strong

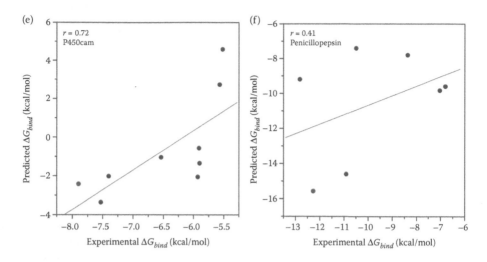

FIGURE 9.2 (Continued)
Correlations between the MM/PBSA binding affinities and the experimental values for (a) a-thrombin, (b) avidin, (c) cytochrome c peroxidase, (d) neuraminidase, (e) P450cam, and (f) penicillopepsin. (Reprinted with permission from Hou, T. et al. 2011. Assessing the performance of the MM/PBSA and MM/GBSA Methods. 1. The accuracy of binding free energy calculations based on molecular dynamics simulations. *J. Chem. Inf. Model.* 51(1): 69–82. Copyright 2011, American Chemical Society.)

polar–polar interactions between ligand and receptor as a valuable guide to select the dielectric constant of the solute. Moreover, this study also concluded that inclusion of conformational entropy is crucial for predicting absolute binding free energies, but not for ranking the binding affinities of similar ligands.

Similar studies have been performed for MM-PB(GB)SA calculations for a total of 46 small molecules targeted to five different protein receptors (Xu et al. 2013). Attention was paid to the effect of (i) AMBER force fields (ff99, ff99SB, ff99SB-ILDN, ff03, and ff12SB), (ii) the timescale of MD simulations, and (iii) the impact of four different charge models (RESP, ESP, AM1-BCC, and Gasteiger) for small molecules.

In a separate work, Swanson et al. (2005) also examined the impact of solute charge, dielectric coefficient, and atomic radii on the accuracy in predicting the solvation-free energies. To this end, a set of 14 polyalanine peptides and a series of 20 nonzwitterionic N-acetyl-X-N'-methylamide dipeptides, with X representing one of the 20 standard amino acids, were subject to explicit solvent simulations, and the charging free energies were determined by means of FEP calculations. These data were then utilized for deriving two optimized sets of atomic radii, which were chosen to define either abrupt or cubic-spline smoother dielectric boundaries, to be used in conjunction with AMBER (parm99) charges. The optimized radii were found to offer increased accuracy of solvation energies and atomic forces in a test set of four protein-like polypeptides. The application of these optimized radii to the binding of peptides to human class II MHC molecules was shown to reflect adequately the distinction between strong and for binding peptides (Cárdenas et al. 2010).

The aim of deriving parameters for implicit solvent models optimized in a system- or atom-specific manner on the basis of experimental data or more rigorous explicit solvent simulations has been adopted in other studies. For instance, the performance of PB calculations with regard to the TIP3P explicit solvent has been examined for a variety of systems of biochemical interest (Tan et al. 2006). The results support the transferability of empirically optimized parameters for the implicit solvent from small training molecules to large testing peptides. However, a computational strategy for optimizing the solute radii on the basis of forces and energies from explicit solvent simulations has been reported in the context of the AMBER partial charges and a spline-smoothed solute surface (Swanson et al. 2007). An alternative approach for deriving optimized radii for PB calculations has been undertaken by Yamagishi et al. (2014). The radii were optimized using results from explicit solvent simulations of amino acid templates and large peptides in the framework of the AMBER protein force field and using a smoothing dielectric function. Moreover, discrimination between radii assigned to N- and C-terminal residues from nonterminal ones was also considered.

In a different approach, Purisima and coworkers have developed the solvated interaction energy (SIE) method, which is an endpoint MM-PBSA-based scoring function that approximates the protein–ligand binding affinity by an interaction energy contribution and a desolvation free energy contribution (Naïm et al. 2007; Cui et al. 2008). Electrostatic solvation effects are calculated with the boundary element solution to the Poisson equation, while nonpolar solvation is based on change in the SAS. As in the single-trajectory approach, the free state is generally obtained by separation of both ligand and receptor from the ligand–receptor complex sampled along the MD trajectory. The SIE method has been carefully calibrated using a diverse set of ligand–protein complexes, including the calibration of parameters such as the dielectric constant, the surface tension coefficient, and the inclusion of an enthalpy–entropy compensating scaling factor. The SIE scoring function leads to a reasonable agreement between predicted and experimental binding affinities, as noted in the external testing against a curated dataset of 343 ligand–protein complexes, leading to a root-mean square error in the predicted binding affinities of 2.5 kcal mol^{-1} (Sulea et al. 2011).

9.2.3 Large-Scale Application of MM-PB(GB)SA Models

The advent of faster computers and automated procedures for preparation of ligands and receptors has promoted the use of MM-PB(GB)SA models in medium- and high-throughput screenings, making them valuable for reranking of docked poses. As an example, Brown and Muchmore (2009) reported a large-scale application to a set of 308 small-molecule ligands in complex with urokinase, PTP-1B, and Chk-1. Briefly, they use a GB implicit solvation model during the computer-intensive ensemble-generating MD runs, whereas in the postproduction process a PB solver that employs a diffuse representation of the dielectric boundary (instead of the more common discrete transition between solute and solvent). Statistically significant correlations to experimentally measured potencies were found, leading to correlation coefficients for the three proteins in the range 0.72–0.83.

Greenidge et al. (2013) have validated an automated implementation of MM-GBSA using a large and diverse selection of 855 protein–ligand complexes. In particular, calculations were performed using the VSGB 2.0 energy model, which features an optimized implicit solvent model that includes physics-based corrections for hydrogen bonding, pi–pi interactions, self-contact interactions and hydrophobic contacts, and parameters were fit to a crystallographic database of 2239 single side chain and 100 11–13 residue loop predictions (Li et al. 2012). Calculations were performed using the KNIME-automated workflow. After carefully removing flawed structures, comparison of calculated and experimental binding affinities showed a significant correlation ($R^2 = 0.63$; Figure 9.3). The study also discussed the impact of ligand strain and water molecules, revealing that while inclusion of water molecules deteriorates the predictive quality, inclusion of ligand strain slightly improves the overall accuracy. In an independent study, the accuracy of the VSGB 2.0 energy model in predicting binding free energies was

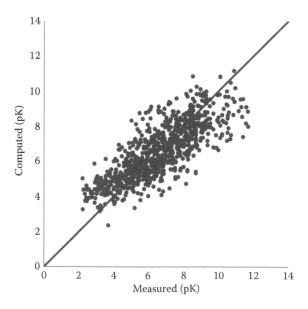

FIGURE 9.3
Comparison of computed and experimental binding affinities. (Reprinted with permission from Greenidge, P. A. et al. 2013. MM/GBSA binding energy prediction on the PDBbind data set: Successes, failures, and directions for further improvement. *J. Chem. Inf. Model.* 53(1): 201–209. Copyright 2013, American Chemical Society.)

also tested for 106 protein–ligand complexes (Mulakala and Viswanadhan 2013). The results indicate that this method may be approaching the accuracy required for absolute binding free energy determination, although through linear regression and without any conformational sampling. Furthermore, given the modest computational cost of these calculations, the MM-GBSA formalism may be poised toward generating physics-based scoring functions for docking.

Very recently, Greenidge et al. (2014) have shown that MM-GBSA can be used as an independent scoring function to assess the energetically preferred pose as generated with multiple scoring functions, and in multiple protein conformations. The results supported the role of MM-GBSA to distinguish between true and decoy poses of a ligand in addition to the rescoring of data sets.

A last example of the progressive large-scale application of MM-PB(GB)SA methods is the high-throughput virtual screening pipeline for *in silico* screening of virtual compound databases using high-performance computing (Zhang et al. 2014). This pipeline involves an automated receptor preparation scheme with unsupervised binding site identification, including receptor/target preparation, ligand preparation, VinaLC docking calculation, and MM-GBSA rescoring. The results demonstrate that MM-GBSA rescoring has higher average receiver operating characteristic (ROC) area under curve (AUC) values and consistently better early recovery of actives than Vina docking alone, though the enrichment performance is target-dependent.

9.3 Per-Residue Decomposition of the MM-PB(GB)SA Free Energy

The decomposition into per-residue and residue-pairwise contributions of the MM-PB(GB)SA binding free energy allows to unravel the network of energetic interactions that stabilize ligand–protein binding, thus providing insight into key features of binding (Gohlke et al. 2003). All the components of the binding affinity (Equation 9.2) can be decomposed with certain degree of approximation into per-residue and also residue-pairwise contributions according to the standard scheme given by Equation 9.10.

$$\Delta G_{bin} = \sum_{i=1}^{n} \Delta G^i = \sum_{i=1}^{n} \sum_{j \neq i}^{n} \Delta G^{i,j} \tag{9.10}$$

where n is the total number of residues, ΔG^i are the per-residue contributions, and $\Delta G^{i,j}$ are the residue-pairwise interaction contributions.

Under this scheme ΔG_{bin} can also be partitioned into the receptor and ligand components by summing the corresponding per-residue contributions of each fragment (Equation 9.11).

$$\Delta G_{bin} = \Delta G^{receptor} + \Delta G^{ligand} \tag{9.11}$$

It is worth noting that only the electrostatic (ΔG_{elec}) and van der Waals (ΔG_{vdW}) terms are strictly residue-pairwise decomposable, so that one-half of the pairwise interaction energy between two residues i and j is attributed to both of them. However, the solvation terms are not inherently decomposable, since the effective Born radii for GB and dielectric boundaries for PB are dependent on the surroundings (Miller et al. 2012).

Regarding the GB polar solvation term, $\Delta G_{sol-p}^{i,j}$, a pairwise descreening approximation was implemented by Onufriev et al. (Onufriev et al. 2000; Tsui and Case 2001) based on the improvement of the standard GB model (Hawkins et al. 1995) as noted in Equation 9.12.

$$\Delta G_{sol-p}^{i,j} = \sum_{l\in i}^{n_i} \sum_{k\in j}^{n_j} -\frac{1}{2}\left(\frac{1}{\varepsilon_{in}} - \frac{e^{-\kappa f_{GB}}}{\varepsilon_{out}} \right) \frac{q_l q_k}{f_{GB}} \tag{9.12}$$

where ε_{in} and ε_{out} are the solute and solvent dielectric constants, κ is the Debye–Hückel screening parameter to account for salt effects at low salt concentrations (Srinivasan et al. 1999).

Since f_{GB} depends on the effective Born radius (Equation 9.8), $\Delta G_{sol-p}^{i,j}$ is inherently nondecomposable, that is, the polar solvation interaction between residues i and j is affected by all other atoms in the system. Therefore, the binding free energies of receptor and ligand (Equation 9.11) become asymmetric, since the effective Born radius yields different values depending on the overall structure of either complex or receptor/ligand. A similar reasoning can be used in relation to the PB dielectric boundary to reach the conclusion that the PB polar solvation energy is neither inherently decomposable nor produces symmetric binding free energies. However, the nonpolar solvation term, ΔG_{sol-np}, also contains intrinsic difficulties in its geometry decomposition due to the nonlocal character of the SASA-dependent term used for its calculation (Gohlke et al. 2003), introducing asymmetry in the binding free energy between the protein and the ligand.

Regarding the configurational entropy, the decomposition at residue or residue-pairwise level remains still to be solved, though attempts to decompose the normal modes that contribute to the vibrational entropy into atomic contributions have been reported (Zoete and Michielin 2007). Generally, the configurational entropy decomposed at the residue level due to the loss of torsional freedom can be computed using the computational scheme adopted by Honig and coworkers (Froloff et al. 1997), which is based on the empirical scale of Pickett and Stemberg (1993). This procedure separates backbone and side-chain components. For the backbone, an entropic penalty of 2 kcal mol^{-1} per residue is considered, whereas a variable value is computed for side-chain component depending on the solvent-exposed surface area (Doig and Sternberg 1995).

The MM-PB(GB)SA fragmental decomposition yields a high number of components that, combined with the systematic application to a set of protein–ligand complexes either from MD simulations or other sampling methods, can form voluminous energy matrices. The amount of data generated for this decomposition is vast and thus impedes univariate exploration. Alternatively, multivariate data analysis techniques such as partial least squares (PLS) or principal component analysis (PCA) have found their applicability to the in-depth exploration of the computed energy matrices in order to find significant residues or residue-pairwise contributions that govern the binding free energy.

The per-residue decomposition methodology has been widely applied to the study of protein–ligand binding free energy (Zoete and Michielin 2007; Berhanu and Masunov 2012; Laurini et al. 2013). However, the residue-pairwise decomposition has been less used, though recently several works have explored its potentiality. For instance, it has been used to elucidate the signal transmission mechanism in the allosteric regulation of protein kinases C by determining the differences in the residue-pairwise interaction profiles among six protein states of the mentioned protein (Seco et al. 2012). Furthermore, Pouplana and Campanera (2015) have used it to determine the relative importance of the hydrophobic fragments of Aβ oligomers in the oligomerization process of such peptides. As shown in the decompostion of the intermonomeric van der Waals free energy in Figure 9.4, the hydrophobic collapse in the formation of these oligomers is caused by hydrophobic interactions between three well-defined hydrophobic fragments: 31–35 (C-terminal hydrophobic region [CTHR]), 17–20 (central hydrophobic region [CHC]), and 12–14 (N-terminal hydrophobic region [NTHR]), ordered according to their importance.

9.4 Quantum Mechanics and Implicit Solvation Models

The use of simplified expressions in classical force fields is understandable in terms of providing an efficient sampling, as well as in facilitating the parametrization of the large number of functional groups that can be incorporated into drug-like molecules. However, these approximations also limit the accuracy of classical force fields in describing the intermolecular interactions that mediate the recognition between ligands and proteins. Thus, besides typical interactions such as salt bridges, standard hydrogen bonds, and van der Waals forces, a wider number of stabilizing interactions

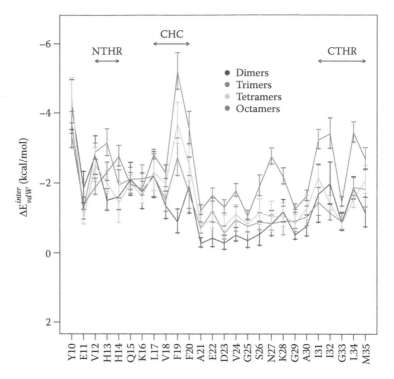

FIGURE 9.4

(See color insert.) Residue decomposition of the intermonomeric total stability free energy (kcal mol⁻¹) of different oligomers of β-amyloid peptide. (Reproduced from Pouplana, R. and J. M. Campanera. 2015. *Phys. Chem. Chem. Phys.* 17(4): 2823–2837. With permission from the PCCP Owner Societies.)

have been characterized in the last decades, including cation-π or anion-π complexes (Frontera et al. 2011), nonstandard hydrogen bonds (Hobza and Havlas 2000), and halogen bonding (Nguyen et al. 2004; Sarwar et al. 2010).

Quantum mechanical (QM) methods are the most accurate approach to the calculations of intermolecular interactions, and they form the basis for the parametrization of force fields. The continued increase in accuracy achieved by QM methods has also stimulated the implementation and usage of QM-based techniques for different applications in the study of ligand–protein complexes. Most of these applications follow the hybrid QM/MM computational scheme (Warshel 2003; Friesner and Guallar 2005), where the Hamiltonian of the whole system can be defined as the sum of three terms (Equation 9.13) corresponding to the QM subsystem ($\hat{H}_{QM}$), the MM subsystem ($\hat{H}_{MM}$), and the coupling between the QM and MM regions ($\hat{H}_{QM/MM}$).

$$\hat{H} = \hat{H}_{QM} + \hat{H}_{MM} + \hat{H}_{QM/MM} \tag{9.13}$$

Although the major goal of QM/MM methods has been the study of reactive processes in condensed media or in enzymes, a wider range of applications is being explored in drug discovery, including the calculation of the ligand–protein interaction energy and the analysis of the energy components, and the rescoring of docking calculations (Hensen et al. 2004; Cho et al. 2005; Illingworth et al. 2008; Cho and Rinaldo 2009; Chaskar et al. 2014).

QM-based strategies have also been developed for the prediction of binding affinities of ligand–protein complexes. To this end, a variety of methodological strategies have been adopted, as will be illustrated by the representative cases presented below (Zhou et al. 2010; Barril and Luque 2012; Ilatovskiy et al. 2013; Mucs and Bryce 2013).

Balaz and coworkers have proposed a four-step strategy for the study of ligand-metalloprotein complexes (Khandelwal et al. 2005). The procedure involves docking of ligands, optimization of the complex, conformational sampling with constrained metal bonds, and a single point QM/MM calculation for the time-averaged structure. Finally, the QM/MM interaction energy, $\Delta\langle E_{QM/MM}\rangle$, is combined with a desolvation term in order to determine the binding free energy (Equation 9.14). After suitable parametrization against experimental data for a set of 28 hydroxamate inhibitors binding to zinc-dependent matrix metalloproteinase 9, Equation 9.14 was able to account for 90% of variance in the inhibition constants.

$$\Delta G_{bin} = \alpha\Delta\langle E_{QM/MM}\rangle + \gamma\Delta\langle SASA\rangle + \kappa \qquad (9.14)$$

where $\Delta\langle SASA\rangle$ denotes the change in SAS upon complexation.

In a distinct study, the ability of QM/MM combined with the PBSA model has been utilized for the calculation of binding affinities for flexible ligands (Gräter et al. 2005). The method was tested for a set of 47 benzamidine derivatives binding to trypsin. The suitability of the computational strategy for automated ligand docking and scoring is supported by the accuracy in predicting the experimental range of binding energies, with a root-mean square error of 1.2 kcal mol^{-1}.

Das et al. (2009) followed a strategy based on the use of protein-polarized QM charges in GBSA calculations for nine protease inhibitors. In this work, the general expression of a GBSA model was adopted, but the ligand was described by assigning either MM charges or the protein-polarized ones as derived from QM/MM calculations. Moreover, attention was paid to the effect of including bridging water molecules that mediate hydrogen bonding with the ligand. The results showed that the binding free energies determined by using those polarized charges (and specific water molecules) showed higher correlation with antiviral IC$_{50}$ data. The importance of including polarization effects through QM/MM methods, combined with a van der Waals correction and a term accounting for desolvation, has also been highlighted for ligands binding to trypsin and cytochrome c peroxidase (Burger et al. 2011).

An elaborate scheme was reported by Raha and Merz (2004, 2005) with the aim to perform a large-scale validation of a QM-based scoring function for predicting the binding affinity of a diverse set of ligands. In this study, the binding affinity was determined as noted in Equation 9.15, where it is decomposed into the gas-phase interaction energy (ΔG_b^{gas}), and the change in solvation-free energy ($\Delta\Delta G_{solv}$) of the complex (ΔG_{solv}^{PL}) relative to protein (ΔG_{solv}^P) and ligand (ΔG_{solv}^L).

$$\Delta G_{bin} = \Delta G_b^{gas} + \Delta\Delta G_{solv} = \Delta G_b^{gas} + \Delta G_{solv}^{PL} - \Delta G_{solv}^P - \Delta G_{solv}^L \qquad (9.15)$$

The gas-phase interaction energy was determined as a sum of electrostatic and nonpolar interaction energies. The former was calculated using the divide-and-conquer method and the semiempirical AM1 or PM3 Hamiltonians, and the latter with the classical attractive component of the Lennard–Jones interaction potential. Furthermore, the entropic term was expressed as the addition of conformational and solvent entropy components. The former was estimated by considering a conformational penalty of 1 kcal mol^{-1} for each rotatable bond of the ligand and in the protein side chains frozen upon formation of the complex. The solvent entropy term accounts for the entropy gained by release of water molecules upon binding, and it was calculated from the buried surface area resulting upon complexation. Finally, the solvation-free energy term was determined using a QM self-consistent reaction field calculation for the complex, ligand, and protein. Finally, the weights of the different components were adjusted by fitting to experimental binding free energies. The method was shown to be effective as scoring function for predicting ligand poses docked to a protein target and for discriminating between native and decoy poses.

A related QM-based scheme based on the semiempirical QM PM6-DH2 method, which includes corrections dispersion energy and hydrogen bonds, has been proposed for the computation of binding affinities (Fanfrlik et al. 2010; Dobes et al. 2011a). Here, the binding affinity is determined by adding the PM6-DH2 interaction enthalpy evaluated in a continuum water environment using the COSMO model. The desolvation of the ligand was further refined by means of solvation model based on density (SMD) continuum calculations. Furthermore, the deformation contribution due to changes in protein and ligand upon binding was also considered. The method was successful in ranking 22 ligands binding to HIV-1 protease, and for the binding of 15 structurally diverse inhibitors to CDK2. Recently, the method has been extended to treat halogen bonding (Dobes et al. 2011b) as well as to treat noncovalent binding in protein–ligand complexes (Fanfrlik et al. 2013).

The MM/QM-COSMO strategy has been adopted to evaluate the binding affinity of phosphopeptide inhibitors of the Lck SH2 domain (Anisimov and Cavasotto 2011). Starting from MD trajectories of the complex, a QM postprocessing is made for a selection of representative snapshots, which were first refined using the PM3 Hamiltonian and the COSMO continuum solvent model. The binding free energy was then determined as noted in Equation 9.16, where the first term in the right-hand side was determined using Equation 9.17, and the entropic term included changes in translational and rotational rigid body component and the change in vibrational entropy.

$$\Delta G_{binding} = \Delta \langle H^{COSMO} \rangle - T \Delta S^{RB} - T \Delta S^{int} \tag{9.16}$$

$$H^{COSMO} = E^{COSMO} + G_{np}^{solv} \tag{9.17}$$

where E^{COSMO} represents the PM3 QM energy (including vacuum and solvation energy components), and the nonpolar contribution (G_{np}^{solv}) is determined using a linear relationship with the change in SAS.

The binding affinities derived from MM/QM-COSMO calculations were compared with the results determined using MM-PBSA and MM-GBSA, as well as the SIE method. The MM/QM-COSMO method showed the best agreement both for absolute (average unsigned error of 0.7 kcal mol^{-1}) and relative binding free energies.

9.5 Conclusion

Despite substantial progresses made in the last years, predicting the binding free energy of ligand to their targets still remains a major challenge for computational chemistry. This conforms to the involvement of different enthalpic and entropic components, each playing a significant contribution, and to the important compensation between these thermodynamic quantities. Furthermore, the need to develop fast, yet accurate estimates of binding affinities, which may discriminate between strong and weak binders and between distinct poses of a given compound, is required for large-scale application in drug discovery. In this context, the use of implicit solvation methods represents a fundamental tool in the path toward novel computational strategies for the high-throughput analysis of ligand–receptor complexes.

In the classical framework, MM-PB(GB)SA methods are *a priori* well suited to attain the preceding goal due to the continuous development of more accurate force fields, and specially to the refinement of the crude approximations inherent in the description of solvent effects through implicit continuum models. Thus, among the wide range of applications achieved by MM-PB(GB)SA methods in the study of biomolecular systems, the large-scale application to virtual screening appears to be especially promising, as these methods are reaching the predictive accuracy that would be required to discriminate among large sets of compounds covering a wide range of binding affinities.

However, the availability of decomposition schemes permits to disclose the contribution of specific molecular determinants (i.e., chemical groups in the ligand or residues in the binding pocket) that play a distinctive role in the binding affinity, thus providing valuable guidelines to assist the structure-based drug design.

The investigation of compounds with small differences in the binding affinity seems still out of the realm of MM-PB(GB)SA methods, partly due to the limitations of the classical force field to account for the interactions formed between a ligand and its target, taking a proper accounting of electrostatic, induction, charge transfer, and dispersion effects, as well as from the simplified description of environmental effects. At this point, QM-based methods used directly for the modeled structures of ligand–protein complexes or in the framework of endpoint sampling techniques represent a promising alternative as a tool to develop and calibrate novel computational strategies designed to provide accurate estimates of binding affinities (Yilmazer and Korth 2013). Furthermore, the development of QM-based strategies can give rise to accurate tools for lead optimization, even though this option is seriously limited by the huge computational cost of high-level QM computations. This explains why most of the QM-based strategies devised for the study of ligand–protein complexes rely on semiempirical methods, often supplemented by suitable correction terms to assure the description of certain types of interactions. On the contrary, current efforts for making quantum chemistry codes more efficient and implementing them in powerful computational resources can be relevant to alleviate the computational requirements of QM-based strategies. Overall, it can be envisaged that QM-based approaches will be an increasingly used and valued tool in computational medicinal chemistry and structure-based drug discovery.

Acknowledgments

This work was supported by the Spanish Ministerio de Innovación y Ciencia (SAF2014-57094-R) and the Generalitat de Catalunya (2014SGR1189). F.J.L. is grateful to Icrea Academia for financial support. W.Z.R. is fellowship from MICITT and CONICIT (Costa Rica).

References

Adler, M. and P. Beroza. 2013. Improved ligand binding energies derived from molecular dynamics: Replicate sampling enhances the search of conformational space. *J. Chem. Inf. Model.* 53(8): 2065–2072.

Anisimov, V. M. and C. N. Cavasotto. 2011. Quantum mechanical binding free-energy calculation for phosphopeptide inhibitors of the Lck SH2 domain. *J. Comput. Chem.* 32(10): 2254–2263.

Barril, X. and F. J. Luque. 2012. Molecular simulation methods in drug discovery: A prospective outlook. *J. Comput.-Aided Mol. Des.* 26(1): 81–86.

Bashford, D. and D. A. Case. 2000. Generalized Born models of macromolecular solvation effects. *Annu. Rev. Phys. Chem.* 51: 129–152.

Berhanu, W. M. and A. E. Masunov. 2012. Unique example of amyloid aggregates stabilized by main chain H-bond instead of the steric zipper: Molecular dynamics study of the amyloidogenic segment of amylin wild-type and mutants. *J. Mol. Model.* 18(3): 891–903.

Bissantz, C., B. Kuhn, and M. Stahl. 2010. A medicinal chemist's guide to molecular interactions. *J. Med. Chem.* 53(14): 5061–5084.

Boukharta, L., H. Gutiérrez-de-Terán, and J. Aqvist. 2014. Computational prediction of alanine scanning and ligand binding in G-protein coupled receptors. *PLoS Comput. Biol.* 10(4): e1003585.

Brandsdal, B. O., F. Österberg, M. Almlöf, I. Feierberg, V. Luzhkov, and J. Aqvist. 2003. Free energy calculations and ligand binding. *Adv. Protein Chem.* 66: 123–158.

Brown, S. P. and S. W. Muchmore. 2009. Large-scale application of high-throughput molecular mechanics with Poisson-Boltzmann surface area for routine physics-based scoring of protein-ligand complexes. *J. Med. Chem.* 52(10): 3159–3165.

Burger, S. K., D. C. Thompson, and P. W. Ayers. 2011. Quantum mechanics/molecular mechanics strategies for docking pose refinement: Distinguishing between binders and decoys in cytochrome c peroxidase. *J. Chem. Inf. Model.* 51(1): 93–101.

Butler, K. T., F. J. Luque, and X. Barril. 2009. Toward accurate relative energy predictions of the bioactive conformation of drugs. *J. Comput. Chem.* 30(4): 601–610.

Cárdenas, C., A. Bidon-Chanal, P. Conejeros, G. Arenas, S. Marshall, and F. J. Luque. 2010. Molecular modelling of class I and II alleles of the major histocompatibility complex of Salmo salar. *J. Comput.-Aided Mol. Des.* 24(12): 1035–1051.

Chang, C. A., W. Chen, and M. K. Gilson. 2007. Ligand configurational entropy and protein binding. *Proc. Natl. Acad. Sci. USA* 104(5): 1534–1539.

Chaskar, P., V. Zoete, and U. F. Röhring. 2014. Toward on-the-fly quantum mechanical/molecular mechanical (QM/MM) docking: Development and benchmark of a scoring function. *J. Chem. Inf. Model.* 54(11): 3137–3152.

Chipot, C. and A. Pohorille. (Eds.), 2007. Free energy calculations. *Theory and Applications in Chemistry and Biology.* Springer Series in Chemical Physics, vol. 86. Berlin: Springer.

Cho, A. E., V. Guallar, B. J. Berne, and R. Friesner. 2005. Importance of accurate charges in molecular docking: Quantum mechanical/molecular mechanical (QM/MM) approach. *J. Comput. Chem.* 26(9): 915–931.

Cho, A. E. and D. Rinaldo. 2009. Extension of QM/MM docking and its applications to metalloproteins. *J. Comput. Chem.* 30(16): 2609–2616.

Csermely, P., R. Palotai, and R. Nussinov. 2010. Inducedfit, conformational selection and independent dynamic segments: An extended view of binding events. *Trends Biochem. Sci.* 35(10): 539–546.

Cui, Q., T. Sulea, J. D. Schrag, C. Munger, M.-N. Hung, M. Naïm, M. Cugler, and E. O. Purisima. 2008. Molecular dynamics—Solvent interaction energy studies of protein-protein interactions: The MP1-p14 scaffolding complex. *J. Mol. Biol.* 379(4): 787–802.

Das, D., Y. Koh, Y. Tojo, A. K. Gosh, and H. Mitsuya. 2009. Prediction of potency of protease inhibitors using free energy simulations with polarizable quantum mechanics based ligand charges and a hybrid water model. *J. Chem. Inf. Model.* 49(12): 2851–2862.

Dobes, P., J. Fanfrlik, J. Rezac, M. Otypeka, and P. Hobza. 2011a. Transferable scoring function based on semiempirical quantum mechanical PM6-DH2 method: CDK2 with 15 structurally diverse inhibitors. *J. Comput.-Aided Mol. Des.* 25(3): 223–235.

Dobes, P., J. Rezac, J. Fanfrlik, M. Otypeka, and P. Hobza. 2011b. Semiempirical quantum mechanical method PM6-DH2X describes the geometry and energetics of CK2-inhibitor complexes involving halogen bonds well, while the empirical potential fails. *J. Phys. Chem. B* 115(26): 8581–8589.

Doig, A. J. and M. J. E. Sternberg. 1995. Side-chain conformational entropy in protein folding. *Prot. Sci.* 4(11): 2247–2251.

Fanfrlik, J., A. K. Bronowska, J. Rezac, O. Prenosil, J. Konvalinka, and P. Hobza. 2010. A reliable docking/scoring scheme based on the semiempirical quantum mechanical PM6-DH2 method accurately covering dispersion and H-bonding: HIV-1 protease with 22 ligands. *J. Phys. Chem. B* 114(39): 12666–12678.

Fanfrlik, J., P. S. Brahmkshatriya, J. Rezac, A. Jilkova, M. Horn, M. Mares, P. Hobza, and M. Lepsik. 2013. Quantum mechanics-based scoring rationalizes the irreversible inactivation of parasitic *Schistosoma mansoni* cysteine peptidase by vinyl sulfone inhibitors. *J. Phys. Chem. B* 117(48): 14973–14982.

Friesner, R. A. and V. Guallar. 2005. Ab initio quantum chemical and mixed quantum mechanics/molecular mechanics (QM/MM) methods for studying enzymatic catalysis. *Annu. Rev. Phys. Chem.* 56: 389–427.

Froloff, N., A. Windemuth, and B. Honig. 1997. On the calculation of binding free energies using continuum methods: Application to MHC class I protein-peptide interactions. *Prot. Sci.* 6(6): 1293–1301.

Frontera, A., D. Quiñonero, and P. M. Deyà. 2011. Cation–π and anion–π interactions. *WIRES Comput. Mol. Sci.* 1(3): 440–459.

Genheden, S. and U. Ryde. 2011. Comparison of the efficiency of the LIE and MM/GBSA methods to calculate ligand-binding affinities. *J. Chem. Theory Comput.* 7(11): 3768–3778.

Gohlke, H. and G. Klebe. 2002. Approaches to the description and prediction of the binding affinity of small-molecule ligands to macromolecular receptors. *Angew. Chem. Int. Ed.* 41(15): 2644–2676.

Gohlke, H., C. Kiel, and D. A. Case. 2003. Insights into protein-protein binding by binding free energy calculation and free energy decomposition for the Ras-Raf and Ras-RalGDS complexes. *J. Mol. Biol.* 330(4): 891–913.

Gräter, F., S. M. Schwarzl, A. Dejaegere, S. Fischer, and J. C. Smith. 2005. Protein/ligand binding free energies calculated with quantum mechanics/molecular mechanics. *J. Phys. Chem. B* 109(20): 10474–10483.

Greenidge, P. A., C. Kramer, J.-C. Mozziconacci, and R. M. Wolf. 2013. MM/GBSA binding energy prediction on the PDBbind data set: Successes, failures, and directions for further improvement. *J. Chem. Inf. Model.* 53(1): 201–209.

Greenidge, P. A., C. Kramer, J.-C. Mozziconacci, and W. Sherman. 2014. Improved docking results via reranking of ensembles of ligand poses in multiple x-ray protein conformations with MM-GBSA. *J. Chem. Inf. Model.* 54(10): 2697–2717.

Harris, R. C., A. H. Boschitsch, and M. O. Fenley. 2013. Influence of grid spacing in Poisson-Boltzmann equation binding energy estimation. *J. Chem. Theory Comput.* 9(8): 3677–3685.

Hawkins, G. D., C. J. Cramer, and D. G. Truhlar. 1995. Pairwise solute descreening of solute charges from a dielectric medium. *Chem. Phys. Lett.* 246(1–2): 122–129.

Hensen, C., J. C. Hermann, K. Nam, S. Ma, J. Gao, and H.-D. Höltje. 2004. A combined QM/MM approach to protein–ligand interactions: Polarization effects of the HIV-1 protease on selected high affinity inhibitors. *J. Med. Chem.* 47(27): 6673–6680.

Hobza, P. and Z. Havlas. 2000. Blue-shifting hydrogen bonds. *Chem. Rev.* 100(11): 4253–4264.

Hou, T., J. Wang, Y. Li, and W. Wang. 2011. Assessing the performance of the MM/PBSA and MM/GBSA Methods. 1. The accuracy of binding free energy calculations based on molecular dynamics simulations. *J. Chem. Inf. Model.* 51(1): 69–82.

Ilatovskiy, A. V., R. Abagyan, and I. Kufareva. 2013. Quantum mechanics approaches to drug research in the era of structural chemogenomics. *Int. J. Quantum Chem.* 113(12): 1669–1675.

Illingworth, C. J. R., G. M. Morris, K. E. B. Parkes, C. R. Snell, and C. A. Reynolds. 2008. Assessing the role of polarization in docking. *J. Phys. Chem. A* 112(47): 12157–12163.

Jorgensen, W. L. 2009. Efficient drug lead discovery and optimization. *Acc. Chem. Res.* 42(6): 724–733.

Khandelwal, A., V. Lukacova, D. Comez, D. M. Kroll, S. Raha, and S. Balaz. 2005. A combination of docking, QM/MM methods, and MD simulation for the binding affinity estimation of metalloprotein ligands. *J. Med. Chem.* 48(17): 5437–5447.

Kongsted, J. and U. Ryde. 2009. An improved method to predict the entropy term with the MM/PBSA approach. *J. Comput.-Aided Mol. Des.* 23(2): 63–71.

Kuntz, I. D., K. Chen, K. A. Sharp, and P. A. Kollman. 1999. The maximal affinity of ligands. *Proc. Natl. Acad. Sci. USA* 96(18): 9997–10002.

Laurini, E., V. Da Col, B. Wünsch, and S. Prici. 2013. Analysis of the molecular interactions of the potent analgesic S1RA with the σ1 receptor. *Bioorg. Med. Chem. Lett.* 23(10): 2868–2871.

Lawrenz, M., R. Baron, Y. Wang, and J. A. McCammon. 2011. Effects of biomolecular flexibility on alchemical calculations of absolute binding free energies. *J. Chem. Theory Comput.* 7(7): 2224–2232.

Li, J., R. Abel, K. Zhu, Y. Cao, S. Zhao, and R. A. Friesner. 2012. The VSGB 2.0 model: A next generation energy model for high resolution protein structure modelling. *Proteins: Struct., Funct., Bioinf.* 79(10): 2794–2812.

Lill, M. A. and J. J. Thompson. 2011. Solvent interaction energy calculations on Molecular Dynamics trajectories: Increasing the efficiency using systematic frame selection. *J. Chem. Inf. Model.* 51(10): 2680–2689.

Merz, K. M. Jr. 2010. Limits of free energy computation for protein-ligand interactions. *J. Chem. Theory Comput.* 6(5): 1769–1776.

Michel, J. and J. W. Essex. 2010. Prediction of protein–ligand binding affinity by free energy simulations: Assumptions, pitfalls and expectations. *J. Comput.-Aided Mol. Des.* 24(8): 639–658.

Miller, B. R., T. D. McGee, J. M. Swails, N. Homeyer, H. Gohlke, and A. E. Roitberg. 2012. MMPBSA.py: An efficient program for end-state free energy calculations. *J. Chem. Theory Comput.* 8(9): 3314–3321.

Mucs, D. and R. A. Bryce. 2013. The application of quantum mechanics in structure-based drug design. *Expert Op. Drug Discov.* 8(3): 263–276.

Mulakala, C. and V. N. Viswanadhan. 2013. Could MM-GBSA be accurate enough for calculation of absolute protein/ligand binding free energies? *J. Mol. Graphics Model.* 46: 41–51.

Naïm, M., S. Bhat, K. N. Rankin, S. Dennis, S. F. Chowdhury, I. Siddiqi, P. Drabik et al. 2007. Solvated Interaction Energy (SIE) for scoring protein–ligand binding affinities. 1. Exploring the parameter space. *J. Chem. Inf. Model.* 47(1): 122–133.

Nguyen, H. L., P. N. Horton, M. B. Hursthouse, A. C. Legon, and D. W. Bruce. 2004. Halogen bonding: A new interaction for liquid crystal formation. *J. Am. Chem. Soc.* 126(1): 16–17.

Onufriev, A., D. Basford, and D. A. Case. 2000. Modification of the Generalized Born model suitable for macromolecules. *J. Phys. Chem B.* 104(15): 3712–3720.

Orozco, M. and F. J. Luque. 2000. Theoretical methods for the description of the solvent effect in biomolecular systems. *Chem. Rev.* 100 (11): 4187–4225.

Pickett, S. D. and M. J. E. Stemberg. 1993. Empirical scale of side-chain conformational entropy in protein folding. *J. Mol. Biol.* 231(3): 825–839.

Pitera, J. W. and W. F. Van Gunsteren. 2002. A comparison of non-bonded scaling approaches for free energy calculations. *Mol. Simul.* 28(1–2): 45–65.

Pliego, J. R., Jr. and J. M. Riveros. 2002. Gibbs energy of solvation of organic ions in aqueous and dimethyl sulfoxide solutions. *Phys. Chem. Chem. Phys.* 4(9): 1622–1627.

Pouplana, R. and J. M. Campanera. 2015. Energetic contributions of residues to the formation of early amyloid-β oligomers. *Phys. Chem. Chem. Phys.* 17(4): 2823–2837.

Raha, K. and K. M. Merz Jr. 2004. A quantum mechanics-based scoring function: Study of zinc ion-mediated ligand binding. *J. Am. Chem. Soc.* 126(4): 1020–1021.

Raha, K. and K. M. Merz Jr. 2005. Large-scale validation of a quantum mechanics based scoring function: Predicting the binding affinity and the binding mode of a diverse set of protein-ligand complexes. *J. Med. Chem.* 48(14): 4558–4575.

Reynolds, C. A. and M. K. Holloway. 2011. Thermodynamics of ligand binding and efficiency. *ACS Med. Chem. Lett.* 2(6): 433–437.

Sarwar, M. G., B. Dragisic, L. J. Salsberg, C. Gouliaras, and M. S. Taylor. 2010. Thermodynamics of halogen bonding in solution: Substituent, structural, and solvent effects. *J. Am. Chem. Soc.* 132(5): 1646–1653.

Seco, J., C. Ferrer-Costa, J. M. Campanera, R. Soliva, and X. Barril. 2012. Allosteric regulation of PKCθ: Understanding multistep phosphorylation and priming by ligands in AGC kinases. *Proteins: Struct., Funct., Bioinf.* 80(1): 269–280.

Sitkoff, D., K. A. Sharp, and B. Honig. 1994. Accurate calculation of hydration free energies using macroscopic solvent models. *J. Phys. Chem.* 98(7): 1978–1988.

Spyrakis, F., A. Bidon-Chanal, X. Barril, and F. J. Luque. 2011. Protein flexibility and ligand recognition: Challenges for molecular modelling. *Curr. Topics Med. Chem.* 11(2): 192–210.

Srinivasan, J., M. W. Trevathan, P. Beroza, and D. A. Case. 1999. Application of a pairwise Generalized Born model to proteins and nucleic acids: Inclusion of salt effects. *Theor. Chem. Acc.* 101(6): 426–434.

Steinbrecher, T., D. L. Mobley, and D. A. Case. 2007. Nonlinear scaling schemes for Lennard-Jones interactions in free energy calculations. *J. Chem. Phys.* 127(21): 214108.

Still, W. C., A. Tempczyk, R. C. Hawley, and T. Hendrickson. 1990. Semianalytical treatment of solvation for molecular mechanics and dynamics. *J. Am. Chem. Soc.* 112(16): 6127–6129.

Stoica, I., S. K. Sadiq, and P. V. Coveney. 2008. Rapid and accurate prediction of binding free energies for saquinavir-bound HIV-1 proteases. *J. Am. Chem. Soc.* 130(8): 2639–2648.

Sulea, T., Q. Cui, and E. O. Purisima. 2011. Solvated Interaction Energy (SIE) for scoring protein–ligand binding affinities. 2. Benchmark in the CSAR-2010 scoring exercise *J. Chem. Inf. Model.* 51(9): 2066–2081.

Swanson, J. M. J., S. A. Adcock, and J. A. McCammon. 2005. Optimized radii for Poisson-Boltzmann calculations with the AMBER force field. *J. Chem. Theory Comput.* 1(3): 484–493.

Swanson, J. M. J., J. A. Wagoner, N. A. Baker, and J. A. McCammon. 2007. Optimizing the Poisson dielectric boundary with explicit solvent forces and energies: Lessons learned with atom-centered dielectric functions. *J. Chem. Theory Comput.* 3(1): 170–183.

Tan, C., L. Yang, and R. Luo. 2006. How well does Poisson-Boltzmann implicit solvent agree with explicit solvent? A quantitative analysis. *J. Phys. Chem. B* 110(37): 18680–18687.

Tirado-Rives, J. and W. L. Jorgensen. 2006. Contribution of conformer focusing to the uncertainty in predicting free energies for protein–ligand binding. *J. Med. Chem.* 49(20): 5880–5884.

Tomasi, J. and M. Persico. 1994. Molecular interactions in solution: An overview of methods based on continuous distributions of the solvent. *Chem. Rev.* 94(7): 2027–2094.

Treesuwan, W. and S. Hannongbua. 2009. Bridge water mediates nevirapine binding to wild type and Y181C HIV-1 reverse transcriptase—Evidence from molecular dynamics simulations and MM/PBSA calculations. *J. Mol. Graphics Model.* 27(8): 921–929.

Tsui, V. and D. A. Case. 2001. Theory and applications of the Generalized Born solvation model in macromolecular simulations. *Biopolymers* 56(4): 275–291.

Wang, J. M., T. J. Hou, and X. Xu. 2006. Recent advances in free energy calculations with a combination of molecular mechanics and continuum models. *Curr. Comput.-Aided Drug Des.* 2(3): 287–306.

Warshel, A. 2003. Computer simulations of enzyme catalysis: Methods, progress, and insights. *Annu. Rev. Biophys. Biomol. Struct.* 32: 425–443.

Weis, A., K. Katebzadeh, P. Söderhjelm, I. Nilsson, and U. Ryde. 2006. Ligand affinities predicted with the MM/PBSA method: Dependence on the simulation method and the force field. *J. Med. Chem.* 49(22): 6596–6606.

Williams, D. H., E. Stephens, D. P. O'Brien, and M. Zhou. 2004. Understanding noncovalent interactions: Ligand binding energy and catalytic efficiency from ligand-induced reductions in motion within receptors and enzymes. *Angew. Chem. Int. Ed.* 43(48): 6596–6616.

Wolfenden, R., L. Andersson, P. M. Cullis, and C. C. B. Southgate. 1981. Affinities of amino acid side chains for solvent water. *Biochemistry* 20(4): 849–855.

Wong, S., R. E. Amaro, and J. A. McCammon. 2009. MM/PBSA captures key role of intercalating water molecules at a protein-protein interface. *J. Chem. Theory Comput.* 5(2): 422–429.

Xu, L., H. Sun, Y. Li, J. Wang, and T. Hou. 2013. Assessing the performance of MM/ PBSA and MM/GBSA methods. 3. The impact of force fields and ligand charge models. *J. Phys. Chem.* B 117(27): 8408–8421.

Yamagishi, J., N. Okimoto, G. Morimoto, and M. Taiji. 2014. A new set of atomic radii for accurate estimation of solvation free energy by Poisson-Boltzmann solvent model. *J. Comput. Chem.* 35(29): 2132–2139.

Yilmazer, N. D. and M. Korth. 2013. Comparison of molecular mechanics, semi-empirical quantum mechanical, and density functional theory methods for scoring protein-ligand interactions. *J. Phys. Chem.* B 117(27): 8075–8084.

Zhang, X., S. E. Wong, and F. C. Lighstone. 2014. Toward fully automated high performance computing drug discovery: A massively parallel virtual screening pipeline for docking and molecular mechanics/generalized born surface area rescoring to improve enrichment. *J. Chem. Inf. Model.* 54(1): 324–337.

Zhou, T., D. Huang, and A. Caflisch. 2010. Quantum mechanical methods for drug design. *Curr. Top. Med. Chem.* 10(1): 33–45.

Zhu, Y.-L., P. Beroza, and D. R. Artis. 2014. Including explicit water molecules as part of the protein structure in MM/PBSA calculations. *J. Chem. Inf. Model.* 54(2): 462–469.

Zoete, V. and O. Michielin. 2007. Comparison between computational alanine scanning and per-residue binding free energy decomposition for protein–protein association using MM-GBSA: Application to the TCR-p-MHC complex. *Proteins: Struct., Funct., Bioinf.* 67(4): 1026–1047.

Section II

Advanced Techniques

10

Toward Complete Cellular Pocketomes and Predictive Polypharmacology

Ruben A. Abagyan and Bryn Taylor

CONTENTS

10.1 Introduction

Predicting molecular binding by docking is a challenging task because of the binding site flexibility, imperfections of the molecular mechanics force field, and sampling limitations. Yet, just as the laws of physics can predict the locations of planets, stars, and asteroids, the laws of molecular physics should be able to derive the conformations and interactions of molecules in an organism from three-dimensional (3D) models and molecular mechanics laws of interaction energetics.

Despite inconsistent funding of structural biology projects, crystal structure entries in the Protein Data Bank (PDB) continue to increase at a consistent rate. Although the structural coverage of the human proteome is estimated to be merely 10%, homology modeling, functional state predictions, and flexibility analysis expand this knowledge and create a possibility for structure-based drug discovery and repurposing. Analyzing the structural composition of proteomes allows us to examine and rank different binding sites for drug targeting. The development of the pocketome, a comprehensive encyclopedia of conformational ensembles of druggable binding sites in proteins, enhanced the drug research field by providing data to investigate interactions of drugs with specific proteins of interest. The significance of the pocketome database is that all structurally significant transient binding sites are automatically derived, and all structural information about each site is collected in one place for further analysis and docking model derivation. Previously, we developed rules for finding an optimal subset of conformational variants to represent induced fit (Rueda et al. 2012) that increases recognition performance of the models dramatically and allows us to apply 4D approaches for docking and other ensemble-based methods.

The rapidly growing catalog of structures, coupled with the increasing sophistication of docking methods, provides a plethora of information and tools to predict molecular binding, identify ligands, and repurpose known drugs or predict their polypharmacological profile. Here, we describe how the crystallographic pocketome is derived, how new allosteric pockets can be predicted, how models by homology or loop simulations can be used to generate pocket models for not-yet crystallized proteins or domains, and demonstrate practical applications of these concepts.

10.1.1 The PDB Is Growing but the Proteome Coverage Is Still Small

The protein structure at atomic resolution provides the ultimate view into molecular interactions between cell metabolites and signaling molecules, drugs, environmental chemicals, toxins, and cellular or excreted proteins performing various functions. The rapid expansion of crystallographic information of proteins and binding sites in the PDB coupled with computational prediction of novel protein–ligand interactions creates an exceptional opportunity to enhance drug research pipelines. Since its inception in 1970, the PDB has grown to over 100,000 files, 84% of which are crystallographic structures with the median x-ray resolution of 2.1 Å and the standard deviation of the resolution of 0.7 Å. Despite the steady growth of the PDB, it is still glaringly incomplete. *Homo sapiens* is the most well-characterized organism in the PDB, but even this data is lacking. For instance, the PDB only covers 10% of human amino acid sequences, 21% (of 20,193) of Uniprot-annotated human proteins with various coverage, and 3% of GPCRs. Only one-quarter of those 21% of solved protein fragments cover the entire protein sequence. In conclusion, a whopping 4/5th of the human proteins have no high-resolution structure at all, while three-quarters of the known 1/5th have incomplete coverage.

PDB coverage of bacteria, viruses, and other organisms is even less complete. This partial coverage necessitates homology modeling to create structural models that are unavailable in the database. X-ray crystallography is the most accurate source of structural "snapshots," but the next best option is modeling by homology to determine binding pockets and perform docking studies and ligand screens. Small molecule interactions with these pockets are particularly interesting to investigate because the sites also tend to be binding sites for toxic or therapeutic chemicals.

10.1.2 The Pocketome of an Organism

Imagine a small molecule floating about the cytoplasm, plasma, or intercellular lymph. If the small molecule is charged, it is additionally driven by electrostatic gradients and carried around by fluid currents. Instead of bumping into proteins or nucleic acids on its journey, the small molecule interacts with sites known as "pockets." These pockets are found on single protein domains, between domains, and at the interface of a homo- or hetero-oligomeric complexes and molecular assemblies. Pockets may include firmly bound cofactors (e.g., heme), metals, and structural waters in addition to the usual amino acid residues from the pocket-forming proteins or groves of DNA and RNA. For example, a ribosome has drug-binding pockets that are formed between proteins and RNAs. Likewise, there are drug-binding pockets at various interfaces of GABA hetero-pentameric receptors. These pockets are real entities that can be named, described, and used as a distinct possible destination a small molecule may act upon.

To enhance understanding of flexible macromolecular ligand interactions, we developed the notion of the "Pocketome" of a cell (term first introduced in An et al. [2005]). The pocketome is a comprehensive set of binding pockets of small molecules that can be cataloged and described by geometrical and physicochemical characteristics. Ideally, each pocket is confirmed by experimental crystallographic observations where the binding pose and the pocket location can be unambiguously identified (the so-called "Experimental" or "Observed" Pocketome).

However, in many cases these cocrystal structures are not available and the pockets need to be predicted. The pockets range in "druggability" from shallow, open, and poor to deep and druggable. The druggability can be loosely defined by our ability to find a small molecule binder that binds to that location with single- or double-digit nanomolar binding constant. There are several algorithms that use geometrical and property criteria to predict the druggable binding pockets. Geometric algorithms such as SURFNET, LigSite, PASS, Roll, and fPocket find and analyze cavities on protein surfaces. SURFNET investigates the spaces between protein atoms by fitting spheres in the gap regions, displaying the clefts of the protein (Laskowski 1995). LigSite places the protein in a Cartesian grid and scans along the x, y, and z axes and the cubic diagonals for cavities contained by the protein (Hendlich et al. 1997). PASS uses spherical probes to coat the surface of the protein to identify active site points, and then filters out the probes that are not adequately buried or collide with the protein (Brady and Stouten 2000). Roll is an algorithm implemented in POCASA that detects cavities of proteins by means of a rolling sphere (Yu et al. 2010). FPocket identifies pockets using alpha sphere theory, by way of Voronoi tessellation (Le Guilloux et al.

2009). Two other approaches, APROPOS (Peters et al. 1996) and CAST (Liang et al. 1998), identify pockets by employing the α-shaped algorithm that compares protein surfaces at varying detail.

Our algorithm, PocketFinder, predicts the location of the "good" binding pockets using a Gaussian convolution of the van der Waals potential (An et al. 2005). PocketFinder is fast, sensitive, and specific, similar to the geometric algorithms just discussed. In addition to identification of straightforward binary protein–ligand interactions, this algorithm enables automatic recognition of sites containing metal ions or bound cofactors, or sites located at multimer assembly interfaces. Furthermore, the algorithm facilitates accurate ligand–residue interaction maps, performs conformational clustering, and quantification of cross compatibility between pockets and ligands from different structures. This concept of druggability of "good" binding pockets was further developed a few years later by the introduction of the "drug-like" density (DLID). The DLID represents the likeliness that pocket will bind a drug-like molecule (Sheridan et al. 2010), and corresponds with the "druggability" described by Cheng et al. (2007). The algorithm uses a transformation of the Lennard–Jones potential calculated from a 3D protein structure that does not require any prior knowledge about a potential ligand molecule, thus allowing for pocket identification in both apo- and bound structures. PocketFinder can be used to predict ligand-binding pockets of uncharacterized protein structures, suggest new allosteric pockets, evaluate feasibility of protein–protein interaction inhibition, and prioritize molecular targets. The predicted binding envelopes that could be targeted by small "druglike" compounds are hierarchically assembled into the known pocketome of that particular organism. After identification and collection of potential small molecule binding envelopes in a structural proteome, the next step is to cluster them into classes and categories according to their size, shape, and physicochemical properties and compare with a collection of chemical substrates or ligands (An et al. 2005).

In summary, the real pocketome is a set of pockets in an organism that can be targeted with appreciable binding free energy directly related to the log of the dissociation constant, K_d. The most important fraction of the real pocketome has already been characterized through crystallography and can be derived with the "Site-Finder" procedure described in Kufareva et al. (2012a,b). Additionally, pockets can be discovered by the usual process of prediction followed by experimental validation.

10.1.3 The Visible Crystallographic Pocketome: Multiple Species

The pocketome contains 3000 entries derived from dozens of different organisms. The distribution of the pockets derived for a particular organism directly (without borrowing homologous or identical pockets from other species) is as follows.

The Human pocketome is the most comprehensive collection, consisting of 906 entries to date. We expect the pocketomes to grow along with the structural proteomes and the improvements of the envelope prediction and classification methods. The PDB and Uniprot knowledgebase feeds the pocketome regularly and automatically from the current releases of those databases. This information is complemented by manually provided seed ligand locations. The pocketome website (pocketome.org) equips the user with annotated structural ensembles of the binding sites, contact maps for individual pockets, and overall binding site and pairwise comparison matrices clustered by ligand-pocket compatibility. Structures are available to be downloaded in interactive datapacks in ICB format (works with free ICM-browser) and also can be viewed and manipulated online with free Molsoft ActiveICM browser plug-in ([both available for three major desktop platforms at molsoft.com] [Raush et al. 2009]).

10.1.4 The Predicted Pocketome and the Observed Pocketome

There are two types of pocketomes: observable and predicted. The observable pocketome contains binding sites on proteins that are either known to bind ligands, or are determined by crystal structures that have been cocrystallized with ligands. The predicted pocketome is a collection of potential small molecule binding sites that is identified by PocketFinder based on crystal structures or homology models.

A binding pocket is an individual set of residues in a particular protein ligand complex, whereas a binding site is a superset of overlapping pockets for a particular protein. A single binding site may interact with several different ligands (as shown in Figure 10.1). The intrinsic flexibility of binding sites, which allows accommodation of a variety of binding partners essential for maintaining biological function, makes it challenging to predict interactions of ligands.

Small molecules vary widely in terms of the shape, hydrophobicity, distribution of charges, and polar groups. Any molecule that binds tightly (i.e., the K_d required for its biological action) must have optimal van der Waals interactions with the protein. Sufficient binding of a ligand to a pocket is in the 10–40 nM range (Bickerton et al. 2012). This binding affinity is one of the parameters involved in docking ligands to a pocket. These pockets have been traditionally identified by cocrystallization with a known ligand; if no cocrystallization is possible, then alternate methods can be explored. One option is computational structural analysis, which has been shown to detect greater than 95% of ligand-binding sites (An et al. 2005). This functional information, after ligand-binding sites are identified, docked, and scored, can then be translated into structure-based drug design. The next question that should be addressed is whether small molecule binding will interfere with protein function: this can be determined by examining

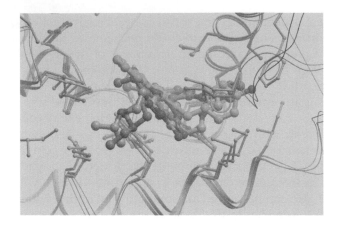

FIGURE 10.1

(See color insert.) Phosphodiesterase 5A (PDE5A) can interact with many different ligands. For clarity, three out of 41 cocrystal ligand structures were arbitrarily selected and displayed: 3TGG chain A (Hughes, R. O., T. Maddux, D. Joseph Rogier et al. 2011. *Bioorg. Med. Chem. Lett.* 21(21): 6348–6352.), 4MDG chain A (Brynda, J., P. Mader, V. Sicha et al. 2013. *Angew. Chem. Int. Ed. Engl.* 52(51): 13760–13763.), and 2CHM chain A (Allerton, C. M., C. G. Barber, K. C. Beaumont et al. 2006. *J. Med. Chem.* 49(12): 3581–3594.), to demonstrate how the receptor changes conformation in response to distinct ligand binding. Although the backbone deviations are minimal, the side chains undergo induced changes upon binding to adjust for the fit of each ligand. Carbons are colored by cocrystal structure, and ligands are represented by the thicker balls and sticks.

the functional significance of the protein region through homology and sequence conservations (Chelliah et al. 2004).

10.2 The Observable Pocket Definition

While prediction of druggable pockets from the structure of proteins or protein complexes still needs to be confirmed by actually finding a small molecule that binds to this pocket with appreciable binding constant (say, under 100 nM), an alternative is to enumerate all the locations that were observed in cocrystallization experiments as (i) available for small molecule binding; and (ii) promiscuous, that is, not requiring a permanent molecular partner (e.g., a heme binding pocket in a cytochrome will always contain a heme unless the protein is engineered to fold without it).

A procedure to derive the observable pocketome from every growing set of protein structures was described in 2012 and made available ([Kufareva et al. 2012a,b] see also, http://pocketome.org). This algorithm, based on the idea of a consistent structural ensemble, does not cover some cases where only one cocrystal structure is available, yet it is known that the binding site can indeed bind various small molecules with high affinity. These singletons are added via a manually curated list of binding sites as a supplementary input to the fully automated pipeline.

10.3 The Envelope Prediction Algorithm

The structure-based derivation algorithm introduced in 2004 was based on a transformation of the short acting Lennard Jones potential P^0 on a set of grid points with contributions from all atoms. The P^0 potential by itself is totally uncharacteristic, but when convoluted with an appropriate kernel that aggregates it in space and filtered from small chunks, it yields the envelopes and binding sites that correspond near perfectly to the actual binding sites. The function looks as follows:

$$P^0(\vec{r}) = \sum_a \frac{A_{aC}}{r_{ag}^{12}} - \frac{B_{aC}}{r_{ag}^6}$$

$$P(\vec{r}) = \int e^{-((\vec{\rho}-\vec{r})/\lambda)^2} P^0(\vec{\rho}) \, d\vec{\rho}$$

$$\lambda = 2.6A$$

The predicted pocketome is a compilation of binding sites that have the potential to bind small molecules. PocketFinder was found to match the experiment best with the value of space lambda parameter near 2.6 Å. At this value the PocketFinder method predicts pockets successfully: 96.8% of known binding sites were correctly identified when 5616 protein-ligand binding sites of complexes were tested (An et al. 2005). Additionally, 85.7% of the binding sites showed coverage of the known contact area higher than 80%. After using this algorithm and identifying potential small molecule binding envelopes in a structural proteome, we can categorize and compare the pockets to small molecules, chemical substrates, or ligands, for a docking screen for drug repurposing. Characterization of the predicted envelope can also direct ligand design for drug development. This information can also be used to identify locations for orphan receptors to bind, or for uncharacterized secondary binding sites of known receptors. Protein–protein interaction inhibition can also be evaluated at the interface patches on protein subunits after application of the algorithm.

We used this pocket prediction approach several times to find drugs that address both diseases and pathogens. A rational structure-based drug design was performed to treat the formation of intrahepatic polymers that aggregate as inclusions in liver disease associated with the Z allele mutant (Glue342Lys) of alpha1-antitrypsin (Mallya et al. 2007). This disease affects 1:1700 of North American Caucasians, with a 2–3% death rate. Low plasma alpha-antitrypsin levels lead to emphysema and higher risk of lung cancer.

After prediction of a pocket involved in polymerization, a virtual ligand screen with 1.2 million small molecules detected potential modulator compounds. Testing *in vitro* revealed six compounds that reduced polymer formation. Additional ligand binding on the cavity was modeled and 10 more compounds were found that blocked polymerization entirely. This process of pocket prediction and virtual compound docking followed by *in vitro* confirmation provided modulators that successfully enhance clearance of intracellular aggregates.

A second example of using pocket prediction and *in silico* screening involved determining the mechanism by which *allosteric* enhancers slow the dissociation of orthosteric agonists but not antagonists (Kennedy et al. 2014). Allosteric enhancers are attractive pharmacological agents because of their space and time resolution that is defined by the native hormone, mediator, or signaling molecule. For the enhancer to be active, an orthosteric site must be occupied by an agonist, which confers specificity to stressed tissues that produce adenosine. *In silico* screening of an allosteric enhancer library combined with homology modeling of the A1 receptor suggested a structure–activity relationship in which the allosteric enhancers bind to a certain pocket in a loop.

Emerging resistance to drugs that target common and critical infectious diseases is a serious problem. To address this issue of resistance and investigate other drug candidates, it is useful to identify and prioritize potential drug target sites on pathogens. The pocketome of a particular virus, bacterium, protozoan, fungus, or parasitic worm is a source for either a drug discovery/screening campaign or a drug repurposing effort. This kind of approach may be a good starting point in identifying or prioritizing the targets, since every pocket can be assigned a set "druggability" properties including pocket size, solvent exposure, hydrophobicity, uniqueness, and sequence conservation for rapidly mutating pathogens.

Nicola et al. (2008) applied this method of computational evaluation of small-molecule binding sites across a genome to malaria, and then used this information for structure-based drug design. Resistance has emerged to drugs (chloroquine and sulfadoxine) that target malaria, a parasitic disease that causes over 1 million deaths per year (UNICEF and Global Partnership to Roll Back Malaria 2005). *Plasmodium falciparum* is the causal agent of the majority of all deadly malarial cases. Many of the *P. falciparum* proteins have been crystallized, and thus are a good target for examining the structural proteome and identifying novel drugs. In 2008, Nicola et al. did just that, identifying prime inhibitor candidates for virtual screening by analyzing the structural genome and pockets. Specifically, the group selected enoyl-acyl carrier protein reductase that was a potential inhibitor ready for subsequent screening and validation *in vitro* (Nicola et al. 2008).

Our most recent example of pocket prediction and *in silico* screening is with regard to the Ebola virus, which was examined due to the urgency of the recent outbreak in West Africa. The Ebola virus is the causative agent of the Ebola hemorrhagic fever, which has a severe fatality rate of up to 90% (Dixon et al. 2014). The 2014 Ebola epidemic is the largest in history and there are currently no approved pharmaceuticals or vaccines for treatment, nor are the structural domains of virus proteins at atomic resolution sufficiently characterized. In order to create or identify an effective pharmaceutical treatment, a better understanding of the basic structure and chemical biology of Ebola proteins is critical. The Ebola virus has a small proteome consisting of seven proteins, with good structural coverage of five out of seven of those proteins. Modulating the function of these proteins may render the virus inactive. Thus, it is useful to investigate the structure of each protein and determine locations available for small molecule binding as a means of targeting multiple mechanisms of the virus. We are currently creating the Ebola virus pocketome. We identified three pockets on the VP40 matrix protein and determined that they are likely candidates for binding ligands (one pocket is highlighted in Figure 10.2). We docked 4550 of NCAT's Pharmaceutical Collection of approved drugs against these three pockets to collect a list of chemicals that are predicted to bind favorably. Pockets may also be identified on the remaining six proteins and the same list of chemicals will be docked and ranked with the hope of identifying compounds that will modulate the

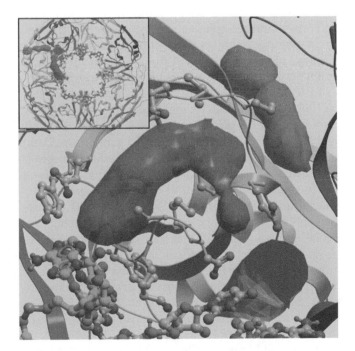

FIGURE 10.2
(**See color insert.**) Druggable pocket analysis reveals this (blue) pocket on the surface of the Ebola virus protein VP40. A small molecule binding to this pocket is predicted to interfere with assembly of the octomer (see inset) or disrupt the correct positioning of the viral RNA, perhaps inhibiting viral function.

function of the proteins. The compounds will have to be now tested *in vitro* to validate the binding event and evaluate the binding constant. Because the FDA has already approved the screened drugs, they can bypass stage 1 and 2 clinical trials and have an expedited time to actual treatment of patients. This technique and method of investigation can be applied to other pathogens, including viruses, bacteria, parasites, protozoans, and fungi.

10.4 Docking against a Pocketome Ensemble

One of the major problems in ligand docking is the conformational flexibility of the pockets and ligand-specific induced fit (e.g., Cavasotto and Abagyan 2004; Cavasotto et al. 2005). The compilation of the structural binding sites together with their conformational variability exemplified by the multiple cocrystal structures and together with the cocrystallized small molecule modulators opens an opportunity for large-scale proteome-wide docking and screening. Here, we will focus on the methods developed within the internal coordinate mechanics framework but the general principles may be transferable to other kinds of approaches (e.g., molecular dynamics).

The docking technique requires (i) a definition of the pocket and its flexibility, (ii) a search algorithm that will predict a binding pose of a flexible ligand along with the induced fit, and (iii) a scoring function that will assign an estimate of the binding free energy to each pose of each ligand. For the search algorithm to be successful it must take into account poses and conformations, allowing for flexibility of both the protein and the ligand, but with sufficient efficiency to enable large-scale screening (Damm-Ganamet et al. 2013). Ligand binding induces conformational changes that need to be accounted for in order to correctly predict binding, because even minute changes in conformation can significantly alter the outcome. The experimental pocketome compilations offer the multiple cocrystallized pocket conformations to be used as a surrogate for real flexibility. That surrogate is highly efficient especially when used with the four-dimensional (4D) docking protocol (Bottegoni et al. 2009). Receptor flexibility in the 4D ligand docking protocol allows for the pocket flexibility to be a single discrete variable. Self-docking is the process of docking a complex crystal structure with its cognate ligand, which is 91% successful (Neves et al. 2012). Cross-docking uses the same protein in several different conformations, and correctly docks ligands less than 50% of the time.

There are three possible methods to overcome this humble success rate of a single pocket conformation cross-docking exercise: Multiple Experimental Conformations (MRC) with a conformational ensemble (Totrov and Abagyan 2008), 4D docking (concurrent sampling against multiconformational grids) (Bottegoni et al. 2009), or systematic omit models and refinement (SCan

Alanines and REfine: SCARE) (Bottegoni et al. 2008). The 4D docking, which incorporates receptor conformational ensembles in a single-docking simulation, maintains the accuracy of traditional ensemble docking while decreasing the sampling time. The "fourth-dimension" refers to the multiplicity of pockets within each ensemble that expands the pocketome data. Using all available pocket conformations may not be the best strategy since too many pocket alternatives increase both the noise and the signal. Several articles have formulated the optimal strategy for selection of a subset of conformers for the docking and screening applications (Rueda et al. 2010; Bottegoni et al. 2011). The ligand information can also be used to select an optimal subset and/or improve the pocket conformations of a homology model (Cavasotto et al. 2008; Katritch et al. 2012; Rueda et al. 2012).

If the crystallographic source of the receptor variations is insufficient, computationally generated models can be used to generate this conformational ensemble. One application of computationally generated receptor variants is the novel rearrangements of the binding pocket (Bottegoni et al. 2009) that increase the chance of identifying new ligands.

10.5 Screening against the Pocketome

Screening against multiple pockets represents the newest direction in docking. Traditionally, the docking was used to screen a large set of chemicals against one or several targets to identify new chemical leads (e.g., McRobb et al. 2014). The screen of the KEGG metabolites against the rhodopsin and bacteriorhodopsin is a good early illustration of that power (Cavasotto et al. 2003). However, the availability of precompiled and annotated ensembles ready for docking enables a novel twist for the docking screens: screening of one or several ligands against multiple targets. The first applications of docking to target screening have been done for the kinases (Kufareva and Abagyan 2008) and nuclear receptors (Park et al. 2010). The transition from a ligand screen to a target screen is not trivial because it imposes two new requirements on the docking models: (i) high sensitivity and specificity; and (ii) comparability of the docking scores between different target models. In contrast, a traditional ligand screen against a single model allows for a large fraction of false negatives, because it is not necessary to fish out *all* hits from the multimillion chemical library, as long as some binders/activators are identified with the screening model. We also do not care about the relative scale of the scores for the single target screening application.

The first challenge in the target profiling can be addressed to some degree with the optimal set of the experimentally determined conformations (e.g., Rueda et al. 2012). The second one can be addressed by either finding a transformation of the scores from experimental data on binding (Kufareva and

Abagyan 2008; Park et al. 2010), or by normalizing against a large collection of drug-like molecules (i.e., the set of marketed small molecule drugs).

It is worth mentioning that the target can be represented not only by the pocket models but also from the averaged atom property fields of the cocrystallized ligands (Totrov and Abagyan 2008; Chen et al. 2014). These models may achieve even higher area-under-curve (AUC) values for the activity benchmarks, as demonstrated in Abagyan et al. (2012) and Kufareva et al. (2012a, b) but they do have some level of historical chemical memory, even though it has been substantially reduced through the use of exact bound poses and ensemble averaging. A comparison of two main docking-based target screens has been published recently (Chen et al. 2014). These screens enable the following applications:

- Deorphanization, or predicting targets of leads from a phenotypic/cell assay
- Discovering biological targets for common cellular metabolites by screening and validating their multitarget profile
- Predicting adverse effects of drugs and environmental compounds

The first screens show serious promise, as they have been benchmarked for their ability to determine a multitarget profile of any compound. In this type of target panels, different target models may have highly variable benchmark performance. Therefore, they should be considered and evaluated individually and used according to specific performance values such as AUC.

10.6 Conclusion

With the introduction of the pocketome of an organism, combined with the pocketome database, a new type of screen emerged. This is a docking screen of one or several chemicals against a large collection of 3D models of binding sites of macromolecules of an organism. The models can be built from cocrystallized ligand information, or from the basis of the pockets and their flexibility. These target models are used to discover a complex multitarget profile of chemicals with applications for basic biology, drug discovery, and determination of adverse effects.

References

Abagyan, R., W. Chen, and I. Kufareva. 2012. Docking, screening and selectivity prediction for small-molecule nuclear receptor modulators. In: *Computational*

Approaches to Nuclear Receptors, P. Cozzini and G. E. Kellogg, (eds.). Cambridge: RSC, pp. 84–109.

Allerton, C. M., C. G. Barber, K. C. Beaumont et al. 2006. A novel series of potent and selective PDE5 inhibitors with potential for high and dose-independent oral bioavailability. *J. Med. Chem.* 49(12): 3581–3594.

An, J., M. Totrov and R. Abagyan. 2005. Pocketome via comprehensive identification and classification of ligand binding envelopes. *Mol. Cell Proteomics* 4(6): 752–761.

Bickerton, G. R., G. V. Paolini, J. Besnard, S. Muresan, and A. L. Hopkins. 2012. Quantifying the chemical beauty of drugs. *Nat. Chem.* 4(2): 90–98.

Bottegoni, G., I. Kufareva, M. Totrov, and R. Abagyan. 2008. A new method for ligand docking to flexible receptors by dual alanine scanning and refinement (SCARE). *J. Comput. Aided. Mol. Des.* 22(5): 311–325.

Bottegoni, G., I. Kufareva, M. Totrov, and R. Abagyan. 2009. Four-dimensional docking: A fast and accurate account of discrete receptor flexibility in ligand docking. *J. Med. Chem.* 52(2): 397–406.

Bottegoni, G., W. Rocchia, M. Rueda, R. Abagyan, and A. Cavalli. 2011. Systematic exploitation of multiple receptor conformations for virtual ligand screening. *PLoS One* 6(5): e18845.

Brady, G. P., Jr. and P. F. Stouten. 2000. Fast prediction and visualization of protein binding pockets with PASS. *J. Comput. Aided. Mol. Des.* 14(4): 383–401.

Brynda, J., P. Mader, V. Sicha et al. 2013. Carborane-based carbonic anhydrase inhibitors. *Angew. Chem. Int. Ed. Engl.* 52(51): 13760–13763.

Cavasotto, C. N. and R. A. Abagyan. 2004. Protein flexibility in ligand docking and virtual screening to protein kinases. *J. Mol. Biol.* 337(1): 209–225.

Cavasotto, C. N., J. A. Kovacs, and R. A. Abagyan. 2005. Representing receptor flexibility in ligand docking through relevant normal modes. *J. Am. Chem. Soc.* 127(26): 9632–9640.

Cavasotto, C. N., A. J. Orry, and R. A. Abagyan. 2003. Structure-based identification of binding sites, native ligands and potential inhibitors for G-protein coupled receptors. *Proteins* 51(3): 423–433.

Cavasotto, C. N., A. J. Orry, N. J. Murgolo et al. 2008. Discovery of novel chemotypes to a G-protein-coupled receptor through ligand-steered homology modeling and structure-based virtual screening. *J. Med. Chem.* 51(3): 581–588.

Chelliah, V., L. Chen, T. L. Blundell, and S. C. Lovell. 2004. Distinguishing structural and functional restraints in evolution in order to identify interaction sites. *J. Mol. Biol.* 342(5): 1487–1504.

Chen, Y. C., M. Totrov, and R. Abagyan. 2014. Docking to multiple pockets or ligand fields for screening, activity prediction and scaffold hopping. *Future Med. Chem.* 6(16): 1741–1755.

Cheng, A. C., R. G. Coleman, K. T. Smyth et al. 2007. Structure-based maximal affinity model predicts small-molecule druggability. *Nat. Biotech.* 25(1): 71–75.

Damm-Ganamet, K. L., R. D. Smith, J. B. Dunbar, Jr., J. A. Stuckey, and H. A. Carlson. 2013. CSAR benchmark exercise 2011–2012: Evaluation of results from docking and relative ranking of blinded congeneric series. *J. Chem. Inf. Model.* 53(8): 1853–1870.

Dixon, M. G., I. J. Schafer, Control Centers for Disease, and Prevention. 2014. Ebola viral disease outbreak—West Africa, 2014. *MMWR Morb Mortal Wkly Rep* 63(25): 548–551.

Hendlich, M., F. Rippmann, and G. Barnickel. 1997. LIGSITE: Automatic and efficient detection of potential small molecule-binding sites in proteins. *J. Mol. Graph. Model.* 15(6): 359–363, 389.

Hughes, R. O., T. Maddux, D. Joseph Rogier et al. 2011. Investigation of the pyrazinones as PDE5 inhibitors: Evaluation of regioisomeric projections into the solvent region. *Bioorg. Med. Chem. Lett.* 21(21): 6348–6352.

Katritch, V., M. Rueda, and R. Abagyan. 2012. Ligand-guided receptor optimization. *Methods Mol. Biol.* 857: 189–205.

Kennedy, D. P., F. M. McRobb, S. A. Leonhardt et al. 2014. The second extracellular loop of the adenosine A1 receptor mediates activity of allosteric enhancers. *Mol. Pharmacol.* 85(2): 301–309.

Kufareva, I. and R. Abagyan. 2008. Type-II kinase inhibitor docking, screening, and profiling using modified structures of active kinase states. *J. Med. Chem.* 51(24): 7921–7932.

Kufareva, I., Y. C. Chen, A. V. Ilatovskiy, and R. Abagyan. 2012a. Compound activity prediction using models of binding pockets or ligand properties in 3D. *Curr. Top. Med. Chem.* 12(17): 1869–1882.

Kufareva, I., A. V. Ilatovskiy, and R. Abagyan. 2012b. Pocketome: An encyclopedia of small-molecule binding sites in 4D. *Nucleic Acids Res.* 40(Database issue): D535–D540.

Laskowski, R. A. 1995. SURFNET: A program for visualizing molecular surfaces, cavities, and intermolecular interactions. *J. Mol. Graph.* 13(5): 323–330, 307–308.

Le Guilloux, V., P. Schmidtke, and P. Tuffery. 2009. Fpocket: An open source platform for ligand pocket detection. *BMC Bioinformatics* 10: 168.

Liang, J., H. Edelsbrunner, and C. Woodward. 1998. Anatomy of protein pockets and cavities: Measurement of binding site geometry and implications for ligand design. *Protein Sci.* 7(9): 1884–1897.

Mallya, M., R. L. Phillips, S. A. Saldanha et al. 2007. Small molecules block the polymerization of Z alpha1-antitrypsin and increase the clearance of intracellular aggregates. *J. Med. Chem.* 50(22): 5357–5363.

McRobb, F. M., I. Kufareva, and R. Abagyan. 2014. *In silico* identification and pharmacological evaluation of novel endocrine disrupting chemicals that act via the ligand-binding domain of the estrogen receptor alpha. *Toxicol. Sci.* 141(1): 188–197.

Neves, M. A., M. Totrov, and R. Abagyan. 2012. Docking and scoring with ICM: The benchmarking results and strategies for improvement. *J. Comput. Aided. Mol. Des.* 26(6): 675–686.

Nicola, G., C. A. Smith, and R. Abagyan. 2008. New method for the assessment of all drug-like pockets across a structural genome. *J. Comput. Biol.* 15(3): 231–240.

Park, S. J., I. Kufareva, and R. Abagyan. 2010. Improved docking, screening and selectivity prediction for small molecule nuclear receptor modulators using conformational ensembles. *J. Comput. Aided. Mol. Des.* 24(5): 459–471.

Peters, K. P., J. Fauck, and C. Frommel. 1996. The automatic search for ligand binding sites in proteins of known three-dimensional structure using only geometric criteria. *J. Mol. Biol.* 256(1): 201–213.

Raush, E., M. Totrov, B. D. Marsden, and R. Abagyan. 2009. A new method for publishing three-dimensional content. *PLoS One* 4(10): e7394.

Rueda, M., G. Bottegoni, and R. Abagyan. 2010. Recipes for the selection of experimental protein conformations for virtual screening. *J. Chem. Inf. Model.* 50(1): 186–193.

Rueda, M., M. Totrov, and R. Abagyan. 2012. ALiBERO: Evolving a team of complementary pocket conformations rather than a single leader. *J. Chem. Inf. Model.* 52(10): 2705–2714.

Sheridan, R. P., V. N. Maiorov, M. K. Holloway, W. D. Cornell, and Y. D. Gao. 2010. Drug-like density: A method of quantifying the "bindability" of a protein target based on a very large set of pockets and drug-like ligands from the Protein Data Bank. *J. Chem. Inf. Model.* 50(11): 2029–2040.

Totrov, M. and R. Abagyan. 2008. Flexible ligand docking to multiple receptor conformations: A practical alternative. *Curr. Opin. Struct. Biol.* 18(2): 178–184.

UNICEF, and Global Partnership to Roll Back Malaria. 2005. *World Malaria Report: 2005.* Geneva: World Health Organization.

Yu, J., Y. Zhou, I. Tanaka, and M. Yao. 2010. Roll: A new algorithm for the detection of protein pockets and cavities with a rolling probe sphere. *Bioinformatics* 26(1): 46–52.

11

MM-GB/SA Rescoring of Docking Poses: Tricks of the Trade

Cristiano R. W. Guimarães

CONTENTS

11.1 Introduction

The computational methodologies used to understand structural and energetic relationships to binding vary in speed and accuracy. The molecular dynamics (MD) and Monte Carlo (MC) simulations coupled with free-energy perturbation (FEP) or thermodynamic integration (TI) calculations are the most rigorous computational approaches currently used to estimate relative binding affinities (Guimarães et al. 2005; Jorgensen 1989, 1998; Kollman 1993; Pearlman and Charifson 2001; Simonson et al. 2002). Although these methods have provided impressive results for several protein–ligand systems, they are computationally intensive and have generally been applied to study a small number of ligands in a congeneric series (Boyce et al. 2009; Deng and Roux 2006; Guimarães 2011; Luccarelli et al. 2010; Michel et al. 2006; Michel and Essex 2008; Mobley et al. 2007).

Small-molecule docking is designed to orient and score a large number of molecules for complementarity against a macromolecular binding site in a short period of time (Alvarez 2004; Powers et al. 2002; Schapira et al. 2003; Shoichet et al. 2002; Shoichet 2004; Taylor et al. 2002; Walters et al. 1998). The critical issues in docking include the prediction of the correct binding pose and the accurate estimation of the corresponding binding affinity. Despite the enormous size of the conformational space for the ligands, different docking methodologies, for example, force field-based, empirical, and knowledge-based, have all been successful in reproducing the crystallographic binding modes (Friesner et al. 2004; Jones et al. 1997; Kuntz et al. 1982; Muegge and Martin 1999; Rarey et al. 1996). However, the accuracy in predicting binding affinities is quite poor for all of them (Charifson et al. 1999; Perola et al. 2004; Stahl and Rarey 2001; Warren et al. 2006). The computational errors may be attributed to many approximations employed in the scoring functions, particularly the ones that lead to poor estimation of the desolvation, intramolecular, and entropy penalties for the ligands upon binding. Since the docking algorithms provide good-quality binding poses, an energy function with more physically reasonable description of binding contributions can be employed to rescore the docking results.

MM-based scoring methods, using all atom force fields coupled with Poisson–Boltzman (MM-PB/SA) (Barril et al. 2001) or Generalized Born calculations (MM-GB/SA) (Kuhn and Kollman 2000) to model solvation, have recently seen an upsurge in popularity. Although the latter has been collectively referred to as MM-GB/SA, there are in fact many flavors in the literature differing in the force fields and GB/SA solvation models employed, use of a single energy-minimized structure or an ensemble of conformations extracted from MD/MC simulations or conformational search methods for the unbound and bound states, and exclusion or not of binding contributions that deteriorate the method accuracy. Overall, when compared to docking scoring functions, the physics-based methods provide improved enrichment in the virtual screening of databases and better correlation between calculated binding affinities and experimental data (Foloppe and Hubbard 2006; Haider et al. 2011; Hou et al. 2011; Huang et al. 2006a,b; Lee and Sun 2007; Lyne et al. 2006).

In the case of our own flavor of MM-GB/SA (Guimarães and Cardozo 2008), when rescoring docking poses of congeneric series for pharmaceutically relevant targets, we observed correlations with experimental data that were far superior to the ones obtained with the Glide XP scoring function (Friesner et al. 2004, 2006). In one test case, the results obtained with the physics-based scoring were even competitive with the computationally intensive FEP methods (Guimarães 2011). The aim of this work is to describe the foundations of the original methodology and improvements that followed.

11.2 MM-GB/SA Rescoring

In our implementation of the MM-GB/SA rescoring (Figure 11.1), a conformational search for the inhibitors in the unbound state and energy minimization for the complexes using OPLS_2005 (Jorgensen et al. 1996; Kaminski

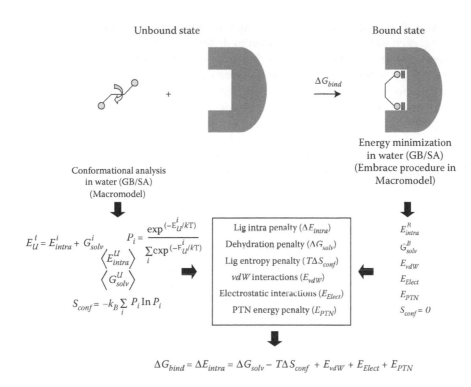

FIGURE 11.1
Schematic representation of the MM-GB/SA rescoring procedure.

et al. 2001) and GB/SA within Macromodel (MacroModel 2005) were performed. In the unbound state, all conformers within 5.0 kcal/mol from the lowest energy conformer were retained. A root-mean-square deviation (RMSd) value of 0.3 Å for heavy atoms and hydrogens connected to heteroatoms was used to obtain unique conformations. Assuming a Boltzmann distribution, the probabilities for each conformer (P_i) were calculated and the average intramolecular and solvation energies for each compound obtained. The conformational entropies (S_{conf}) were computed from the probabilities using Equation 11.1, where k_B is the Boltzmann constant.

$$S_{conf} = -k_B \sum_{i=i}^{n} P_i \ln P_i \qquad (11.1)$$

To better account for the protein flexibility, the best pose for each inhibitor was energy-minimized in the bound state. In energy minimization, no constraints were applied to residues within 5 Å from the center of the system. A second shell of 3 Å around the first shell was defined and constraints of 50 kcal/mol Å² applied to the residues therein. The remaining residues were held fixed.

This was done with the purpose of reducing the aforementioned noise in the scoring; each complex could be driven to different local minima in a fully flexible energy minimization step. After the energy minimization step, the protein energy (E_{PTN}) values for all complexes were extracted. This term describes the protein deformation imposed by each ligand. Besides E_{PTN}, the energy-minimized structures for the complexes provided the intramolecular and solvation energies for the ligands in the protein environment, and the protein–ligand intermolecular van der Waals (E_{vdW}) and electrostatic (E_{Elect}) interaction energies. In the bound state, it was assumed that there was only one conformation accessible to each ligand; its conformational entropy is therefore zero. In this manner, the binding energy (ΔG_{bind}) was calculated as shown in Equation 11.2.

$$\Delta G_{bind} = \Delta E_{intra} + \Delta G_{solv} - T\Delta S_{conf} + E_{vdW} + E_{Elect} + E_{PTN} \qquad (11.2)$$

In Equation 11.2, ΔE_{intra} and ΔG_{solv} are the intramolecular and desolvation penalties for each ligand upon binding. These penalties reflect how their intramolecular and solvation energies change upon transfer from the unbound to the bound state. Similarly, $-T\Delta S_{conf}$ is the ligand conformational entropy penalty, multiplied by the temperature to convert it into free energy. The final ranking was obtained by calculating relative binding energies ($\Delta\Delta G_{bind}$) using the top-scoring inhibitor of each target as reference.

11.3 Learnings

One of the main advantages of our scoring approach is that the calculated binding contributions are separated. This provides interpretation of SAR data when the method is used retrospectively or allows modulation of specific binding contributions to gain affinity when used prospectively. The separation also enables diagnose of terms that improve or deteriorate the correlation with experimental data. The calculated contributions that are consistently harmful to the accuracy of the method were permanently excluded from our MM-GB/SA scoring equation. Equation 11.2 provides the best results across a series of targets and their respective ligands. However, one should keep in mind that the equation and its terms are not perfect; some of their strengths and weakness are outlined below:

a. Force fields perform reasonably well at calculating the relative energies between different energy minima but they tend to overestimate energy barriers. As the bound conformation for the ligand is not at any particular energy minimum since it is deformed by the protein, the ΔE_{intra} values tend to be more positive than what would be expected using a quantum-mechanical method. This problem should be minimized when scoring a congeneric series;

b. In most cases, ΔE_{intra}, the ligand intramolecular penalty upon binding, is a positive number but there are few cases when it is negative. One classic example is when the compound forms an intramolecular hydrogen bond in the bound state but not in solution due to competition with the solvent. In this case, ΔG_{solv} will be very unfavorable. In any event, the sum between ΔE_{intra} and ΔG_{solv} is always positive;

c. ΔE_{intra} is highly correlated with the sum between protein–ligand E_{vdW} and E_{Elect} interactions; ligands are deformed as much as possible to maximize intermolecular interactions with the protein;

d. $-T\Delta S_{conf}$, as described above, which assumes a Boltzmann distribution in solution, is the correct way of estimating the ligand conformational entropy penalty upon binding. A common approach used in the literature, which penalizes each rotatable bond in the ligand that becomes "frozen" upon binding by +0.65 kcal/mol, considerably overestimates the entropy loss. This is because this approach assumes that each rotatable bond has three degenerate conformations, giving a total of 3N possible conformations, all equal in energy, for a molecule with N rotatable bonds;

e. $-T\Delta S_{conf}$ for a congeneric series has a typical dynamic range of approximately 1 kcal/mol, and it does not have an appreciable impact on the MM-GB/SA scoring;

f. The protein–ligand E_{vdW} interaction term generally dominates the binding energy differences; it is the term with the best correlation when plotted individually against experimental activities.

g. The protein–ligand E_{Elect} interaction term is important but somewhat problematic. The application of a protein dielectric constant of 1 in a model where protein motions are not taken into account and the use of a fixed charged force field cause overestimation of electrostatic attractions and repulsions due to the lack of shielding effects. Shielding from the solvent as estimated by the GB method alleviates this problem but this term tends to be noisy and is generally excluded from the scoring equation. Hence, one should be careful when scoring ligands that form hydrogen bonds with the protein; they tend to have very favorable scores since the desolvation penalty term ΔG_{solv} is not enough to offset the overestimated E_{Elect} term. Depending on the makeup of the congeneric series being scored, E_{Elect} might adversely affect the correlation with the experiment, especially if the ability to form hydrogen bonds with the protein is limited to only few ligands in the series and the hydrogen bonds are nonproductive, as indicated by the experimental data.

h. Applying energy minimization for the complexes rather than MD simulations greatly increases computational efficiency and provides a method with a timescale compatible with synthetic chemistry–biological test cycles. However, lack of sampling could in theory pose a significant limitation on the method since the protein would not be able to relax to accommodate different scaffolds after docking. This problem should be minimized when scoring a congeneric series. In addition, a recent study suggests that a single, relaxed structure for each complex provides superior results when compared to the standard averaging over MD trajectories (Kuhn et al. 2005). A possible explanation for this is the introduction of noise in the scoring as each complex could be visiting different regions of the phase space due to short trajectories.

i. E_{PTN} also suffers from the lack of electrostatic shielding mentioned above. This is evident in cases where ligands disturb neighboring salt bridges within the protein at different degrees; kinases are a classic example with the salt bridges between the catalytic Lys and the Glu residue from the C-helix and/or the Asp residue from the DFG loop adopt different geometries for each ligand. As a consequence, E_{PTN} can get very noisy. One solution for this is to reduce the shell of flexible residues in the energy minimization from 5 to 3 Å.

j. Entropy contributions such as the changes in translational, rotational, and vibrational entropies for the ligand and protein upon binding are ignored. The inclusion of such contributions for ligands in a congeneric series using the rigid rotor harmonic oscillator (RRHO) approximation as implemented in Macromodel has little to no impact on the rank ordering. The contributions for the protein are assumed to be relatively constant within a series.

k. Another entropic contribution ignored here is associated with the narrowing of the torsional energy wells for the ligands and the protein when forming the complex compared to solution (Chang et al. 2007). The restriction of torsional motions is possibly the entropic contribution that affects rank ordering the most. However, its calculation is extremely intensive and typically requires 1–2 days per compound on a single CPU; the MM-GB/SA score for 50–100 ligands takes few hours on a single CPU, an acceptable turnaround in the pharmaceutical industry.

l. The scoring terms of our MM-GB/SA protocol are now obtained very easily using Knime Extensions as depicted in Figure 11.2. Knime is a modular, highly configurable framework for easy workflow automation and data analysis (Knime 2008).

m. Solvent effects are included in the protein–ligand complex geometry optimization using GB/SA, but the protein desolvation term calculated by the continuum model (ΔG_{solv}^{PTN}) is excluded from the scoring since it consistently deteriorates the correlation with experimental results (Guimarães and Mathiowetz 2010).

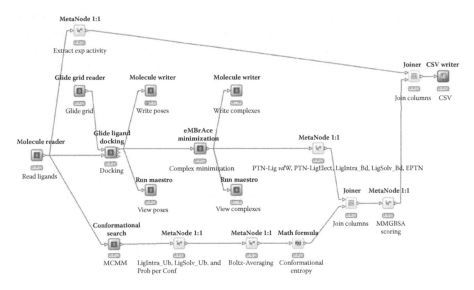

FIGURE 11.2
Automated MM-GB/SA rescoring with Knime.

11.4 Further Investigations

11.4.1 MM-GB/SA Augmented by Watermap

The GB model has been shown to give solvation-free energies in agreement with experiment for small molecules (Jorgensen et al. 2004; Still et al. 1990). However, the performance of this model for simulations of large biomolecules is questionable at best (Roe et al. 2007). As for the nonpolar components of solvation in GB/SA, the empirical parametrization of the nonpolar components of hydration-free energies based solely on the solvent accessible surface area is insufficient; favorable vdW dispersion between interior atoms of the solute and the solvent, insignificant for small molecules, is an important effect in the solvation of large solutes such as biopolymers, and not well captured in a simple surface-area dependent term (Gallicchio et al. 2000; Pitera and van Gunsteren 2001). This is particularly problematic when protein systems differ significantly in the number of buried and solvent-exposed atoms, which is the case when estimating the different protein desolvation contributions caused by each ligand.

The explicit consideration of water molecules in protein-binding sites is then an interesting alternative to improve the quality of scoring methods that are based on the implicit description of solvent effects. One such method is the one developed by Abel and coworkers called WaterMap (Abel et al. 2008). In this method, the hydration site locations in the binding-site cavity are obtained using a clustering technique applied to an MD simulation of explicit water molecules solvating a rigid protein structure. The thermodynamic properties of the hydration sites, specifically enthalpy and entropy changes with respect to bulk water, are obtained from averaging solvent–solvent and protein–solvent interaction energies and application of inhomogeneous solvation theory, respectively. A displaced-solvent functional was then derived to estimate the free energy liberation (ΔG_{WM}) when a ligand that is suitably complementary to the binding site displaces the waters therein into an assumed-to-preexist cavity in bulk solution, previously occupied by the ligand. In order to accommodate ligand binding, the binding site waters get displaced to the cavity in solution leaving a cavity of identical size and shape in the protein (Figure 11.3). The WaterMap method then represents an attempt to isolate the free energy associated with transferring the solvent cavity from the bulk to the binding site from all other contributions to binding and provides, in other words, an estimate for the hydrophobic effect.

The functional depends on the degree of overlap between the ligand heavy atoms and the hydration sites and the energetics of the waters that are displaced. Specifically, the functional considers that a water molecule is completely displaced and therefore its full energy is liberated when the distance between the hydration site center and the ligand heavy atom approaches zero. The energy of hydration site displacement then decreases linearly to a value of zero when the distance between the two atoms is equal to 80% the sum of their *vdW* radii, beyond which there is no displacement. Multiple ligand atoms may contribute to the displacement of a given hydration site; however, these contributions cease once total displacement is achieved. The *ab initio* form of the displaced-solvent functional as described by Abel and coworkers was employed in this work (Abel et al. 2008).

Incorporation of ΔG_{WM} into our MM-GB/SA equation improves the scoring, but only modestly (Guimarães and Mathiowetz 2010). It is possible that part of that is due to the fact that the combined method is approaching the maximum R^2 value a model can obtain given the properties of the data sets studied, as suggested by Brown and coworkers (Brown et al. 2009). The small improvement can also be explained by the high correlation between the

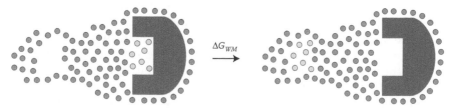

FIGURE 11.3

(See color insert.) Schematic representation of the process simulated by WaterMap. The white area represents the cavity in the bulk that is transferred to the protein binding site. The orange dots represent the binding site waters that get displaced into the bulk solution. WaterMap estimates the free energy liberation (ΔG_{WM}) for the displaced waters.

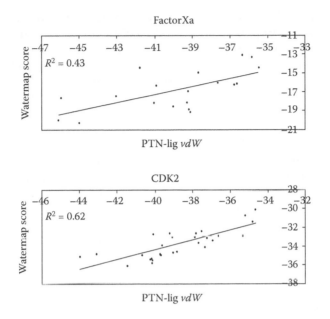

FIGURE 11.4
Correlation between protein–ligand vdW interactions and WaterMap free energy liberation term.

ΔG_{WM} term and the protein–ligand E_{vdW} interaction term, the former a measure of the hydrophobic effect and the latter of hydrophobic-like interactions. This is illustrated in Figure 11.4 for two test cases, factor Xa and CDK2.

11.4.2 Large Dynamic Range in MM-GB/SA: Comparison with FEP Results

Although the MM-GB/SA scoring equation provides good correlation with experimental data and accurate rank ordering, the scores display a large dynamic range (15–20 kcal/mol) with respect to the experimental range, typically around 4–5 kcal/mol. This can have enthalpic as well as entropic origins. As for the enthalpic effects, it is possible that the wider scoring spread is due to (i) the lack of shielding of electrostatic interactions between the protein and ligands that cause overestimation of electrostatic attractions and repulsions, (ii) the lack of thermal effects as only one energy-minimized structure for each complex is considered resulting in overly optimal protein–ligand interactions, and (iii) the lack of complete protein relaxation/ strain introduced by different ligands; the ligands that interact more favorably with the protein might deform it at a larger extent than what is captured by just a constrained energy minimization. Another potential explanation for the wider scoring spread is associated with the incomplete description of enthalpy–entropy compensation such as (i) more significant vibrational entropy penalties for complexes displaying more favorable protein–ligand interactions, (ii) greater loss of translational and rotational entropies upon binding for ligands with higher molecular weight, which tend to exhibit more favorable hydrophobic effect and *vdW* interactions with the protein, and (iii) a more significant loss of torsional vibrational entropy for the complexes between the protein and the more flexible ligands, which have more opportunities to maximize their intermolecular interactions.

Figure 11.5 shows a large dynamic range for the MM-GB/SA method (~15 kcal/mol) compared to the experimental range (~1.8 kcal/mol) when scoring a series of human Carbonic Anhydrase (hCAII) inhibitors (Scott et al. 2009). The experimental binding free energies were obtained by Isothermal Titration Calorimetry (ITC). To evaluate the origin of the large dynamic range in MM-GB/SA, a computational Van't Hoff analysis was conducted for two pairs of ligands, benzenesulfone to 4-Cl-benzenesulfone (H → 4-Cl) and benzenesulfone to 4-NH_2-benzenesulfone (H → 4-NH_2), by running FEP simulations with MCPRO+ (MCPRO+ 2008) and Desmond (Desmond 2009) at 298 K and at ±30 K. In the analysis, it was assumed that the heat capacity remains unchanged over the temperature interval (Prabhu and Sharp 2005). The assumption here is that the results obtained with MCPRO+, with its restricted sampling, can be extrapolated to MM-GB/SA, which uses only one energy-minimized structure to describe the protein–ligand complex. In MCPRO+, only the side chains of residues with any atom within 10 Å from the ligands are varied and the protein backbone is fixed. Although the ligand is free to move in MC simulations of the unbound state, one should not expect that all accessible conformations and the full range of dihedral angle values for each torsional well are visited, even for very long simulations. This implies that the description of entropic contributions, shielding of electrostatic interactions, thermal effects, and protein relaxation/strain will

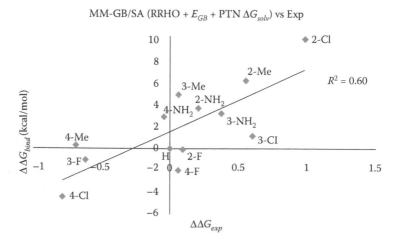

FIGURE 11.5
Correlation between MM-GB/SA scores ($\Delta\Delta G_{bind}$) and ITC values ($\Delta\Delta G_{exp}$) for a series of hCAII inhibitors.

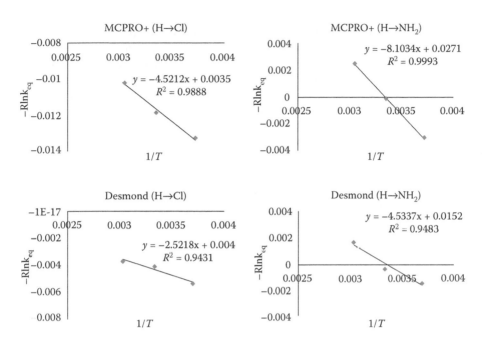

FIGURE 11.6
Van't Hoff plots obtained with MCPRO+ (top) and Desmond (bottom) for the H → 4-Cl and H → 4-NH$_2$ pairs.

be, like in MM-GB/SA, somewhat incomplete in the FEP results obtained with MCPRO+.

Figure 11.6 compares the Van't Hoff plots for the H → 4-Cl and H → 4-NH$_2$ pairs obtained with Desmond and MCPRO+. The experimental and calculated enthalpic and entropic contributions to the relative binding free energies are shown in Table 11.1. Although the $\Delta\Delta G_{bind}$ values obtained with

TABLE 11.1

Enthalpic and Entropic Contributions Extracted from Van't Hoff Plots Obtained with MCPRO+ and Desmond (Values in kcal/mol)

	H → 4-Cl			H → 4-NH$_2$		
	$\Delta\Delta H_{bind}$	$-T\Delta\Delta S_{bind}$	$\Delta\Delta G_{bind}$	$\Delta\Delta H_{bind}$	$-T\Delta\Delta S_{bind}$	$\Delta\Delta G_{bind}$
MM-GB/SA	–	–	−4.50	–	–	+2.93
MCPRO+	−4.52 ± 0.19	+0.97 ± 0.24	−3.55 ± 0.12	−8.10 ± 0.14	+8.06 ± 0.17	−0.04 ± 0.09
Desmond	−2.52 ± 0.26	+1.28 ± 0.30	−1.24 ± 0.15	−4.53 ± 0.20	+4.43 ± 0.23	−0.10 ± 0.12
ITC[a]	−0.29	−0.76	−1.05 (−0.78)[b]	+0.99	−0.49	+0.50 (−0.05)[b]

[a] ITC $\Delta\Delta H_{bind}$ and $-T\Delta\Delta S_{bind}$ values (see Scott, A. D. et al. 2009. *Chem. Med. Chem.* 4(12): 1985–1989.)

[b] Values in parenthesis were corrected (see Guimarães, C. R. W. 2011. *J. Chem. Theory Comput.* 7(7): 2296–2306.)

MCPRO+ and Desmond match the experimental values reasonably well, the enthalpic and entropic contributions do not agree with the ITC data. A possible explanation is that, of the parameters measured directly by ITC, the free energy $\Delta G°$ has the lowest signal-to-noise ratio, as measured values fall in a relatively narrow range. The enthalpic contribution ($\Delta H°$) has a higher signal to noise, with the entropic contribution ($\Delta S°$) being even less precise since errors are compounded; $\Delta S°$ is calculated as the difference between $\Delta H°$ and $\Delta G°$. Alternatively, it is possible that the lack of agreement is due to the fact that the experimental $\Delta\Delta H_{bind}$ and $-T\Delta\Delta S_{bind}$ values still contain the ionization step for the inhibitor before binding to hCAII. The sulfonamide group binds to hCAII in its deprotonated state and were simulated that way. In order to compare with the calculated $\Delta\Delta G_{bind}$ values, the free energies associated with the ionization step were removed from the experimental ITC values since the pK_a of the molecules and pH of the experiment were known, but that was not possible for the experimental $\Delta\Delta H_{bind}$ and $-T\Delta\Delta S_{bind}$ values.

If the analysis is focused on the difference between the FEP methods, it is clear that MCPRO+ provides enthalpic contributions that are exaggerated compared to those from Desmond. In the case of H → 4-Cl, it is unlikely that this is due to diminished shielding of electrostatic interaction between the 4-Cl analog and the protein; the substituent is in close contact with a Phe residue (F129) (Figure 11.7). More plausible explanations are either associated with reduced thermal effects that might lead to too favorable *vdW* interactions and/or limited protein deformation that does not offset the gain in interactions for 4-Cl due to restriction of degrees of freedom in the MC simulations.

It is interesting to see that the MCPRO+ $\Delta\Delta H_{bind}$ between H and 4-Cl matches their MM-GB/SA relative score of −4.50 kcal/mol, which despite few entropic contributions included is mostly dominated by enthalpic terms. A more significant entropy loss of +0.97 kcal/mol for the 4-Cl derivative compared to the unsubstituted analog results in a $\Delta\Delta G_{bind}$ of −3.55 kcal/mol obtained with MCPRO+. The increased sampling in Desmond generates a $-T\Delta\Delta S_{bind}$ value of +1.28 kcal/mol, just slightly more positive than the value reported by MCPRO+ (Table 11.1). Thus, the larger free energy gap for the H → 4-Cl transformation caused by restricted sampling is almost purely enthalpic.

A somewhat different scenario is seen for the H → 4-NH$_2$ pair. Table 11.1 shows that $\Delta\Delta H_{bind}$ obtained with MCPRO+ is also exaggerated when compared to Desmond, but differently from the H → 4-Cl case, the $-T\Delta\Delta S_{bind}$ contribution completely offsets that; $-T\Delta\Delta S_{bind}$ values of +8.06 and +4.43 kcal/mol obtained with MCPRO+ and Desmond, respectively, lead to almost identical $\Delta\Delta G_{bind}$. Figure 11.7 sheds some light on the enthalpy–entropy compensation observed for the 4-NH$_2$ analog. It shows that the NH$_2$ group has the ability to interact with Asn61, Asn66, and Gln91 via water-mediated hydrogen bonds. It is then plausible that in this case the enthalpic and entropic contributions are affected by the different structural and thermodynamic properties of the water molecules in the binding site as a result of restricted versus full protein sampling. A less mobile protein, and consequently less mobile

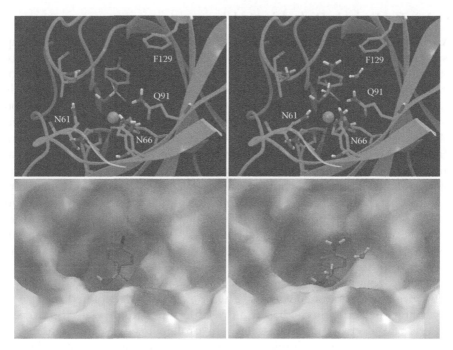

FIGURE 11.7
(**See color insert.**) Representative theoretical structures of the complexes between hCAII and the 4-Cl (left) and 4-NH$_2$ (right) substituted benzene sulfonamide inhibitors. Molecular surface representations are also shown at the bottom.

water molecules, in MCPRO+ leads to overly favorable electrostatic interactions for the 4-NH$_2$ analog due to reduced shielding and thermal effects. The less fluid hydrogen bond network for the 4-NH$_2$ analog would also result in a greater entropy loss upon binding estimated by MCPRO+. The results obtained with the MC and MD simulations in explicit solvent also explain why the MM-GB/SA relative score for H $\rightarrow$ 4-NH$_2$ pair underpredicts the binding energy of the latter; the continuum solvation model is unable to describe the water-mediated hydrogen bonds with the protein that contribute to the binding of the 4-NH$_2$ analog.

If the implications of MCPRO+ restricted sampling on enthalpic and entropic contributions to binding are extrapolated to MM-GB/SA, a reasonable hypothesis for the large dynamic range in MM-GB/SA is obtained. The scoring spread is not only affected by ignored entropic contributions, that is, all for the protein and the torsional entropy changes for the ligand, but also exaggerated enthalpic separation between the weak and potent compounds due to the lack of sampling. The resolution of whether this is caused by diminished shielding of electrostatic interactions, thermal effects, or protein relaxation/strain is complex, especially because it seems to be dependent on the case.

11.4.3 The Variable Dielectric Model

As mentioned above, one plausible cause for the exaggerated enthalpic gap is the application of an internal dielectric constant (ε_{in}) of 1 in a model where protein motions and polarization are not taken into account. Hence, electrostatic interactions are not shielded enough and protein–ligand electrostatic attractions and repulsions are overestimated, causing the large separation between potent and weak compounds (Guimarães 2011; Guimarães and Mathiowetz 2010). As previously described, when the protein permanent dipoles are included explicitly but their relaxation, that is, the protein reorganization, and the protein-induced dipoles are considered implicitly, the value of ε_{in} is not well defined (Schutz and Warshel 2001). Warshel and coworkers suggest that ε_{in} should be between 4 and 6 for dipole–charge interactions and 10 for charge–charge interactions (Muegge et al. 1996; Sham et al. 1998). More recently, a variable dielectric model has been developed to increase the accuracy in protein side chain and loop predictions (Zhu et al. 2007). The authors introduced an energy model where ε_{in} is allowed to vary as a function of the interacting residues.

Inspired by Zhu and coworkers (Zhu et al. 2007), we explored the use of a variable dielectric model based on residue types to alleviate the overestimation of electrostatic effects between protein residues and ligands for improved MM-GBSA scoring. Since poor description of protein–ligand electrostatic interactions could not only result in a wider scoring spread but also affect the correlation with experiment, we decided to use binding data to derive the set of variable dielectric constants. Specifically, the pharmaceutically relevant targets CDK2, FactorXa, p38 (p38_a), and PDE10A and respective congeneric series were considered in the optimization process that led to the set of variable dielectric constants, subsequently tested on two additional datasets, the hCAII and a second p38 chemical series (p38_b) (Ravindranathan et al. 2011).

The focus of that work was to obtain a set of dielectric constants based on residue types that improves MM-GB/SA scoring. A specific dielectric constant is assigned for the interactions between all atoms belonging to a residue type and the ligand atoms. The side chains for all polar (Ser, Thr, Asn, Gln) and ionizable residues (His, Lys, Arg, Asp, Glu), which are expected to be more polarizing, were considered individually in the optimization. All remaining residue side chains and backbone atoms were bundled in a group called "other." For simplicity, neutral and protonated states of the ionizable residues were not treated separately. The dielectric constant for a given residue–ligand pair was the same whether the residue interacts with a neutral or charged ligand.

Five different values (1, 2, 4, 8, and 20) were considered for every residue type (Ser, Thr, Asn, Gln, His, Lys, Arg, Asp, Glu, and other). The performance of all possible combinations of dilectric constants against the experimental data was judged based on correlation coefficients (R^2) and predictive indices (PI). The latter is a measure of how accurate the predicted rank order is compared to the experiment, with –1, 0, and +1 meaning opposite, random, or perfect predictions, respectively. Table 11.2 illustrates the combinations for each target that maximized R^2 and PI separately. Although the combinations listed on Table 11.2 are the very best for each system according to each metric, there were few other solutions that provided just slightly worse results. The set of optimal dielectrics constants for all targets simultaneously was derived by verifying the combination whose R^2 and PI values deviated the least from each individual's best (Table 11.2).

Arg and Glu have the largest values, 20 and 8, respectively, which seems reasonable since those residues, very flexible and polarizing, can be more easily shielded. The optimal value for Asp, with a shorter side chain and reduced flexibility when compared to Glu, is 2. Interestingly, a much smaller dielectric constant was obtained for Lys in contrast to the one for Arg. In a study of residue density in proteins (Baud and Karlin 1999), it became evident that in spite of evolutionary relatedness, Arg is more buried, more frequently involved in salt bridges, hydrogen bonds, and cationic-aromatic contacts. It is then plausible that a larger $\varepsilon_{in}(k)$ value than Lys emerges for Arg in the optimization process. In the case of the polar and the ionizable His residues, found to be in its neutral state in the majority of the cases here, the values are fairly small, ranging from 1 to 4. For three of the five residues, the dielectric constants seem to be correlated with the magnitude of the side chain dipole moments, with the value for His>Asn>Ser. As for Gln and Thr, the dielectric constants obtained seem to be counterintuitive when compared to their closest analogs, Asn and Ser, respectively. The optimal value for the more flexible side chain of the pair is actually smaller; this might be a function of the specific residue distributions for the targets in the training set. Finally, the $\varepsilon_{in}(k)$ value of 4 for the set that contains all remaining side chains might be somewhat high because it also contains all backbone atoms.

TABLE 11.2

Optimal Set of Residue-Based Dielectric Constants for the Targets Individually and Best Overall

Res Type	CDK2		FactorXa		PDE10A		p38_a		Optimal
Ser	20	1	1	1	20	1	20	20	1
Thr	20	2	20	2	1	2	1	1	4
Asn	1	1	20	1	20	8	1	4	2
Gln	1	1	1	20	4	2	1	1	1
His	20	1	20	20	20	1	1	20	4
Lys	2	2	20	1	20	20	1	1	2
Arg	1	1	1	1	2	1	20	20	20
Asp	1	8	20	20	2	20	20	20	2
Glu	20	20	1	1	1	1	20	20	8
Other	1	1	4	8	20	4	20	2	4
	$R^2 = 0.56$ PI = 0.76		$R^2 = 0.68$ PI = 0.90		$R = 0.53$ PI = 0.71		$R^2 = 0.58$ PI = 0.75		

TABLE 11.3

MM-GB/SA Results Using Standard and Variable Dielectric Protein–Ligand Electrostatics

Target	R^2 STD	R^2 VAR	PI STD	PI VAR	DR STD	DR VAR
CDK2	0.48	0.52	0.69	0.73	17.6	13.1
FactorXa	0.59	0.66	0.84	0.87	14.8	9.3
PDE10A	0.47	0.51	0.65	0.67	8.3	7.1
p38_a	0.33	0.55	0.46	0.71	20.9	21.9
hCAII	0.32	0.58	0.63	0.75	11.9	7.8
p38_b	0.41	0.43	0.68	0.70	10.5	10.5

Table 11.3 illustrates the R^2 and PI values obtained using the standard (STD) and variable (VAR) dielectric MM-GB/SA scoring procedures, the latter using the optimal dielectric values in Table 11.2. It is clear that the variable dielectric approach improves the description of protein–ligand electrostatics. It performs better than standard dielectrics in all cases, including the two systems in the test set, hCAII and p38_b. One should note that the variable dielectric approach will not necessarily provide significant improvements over the standard electrostatic treatment for all cases. This is illustrated in Table 11.3 for a couple of systems, PDE10A and p38_b. In those instances, the residues around the ligand are mostly nonpolar, and the electrostatic interactions between them are not appreciably large. Finally, Table 11.3 indicates that the variable dielectric approach reduces the score dynamic range (DR) in four of the six systems, although no attempt has been made to improve DR in the optimization process. This supports the view that the exaggerated protein–ligand electrostatic interaction due to the lack of shielding effects in the standard MM-GB/SA model is indeed a key factor in its wide scoring spread.

Acknowledgment

The author thanks Alan Mathiowetz and Mario Cardozo, who greatly contributed to the development of the MM-GB/SA protocol described in this work.

References

Abel, R., T. Young, R. Farid, B. J. Berne, R. A. Friesner. 2008. Role of the active-site solvent in the thermodynamics of factor Xa ligand binding. *J. Am. Chem. Soc.* 130(9): 2817–2831.

Alvarez, J. C. 2004. High-throughput docking as a source of novel drug leads. *Curr. Opin. Chem. Biol.* 8(1): 1–6.

Barril, X., J. L. Gelpí, J. M. López, M. Orozco, F. J. Luque. 2001. How accurate can molecular dynamics/linear response and Poisson–Boltzmann/solvent accessible surface calculations be for predicting relative binding affinities? Acetylcholinesterase huprine inhibitors as a test case. *Theor. Chem. Acc.* 106(1/2): 2–9.

Baud, F. and S. Karlin. 1999. Measures of residue density in protein structures. *Proc. Natl. Acad. Sci. USA* 96(22): 12494–12499.

Boyce, S. E., D. L. Mobley, G. J. Rocklin, A. P. Graves, K. A. Dill, B. K. Shoichet. 2009. Predicting ligand binding affinity with alchemical free energy methods in a polar model binding site. *J. Mol. Biol.* 394(4): 747–763.

Brown, S. P., S. W. Muchmore, P. J. Hajduk. 2009. Healthy skepticism: Assessing realistic model performance. *Drug Discov. Today* 14(7/8): 420–427.

Chang, C. A., W. Chen, M. K. Gilson. 2007. Ligand configurational entropy and protein binding. *Proc. Natl. Acad. Sci. USA* 104(5): 1534–1539.

Charifson, P. S., J. J. Corkey, M. A. Murcko, W. P. Walters. 1999. Consensus scoring: A method for obtaining improved hit rates from docking databases of three-dimensional structures into proteins. *J. Med. Chem.* 42(25): 5100–5109.

Deng, Y. and B. Roux. 2006. Calculation of standard binding free energies: Aromatic molecules in the T4 lysozyme L99A mutant. *J. Chem. Theory Comput.* 2(5): 1255–1273.

Desmond, version 2.2, Schrödinger, LLC, New York, NY, 2009.

Foloppe, N. and R. Hubbard. 2006. Towards predictive ligand design with free-energy based computational methods? *Curr. Med. Chem.* 13(29): 3583–3608.

Friesner, R. A., J. L. Banks, R. B. Murphy, T. A. Halgren, J. J. Klicic, D. T. Mainz, M. P. Repasky et al. 2004. Glide: A new approach for rapid, accurate docking and scoring. 1. Method and assessment of docking accuracy. *J. Med. Chem.* 47(7): 1739–1749.

Friesner, R. A., R. B. Murphy, M. P. Repasky, L. L. Frye, J. R. Greenwood, T. A. Halgren, P. C. Sanschagrin, D. T. Mainz. 2006. Extra precision Glide: Docking and scoring incorporating a model of hydrophobic enclosure for protein-ligand complexes. *J. Med. Chem.* 49(21): 6177–6196.

Gallicchio, E., M. M. Kubo, R. M. Levy. 2000. Enthalpy-entropy and cavity decomposition of alkane hydration free energies: Numerical results and implications for theories of hydrophobic solvation. *J. Phys. Chem. B* 104(26): 6271–6285.

Guimarães, C. R. W. 2011. A direct comparison of the MM-GB/SA scoring procedure and free-energy perturbation calculations using Carbonic Anhydrase as a test case: Strengths and pitfalls of each approach. *J. Chem. Theory Comput.* 7(7): 2296–2306.

Guimarães, C. R. W., D. L. Boger, W. L. Jorgensen. 2005. Elucidation of fatty acid amide hydrolase inhibition by potent α-ketoheterocycle derivatives from Monte Carlo simulations. *J. Am. Chem. Soc.* 127(49): 17377–17384.

Guimarães, C. R. W. and M. Cardozo. 2008. MM-GB/SA rescoring of docking poses in structure-based lead optimization. *J. Chem. Inf. Model.* 48(5): 958–970.

Guimarães, C. R. W. and A. M. Mathiowetz. 2010. Addressing limitations with the MM-GB/SA scoring procedure using the WaterMap method and free-energy perturbation calculations. *J. Chem. Inf. Model.* 50(4): 547–559.

Haider, M. K., H.-O. Bertrand, R. E. Hubbard. 2011. Predicting fragment binding poses using a combined MCSS MM-GBSA approach. *J. Chem. Inf. Model.* 51(5): 1092–1105.

Hou, T., J. Wang, Y. Li, W. Wang. 2011. Assessing the performance of the MM/PBSA and MM/GBSA methods. 1. The accuracy of binding free energy calculations based on molecular dynamics simulations. *J. Chem. Inf. Model.* 51(1): 69–82.

Huang, N., C. Kalyanaraman, K. Bernacki, M. P. Jacobson. 2006a. Molecular mechanics methods for predicting protein–ligand binding. *Phys. Chem. Chem. Phys.* 8(44): 5166–5177.

Huang, N., C. Kalyanaraman, J. J. Irwin, M. P. Jacobson. 2006b. Physics-based scoring of protein-ligand complexes: Enrichment of known inhibitors in large-scale virtual screening. *J. Chem. Inf. Model.* 46(1): 243–253.

Jones, G., P. Willet, R. C. Glen, A. R. Leach, R. Taylor. 1997. Development and validation of a genetic algorithm for flexible docking. *J. Mol. Biol.* 267(3): 727–748.

Jorgensen, W. L. 1989. Free energy calculations: A breakthrough for modeling organic chemistry in solution. *Acc. Chem. Res.* 22(5): 184–189.

Jorgensen, W. L. 1998. Free energy changes in solution. In: *Encyclopedia of Computational Chemistry.* Schleyer, P. v. R., (ed.), Wiley: New York, vol. 2, pp. 1061–1070.

Jorgensen, W. L., D. S. Maxwell, J. Tirado-Rives. 1996. Development and testing of OPLS all-atom force field on conformational energetics and properties of organic liquids. *J. Am. Chem. Soc.* 118(45): 11225–11235.

Jorgensen, W. L., J. P. Ulmschneider, J. Tirado-Rives. 2004. Free energies of hydration from a generalized Born model and an all-atom force Field. *J. Phys. Chem. B* 108(41): 16264–16270.

Kaminski, G. A., R. A. Friesner, J. Tirado-Rives, W. L. Jorgensen. 2001. Evaluation and reparametrization of the OPLS-AA force field for proteins via comparison with accurate quantum chemical calculations on peptides. *J. Phys. Chem. B* 105(28): 6474–6487.

Knime, 2008. version 1.2, Schrödinger, LLC, New York, NY.

Kollman, P. A. 1993. Free energy calculations: Applications to chemical and biochemical phenomena. *Chem. Rev.* 93(7): 2395–2417.

Kuhn, B., P. Gerber, T. Schulz-Gasch et al. 2005. Validation and use of the MM-PBSA approach for drug discovery. *J. Med. Chem.* 48(12): 4040–4048.

Kuhn, B. and P. A. Kollman. 2000. Binding of a diverse set of ligands to avidin and streptavidin: An accurate quantitative prediction of their relative affinities by a combination of molecular mechanics and continuum solvent models. *J. Med. Chem.* 43(20): 3786–3791.

Kuntz, I. D., J. M. Blaney, S. J. Oatley, R. Langridge, T. E. Ferrin. 1982. A geometric approach to macromolecule-ligand interactions. *J. Mol. Biol.* 161(2): 269–288.

Lee, M. R. and Y. Sun. 2007. Improving docking accuracy through molecular mechanics generalized Born optimization and scoring. *J. Chem. Theory Comput.* 3(3): 1106–1119.

Luccarelli, J., J. Michel, J. Tirado-Rives, W. L. Jorgensen. 2010. Effects of water placement on predictions of binding affinities for p38alpha MAP kinase. *J. Chem. Theory Comput.* 6(12): 3850–3856.

Lyne, P. D., M. L. Lamb, J. C. Saeh. 2006. Accurate prediction of the relative potencies of members of a series of kinase inhibitors using molecular docking and MM-GBSA scoring. *J. Med. Chem.* 49(16): 4805–4808.

MacroModel. 2005. version 9.0, Schrödinger, LLC, New York, NY.

MCPRO+. 2008. version 1.36, Schrödinger, LLC, New York, NY.

Michel, J. and J. W. Essex. 2008. Hit identification and binding mode predictions by rigorous free energy simulations. *J. Med. Chem.* 51(21): 6654–6664.

Michel, J., M. L. Verdonk, J. W. Essex. 2006. Protein-ligand binding affinity predictions by implicit solvent simulations: A tool for lead optimization? *J. Med. Chem.* 49(25): 7427–7439.

Mobley, D. L., A. P. Graves, J. D. Chodera, A. C. Reynolds, B. K. Shoichet, K. A. Dill. 2007. Predicting absolute ligand binding free energies to a simple model site. *J. Mol. Biol.* 371(4): 1118–1134.

Muegge, I. and Y. C. Martin. 1999. A general and fast scoring function for protein-ligand interactions: A simplified potential approach. *J. Med. Chem.* 42(5): 791–804.

Muegge, I., T. Schweins, R. Langen, A. Warshel. 1996. Electrostatic control of gtp and gdp binding in the oncoprotein p21 ras. *Structure* 4(4): 475–489.

Pearlman, D. A. and P. S. Charifson. 2001. Are free energy calculations useful in practice? A comparison with rapid scoring functions for the p38 MAP kinase protein system. *J. Med. Chem.* 44(21): 3417–3423.

Perola, E., W. P. Walters, P. S. Charifson. 2004. A detailed comparison of current docking and scoring methods on systems of pharmaceutical relevance. *Proteins* 56(2): 235–249.

Pitera, J. W. and W. F. van Gunsteren. 2001. The importance of solute-solvent van der Waals interactions with interior atoms of biopolymers. *J. Am. Chem. Soc.* 123(13): 3163–3164.

Powers, R. A., F. Morandi, B. K. Shoichet. 2002. Structure-based discovery of a novel, noncovalent inhibitor of AmpC beta-lactamase. *Structure* 10(7): 1013–1023.

Prabhu, N. V. and K. A. Sharp. 2005. Heat capacity in proteins. *Annu. Rev. Phys. Chem.* 56: 521–548.

Rarey, M., B. Kramer, T. Lengauer, G. Klebe. 1996. A fast flexible docking method using an incremental construction algorithm. *J. Mol. Biol.* 261(3): 470–489.

Ravindranathan, K., J. Tirado-Rives, W. L. Jorgensen, C. R. W. Guimarães. 2011. Improving MM-GB/SA Scoring through the application of the variable dielectric model. *J. Chem. Theory Comput.* 7(12): 3859–3865.

Roe, D. R., A. Okur, L. Wickstrom et al. 2007. Secondary structure bias in generalized Born solvent models: Comparison of conformational ensembles and free energy of solvent polarization from explicit and implicit solvation. *J. Phys. Chem. B* 111(7): 1846–1857.

Schapira, M., R. Abagyan, M. Totrov. 2003. Nuclear hormone receptor targeted virtual screening. *J. Med. Chem.* 46(14): 3045–3059.

Schutz, C. N. and A. Warshel. 2001. What are the dielectric "constants" of proteins and how to validate electrostatic models? *Proteins* 44(4): 400–417.

Scott, A. D., C. Phillips, A. Alex, M. Flocco, A. Bent, A. Randall, R. O'Brien, L. Damian, L. H. Jones. 2009. Thermodynamic optimisation in drug discovery: A case study using Carbonic Anhydrase inhibitors. *Chem. Med. Chem.* 4(12): 1985–1989.

Sham, Y. Y., I. Muegge, A. Warshel. 1998. The effect of protein relaxation on charge—Charge interactions and dielectric constants of proteins. *Biophys. J.* 74(4): 1744–1753.

Shoichet, B. K. 2004. Virtual screening of chemical libraries. *Nature* 432(7019): 862–865.

Shoichet, B. K., S. L. McGovern, B. Wei, J. J. Irwin. 2002. Lead discovery using molecular docking. *Curr. Opin. Chem. Biol.* 6(4): 439–446.

Simonson, T., A. Georgios, M. Karplus. 2002. Free energy simulations come of age: Protein-ligand recognition. *Acc. Chem. Res.* 35(6): 430–437.

Stahl, M. and M. Rarey. 2001. Detailed analysis of scoring functions for virtual screening. *J. Med. Chem.* 44(7): 1035–1042.

Still, W. C., A. Tempczyk, R. C. Hawley et al. 1990. Semianalytical treatment of solvation for molecular mechanics and dynamics. *J. Am. Chem. Soc.* 112(16): 6127–6129.

Taylor, R. D., P. J. Jewsbury, J. W. Essex. 2002. A review of protein-small molecule docking methods. *J. Comput.-Aided Mol. Des.* 16(3): 151–166.

Walters, W. P., M. T. Stahl, M. A. Murcko. 1998. Virtual screening—An overview. *Drug Discov. Today* 3(4): 160–178.

Warren, G. L., C. W. Andrews, A.-M. Capelli et al. 2006. A critical assessment of docking programs and scoring functions. *J. Med. Chem.* 49(20): 5912–5931.

Zhu, K., M. R. Shirts, R. A. Friesner. 2007. Improved methods for side chain and loop predictions via the protein local optimization program: Variable dielectric model for implicitly improving the treatment of polarization effects. *J. Chem. Theory Comput.* 3(6): 2108–2119.

12

Free Energy Calculations of Ligand–Protein Binding

Rainer Bomblies, Manuel Luitz, and Martin Zacharias

CONTENTS

12.1 Introduction

The binding free energy is the central quantity to evaluate a given ligand–receptor complex. Hence, accurate calculation or prediction of binding free energies is one of the most important tasks of computational drug discovery. The binding free energy is directly related to the work of bringing a ligand from an unbound state in solution to a bound state in complex with a receptor molecule. It is influenced by direct interactions between ligand and receptor but also by the interaction of both binding partners with the surrounding solvent. Furthermore, changes in average conformation and of conformational fluctuations of the binding partners also contribute to the binding free energy.

The *in silico* identification of possible ligands of a given receptor target molecule, often a protein but sometimes also other types of biomolecules such as nucleic acids, can be separated into two steps: An initial search step involves the identification of putative binders and possible binding sites on the surface of the receptor (Leis et al. 2010). This step typically employs docking programs that rapidly provide many putative complexes and rank these based on surface complementarity or empirical scoring functions (Brooijmans and Kuntz 2003; Kitchen et al. 2004). Since many thousand putative ligands and ligand placements need to be considered, the flexibility of binding partners, conformational entropy, or solvent contributions are neglected or only approximately considered (Leis and Zacharias 2012). Hence, the calculated docking score can usually only be considered as an approximate estimate of the interaction of ligand and receptor. Often in a second evaluation step, more sophisticated scoring schemes are applied to selected complexes. This can involve molecular dynamics (MD) simulations of complexes in explicit solvent and the generation of ensembles of ligand–receptor conformations (Carlson 2002).

Typically, during the evaluation of the ensemble an implicit solvent model such as the finite-difference Poisson–Boltzmann approach or the Generalized Born approach is employed to account for solvation effects (Roux and Simonson 1999; Wang and Wade 2003; Cavasotto 2012). The methodology is frequently referred to as MM/PBSA (molecular mechanics Poisson–Boltzmann surface area) approach and can result in an improved scoring compared to scoring based on single representative structure for each docked complex (Miller et al. 2012). Although sometimes misleadingly called free energy endpoint method, the MM/PBSA approach does not per se provide a free energy of binding but only a mean (ensemble-averaged) energy of binding.

In contrast to docking scoring or methods that evaluate ensembles of representative complex structures, there is a different class of approaches for rigorous calculation of free energy differences. It is based on a simulation process to create or annihilate the ligand (or part of it) or to dissociate the ligand from the binding site and to evaluate the associated work (=free energy). Free energy simulations employ MD or in some cases also Monte Carlo (MC) approaches as techniques to generate appropriate ensembles of states. Within the limitations of the underlying force field such free energy simulation techniques allow, in principle, the accurate calculation of free energy differences including both energetic as well as entropic contributions. It is the aim of the present review to provide an overview of available methods to extract free energy differences from simulation data and to discuss applications in the field of ligand–receptor interactions.

As will be further discussed, a perquisite of accurate free energy simulations is the appropriate sampling of relevant conformational states of a given system, which requires in many cases a series of extensive simulations. Hence, the computational demand of free energy simulations goes much beyond simple scoring of docked ligand–receptor complexes. Even with the steady improvement of computer performance, the systematic screening of large sets of docked complexes with such computationally demanding approaches is still out of reach for routine applications (Chodera et al. 2011). In practice, the application of free energy simulation techniques is largely restricted to absolute free energy calculation of small sets of ligand–receptor complexes or to the calculation of relative free energies associated with chemical modifications of a ligand molecule compared to a reference ligand with known binding affinity. It should also be emphasized that current free energy simulations are not truly predictive in the sense that such simulations make the experimental binding affinity determination obsolete (Fujitani et al. 2005; Shirts 2012). In part this can be due to insufficient sampling, which limits the convergence of calculated free energy differences. Recent methodological improvements and steadily increasing computer performance, however, have provided progress in this direction. The second important limitation is due to the accuracy of current molecular mechanics force fields used to describe molecular interactions. For proteins and nucleic acids fairly accurate force fields have been designed in the course of many years. For the many possible organic drug-like molecules that may bind to biomolecules, in contrast, significantly less experience and testing results are available (Wang et al. 2004; Vanommeslaeghe et al. 2010). However, even within these limitations numerous useful applications are possible, ranging from qualitative predictions on ligand binding, which can help in drug design efforts to offering explanations at the molecular level for the binding behavior of a ligand or its alteration due to chemical modification. In the first part of the review, free energy simulation techniques for alchemical transformations will be reviewed followed by discussion on alternative approaches of induced dissociation of the ligand–receptor complexes combined with the calculation of the associated free energy change. Recent methods to accelerate the simulation process and reduce computational costs will be introduced. Finally, recent methodological advancements, applications, and possible future developments will be discussed.

12.2 Extraction of Free Energies from Molecular Simulations

Over decades the determination of free energies in biomolecular systems has been a major focus of MD simulations. The thermodynamic concept of free energy gives an overall measure for the distribution of available states over a multidimensional energy landscape. A microscopic state in classical MD simulations is thereby given by the Cartesian coordinates for all atoms of the system as well as their momenta. Considering the representation of a biomolecular system in MD simulations, one typically refers to a biomolecule or biomolecular complex that is solvated in a finite-sized box of water molecules and surrounding ions. During the simulation the system is kept under constant volume V or pressure p and the temperature T can be controlled with a thermostat representing a thermal heat bath. Such a system corresponds to the canonical or in case of constant pressure to the isobaric ensemble. The Hamiltonian, or energy function, of the system consists of a kinetic energy term and a potential energy function. The potential energy function is represented by a force field description with energy contributions from bonded and nonbonded particle interactions. It usually does not depend on the momenta of the particles so kinetic and position-dependent (configurational) contributions can be separated. In the same way, it is also possible to separate kinetic and configurational contributions to the partition function Q and to the free energy F of the system. With $\beta = 1/k_bT$, k_b being the Boltzmann constant, Q and F can be written as

$$Q = \iint e^{-\beta H(r,p)} dr\, dp \tag{12.1}$$

$$F = -\frac{1}{\beta} \ln Q \tag{12.2}$$

In common applications for MD simulations on biomolecules, it is impossible to explore the phase space and to calculate the complete associated partition function in its entirety due to the high dimensionality of the system. Free energy calculations in practice aim to reduce the need to explore the complete phase space with the help of expressions of free energy differences between two systems A and B:

$$\Delta F = -\frac{1}{\beta} \ln \frac{Q_A}{Q_B} \tag{12.3}$$

The systems A and B can, for example, refer to the receptor with a bound ligand and without a ligand or may correspond to two different conformational regimes of a protein molecule. To determine the difference in free energy between systems A and B, it is only necessary to sample those regions in phase space which differ among the systems. In the following paragraph, the systems A and B differ chemically and are represented by different force field descriptions.

12.2.1 Deriving Free Energy Changes from Simulations in Alchemical Transformations

Various methods have been suggested to estimate the free energy difference between two systems or distinct system states A and B from MD or MC simulations. In case of free energy simulations on ligand binding, one is interested in the absolute binding free energy of a ligand or in the relative binding affinity of two ligands that differ, for example, in a chemical group. Hence, the states A and B can correspond to a state with ligand absent (A) or present (B) in the receptor binding pocket or in case of considering relative free energy differences the states A or B represent absence or presence of a chemical group in the ligand, respectively. The presence or absence of the ligand or chemical modification can be represented by a difference in the force field description of each system. According to the thermodynamic cycle shown in Figure 12.1 for calculating the contribution to the binding free energy, it is necessary to not only calculate the free energy change with the ligand bound to the receptor but also in the unbound state of the ligand (in the bulk solvent).

Zwanzig introduced the free energy perturbation (FEP) formula as an ensemble average over the Boltzmann factor for the energy difference between the two states calculated in the ensemble of A (Zwanzig 1954). Hence, it is possible to calculate the free energy change due to a change of the system (a perturbation B, for example, change in the force field such as an annihilation or addition of a force field term representing a chemical group of the ligand) from the ensemble average of system A (the unperturbed system):

$$\Delta F_{AB} = -\frac{1}{\beta}\ln\left\langle e^{-\beta \Delta V_{BA}} \right\rangle_A \tag{12.4}$$

The one-sided perturbation is, however, biased by the exclusive sampling of states in only ensemble A. In order to eliminate this bias, information of both ensembles can be combined with a two-sided perturbation approach

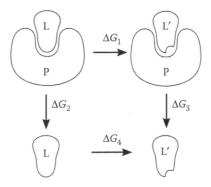

FIGURE 12.1
The thermodynamic cycle for calculating the binding free energy change upon ligand modification. The indicated free energy pathways can be calculated from simulations with different approaches. The horizontal pathways (ΔG_1, ΔG_4) involve a change in the system topology as ligand L morphs into L′ and are accessible from (alchemical) free energy calculations. Vertical pathways (ΔG_2, ΔG_3) involve a change in the association state indicating the binding event of L and L′, respectively, and can be derived from US calculations. Typically, one is interested in the difference free energy of association, which can be obtained from $\Delta\Delta G = \Delta G_1 - \Delta G_4 = \Delta G_2 - \Delta G_3$.

where data from both systems are included. The drawback of this approach is the need to generate trajectories for both ensembles A and B, which in general doubles the computational cost. With the two simulations, the free energy can then be calculated as

$$\Delta F_{AB} = -\frac{1}{\beta} \ln \frac{\left\langle e^{-\beta V_B} \right\rangle_A}{\left\langle e^{-\beta V_A} \right\rangle_B} \tag{12.5}$$

In order to decrease the statistical error of the one- and two-sided FEP methods, Charles H. Bennett came up with a formulation of the free energy difference between two systems as the acceptance ratio of switching the Hamiltonian function from A to B (Bennett 1976). In contrast to Metropolis who formulated a criterion to describe the acceptance of a set of phase space coordinates in MC simulations, Bennett asked for an acceptance criterion which provides minimal error for the calculated free energy difference. For this he expanded the fraction of partition functions, which forms the core of difference free energy estimates,

$$\frac{Q_A}{Q_B} = \frac{\left\langle W(q) \exp[-\beta V_A] \right\rangle_B}{\left\langle W(q) \exp[-\beta V_B] \right\rangle_A} \tag{12.6}$$

where W can be an arbitrary weighting function. Applying Lagrange multipliers, he found that the weighting function that provides the smallest errors for a given set of sampling points for both systems is the Fermi Dirac distribution function $f(x) = 1/(1 + \exp(\beta x))$. With a simple efficiency argument, he further showed that the choice for the number of probes in A and B should be equal in case that the computational effort for the creation of one sample equals in both systems. The Bennett acceptance ration (BAR) for the free energy is thus

$$\Delta F_{AB} = \frac{1}{\beta} \ln \frac{\left\langle f(V_A - V_B + C) \right\rangle_A}{\left\langle f(V_B - V_A - C) \right\rangle_B} + C \tag{12.7}$$

The constant C has to be determined in a postprocessing step after the simulation with the additional condition

$$\sum_A f(V_A - V_B + C) = \sum_B f(V_B - V_A - C) \tag{12.8}$$

By the time of its invention, the postprocessing minimization of C was seen as a drawback of the BAR method but has become a negligible effort in recent free energy calculation protocols (De Ruiter et al. 2013).

In the limit of exhaustive sampling, the perturbation method gives the exact free energy change associated with the perturbation. However, the efficiency or convergence of calculated free energies depends on how well the sampled states for the unperturbed system represent relevant states (those with high Boltzmann probability) of the perturbed system. In order to solve this problem in practical applications, one often splits the process into a series of N small perturbations and controls the switch from A to B with a coupling coordinate λ. At $\lambda = 0$ the system is represented by a Hamiltonian H_A representing state A and at $\lambda = 1$ by Hamiltonian H_B representing state B. At each stage, the free energy change associated with a perturbation step is calculated using the force field change up to a given stage as reference. In this way, the total free energy change of going from state A to B is given by the sum over all perturbation steps:

$$\Delta F_{AB} = \sum_{i=0}^{N-1} \Delta F_{\lambda_i, \lambda_{i+1}} \qquad (12.9)$$

The $\Delta F_{\lambda_i, \lambda_{i+1}}$ represents the free energy changes associated with the transition from intermediate state λ_i to λ_{i+1}. The parameter λ can be coupled in various ways to the change in the Hamiltonian as discussed in the next section. Whenever a smooth transition coordinate λ for transforming the Hamiltonian from system A to B is defined, the thermodynamic integration (TI) (Kirkwood 1935; Barker and Henderson 1976; Beveridge and DiCapua 1989) method is applicable, which is probably the most common method to extract free energy differences from simulations. It requires the derivative of the Hamiltonian with respect to a control parameter λ associated with the transition for a force field representing state A and state B. The ensemble average of the derivative of the Hamiltonian versus the control parameter λ corresponds to the derivative of the free energy versus λ. Often, the analytic λ derivative of the force field can be calculated. By integration of the ensemble average, one can calculate the total free energy change for the transition from A to B:

$$\Delta F_{AB} = \int_0^1 \left\langle \frac{\partial H(\lambda)}{\partial \lambda} \right\rangle_\lambda d\lambda \qquad (12.10)$$

The numerical integration can be performed with different methods, for example, trapezoidal, Simpson, or Clenshaw–Curtis integration (De Ruiter et al. 2013) for which the continuous coupling coordinate λ needs to be discretized and the system to be sampled at each of the intermediate Hamiltonians as it is done for FEP in Equation 12.9. Several variants of the TI scheme are available. For example, in the slow growth method the coupling parameter increases with time during a single trajectory, starting from system A and transforming to system B. If the increment of λ is performed too fast, the system may not be in equilibrium and bias from previous λ steps is observed. This is a general problem of the slow growth method and results in a hysteresis when performing the switching in both directions $\lambda(0 \to 1)$ and $\lambda(1 \to 0)$. However, as the free energy is a thermodynamic state function, its absolute value should be independent of the direction of the pathway.

In standard TI simulations, one tries to equilibrate the simulation system at each discrete λ in order to calculate an ensemble average for the equilibrated system. The influence of different numerical integration methods on the efficiency and accuracy of TI, that is, Simpson, trapezoidal, and Clenshaw–Curtis in comparison with the BAR method, has recently been investigated by Oostenbrink et al. for the serine protease trypsin with four benzamidine-like inhibitors (De Ruiter et al. 2013). BAR was found to better handle fewer intermediate steps compared to TI wherein Simpson was found superior to trapezoidal integration. The benefit of nonequidistant spaced intermediate steps as required by the Clenshaw–Curtis integration method depends strongly on the functional form of the integrand $dH/d\lambda$. Overall BAR should be preferred over TI calculations because of its efficiency and robustness with respect to the choice of intermediate steps between A and B (Bruckner and Boresch 2011; De Ruiter et al. 2013).

A different class of free energy calculation methods is based on the non-equilibrium work theorem by Jarzynski (1997). In this approach, transitions from A to B can be performed rapidly without requiring any equilibration of the system. The associated free energy can be obtained from the average Boltzmann weight of the nonequilibrium work for switching on the transformation. It has also been shown that nonequilibrium approaches to calculate free energy differences are not necessarily more efficient than equilibrium methods (Oberhofer et al. 2005; Oostenbrink and van Gunsteren 2006). A number of variants of the basic methodology have been developed in recent years but the method is still less popular compared to standard TI calculations or alternative equilibrium free energy simulation methods (Wu and Kofke 2005).

12.2.2 Defining a Pathway between System States in Alchemical Transformations

Since free energy is a state function, the pathway from thermodynamic state A to B is arbitrary. However, in practice the pathway of transforming the Hamiltonian representing state A to B can have significant influence on the convergence and accuracy of calculated free energy differences. As indicated above, the most simple method is the linear coupling of the change in Hamiltonian with the control parameter λ:

$$H(\lambda) = (1-\lambda)H_A + \lambda H_B \qquad (12.11)$$

In many cases, the free energy change is not uniform along the reaction coordinate λ and it is useful to apply a nonlinear coupling:

$$H(\lambda) = (1-\lambda)^n H_A(\lambda) + \lambda^n H_B(\lambda) \tag{12.12}$$

with free choice of the exponent parameter n. The nonlinear scaling is advantageous for scaling potentials with a steep distance dependence such as a repulsive Lennard–Jones contribution. To increase the phase space overlap of states A and B, the transition Hamiltonian is typically sampled at intermediate steps of λ. An estimate of the free energy difference of neighboring λ simulations can be derived from either FEP or TI. Sufficient simulation time has to elapse among the samples of the derivative Hamiltonian $dH/d\lambda$ for TI or the difference Hamiltonian to neighboring windows ΔH to provide unbiased samples.

Especially at the endpoints of free energy simulations, when potential functions for atoms are created or annihilated, the form of the radial non-bonded interactions results in a singularity of the interaction at close distance between particles. To avoid the associated large forces and large derivatives of the free energy versus λ, the separation-shifted-scaling (Beutler et al. 1994; Zacharias et al. 1994) or soft-core scaling method has become a standard approach. The soft-core interaction function replaces the distance of particles with an effective radius r_A and r_B to remove the singularity in the Lennard Jones and Coulomb interactions for λ values close to 1 or 0, so the soft-core Hamiltonian reads as

$$H_{\text{soft-core}}(r) = (1-\lambda)H_A(r_A) + \lambda H_B(r_B)$$
$$r_A = (\alpha\sigma_A^6 \lambda^p + r^6)^{1/6} \tag{12.13}$$
$$r_B = (\alpha\sigma_B^6 (1-\lambda)^p + r^6)^{1/6}$$

The soft-core power p, the interaction radius σ, and the scaling factor α are parameters to adjust the smoothness of the transition pathway. Recently, alternative formulations for the soft-core scaling scheme have been proposed that alleviate spurious additional minima due to the original formulation (Gapsys et al. 2012) or produce a low energy transition pathway (Pham and Shirts 2011).

In case of relative free energy calculations of transforming one chemical group into another, one can distinguish two types of pathways. In the single topology method, atom types representing one chemical group (e.g., thermodynamic state A) are transformed into other types that represent state B. Note that for this pathway it may also be necessary to smoothly transform the bonded geometric description of one group into the bonded topology of the target group. In case of a surplus of atoms in one group, it is possible to transform atoms to noninteracting dummies (these dummies still have kinetic energy but all nonbonded interactions are switched off). In contrast,

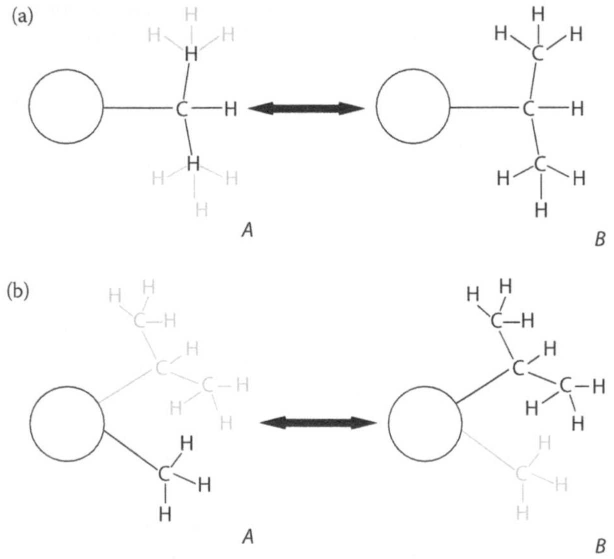

FIGURE 12.2
Alchemical transformation of alanine to valine with the single (a) and dual (b) topology approach. With a single topology, the atoms extending alanine to valine are gradually turned on. For the dual topology, the side chains of valine and alanine are linked to the backbone concurrently. In state *A* the valine side chain exists as a noninteracting dummy, and interactions with the rest of the system are turned on while switching the system to state *B*. Interactions between both side chains are excluded.

in the dual topology method all atoms representing one group are transformed to dummy atoms and simultaneously atoms of the target group are created (starting from noninteracting dummies, see Figure 12.2b). Due to the unphysical transition pathway between *A* and *B*, this method is often termed alchemical free energy calculation.

12.2.3 Free Energies of Binding from Umbrella Sampling along a Ligand–Receptor Dissociation Pathway

Besides alchemical transformations to calculate the relative binding free energy of a ligand bound to a receptor molecule, it is also possible to obtain absolute binding free energies from a simulation of the association or dissociation process itself. From the perspective of the thermodynamic cycle, we follow then in principle the natural pathway of studying biomolecular interactions that is the spatial separation of both binding partners, corresponding as the vertical pathways in Figure 12.1.

Instead of a reaction coordinate λ that annihilates or creates the interaction between ligand and receptor, a spatial reaction coordinate is chosen to dissociate the ligand–receptor complex. The integration of the generalized mean force along such reaction coordinate yields the potential of mean force (PMF) or work of dissociation. Together with the free energy of release of the ligand into the bulk, it allows the calculation of absolute binding free energies. Historically, the PMF was defined as the reversible work supplied to bring two solvated particles from infinite separation to a contact distance (Chandler 1987):

$$w(r) = -\frac{1}{\beta} \ln(g(r)) \tag{12.14}$$

with $g(r)$ being the pair correlation function of the two particles. The term PMF has since been used for numerous different reaction coordinates, many of which are more intricate than distances. A more general definition (Hénin and Chipot 2004) of the PMF as used today is the free energy of a state defined by a particular reaction coordinate:

$$W(\xi) = -\frac{1}{\beta} \ln P_\xi + W_0 \tag{12.15}$$

where W_0 is a constant and P_ξ is the probability of the system to be in state ξ. The free energy difference in direction ξ can be expressed as the difference of PMF values:

$$\Delta W(\xi_1 \rightarrow \xi_2) = W(\xi_2) - W(\xi_1) \tag{12.16}$$

From an MD or MC simulation of a system the free energy difference for a ligand binding to a binding site from the bulk can be calculated as a fraction of Boltzmann weighted states, that is, probabilities of states:

$$\Delta G_{bind} = -\frac{1}{\beta} \ln \int_{site} dr e^{-\beta H(r)} - \frac{1}{\beta} \ln \int_{bulk} dr e^{-\beta H(r)} \tag{12.17}$$

$$\Delta G_{bind} = \frac{1}{\beta} \ln \frac{\int_{site} dr e^{-\beta H(r)}}{\int_{bulk} dr e^{-\beta H(r)}} \tag{12.18}$$

If the ligand is moved solely along the reaction coordinate and the impact of the surroundings along orthogonal coordinates is averaged out, then the free energy of the system, and consequently the probability of states, can be expressed using the PMF:

$$\Delta G_{bind} = \frac{1}{\beta} \ln \left(\frac{\int_{site} d\xi e^{-\beta W(\xi)}}{\int_{bulk} d\xi e^{-\beta W(\xi)}} \right) \tag{12.19}$$

The PMF can be calculated (den Otter and Briels 1998; Darve and Pohorille 2001; Hénin and Chipot 2004) as the potential generating the average force acting in the direction ξ. Forces have to be calculated every step in MD simulations and, are thus readily accessible and can be projected onto the direction of ξ. Commonly, the instantaneous forces F_ξ are collected in small bins and the PMF can be obtained through numerical integration. This approach is equivalent to TI discussed above for the case of alchemical transformation.

Instead of integration of an average force, the PMF can also be obtained directly (Roux 1995; Doudou et al. 2009) from the probability distribution of states along the coordinate ξ:

$$W(\xi^*) = -\frac{1}{\beta}\ln(P_{\xi^*}) + W_0 = W_0 - \frac{1}{\beta}\ln\left(\frac{\int dr\, \delta\left(\xi(r) - \xi^*\right) e^{-\beta U(r)}}{\int dr\, e^{-\beta U(r)}}\right) \quad (12.20)$$

Unfortunately, for most systems it is impossible to sample the full conformational space by a single MD simulation on a feasible timescale. Transitions from the bound to the unbound state, if separated by a large energy barrier, will rarely ever occur. If the starting point is chosen in the bound state, the ligand will not leave the binding site in most simulations and yield no information on the PMF outside of the binding pocket. So, simulating all regions of the reaction coordinate for roughly the same time is desirable. To improve sampling along the reaction coordinate, the Umbrella Sampling (US) method (Torrie and Valleau 1974; Patey and Valleau 1975) simulates the system with a biased potential. Multiple simulations are run with different potentials u_i. Commonly, these potentials are "umbrella-shaped" simple harmonic potentials $u_i = k(\xi - \xi_i)^2$. Every simulation will restrain the ligand to a small area around the umbrella minimum and will only yield reliable information in that area. Combining these windows then gives a full and effective sampling of the entire association or dissociation pathway along the reaction coordinate. Subtraction of the contribution due to the penalty potential allows the extraction of a free energy within each umbrella window except for a free energy offset between each window. The standard technique to obtain the full free energy change along the coordinate ξ is the iterative weighted histogram analysis method (WHAM) (Kumar et al. 1992). Recently, alternative methods have been developed either based on calculating the derivative of the PMF versus coordinate ξ in each window (Kästner and Thiel 2006) or by fitting the sampled data to a free energy curve as a spline function representation (Lee et al. 2013).

12.2.4 Restraining Ligand Orientation and Conformation to Improve Umbrella Sampling

In general, because the conformational space orthogonal to the sampling path ξ is large, convergence of free energies calculated with US is slow.

A solution suggested by Woo and Roux (2005) substantially shrinks this space by restraining the ligand to a defined conformation (c), orientation (r), and axis (a) leading from the binding site to the bulk. The conformation is approximately kept fixed by a harmonic potential for the RMSD of the ligand. For orientation and position restraints, a coordinate system is introduced based on three centers in the protein and ligand each. The PMF calculation is then performed in umbrella windows pulling the constrained ligand from the bound position into the bulk along the axis. Due to the restraints, it is not necessary for each point along the PMF sampling path to sample all possible conformations and orientations of the ligand, which accelerates the PMF convergence. The contributions from the added restraining potentials need to be evaluated at the endpoints of the PMF calculation, that is, the ligand being at the binding site and in the bulk. The total free energy of binding is then given by (see Figure 12.3)

$$\Delta G_{bind} = -\Delta G_c^{site} - \Delta G_r^{site} - \Delta G_a^{site} + \Delta G_{PMF} + \Delta G_a^{bulk} + \Delta G_r^{bulk} + \Delta G_c^{bulk} \qquad (12.21)$$

The release of the orientational and axial restraining in the bulk can be calculated analytically, whereas other contributions need to be evaluated by numerical FEP free energy simulations. Details on how to best calculate the contributions are given in Woo and Roux (2005) and Deng and Roux (2009).

The calculation of absolute free energies of binding using the PMF method along a spatial dissociation pathway does not require the annihilation of the ligand in the binding site and in the bulk solvent. The latter two calculations are necessary when choosing the alchemical transformation pathway for absolute binding free energy calculations (see previous paragraph) and depending on the size and properties may result in fairly large calculated free energies. The binding free energy is then obtained as a difference between these two large numbers, which may cause significant errors in the calculated free energy. On the down side the PMF approach requires a sterically possible pathway for dissociation. Otherwise large free energy barriers may also cause errors in the calculated PMFs. Nevertheless, the PMF approach and several methodological variants have been increasingly applied in recent years (Jiang and Roux 2010; Gumbart et al. 2012; Jiang et al. 2012; Huang and Garcia 2013; Velez-Vega and Gilson 2013; Zeller and Zacharias 2014).

12.2.5 Force Field Representation and Setup of Free Energy Simulations

In principle, if appropriately performed the methods discussed in the previous paragraph allow accurate extraction of free energy differences from molecular simulations. However, as indicated in the introduction, there are several obstacles that limit the applicability and accuracy of free energy simulations. The underlying force field description is one major limitation. For proteins and nucleic acids fairly accurate force fields are available and are evaluated and improved continuously by a large community of users.

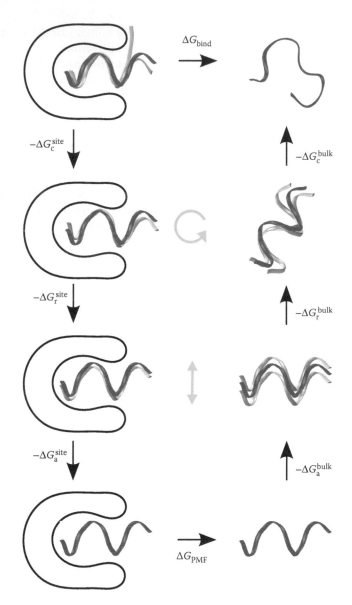

FIGURE 12.3
Contributions for calculating the free energy using a PMF approach and restraining conformation (c), rotation (r) and position relative to an axis (a). The left side shows the ligand in the binding pocket, on the right side the ligand is far enough in the bulk that interactions with the protein are negligible. Contributions to the free energy of binding are illustrated only for the ligand. Note that similar additional contributions also need to be evaluated for the unbound protein.

The availability of force field parameters for organic drug-like molecules, however, is much more limited. In recent years, several approaches for an automatic design and setup of force field parameters for organic molecules have been developed (Wang et al. 2004; Vanommeslaeghe et al. 2010). The availability of such approaches is a prerequisite for a greater applicability of free energy simulations to evaluate ligand binding and the effect of ligand modification on binding properties. Although most of the common software packages for performing molecular mechanics and MD simulations of bio-molecules such as Amber (Case et al. 2012), Charmm (Brooks et al. 2009), Gromacs (Pronk et al. 2013), or NAMD (Phillips et al. 2005) include the necessary code for free energy calculation, the initiation and setup can be quite complicated, which may also prevent users from applying free energy simulations (Chodera et al. 2011). Several efforts to simplify the setup of free energy simulations have been made (Jo et al. 2013; Christ and Fox 2014).

12.2.6 Improving the Sampling in Free Energy Simulations

One prerequisite for the accurate calculation of free energy differences is the appropriate sampling of relevant conformational states at each step of the control parameter λ. Advanced sampling methods can be employed to improve the search for relevant conformations at each step along the reaction coordinate. One of the most common techniques to improve sampling is the replica exchange or parallel tempering method (T-REMD). In the standard setup, several parallel simulations are running at slightly different temperatures and frequent exchanges of conformations between simulations at neighboring temperatures are attempted according to a Metropolis criterion, reviewed for example by Ostermeir and Zacharias (2013). The simulations at higher temperatures can help to overcome energy barriers and through exchanges can also help to improve the sampling at lower temperature replicas. Usually, the lowest temperature reference replica corresponds to the target temperature of interest. Depending on the system size the T-REMD technique can require a significant number of temperature replicas (typically between 8 and 128 replicas). Since the free energy simulation itself consists of several steps along the reaction coordinate, the computational cost is quite significant for such an approach (Ostermeir and Zacharias 2013). However, since all simulations run independently, it is possible to use many parallel simulations on a cluster with little interprocess communication.

The control parameter itself can restrict the sampling of relevant states. For example, in case of US a penalty potential is applied to limit the sampling to a certain interval along the reaction coordinate (equivalent to the λ in case of alchemical transformations). The penalty potential itself may create barriers in the system that prevent easy transitions between regimes relevant for a given interval along the reaction coordinate. Similarly, in alchemical transformations the sampling at a given λ might be trapped in a certain conformational regime, which differs from the regimes sampled in neighboring λ steps. One method to improve the sampling along a reaction coordinate (or λ in case of alchemical transformations) is the Hamiltonian replica exchange method (H-REMD) (Woods et al. 2003). At frequent intervals conformations in neighboring windows of the reaction coordinate are swapped and exchanges are accepted or rejected according to a Metropolis criterion,

$$\min\left(1, \exp\left\{ -\frac{1}{k_B T}\left(H_{\lambda_n}(j) - H_{\lambda_n}(i) - H_{\lambda_{n+1}}(j) + H_{\lambda_{n+1}}(i)\right)\right\}\right)$$

The difference in Hamiltonian is given by either the λ-dependent force field term, in case of alchemical transformations, or by the penalty potential associated with the reaction coordinate in case of US simulations. Exchanges of conformational states between US intervals or λ steps can improve sampling at each step and consequently result in better convergence of the calculated free energy change. The H-REMD methodology comes at no additional computational costs and can improve the convergence of free energy simulations considerably (Kokubo et al. 2011; Luitz and Zacharias 2013). It has been used both in PMF-based free energy simulations to dissociate a ligand from a receptor (Jiang and Roux 2010; Zeller and Zacharias 2014) and also in alchemical free energy simulations (Woods et al. 2003; Luitz and Zacharias 2013), and becomes more and more a standard approach in free energy simulations. A combination of H-REMD and T-REMD protocols along the one-dimensional (1D) λ coordinate has been proposed by Wang et al. (2012), where the temperature in the transition λ values was gradually increased compared to the endpoints in order to improve the transition of global configurations.

It is also possible to use λ itself in a free energy simulation as an additional dynamical variable associated with a mass and kinetic energy (Guo et al. 2003; Mongan and Case 2005; Knight and Brooks 2009). In the λ-dynamics approach, the reaction coordinate λ is not constant but can vary in between boundaries (usually 0 and 1 for λ) during a single MD simulation (Knight and Brooks 2009). The free energy change along the coordinate can be obtained by integrating the generalized force along the coordinate during the simulation (similar to TI). It is, however, necessary to guarantee sufficient sampling of all relevant λ-values. This may involve appropriate biasing potentials or special sampling techniques (Knight and Brooks 2009). The approach has been applied successfully in a number of examples (Guo et al. 2003; Mongan and Case 2005).

In the meta-dynamics methodology (Laio and Parrinello 2002; Barducci et al. 2008, 2011; Limongelli et al. 2012), small Gaussian functions are continuously added along the reaction coordinate to destabilize the currently sampled states. Eventually, this results in a flat free energy surface along the reaction coordinate and the sum of the Gaussian functions represents the free energy curve along the reaction coordinate (with opposite sign). The convergence to a well-defined free energy surface depends on rapid final diffusion along the reaction coordinate. In order to improve convergence it has been coupled with other advanced sampling techniques such as T-REMD (Jiang and Roux 2010). The technique has been used in many applications with spatial reaction coordinates representing association and dissociation pathways for ligand–receptor complexes or different conformational states but not in alchemical transformations. Other approaches to improve the sampling of relevant states are based on the inspection of the calculated free energy with respect to the reaction coordinate. A biasing force can be calculated to offset the free energy change (or derivative) along the reaction coordinate. The adaptive biasing force (ABF) reduces the overall free energy gradients along the reaction coordinate resulting in a smoother free energy surface and in more rapid convergence (Darve and Pohorille 2001; Hénin and Chipot 2004; Babin et al. 2008). In combination with the restraint PMF-methodology described above, the technique has been used to calculate free energies of protein–ligand (Woo and Roux 2005; Gumbart et al. 2012) and protein–protein binding (Gumbart et al. 2013) along a putative dissociation pathway in good agreement with experiment. With a related technique employing an adaptive biasing potential and H-REMD along the reaction coordinate, it has been possible to accurately calculate the binding free energy of a DNA-ligand system resulting in quantitative agreement of free energies from dissociation and association processes and excellent agreement with experimental affinities (Zeller and Zacharias 2014).

12.2.7 One-Step Perturbation for Free Energy Difference Calculation

As indicated above a typical free energy simulation to obtain binding free energy differences due to ligand modifications involves a stepwise transformation with several simulations of intermediate states. It is desirable to reduce the number of intermediate steps in order to reduce the computational demand. Ideally, a transformation should involve only one step. For a one-step transformation (based on one reference state), it would be possible to evaluate several possible modifications simultaneously. Employing the FEP formalism just one simulation of the unperturbed reference state is in principle sufficient to evaluate any modification if the system perturbation is "small" enough to guarantee sufficient overlap with the sampling of states in the reference simulation. The reference state does not need to be an unmodified ligand but can also be an unphysical reference state. The main challenge is here to identify a best possible reference state. Starting in 1996, the van Gunsteren and Oostenbrink groups have put considerable effort into designing efficient schemes for single-step perturbation-free energy calculations of ligand–receptor systems (Liu et al. 1996; Oostenbrink and van Gunsteren 2005; Hritz et al. 2010). Typically, soft core centers attached to the unmodified centers are used as reference states since they allow for some overlap of the region that is, for example, accessible in the unmodified ligand and potentially completely inaccessible in the modified ligand with an added chemical group. Depending on the choice of the reference state and on the type of modification, quite accurate estimates of the free energy associated with a chemical modification of a ligand can be achieved (Oostenbrink 2012). The great advantage is that it is possible to estimate the effect of various possible modifications (e.g., different chemical groups in the ligand), simultaneously. Each modification represents a perturbation of the chosen reference state. In order to correct for the drawback of a single-sided FEP approach to include only information of one system, a method has been devised to combine information of both systems A and B for the free energy difference estimate (Oostenbrink 2012).

Statistical averages are taken for the exponential energy of system B sampled under the Hamiltonian of A and vice versa. The two-sided approach, however, doubles the computational demand because trajectories for both systems have to be generated.

12.3 Conclusions

The accurate calculation of binding free energies is one of the central goals of molecular simulation approaches. Several methods are available to accurately and efficiently extract free energy changes from molecular simulations. The reliable calculation of free energies requires extensive sampling of relevant states and limits the applicability for systematic studies or evaluation of a larger number of ligands or ligand modifications. However, the steady increase in available computer resources and improved sampling techniques will likely reduce this bottleneck in the foreseeable future. The preparation, setup, and analysis of free energy simulations is also more demanding than just performing a rescoring of docking solutions with another scoring function. The most common molecular mechanics simulation packages include the possibility of performing free energy simulations. It is hoped that standardized protocols and setups of free energy simulations will be developed and included in common packages so that a broader range of users may utilize these approaches (Jo et al. 2013; Christ and Fox 2014). A possible route for utilizing free energy calculations in drug design could be the combination of scoring a large set of putative ligands or ligand modifications in complex with a receptor target to preselect promising candidates. High scoring compounds can then be evaluated using more costly free energy simulation methods. Probably the most difficult bottleneck for transforming free energy simulations into a truly predictive simulation methodology is the availability of accurate force field descriptions for the binding partners. It is possible that current force field models are in general not accurate enough for principle reasons because important physical effects are not covered. For example, in current force fields electronic polarizability of the electron clouds is not explicitly included. However, several new force fields have been developed in recent years to include electronic polarizability at least approximately (Banks et al. 1999; Halgren and Damm 2001; Kaminski et al. 2002; Ren and Ponder 2002). It remains to be seen whether such improvements also result in more accurate calculated free energies of ligand–receptor binding. Finally, it should be emphasized that force field improvement and the sampling problem of relevant states are closely coupled. A force field modification can only be evaluated if the sampling algorithm covers all relevant states for the system. Hence, improvements in either of these areas will be beneficial for the realistic prediction of ligand–receptor affinities based on free energy simulations.

Acknowledgment

The authors gratefully acknowledge the financial support by grant SFB1035/B02 of Deutsche Forschungsgemeinschaft.

References

Babin, V., C. Roland, and C. Sagui. 2008. Adaptively biased molecular dynamics for free energy calculations. *J. Chem. Phys.* 128(13): 134101.

Banks, J. L., G. A. Kaminski, R. Zhou, D. T. Mainz, B. J. Berne, and R. A. Friesner. 1999. Parametrizing a polarizable force field from ab initio data. I. The fluctuating point charge model. *J. Chem. Phys.* 110(2): 741–754.

Barducci, A., M. Bonomi, and M. Parrinello. 2011. Metadynamics. *Wiley Interdiscip. Rev. Comput. Mol. Sci.* 1(5): 826–843.

Barducci, A., G. Bussi, and M. Parrinello. 2008. Well-tempered metadynamics: A smoothly converging and tunable free-energy method. *Phys. Rev. Lett.* 100(2): 020603.

Barker, J. A. and D. Henderson. 1976. What is "liquid?" Understanding the states of matter. *Rev. Mod. Phys.* 48(4): 587–671.

Bennett, C. H. 1976. Efficient estimation of free energy differences from Monte Carlo data. *J. Comput. Phys.* 22: 245–268.

Beutler, T. C., A. E. Mark, R. C. van Schaik, P. R. Gerber, and W. F. van Gunsteren. 1994. Avoiding singularities and numerical instabilities in free energy calculations based on molecular simulations. *Chem. Phys. Lett.* 222: 529–539.

Beveridge, D. L. and F. M. DiCapua. 1989. Free energy via molecular simulation: Applications to chemical and biomolecular systems. *Annu. Rev. Biophys. Biophys. Chem.* 18(1): 431–492.

Brooijmans, N. and I. D. Kuntz. 2003. Molecular recognition and docking algorithms. *Annu. Rev. Biophys. Biomol. Struct.* 32(1): 335–373.

Brooks, B. R., C. L. Brooks, A. D. MacKerell et al. 2009. CHARMM: The biomolecular simulation program. *J. Comput. Chem.* 30(10): 1545–1614.

Bruckner, S. and S. Boresch. 2011. Efficiency of alchemical free energy simulations. II. Improvements for thermodynamic integration. *J. Comput. Chem.* 32(7): 1320–1333.

Carlson, H. A. 2002. Protein flexibility and drug design: How to hit a moving target. *Curr. Opin. Chem. Biol.* 6(4): 447–452.

Case, D., T. Darden, T. Cheatham III et al. 2012. *AMBER 12.* University of California, San Francisco.

Cavasotto, C. N. 2012. Binding free energy calculation and scoring in small-molecule docking. In: *Physico-Chemical and Computational Approaches to Drug Discovery*, F. Javier Luque and Xavier Barril (eds.). The Royal Society of Chemistry Publishing, pp. 195–222.

Chandler, D. 1987. *Introduction to Modern Statistical Mechanics.* Oxford University Press, New York, p. 288.

Chodera, J. D., D. L. Mobley, M. R. Shirts, R. W. Dixon, K. Branson, and V. S. Pande. 2011. Alchemical free energy methods for drug discovery: Progress and challenges. *Curr. Opin. Struct. Biol.* 21(2): 150–160.

Christ, C. D. and T. Fox. 2014. Accuracy assessment and automation of free energy calculations for drug design. *J. Chem. Inf. Model.* 54(1): 108–120.

Darve, E. and A. Pohorille. 2001. Calculating free energies using average force. *J. Chem. Phys.* 115(20): 9169–9183.

De Ruiter, A., S. Boresch, and C. Oostenbrink. 2013. Comparison of thermodynamic integration and Bennett acceptance ratio for calculating relative protein-ligand binding free energies. *J. Comput. Chem.* 34(12): 1024–1034.

Den Otter, W. K. and W. J. Briels. 1998. The calculation of free-energy differences by constrained molecular-dynamics simulations. *J. Chem. Phys.* 109(11): 4139–4146.

Deng, Y. and B. Roux. 2009. Computations of standard binding free energies with molecular dynamics simulations. *J. Phys. Chem. B* 113(8): 2234–2246.

Doudou, S., N. A. Burton, and R. H. Henchman. 2009. Standard free energy of binding from a one-dimensional potential of mean force. *J. Chem. Theory Comput.* 5(4): 909–918.

Fujitani, H., Y. Tanida, M. Ito et al. 2005. Direct calculation of the binding free energies of FKBP ligands. *J. Chem. Phys.* 123(8): 084108-1–084108-5.

Gapsys, V., D. Seeliger, and B. L. de Groot. 2012. New soft-core potential function for molecular dynamics based alchemical free energy calculations. *J. Chem. Theory Comput.* 8(7): 2373–2382.

Gumbart, J. C., B. Roux, and C. Chipot. 2012. Standard binding free energies from computer simulations: What is the best strategy? *J. Chem. Theory Comput.* 9(1): 794–802.

Gumbart, J. C., B. Roux, and C. Chipot. 2013. Efficient determination of protein–protein standard binding free energies from first principles. *J. Chem. Theory Comput.* 9(8): 3789–3798.

Guo, Z., J. Durkin, T. Fischmann et al. 2003. Application of the λ-dynamics method to evaluate the relative binding free energies of inhibitors to HCV protease. *J. Med. Chem.* 46(25): 5360–5364.

Halgren, T. A. and W. Damm. 2001. Polarizable force fields. *Curr. Opin. Struct. Biol.* 11(2): 236–242.

Hénin, J. and C. Chipot. 2004. Overcoming free energy barriers using unconstrained molecular dynamics simulations. *J. Chem. Phys.* 121(7): 2904–2914.

Hritz, J., T. Läppchen, and C. Oostenbrink. 2010. Calculations of binding affinity between C8-substituted GTP analogs and the bacterial cell-division protein FtsZ. *Eur. Biophys. J.* 39(12): 1573–1580.

Huang, K. and A. E. Garcia. 2013. Free energy of translocating an arginine-rich cell-penetrating peptide across a lipid bilayer suggests pore formation. *Biophys. J.* 104(2): 412–420.

Jarzynski, C. 1997. Nonequilibrium equality for free energy differences. *Phys. Rev. Lett.* 78(14): 2690–2693.

Jiang, W., Y. Luo, L. Maragliano, and B. Roux. 2012. Calculation of free energy landscape in multi-dimensions with Hamiltonian-exchange umbrella sampling on petascale supercomputer. *J. Chem. Theory Comput.* 8(11): 4672–4680.

Jiang, W. and B. Roux. 2010. Free energy perturbation Hamiltonian replica-exchange molecular dynamics (FEP/H-REMD) for absolute ligand binding free energy calculations. *J. Chem. Theory Comput.* 6(9): 2559–2565.

Jo, S., W. Jiang, H. S. Lee, B. Roux, and W. Im. 2013. CHARMM-GUI ligand binder for absolute binding free energy calculations and its application. *J. Chem. Inf. Model.* 53(1): 267–277.

Kaminski, G. A., H. A. Stern, B. J. Berne et al. 2002. Development of a polarizable force field for proteins via ab initio quantum chemistry: First generation model and gas phase tests. *J. Comput. Chem.* 23(16): 1515–1531.

Kästner, J. and W. Thiel. 2006. Analysis of the statistical error in umbrella sampling simulations by umbrella integration. *J. Chem. Phys.* 124(23): 234106-1–234106-7.

Kirkwood, J. G. 1935. Statistical mechanics of fluid mixtures. *J. Chem. Phys.* 3(5): 300–313.

Kitchen, D. B., H. Decornez, J. R. Furr, and J. Bajorath. 2004. Docking and scoring in virtual screening for drug discovery: Methods and applications. *Nat. Rev. Drug Discov.* 3(11): 935–949.

Knight, J. L. and C. L. Brooks. 2009. λ-Dynamics free energy simulation methods. *J. Comput. Chem.* 30(11): 1692–1700.

Kokubo, H., T. Tanaka, and Y. Okamoto. 2011. Ab Initio prediction of protein–ligand binding structures by replica-exchange umbrella sampling simulations. *J. Comput. Chem.* 32(13): 2810–2821.

Kumar, S., J. M. Rosenberg, D. Bouzida, R. H. Swendsen, and P. A. Kollman. 1992. The weighted histogram analysis method for free-energy calculations on biomolecules I. The method. *J. Comput. Chem.* 13(8): 1011–1021.

Laio, A. and M. Parrinello. 2002. Escaping free-energy minima. *Proc. Natl. Acad. Sci. USA* 99(20): 12562–12566.

Lee, T.-S., B. K. Radak, A. Pabis, and D. M. York. 2013. A new maximum likelihood approach for free energy profile construction from molecular simulations. *J. Chem. Theory Comput.* 9(1): 153–164.

Leis, S. and M. Zacharias. 2012. Accounting for target flexibility during ligand-receptor docking. In: *Physico-Chemical and Computational Approaches to Drug Discovery*, F. Javier Luque and Xavier Barril (eds.). The Royal Society of Chemistry Publishing, pp. 223–243.

Leis, S., S. Schneider, and M. Zacharias. 2010. *In silico* prediction of binding sites on proteins. *Curr. Med. Chem.* 17(15): 1550–1562.

Limongelli, V., L. Marinelli, S. Cosconati et al. 2012. Sampling protein motion and solvent effect during ligand binding. *Proc. Natl. Acad. Sci. USA* 109(5): 1467–1472.

Liu, H., A. E. Mark, and W. F. van Gunsteren. 1996. Estimating the relative free energy of different molecular states with respect to a single reference state. *J. Phys. Chem.* 100(22): 9485–9494.

Luitz, M. P. and M. Zacharias. 2013. Role of tyrosine hot-spot residues at the interface of colicin E9 and immunity protein 9: A comparative free energy simulation study. *Proteins: Struct., Funct., Bioinf.* 81(3): 461–468.

Miller, B. R., T. D. McGee, J. M. Swails, N. Homeyer, H. Gohlke, and A. E. Roitberg. 2012. MMPBSA.py: An efficient program for end-sate free energy calculations. *Journal of Chemical Theory and Computation* 8(9): 3314–3321.

Mongan, J. and D. A. Case. 2005. Biomolecular simulations at constant pH. *Curr. Opin. Struct. Biol.* 15(2): 157–163.

Oberhofer, H., C. Dellago, and P. L. Geissler. 2005. Biased sampling of nonequilibrium trajectories: Can fast switching simulations outperform conventional free energy calculation methods? *J. Phys. Chem. B* 109(14): 6902–6915.

Oostenbrink, C. 2012. Free energy calculations from one-step perturbations. In: *Computational Drug Discovery and Design*. Springer: New York, pp. 487–499.

Oostenbrink, C. and W. F. van Gunsteren. 2005. Free energies of ligand binding for structurally diverse compounds. *Proc. Natl. Acad. Sci. USA* 102(19): 6750–6754.

Oostenbrink, C. and W. F. van Gunsteren. 2006. Calculating zeros: Non-equilibrium free energy calculations. *Chemical Physics* 323(1): 102–108.

Ostermeir, K. and M. Zacharias. 2013. Advanced replica-exchange sampling to study the flexibility and plasticity of peptides and proteins. *Biochim. Biophys. Acta, Proteins Proteomics* 1834(5): 847–853.

Patey, G. N. and J. P. Valleau. 1975. A Monte Carlo method for obtaining the interionic potential of mean force in ionic solution. *J. Chem. Phys.* 63(6): 2334–2339.

Pham, T. T. and M. R. Shirts. 2011. Identifying low variance pathways for free energy calculations of molecular transformations in solution phase. *J. Chem. Phys.* 135(3): 034114-1–034114-22.

Phillips, J. C., R. Braun, W. Wang et al. 2005. Scalable molecular dynamics with NAMD. *J. Comput. Chem.* 26(16): 1781–1802.

Pronk, S., S. Páll, R. Schulz et al. 2013. GROMACS 4.5: A high-throughput and highly parallel open source molecular simulation toolkit. *Bioinformatics* 29(7): 845–854.

Ren, P. and J. W. Ponder. 2002. Consistent treatment of inter- and intramolecular polarization in molecular mechanics calculations. *J. Comput. Chem.* 23(16): 1497–1506.

Roux, B. 1995. The calculation of the potential of mean force using computer simulations. *Comput. Phys. Commun.* 91(1–3): 275–282.

Roux, B. and T. Simonson. 1999. Implicit solvent models. *Biophys. Chem.* 78(1–2): 1–20.

Shirts, M. R. 2012. Best practices in free energy calculations for drug design. In: *Computational Drug Discovery and Design*. Springer: New York, pp. 425–467.

Torrie, G. M. and J. P. Valleau. 1974. Monte Carlo free energy estimates using non-Boltzmann sampling: Application to the sub-critical Lennard-Jones fluid. *Chem. Phys. Lett.* 28(4): 578–581.

Vanommeslaeghe, K., E. Hatcher, C. Acharya et al. 2010. CHARMM general force field: A force field for drug-like molecules compatible with the CHARMM all-atom additive biological force fields. *J. Comput. Chem.* 31(4): 671–690.

Velez-Vega, C. and M. K. Gilson. 2013. Overcoming dissipation in the calculation of standard binding free energies by ligand extraction. *J. Comput. Chem.* 34(27): 2360–2371.

Wang, L., B. Berne, and R. A. Friesner. 2012. On achieving high accuracy and reliability in the calculation of relative protein–ligand binding affinities. *Proc. Natl. Acad. Sci. USA* 109(6): 1937–1942.

Wang, T. and R. C. Wade. 2003. Implicit solvent models for flexible protein–protein docking by molecular dynamics simulation. *Proteins: Struct., Funct., Bioinf.* 50(1): 158–169.

Wang, J., R. M. Wolf, J. W. Caldwell, P. A. Kollman, and D. A. Case. 2004. Development and testing of a general amber force field. *J. Comput. Chem.* 25(9): 1157–1174.

Woo, H.-J. and B. Roux. 2005. Calculation of absolute protein–ligand binding free energy from computer simulations. *Proc. Natl. Acad. Sci. USA* 102(19): 6825–6830.

Woods, C. J., J. W. Essex, and M. A. King. 2003. The development of replica-exchange-based free-energy methods. *J. Phys. Chem. B* 107(49): 13703–13710.

Wu, D. and D. A. Kofke. 2005. Phase-space overlap measures. II. Design and implementation of staging methods for free-energy calculations. *J. Chem. Phys.* 123: 84109.

Zacharias, M., T. P. Straatsma, and J. A. McCammon. 1994. Separation–shifted scaling, A new scaling method for Lennard–Jones interactions in thermodynamic integration. *J. Chem. Phys.* 100(12): 9025–9031.

Zeller, F. and M. Zacharias. 2014. Adaptive biasing combined with Hamiltonian replica exchange to improve umbrella sampling free energy simulations. *J. Chem. Theory Comput.* 10: 703–710.

Zwanzig, R. W. 1954. High-temperature equation of state by a perturbation method. I. Nonpolar gases. *J. Chem. Phys.* 22(8): 1420–1426.

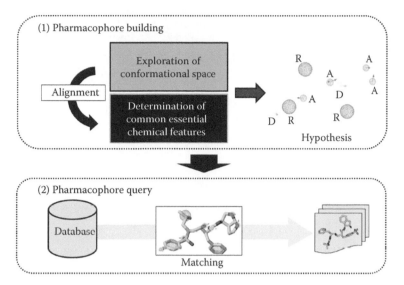

FIGURE 4.1
Schematic showing how a 3D pharmacophore hypothesis is built and then used as a query for database searching. A: hydrogen bond acceptor; D: hydrogen bond donor; R: aromatic.

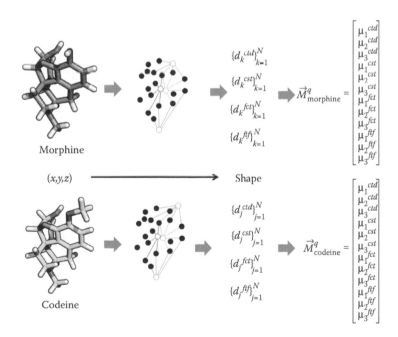

FIGURE 4.2
Ultra-shape recognition. An example of how the shapes and sizes of two molecules, morphine and codeine, can be encoded as two sets of 12 distance descriptors (μ) that make up the vectors $\vec{M}^q_{\text{morphine}}$ and $\vec{M}^q_{\text{codeine}}$, which can be used in a similarity calculation. The locations of *ctd*, *cst*, *fct*, and *ftf* are depicted by hollow circles and, for simplicity, only some distances are shown (see text for details).

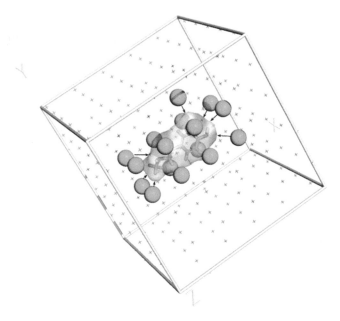

FIGURE 4.3
Representation of a set of observation points (green) around the surface enveloping the adren-aline molecule (sticks). The shortest distances are shown as arrows from some selected points within a cutoff radius of 5 Å.

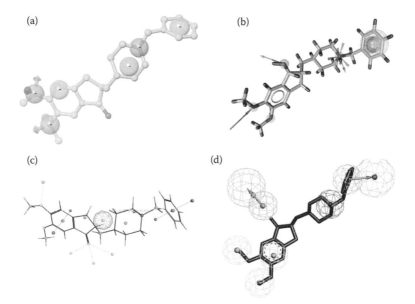

FIGURE 5.1
Pharmacophore models generated by four different software packages using the crystal structure of the aricept–acetylcholinesterase complex (PDB entry 1EVE). (From Kryger, G., I. Silman, and J. L. Sussman. *Structure* 7(3): 297–307.) (a) Pharmacophore hypothesis generated by Phase. (From Dixon, S. L. et al. 2006. *J. Comput. Aided Mol. Des.* 20(10–11): 647–671.) Red sphere = hydrogen bond acceptor, blue sphere = positively ionizable group, and green sphere = hydrophobic group. (b) Pharmacophore query from LigandScout. (From Wolber, G. and T. Langer. 2005. *J. Chem. Inf. Model.* 45(1): 160–169.) Green arrow = hydrogen bond donor, red arrow = hydrogen bond acceptor, yellow sphere = hydrophobic contact, blue star = positively ionizable group, and blue rings = aromatic interaction. (c) Pharmacophore model developed by MOE. (From MOE version 2010.10. Chemical Computing Group Inc., Montreal, Canada.) Yellow sphere = hydrophobic interaction, cyan line = hydrogen bond acceptor, orange line = aromatic ring, green dots = hydrophobic feature. (d) Pharmacophore query generated by Discovery Studio. (From Sprague, P. W. 1995. *Perspect. Drug Discov. Des.* 3(1): 1–20.) Cyan sphere = hydrophobic group, orange sphere = aromatic ring, green sphere = hydrogen bond acceptor, and red sphere = positively ionizable group.

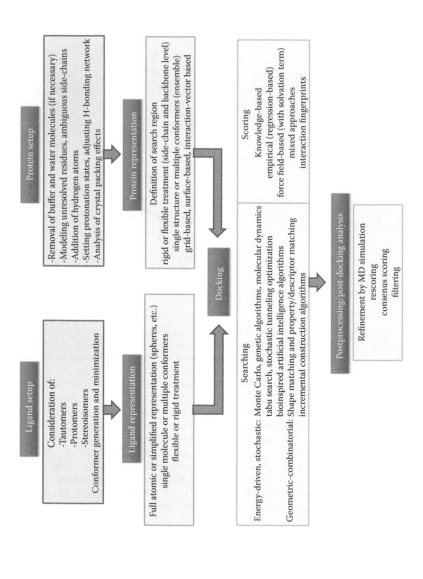

FIGURE 6.1

Simplified overview of the docking workflow, illustrating the major components, the required steps in ligand and protein setup, and the available approaches for solving the docking problem with respect to "representing molecular structures," "searching," and "scoring." The individual items are explained in Section 6.2.

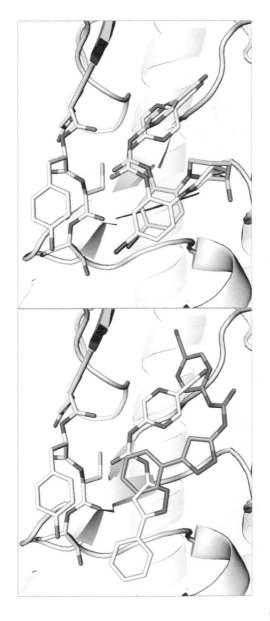

FIGURE 6.2

Illustration of CHK1 docking results for closely related urea derivatives (CHK1_34 und CHK1_36) of the CSAR challenge (Damm-Ganamet et al. 2013; Zilian and Sotriffer 2013). Even though the ligands are very similar, docking with Glide led to top-ranked poses of very different quality. In the case of CHK1_36 (right figure), the top-ranked docking result (shown with green carbon atoms) differs only 1.1 Å from the crystal structure (shown with light gray carbon atoms); moreover, all 10 generated poses were found to be very similarly placed and equally well acceptable. In contrast, for CHK1_34 (left figure) the 10 generated docking poses show very different binding modes, but never the crystallographically observed one; rather, an RMSD of 5.2 Å is measured for the top-ranked pose (light blue carbon atoms) with respect to the crystal structure. The figures were generated with Pymol (The PyMOL Molecular Graphics System, Version 1.3, Schrödinger, LLC).

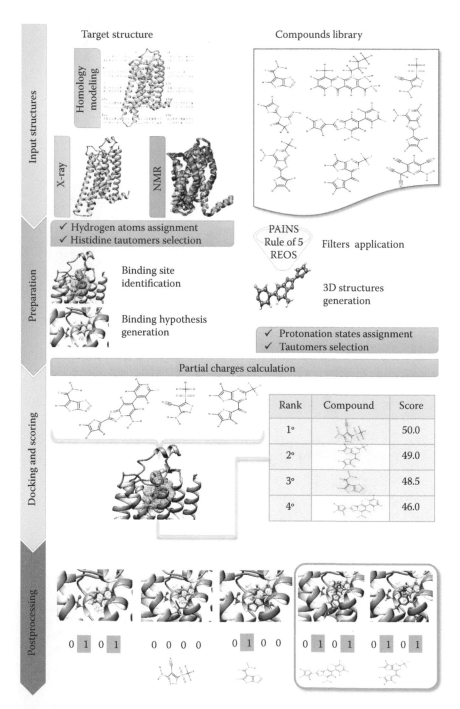

FIGURE 7.1
General workflow of a VS experiment.

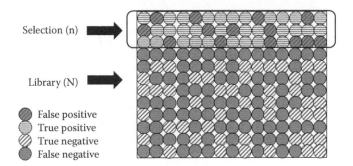

FIGURE 7.4
Selection of n compounds from a library of N entries.

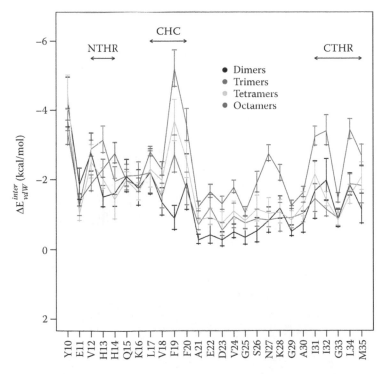

FIGURE 9.4
Residue decomposition of the intermonomeric total stability free energy (kcal mol⁻¹) of different oligomers of β-amyloid peptide. (Reproduced from Pouplana, R. and J. M. Campanera. 2015. *Phys. Chem. Chem. Phys.* 17(4): 2823–2837. With permission from the PCCP Owner Societies.)

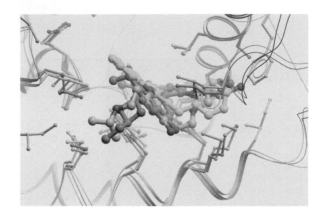

FIGURE 10.1

Phosphodiesterase 5A (PDE5A) can interact with many different ligands. For clarity, three out of 41 cocrystal ligand structures were arbitrarily selected and displayed: 3TGG chain A (Hughes, R. O., T. Maddux, D. Joseph Rogier et al. 2011. *Bioorg. Med. Chem. Lett.* 21(21): 6348–6352.), 4MDG chain A (Brynda, J., P. Mader, V. Sicha et al. 2013. *Angew. Chem. Int. Ed. Engl.* 52(51): 13760–13763.), and 2CHM chain A (Allerton, C. M., C. G. Barber, K. C. Beaumont et al. 2006. *J. Med. Chem.* 49(12): 3581–3594.), to demonstrate how the receptor changes conformation in response to distinct ligand binding. Although the backbone deviations are minimal, the side chains undergo induced changes upon binding to adjust for the fit of each ligand. Carbons are colored by cocrystal structure, and ligands are represented by the thicker balls and sticks.

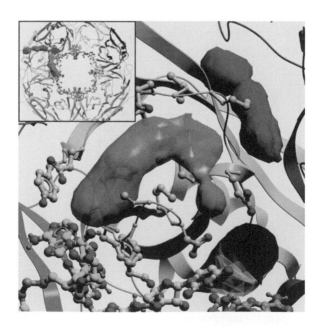

FIGURE 10.2

Druggable pocket analysis reveals this (blue) pocket on the surface of the Ebola virus protein VP40. A small molecule binding to this pocket is predicted to interfere with assembly of the octomer (see inset) or disrupt the correct positioning of the viral RNA, perhaps inhibiting viral function.

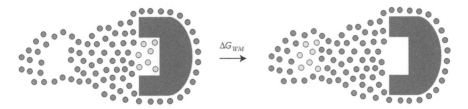

FIGURE 11.3
Schematic representation of the process simulated by WaterMap. The white area represents the cavity in the bulk that is transferred to the protein binding site. The orange dots represent the binding site waters that get displaced into the bulk solution. WaterMap estimates the free energy liberation (ΔG_{WM}) for the displaced waters.

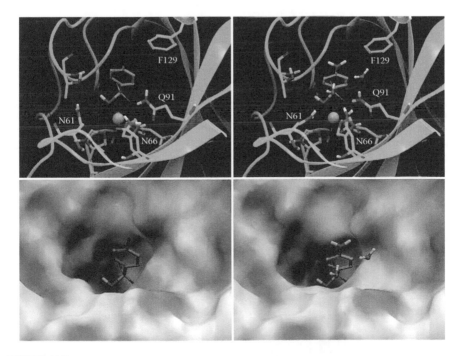

FIGURE 11.7
Representative theoretical structures of the complexes between hCAII and the 4-Cl (left) and 4-NH$_2$ (right) substituted benzene sulfonamide inhibitors. Molecular surface representations are also shown at the bottom.

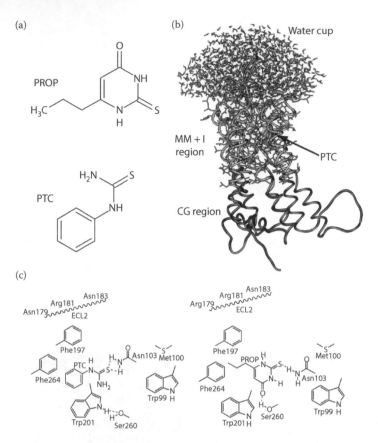

FIGURE 13.3

(a) Schematic structure of PTC and PROP, agonists of the TAS2R38 receptor. (b) MM/CG representation of the TAS2R38 receptor in complex with PTC. Water molecules and residues belonging to the MM and I regions are represented as lines. PTC atoms are represented as spheres. (c) Binding of PTC and PROP to the TAS2R38 bitter receptor as emerging from MM/CG simulations and experiments. (Adapted from Marchiori, A., L. Capece, A. Giorgetti et al. 2013. *PLoS One* 8(5): e64675.)

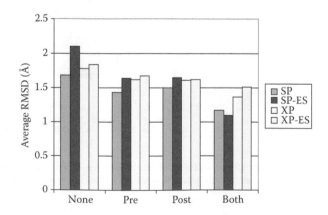

FIGURE 14.2

Docking accuracy obtained by different protocols in self-docking mode. (Adapted with permission from Sándor, M. et al. 2010. *J. Chem. Inf. Model.* 50(6): 1165–1172. Copyright 2010, American Chemical Society.)

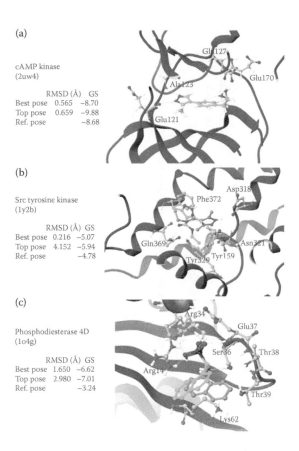

(a)

cAMP kinase
(2uw4)

	RMSD (Å)	GS
Best pose	0.565	−8.70
Top pose	0.659	−9.88
Ref. pose		−8.68

Glu127
Ala123
Glu170
Glu121

(b)

Src tyrosine kinase
(1y2b)

	RMSD (Å)	GS
Best pose	0.216	−5.07
Top pose	4.152	−5.94
Ref. pose		−4.78

Asp318
Phe372
Gln369
Asn321
Tyr329 Tyr159

(c)

Phosphodiesterase 4D
(1o4g)

	RMSD (Å)	GS
Best pose	1.650	−6.62
Top pose	2.980	−7.01
Ref. pose		−3.24

Arg34
Glu37
Ser36
Thr38
Arg1∗
Thr39
Lys62

FIGURE 14.3
Typical examples for accurate docking (a), scoring error (b), and sampling error (c) obtained by Glide SP docking with pre- and postprocessing in self-docking mode. (Adapted with permission from Sándor, M. et al. 2010. *J. Chem. Inf. Model.* 50(6): 1165–1172. Copyright 2010, American Chemical Society.)

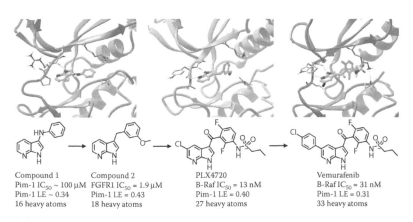

Compound 1
Pim-1 IC$_{50}$ ~ 100 μM
Pim-1 LE ~ 0.34
16 heavy atoms

Compound 2
FGFR1 IC$_{50}$ = 1.9 μM
Pim-1 LE = 0.43
18 heavy atoms

PLX4720
B-Raf IC$_{50}$ = 13 nM
Pim-1 LE = 0.40
27 heavy atoms

Vemurafenib
B-Raf IC$_{50}$ = 31 nM
Pim-1 LE = 0.31
33 heavy atoms

FIGURE 14.4
Structure-guided optimization of Vemurafenib.

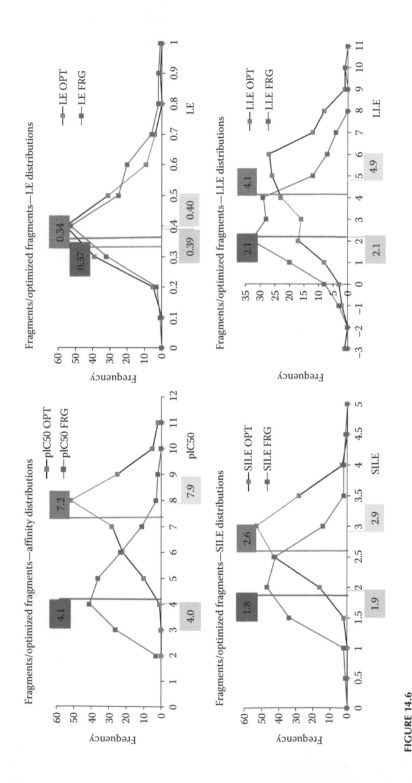

FIGURE 14.6
Distribution of affinity, LE, SILE, and LLE of fragment hits and optimized compounds. (Adapted with permission from Ferenczy, G. G. and G. M. Keserű. 2013. *J. Med. Chem.* 56(6): 2478–2486. Copyright 2013, American Chemical Society.)

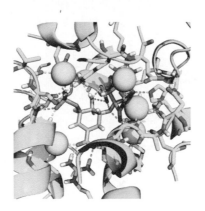

FIGURE 15.1
Strong and important mediation of tightly bound waters in protein–ligand binding shown by
a cyclohexene ligand in cocrystal with a phosphate synthase protein.

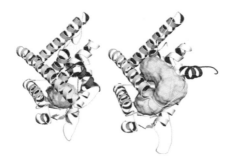

FIGURE 16.1
The close and open ER α conformations. H12 is colored in red, while the binding site volume
is shown in yellow.

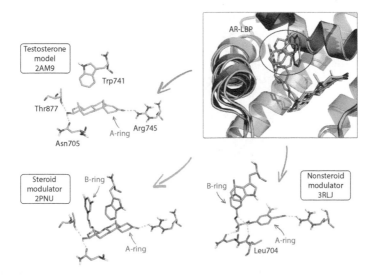

FIGURE 16.3
Model of ligand–protein interaction for testosterone (green, PDB code 2AM9), steroidal modulator EM-5744 (yellow, PDB code 2PNU), nonsteroidal modulator SARM-S22 (violet, PDB code
3RLJ). The presence of a bulky protruding B-ring induces conformational rearrangement of
Trp741 side chain and of other two methionine residues (not showed).

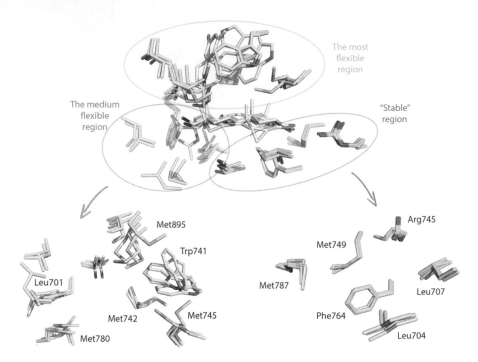

FIGURE 16.4

Superimposition of different AR structure: the most flexible (green-circled), medium flexible (blue-circled), and "stable" (red-circled) regions are shown. All different ligands are represented in gray. Backbone atoms are not reported for clarity. (PDB codes 2AM9, 3RLJ, 2PNU, and 2OZ7.)

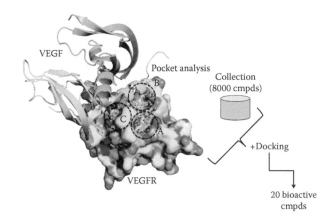

FIGURE 17.3

VEGF-VEGFR binding pockets. The crystal structure of residues 8–109 of VEGF (cartoon diagram) in complex with VEGFR-1 D2 domain (shown here in solid surface representation; yellow, hydrophobic/aromatic; red, oxygen atom and/or negatively charged; blue, nitrogen atom and/or positively charged) is shown. A probe-mapping algorithm was used to analyze the interface area (green sphere highlights regions where carbon atoms can bind with reasonable affinity, blue spheres represent nitrogen atoms and red spheres, carbonyl groups). Three subpockets, A, B, and C, could be identified and are shown as dashed circles. Structure-based virtual screening was carried out over this entire zone and 20 molecules were identified. The best compound binds directly to the VEGFR-1 D2 domain and inhibits PPI.

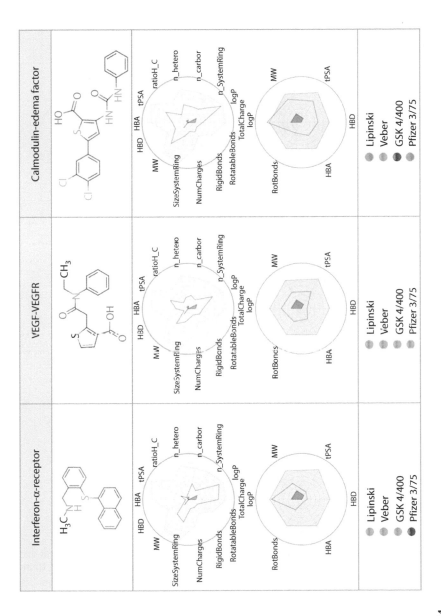

FIGURE 17.4

Analysis of three PPI inhibitors. 2D structures and ADME-Tox properties evaluation (computed with FAF-Drugs) for the three best PPI inhibitors discussed in the success story section (see text for further explanations about the rules).

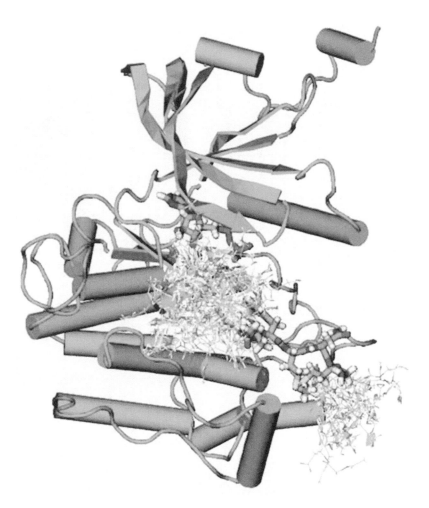

FIGURE 18.2
The hexapeptide GDYMNM (shown in line model) utilizes two distinct sites to enter or exit the catalytic domain of the insulin receptor tyrosine kinase (shown in cartoon). (Reproduced from Huang, Z. and C. F. Wong. 2012b. *Proteins Struct. Funct. and Bioinformat.* 80(9):2275–2286.)

13

Molecular Mechanics/Coarse-Grained Simulations as a Structural Prediction Tool for GPCRs/Ligand Complexes

Francesco Musiani, Alejandro Giorgetti, and Paolo Carloni

CONTENTS

13.1 Introduction

G protein-coupled receptors (GPCRs) form the largest membrane-bound receptor family expressed by humans (encompassing ca. 4% of the protein-coding genome) (Schoneberg et al. 2004). They are of paramount importance for pharmaceutical intervention (ca. 40% of currently marketed drugs target GPCRs) (Overington et al. 2006). GPCRs are located in the plasma membrane and transduce signals through their interactions with both extracellular ligands (or light in the case of rhodopsin) and intracellular heterotrimeric guanine nucleotide-binding proteins (G proteins) to initiate signaling cascades that allow cells to react to changes within their environment (Audet and Bouvier 2012). The resulting response regulates a broad range of cellular processes engaged in the control of cell proliferation, differentiation, motility, as well as apoptosis. Chemicals and light sensing also rely on GPCRs signaling. These proteins are also involved in a plethora of inflammatory diseases (Sun and Ye 2012), cardiovascular diseases, neurological disorders, and cancer (Dorsam and Gutkind 2007).

13.2 Structural Determinants of GPCRs

GPCRs share a common scaffold comprising an extracellular N-terminal loop (N-term), followed by seven trans-membrane (TM) α-helices (TM1 to TM7) connected by intracellular (IL), extracellular (EL) loops, and an intra-cellular C-terminal loop (C-term) (Figure 13.1a) (Venkatakrishnan et al. 2013). GPCRs' tertiary structure resembles a barrel, with the seven transmem-brane helices forming a cavity within the plasma membrane that serves as ligand-binding domain, often covered by the EL2. In several cases, they can exist as homo- or hetero-dimers or higher-order oligomers during their life cycle *in vivo* (Gurevich and Gurevich 2008). Currently, the PDB reports 24 unique experimental structures (as of February 2014), of which 18 from *Homo sapiens* (as reported in http://blanco.biomol.uci.edu/mpstruc) (Rosenbaum et al. 2009; Topiol and Sabio 2009; Sprang 2011; Venkatakrishnan et al. 2013). Twenty-one of them belong to the rhodopsin family (Figure 13.1b), one to the frizzled/taste2 family (Wang et al. 2013), and two to the secretin family (Hollenstein et al. 2013; Siu et al. 2013) (Figure 13.1b). A great effort is pres-ently being carried out in order to extend our structural knowledge on this receptor superfamily (i.e., the GPCR network [Stevens et al. 2013]).

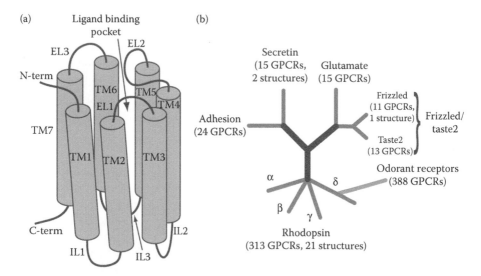

FIGURE 13.1
(a) Representation of GPCR fold. Transmembrane helices (TM) are reported as cylinders. Intracellular (IL) and extracellular (EL) loops are indicated. (b) The human GPCR's phyloge-netic tree according to the GRAFS system (glutamate, rhodopsin, adhesion, frizzled/taste2, secretin). (From Bjarnadottir, T. K. et al. 2006. *Genomics* 88(3): 263–273.) The rhodopsin fam-ily can be divided into four subbranches (named α, β, γ, and δ). The frizzled/taste2 group includes two distinct clusters, the frizzled receptors and the TAS2 receptors. The GRAFS sys-tem excludes the olfactory receptors (located in a subbranch of the rhodopsin δ-branch) and pheromone receptors of type 1.

Molecular dynamics simulations based on experimental structural information are instrumental to gain insights into the dynamical properties of GPCRs based on the crystal structures available so far (see refs. Vanni et al. 2009, 2010, 2011; Dror et al. 2011) for some examples on the adrenergic receptors and Refs. (Provasi et al. 2009, 2010; Scarabelli et al. 2014; Yuan et al. 2013) for the opioid receptors).

Unfortunately, the members of the family for which the structure is known represent just the 3% of human GPCRs. However, the recent array of new structures increase the possibility of developing more accurate homology models of GPCRs. In particular, an accurate modeling of the agonist- and antagonist-bound binding sites is crucial for the successful use of high-throughput docking techniques (Vilar et al. 2011) complemented by the use of adequate set of ligands and decoys (Gatica and Cavasotto 2012). Protein homology modeling is based on the fact that members of the same family share a similar structure (Tramontano et al. 2008). The quality of the models thus strongly depends on the evolutionary distance between the member of the family with known structure (template) and the target protein (Tramontano et al. 2008). Generally speaking, predictions can follow different routes in case closely related evolutionary templates exist or not (Figure 13.1b). In the remaining part of the chapter, we review both types of modeling cases.

13.3 Predictions Based on Closely Related Evolutionary Templates

Several excellent bioinformatics studies have elucidated structure–functions relationships of members of the rhodopsin subfamily (Petrel et al. 2004; Niv et al. 2006; Niv and Filizola 2008; de Graaf and Rognan 2009; Ivanov et al. 2009; Bhattacharya et al. 2010; Kufareva et al. 2011),[*] for which excellent templates exist.

The GPCR Dock assessments (Michino et al. 2009; Kufareva et al. 2011) are community-wide, blind structural predictions of agonist/antagonists in complex with GPCRs (so far human proteins members of the rhodopsin subfamily). The predictions are then compared with the x-ray structures that were released after the assessment. In the first edition, GPCR Dock 2008 (Michino et al. 2009), 29 groups predicted the structure of the human A_{2A} adenosine receptor bound to the ligand ZM241385. Precise modeling of the extracellular loops, together with the location of the disulfide bond and an accurate alignment of the TM regions, has turned out to be crucial ingredients of an accurate prediction. In the last reported competition, GPCR Dock

---

[*] Because of the large number of studies, this section cannot be exhaustive and only some studies will be reported.

2010 (Kufareva et al. 2011), 35 groups predicted the structure of two GPCRs. The first is dopamine D3 receptor in complex with antagonist eticlopride. Its structural determinants were predicted fairly well using the adrenergic receptors as templates (sequence identity [SI] ca. 40%). The second target was CXCR4 in complex with isothiourea IT1t antagonists and CVX15 cyclic peptide antagonist. The available structural templates were distant homologues and not unexpectedly the accuracy of the prediction was less satisfactory. This shows that, indeed, in the absence of a suitable template, GPCRs modeling still remains very challenging. It will be highly interesting to see whether the degree of accuracy in the prediction will increase significantly in the last competition (http://gpcr.scripps.edu/GPCRDock2013).

The power of state-of-the-art structural predictions is shown, for instance, by a recent study of Gutierrez de Teràn and coworkers (Rodriguez et al. 2011). Comparison with experiments shows that their prediction of the A_{2B} adenosine receptor's binding cavity is very accurate. The SI between the target and the templates (A_{2A} adenosine receptor) was around 60%. This approach was recently implemented in the GPCR-ModSim web server (Gutierrez-de-Teran et al. 2013). The same procedure was also used for the successful structural prediction of the human neuropeptide receptor Y2 (Fallmar et al. 2011). In another relevant example, Carlsson and collaborators have docked over 3.3 million molecules against a homology model of the dopamine D3 receptor, before the crystal structure was solved (Carlsson et al. 2011). They have then experimentally tested the 26 molecules with the highest ranking. One of these novel ligands was therefore optimized and followed as a potential drug candidate. This shows that predictions may be reliable for drug design if based on a template of the same subfamily (Carlsson et al. 2011).

13.4 Other Predictions

The SI between most GPCRs and their best templates for homology modeling is lower than 20% (Rayan 2010). These include neglecting all olfactory and taste receptors (overall, more than 400 receptors). In this condition, side chains orientations, including those in the binding site, are poorly predicted (Eswar et al. 2007). This problem adds to difficulties associated with target selection and alignment required for homology modeling, as well limitations of docking procedures. Indeed, standard and automatic docking procedures on homology modeling with such templates, such as those used in Refs. (Garcia-Perez et al. 2011; Kothandan et al. 2012), may suffer from severe limitations. These include and neglecting the presence of explicit solvent (Camacho 2005). This is particularly important for GPCRs, as water molecules can be found in the binding site of these receptors and they may be crucial to stabilize the ligand (Angel et al. 2009; Nygaard et al. 2010). Possible solutions can be molecular simulation-based structural refinement and/or experimental validation (Khafizov et al. 2007; Mobarec et al. 2009; Biarnes et al. 2010; Brockhoff et al. 2010; Slack et al. 2010; Yarnitzky et al., 2010; Carlsson et al. 2011; Levit et al. 2012; Marchiori et al. 2013). In fact, one may identify residues that are important for ligand binding and validate the predictions by agonist/antagonist binding essays on target GPCR's mutants (Costanzi 2013; Marchiori et al. 2013). Section 13.5 focuses on our effort to address this issue.

13.5 A Simulation Approach to Structural Predictions of Targets with Low SI with Their Templates

As discussed in the previous section, we basically do not know where side chains are located when the SI between template and target is about 20% or lower (Tramontano et al. 2008). Hence, it might actually be better not to include them at all in the model rather than including them in wrong orientations. Keeping this in mind, a computational tool aimed to improve the structural prediction quality of GPCRs/ligand complexes was developed. This is a hybrid "Molecular Mechanics/Coarse-Grained" (MM/CG) scheme. In this approach, different parts of the system are modeled at both different levels of theory, taking care in suitably describing the coupling at the interface (Neri et al. 2005, 2008; Leguebe et al. 2012). In other words, the GPCR's ligand, the binding site, and the water molecules around it are treated using an atomistic force field, while the protein frame is described at CG level using a Go-like model (Go and Abe 1981) (Figure 13.2). This model includes only the Cα atoms of the protein. This method is much cheaper than full-atom MD simulations (Leguebe et al. 2012).

13.5.1 Theory of the MM/CG Method

We have adapted to membrane proteins, in particular GPCRs, an approach already developed for enzymes: the MM/CG hybrid method. In this method, different parts of the system to be simulated are modeled concurrently. Indeed, while the region of interest, together with a droplet of water molecules, is considered in an all atom fashion, the rest of the protein is treated at a coarse-grained level. Finally, a coupling scheme is used to connect the boundary of models. Thus, the potential energy function in the MM/CG scheme is split into terms corresponding to different set of atoms, belonging to the MM, CG, MM/I, and CG/I regions:

$$V = E_{MM} + E_I + E_{I/MM} + E_{CG} + E_{CG/I} \qquad (13.1)$$

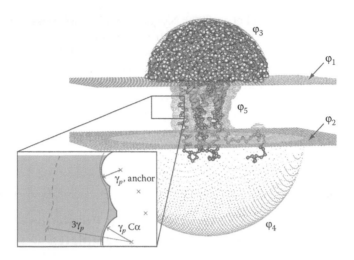

FIGURE 13.2
MM/CG model of human CXCR4; MM and I regions are represented by gray tube, CG region, and waters are shown as spheres. Five walls around the GPCR are used to mimic the presence of lipid bilayer: the planar walls ($\varphi_{1,2}$) are the gray sheets located at the height of the membrane lipids head, the outer walls ($\varphi_{3,4}$) are the two hemispheres, the membrane wall (φ_5) is the surface around the protein. Details of the employed smoothing technique are reported in the figure inset.

where E_{MM}, E_I, and E_{CG} are the potential energy of the all atom (MM) region, the interface (I), and the coarse grained (CG) region, respectively. $E_{I/MM}$ and $E_{CG/I}$ describe the interaction energy between the interface and the MM region, and that between the interface and the CG region, respectively. Atoms in the interface region are considered at the atomistic level, consequently the terms E_I and $E_{I/MM}$ have the same form as E_{MM} and they are characterized by the GROMOS96 force field (Scott et al. 1999), whereas E_{CG} and $E_{CG/I}$ take the form of the Go-like model. $E_{CG/I}$ ensures the integrity of the protein backbone. This term includes the bonded interactions between the CG atoms and the Cα atoms in the interface, as well as the nonbonded interactions between CG atoms and the Cα, Cβ atoms in the interface. E_{CG} is given by

$$E_{CG} = \frac{1}{4}\sum_i K_b\left(|R_i - R_{i+1}|^2 - b_{ii+1}^2\right)^2 + \sum_{i>j} V_0\left\{1 - \exp\left[-B_{ij}(|R_i - R_j| - b_{ij})\right]\right\}^2 \quad (13.2)$$

The first term describes the interaction between consecutive CG beads (the Cα atoms), where K_b is the force constant and b_{ij} is the equilibrium distance corresponding to the native distance between CG atoms. Nonbonded interactions are taken into account in the second term using a Morse-type potential, where $V_0 = 5.3$ kJ mol^{-1} is the well depth and its modulating coefficient is $B_{ij} = 6/b_{ij}$ nm^{-1}. These two parameters have been already employed in investigating both soluble and membrane enzymes (Neri et al. 2005, 2008).

For GPCRs, the same value for V_0 was considered, whereas B_{ij} is set to $5 + 6/b_{ij}$ nm^{-1}. This setup ensures the stability of the protein inside its transmembrane site.

The thermal and viscous solvent effects acting on the system are mimicked by using the Langevin equation with a potential of mean force, $V(r_i)$ (Nadler et al. 1987):

$$m_i \frac{d^2 r_i}{dt^2} = -m_i \gamma_i \frac{dr_i}{dt} + V(r_i) + \eta_i(t) \tag{13.3}$$

where γ_i is the friction coefficient and η_i is a stochastic noise satisfying the relations: $\eta_i(t) = 0$ and $\eta_i(t)\eta_j(t') = \delta_{ij}\delta(t - t')2K_B T\gamma_i$; where K_B is the Boltzmann constant and T is the temperature. If the I and MM regions are solvent exposed, the solvent is treated in an explicit way using the SPC water model (Berweger et al. 1995). In the framework of the MM/CG approach, a drop of water molecule is centered around the MM and I regions and if a molecule exits from the water shell, its velocity is reflected toward the inside. Within this approach, water in proximity of the all-atom region are very similar to those in bulk, but approaching the drop border located approximately at the interface region, the water density lowers, providing a rough approximation to bulk behavior (Neri et al. 2005).

Different to what happens in soluble enzymes, when dealing with GPCRs, we have to take into account the presence of the cell membrane. This is realized by introducing five repulsive walls (φ_i, $i = 1,2,...,5$) into the system (Figure 13.2) (Leguebe et al. 2012). The five walls, around the protein, are described by five corresponding functions using a level-set approach (Osher and Sethian 1988). The region of points r where all the five $\varphi_i(r)$ are positive characterizes the protein site. The wall i itself is formed by the set of points for which φ_i vanishes. Two planar walls (φ_i, $i = 1, 2$) coincide with the height of the heads of membrane lipids. Two hemispheric walls ("outer walls," φ_i, $i = 3, 4$), capping the extracellular and cytoplasmic ends of the protein, are described by the functions $\varphi_i(r) = r_i - r - c_{hi}$ defined only outside the membrane region. The center c_{hi} of each hemisphere is located at the height of the heads of phospholipids, above/under the center of mass of the protein. The radius r_i of each hemisphere is defined such that the minimum distance between any protein atoms and the wall is 15 Å. This creates a droplet of waters around the MM region similar to Ref. (Neri et al. 2005, 2008). The membrane wall φ_5 is defined by $\varphi_5(\mathbf{r}) = r_p - \min_j \mathbf{r} - c_j$, where the distance between the point $\mathbf{r}$ and the closest initial position of Cα atoms c_j is computed, and r_p is a distance parameter with a default value 2.0 Å. Additionally, a smoothing technique (Leguebe et al. 2012) is applied to avoid discontinuities in the wall. In particular, choosing a too small value of r_p around each atom, the whole molecule may be too constrained, and many discontinuities may appear, as well as points inside the protein site. To prevent this, a larger radius (three times the desired distance) is used, around the Cα atoms only, hence significantly smoothing the surface (see inset in Figure 13.2).

Boundary potentials $V_i(d)(i = 1,2,\ldots,5)$ are added to the MM/CG potential energy function. They are defined as functions of distance d between an atom and the corresponding walls:

$$V_i(d) = \frac{1}{d} \quad \text{for } i = 1,2; \tag{13.4}$$

$$V_i(d) = 4\varepsilon\left[\left(\frac{\sigma}{d}\right)^2 - \frac{\sigma}{d}\right] \quad \text{for } i = 3,4,5 \tag{13.5}$$

In particular, the potential applied to an atom is the one corresponding to the closest wall φ_i from that atom, that is, V_i $(i : \min_{r'}(\mathbf{r} - \varphi_i(\mathbf{r}'))) = d$. $V_i(i = 1,2)$ is purely repulsive; $V_i(i = 3,4,5)$ is a softened Lennard-Jones-type potential; ε is the depth of the potential well; and σ is the finite distance at which the potential $V_i(i = 3,4,5)$ is zero. The minimum of the potential is at $d = 2\sigma = r_p$. Waters, Cα atoms of both MM and CG regions, and atoms belonging to external aromatic residues Trp and Tyr are influenced by these potentials. The membrane wall potential V_5 constrains the shape of the protein while providing a good degree of flexibility. This model neither includes electrostatics nor allows distinguishing between different types of bilayers.

The force due to the presence of the wall is derived from the following equations:

$$\vec{F}_i(r) = -\frac{\partial V_i}{\partial d}\nabla d(r) \tag{13.6}$$

The cut-off distance of the force is set to 7 Å for the repelling walls $V_i(i = 1,2)$, and to $1.5r_p$ for the outer and membrane walls $V_i(i = 3,4,5)$. The first value is chosen such that a water molecule cannot pass through this distance during one time step, while the second value guarantees that the force does not affect the MM region. The force is shifted so that it is continuous at the cut-off distance to avoid a sharp disruption. In addition, it is set to a finite value (1000 kJ mol^{-1} nm^{-1}) near the wall to prevent too large forces acting on the system.

13.5.2 Testing and Applying the Method for Structural Predictions

The predictive power of the MM/CG approach has been tested on a system for which the x-ray structure is available. This is the human β2 adrenergic receptor (β2AR) in complex with its inverse agonist S-Carazolol (S-Car) and its agonist R-Isoprenaline (R-Iso) (Cherezov et al. 2007). We performed simulations using (i) directly the β2AR x-ray structure (Leguebe et al. 2012), and then (ii) a β2AR homology model built on squid rhodopsin (PDB id: 2Z73) (Murakami and Kouyama 2008) template that displays a sequence identity of 20% with the target (Marchiori et al. 2013).

i. We have used an all-atom MD simulation performed on the same system by Vanni et al. (2011). The MM/CG simulations were carried out for up to 800 ns. In both MM/CG simulations, the MM region consisted of ca. 10% of the overall systems. This allows to achieve a 15-fold speedup compared to MD simulations of the same system (Leguebe et al. 2012). The MM/CG simulations carried out on the β2AR/S-Car and on the β2AR/R-Iso systems were both in agreement with their corresponding all-atom MD (Leguebe et al. 2012). In a second step of the procedure with the aim of eliminating putative bias due to the original positioning of the ligands and to gain insights into the predictive power of our method, we ran additional simulations in which we have translated and rotated the ligand S-Car in a position different from the crystallographic pose, lacking all the interactions with the residues found in the x-ray structure of β2AR/S-Car complex. In these new simulations, the ligand migrates to the correct pose between 150 and 200 ns, forming key interactions (Leguebe et al. 2012).

ii. In the case of β2AR model structure, after 0.8 μs of MM/CG simulation time, the β2AR structure in complex with S-Car is similar to the x-ray structure (RMSD of the Cα atoms 2 Å). The interactions observed, between the ligand and the protein present in the x-ray structure, are reproduced also in the MM/CG simulation (Marchiori et al. 2013).

The same procedure used in the case of β2AR model structure was then applied to one of the family for which there is no structural template, the T2R family. We focus on the human TAS2R38 (hTAS2R38) receptor in complex with its agonists phenylthiocarbamide (PTC) and propylthiouracil (PROP) (Figure 13.3a) (Marchiori et al. 2013). In this case, two models (A and B) of hTAS2R38 were selected out of 200 built by multitemplate homology modeling. Models A and B were selected on the basis of a clustering approach. The principal difference between the models was the highly variable extracellular loop EL2 (Figure 13.1a). Model A showed a loop conformation closed over the binding cavity while in model B the EL2 loop was in an open conformation far from the binding pocket. To study the interactions with PTC and PROP, the two models were then funneled through a standard docking protocol using the information-driven Haddock program (Marchiori et al. 2013). We have then selected two representative docking poses for each of the models. Although these models largely satisfied the existing experimental data (Biarnes et al. 2010), in order to obtain a more accurate description of the binding poses and the specific receptor–ligand interactions, the four models underwent μs-long MM/CG simulations, each at room temperature

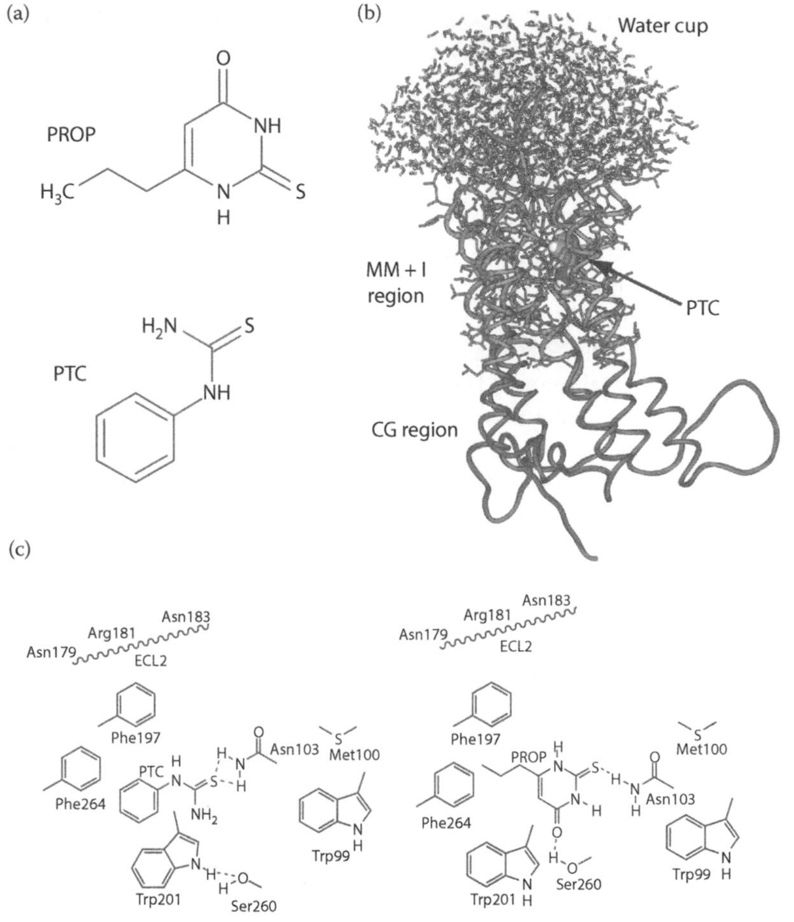

FIGURE 13.3
(**See color insert.**) (a) Schematic structure of PTC and PROP, agonists of the TAS2R38 receptor. (b) MM/CG representation of the TAS2R38 receptor in complex with PTC. Water molecules and residues belonging to the MM and I regions are represented as lines. PTC atoms are represented as spheres. (c) Binding of PTC and PROP to the TAS2R38 bitter receptor as emerging from MM/CG simulations and experiments. (Adapted from Marchiori, A., L. Capece, A. Giorgetti et al. 2013. *PLoS One* 8(5): e64675.)

(Figure 13.3b). MM/CG identified the best binding pose of each agonist. Then, new site-directed mutagenesis experiments were carried out, which confirmed the predicted models (Marchiori et al. 2013). The calculations pointed out key interactions between hTAS2R38 and its agonists, which would have been impossible to capture with the standard bioinformatics/docking approach (Marchiori et al. 2013). Moreover, after MM/CG simulations validated with site-directed mutagenesis experiments, we concluded that the EL2 loop conformation may resemble the open conformation.

The current version of MM/CG code has been implemented within the GROMACS 4.5 code (Berendsen et al. 1995; Lindahl et al. 2001; Van Der Spoel et al. 2005; Hess et al. 2008; Pronk et al. 2013). Multiple systems can be simulated in parallel (Pronk et al. 2013). Hence, massively parallel architectures could be efficiently exploited in HPC-based ligand screening, even performing free energy calculations. To reach this goal, our laboratory is currently implementing grand canonical ensemble simulations.

13.6 Perspectives

In this chapter we have reviewed the efforts undertaken by the scientific community aimed at characterizing the interactions between most GPCRs (for which experimental information is not available) and their cognate agonists. When reliable GPCR templates belonging to the same subfamily of the target can be identified, state-of-the-art approaches of homology modeling, docking, and extensive all-atom MD simulations lead to a high-resolution description of the interaction, even at the level of undertaking a structure-based drug design studies. In all the other cases, which involve the majority of GPCRs at present, state-of-the-art modeling protocols produce just low-resolution models. These can hardly be used as the initial step of successful docking approaches. Indeed, side-chain positioning is likely to be wrong. Extensive MD simulations may be then used to explore the conformational space. Unfortunately, long all-atom MD simulations of a receptor embedded in the membrane are extremely demanding in terms of computational power. In cases like this, multiscale-hybrid approaches may help to a great extent. A protocol combining low-resolution homology modeling, docking, and MM/CG simulations has been developed by us to study the interaction of GPCRs and their cognate agonists, even when the available templates do not belong to the same subfamily. The encouraging results reported so far lead us to suggest that in the near future combined methodologies such as those described here may help structure-based drug design studies for most GPCRs.

References

Angel, T. E., M. R. Chance, and K. Palczewski. 2009. Conserved waters mediate structural and functional activation of family A (rhodopsin-like) G protein-coupled receptors. *Proc. Natl. Acad. Sci. USA* 106(21): 8555–8560.

Audet, M. and M. Bouvier. 2012. Restructuring G-protein-coupled receptor activation. *Cell* 151(1): 14–23.

Berendsen, H. J. C., D. van der Spoel, and R. van Drunen. 1995. GROMACS: A message-passing parallel molecular dynamics implementation. *Comput. Phys. Commun.* 91(1–3): 43–56.

Berweger, C. D., W. F. van Gunsteren, and F. Müller-Plathe. 1995. Force field parametrization by weak coupling. Re-engineering SPC water. *Chem. Phys. Lett.* 232(5–6): 429–436.

Bhattacharya, S., G. Subramanian, S. Hall, J. Lin, A. Laoui, and N. Vaidehi. 2010. Allosteric antagonist binding sites in class B GPCRs: Corticotropin receptor 1. *J. Comput. Aid. Mol. Des.* 24(8): 659–674.

Biarnes, X., A. Marchiori, A. Giorgetti et al. 2010. Insights into the binding of Phenyltiocarbamide (PTC) agonist to its target human TAS2R38 bitter receptor. *PLoS One* 5(8): e12394.

Bjarnadottir, T. K., D. E. Gloriam, S. H. Hellstrand, H. Kristiansson, R. Fredriksson, and H. B. Schioth. 2006. Comprehensive repertoire and phylogenetic analysis of the G protein-coupled receptors in human and mouse. *Genomics* 88(3): 263–273.

Brockhoff, A., M. Behrens, M. Y. Niv, and W. Meyerhof. 2010. Structural requirements of bitter taste receptor activation. *Proc. Natl. Acad. Sci. USA* 107(24): 11110–11115.

Camacho, C. J. 2005. Modeling side-chains using molecular dynamics improve recognition of binding region in CAPRI targets. *Proteins* 60(2): 245–251.

Carlsson, J., R. G. Coleman, V. Setola et al. 2011. Ligand discovery from a dopamine D3 receptor homology model and crystal structure. *Nat. Chem. Biol.* 7(11): 769–778.

Cherezov, V., D. M. Rosenbaum, M. A. Hanson et al. 2007. High-resolution crystal structure of an engineered human beta2-adrenergic G protein-coupled receptor. *Science* 318(5854): 1258–1265.

Costanzi, S. 2013. Modeling G protein-coupled receptors and their interactions with ligands. *Curr. Opin. Struct. Biol.* 23(2): 185–190.

de Graaf, C. and D. Rognan. 2009. Customizing G Protein-coupled receptor models for structure-based virtual screening. *Curr. Pharm. Des.* 15(35): 4026–4048.

Dorsam, R. T. and J. S. Gutkind. 2007. G-protein-coupled receptors and cancer. *Nat. Rev. Cancer* 7(2): 79–94.

Dror, R. O., A. C. Pan, D. H. Arlow et al. 2011. Pathway and mechanism of drug binding to G-protein-coupled receptors. *Proc. Natl. Acad. Sci. USA* 108(32): 13118–13123.

Eswar, N., B. Webb, M. A. Marti-Renom et al. 2007. Comparative protein structure modeling using MODELLER. *Curr. Protoc. Protein Sci.* Chapter 2: Unit 2 9.

Fallmar, H., H. Akerberg, H. Gutierrez-de-Teran, I. Lundell, N. Mohell, and D. Larhammar. 2011. Identification of positions in the human neuropeptide Y/peptide YY receptor Y2 that contribute to pharmacological differences between receptor subtypes. *Neuropeptides* 45(4): 293–300.

Garcia-Perez, J., P. Rueda, J. Alcami et al. 2011. Allosteric model of maraviroc binding to CC chemokine receptor 5 (CCR5). *J. Biol. Chem.* 286(38): 33409–33421.

Gatica, E. A. and C. N. Cavasotto. 2012. Ligand and decoy sets for docking to G protein-coupled receptors. *J. Chem. Inf. Model.* 52(1): 1–6.

Go, N. and H. Abe. 1981. Noninteracting local-structure model of folding and unfolding transition in globular proteins. I. Formulation. *Biopolymers* 20(5): 991–1011.

Gurevich, V. V. and E. V. Gurevich. 2008. GPCR monomers and oligomers: It takes all kinds. *Trends Neurosci.* 31(2): 74–81.

Gutierrez-de-Teran, H., X. Bello, and D. Rodriguez. 2013. Characterization of the dynamic events of GPCRs by automated computational simulations. *Biochem. Soc. Trans.* 41(1): 205–212.

Hess, B., C. Kutzner, D. van der Spoel, and E. Lindahl. 2008. GROMACS 4: Algorithms for highly efficient, load-balanced, and scalable molecular simulation. *J. Chem. Theory Comput.* 4(3): 435–447.

Hollenstein, K., J. Kean, A. Bortolato et al. 2013. Structure of class B GPCR corticotropin-releasing factor receptor 1. *Nature* 499(7459): 438–443.

Ivanov, A. A., D. Barak, and K. A. Jacobson. 2009. Evaluation of homology modeling of G-protein-coupled receptors in light of the A2A adenosine receptor crystallographic structure. *J. Med. Chem.* 52(10): 3284–3292.

Khafizov, K., C. Anselmi, A. Menini, and P. Carloni. 2007. Ligand specificity of odorant receptors. *J. Mol. Model.* 13(3): 401–409.

Kothandan, G., C. G. Gadhe, and S. J. Cho. 2012. Structural insights from binding poses of CCR2 and CCR5 with clinically important antagonists: A combined *in silico* study. *PLoS One* 7(3): e32864.

Kufareva, I., M. Rueda, V. Katritch, R. C. Stevens, and R. Abagyan. 2011. Status of GPCR modeling and docking as reflected by community-wide GPCR dock 2010 assessment. *Structure* 19(8): 1108–1126.

Leguebe, M., C. Nguyen, L. Capece, Z. Hoang, A. Giorgetti, and P. Carloni. 2012. Hybrid molecular mechanics/coarse-grained simulations for structural prediction of G-protein coupled receptor/ligand complexes. *PLoS One* 7(10): e47332.

Levit, A., D. Barak, M. Behrens, W. Meyerhof, and M. Y. Niv. 2012. Homology model-assisted elucidation of binding sites in GPCRs. *Methods Mol. Biol.* 914: 179–205.

Lindahl, E., B. Hess, and D. van der Spoel. 2001. GROMACS 3.0: A package for molecular simulation and trajectory analysis. *J. Mol. Model.* 7(8): 306–317.

Marchiori, A., L. Capece, A. Giorgetti et al. 2013. Coarse-grained/molecular mechanics of the TAS2R38 bitter taste receptor: Experimentally-validated detailed structural prediction of agonist binding. *PLoS One* 8(5): e64675.

Michino, M., E. Abola, GPCR Dock 2008 participants et al. 2009. Community-wide assessment of GPCR structure modelling and ligand docking: GPCR Dock 2008. *Nature Rev.* 8: 455–463.

Mobarec, J. C., R. Sanchez, and M. Filizola. 2009. Modern homology modeling of G-protein coupled receptors: Which structural template to use? *J. Med. Chem.* 52(16): 5207–5216.

Murakami, M. and T. Kouyama. 2008. Crystal structure of squid rhodopsin. *Nature* 453(7193): 363–367.

Nadler, W., A. T. Brunger, K. Schulten, and M. Karplus. 1987. Molecular and stochastic dynamics of proteins. *Proc. Natl. Acad. Sci. USA* 84(22): 7933–7937.

Neri, M., C. Anselmi, M. Cascella, A. Maritan, and P. Carloni. 2005. Coarse-grained model of proteins incorporating atomistic detail of the active site. *Phys. Rev. Lett.* 95(21): 218102.

Neri, M., M. Baaden, V. Carnevale, C. Anselmi, A. Maritan, and P. Carloni. 2008. Microseconds dynamics simulations of the outer-membrane protease T. *Biophys. J.* 94(1): 71–78.

Niv, M. Y. and M. Filizola. 2008. Influence of oligomerization on the dynamics of G-protein coupled receptors as assessed by normal mode analysis. *Proteins* 71(2): 575–586.

Niv, M. Y., L. Skrabanek, M. Filizola, and H. Weinstein. 2006. Modeling activated states of GPCRs: The rhodopsin template. *J. Comput. Aid. Mol. Des.* 20(7–8): 437–448.

Nygaard, R., L. Valentin-Hansen, J. Mokrosinski, T. M. Frimurer, and T. W. Schwartz. 2010. Conserved water-mediated hydrogen bond network between TM-I, -II, -VI, and -VII in 7TM receptor activation. *J. Biol. Chem.* 285(25): 19625–19636.

Osher, S. and J. A. Sethian. 1988. Fronts propagating with curvature-dependent speed–algorithms based on Hamilton-Jacobi formulations. *J. Comput. Phys.* 79(1): 12–49.

Overington, J. P., B. Al-Lazikani, and A. L. Hopkins. 2006. How many drug targets are there? *Nat. Rev. Drug. Discov.* 5(12): 993–996.

Petrel, C., A. Kessler, P. Dauban, R. H. Dodd, D. Rognan, and M. Ruat. 2004. Positive and negative allosteric modulators of the Ca^{2+} sensing receptor interact within overlapping but not identical binding sites in the transmembrane domain. *J. Biol. Chem.* 279(18): 18990–18997.

Pronk, S., S. Pall, R. Schulz et al. 2013. GROMACS 4.5: A high-throughput and highly parallel open source molecular simulation toolkit. *Bioinformatics* 29(7): 845–854.

Provasi, D., A. Bortolato, and M. Filizola. 2009. Exploring molecular mechanisms of ligand recognition by opioid receptors with metadynamics. *Biochemistry* 48(42): 10020–10029.

Provasi, D., J. M. Johnston, and M. Filizola. 2010. Lessons from free energy simulations of delta-opioid receptor homodimers involving the fourth transmembrane helix. *Biochemistry* 49(31): 6771–6776.

Rayan, A. 2010. New vistas in GPCR 3D structure prediction. *J. Mol. Model.* 16(2): 183–191.

Rodriguez, D., A. Pineiro, and H. Gutierrez-de-Teran. 2011. Molecular dynamics simulations reveal insights into key structural elements of adenosine receptors. *Biochemistry* 50(19): 4194–4208.

Rosenbaum, D. M., S. G. Rasmussen, and B. K. Kobilka. 2009. The structure and function of G-protein-coupled receptors. *Nature* 459(7245): 356–363.

Scarabelli, G., D. Provasi, A. Negri, and M. Filizola. 2014. Bioactive conformations of two seminal delta opioid receptor penta-peptides inferred from free-energy profiles. *Biopolymers* 101(1): 21–27.

Schoneberg, T., A. Schulz, H. Biebermann, T. Hermsdorf, H. Rompler, and K. Sangkuhl. 2004. Mutant G-protein-coupled receptors as a cause of human diseases. *Pharmacol. Ther.* 104(3): 173–206.

Scott, W. R. P., P. H. Hunenberger, I. G. Tironi et al. 1999. The GROMOS biomolecular simulation program package. *J. Phys. Chem. A* 103(19): 3596–3607.

Siu, F. Y., M. He, C. de Graaf et al. 2013. Structure of the human glucagon class B G-protein-coupled receptor. *Nature* 499(7459): 444–449.

Slack, J. P., A. Brockhoff, C. Batram et al. 2010. Modulation of bitter taste perception by a small molecule hTAS2R antagonist. *Curr. Biol.* 20(12): 1104–1109.

Sprang, S. R. 2011. Cell signalling: Binding the receptor at both ends. *Nature* 469(7329): 172–173.

Stevens, R. C., V. Cherezov, V. Katritch et al. 2013. The GPCR Network: A large-scale collaboration to determine human GPCR structure and function. *Nat. Rev. Drug Discov.* 12(1): 25–34.

Sun, L. and R. D. Ye. 2012. Role of G protein-coupled receptors in inflammation. *Acta Pharmacol. Sin.* 33(3): 342–350.

Topiol, S. and M. Sabio. 2009. X-ray structure breakthroughs in the GPCR transmembrane region. *Biochem. Pharmacol.* 78(1): 11–20.

Tramontano, A., D. Cozzetto, A. Giorgetti, and D. Raimondo. 2008. The assessment of methods for protein structure prediction. *Methods Mol. Biol.* 413: 43–57.

Van Der Spoel, D., E. Lindahl, B. Hess, G. Groenhof, A. E. Mark, and H. J. C. Berendsen. 2005. GROMACS: Fast, flexible, and free. *J. Comput. Chem.* 26(16): 1701–1718.

Vanni, S., M. Neri, I. Tavernelli, and U. Rothlisberger. 2009. Observation of "ionic lock" formation in molecular dynamics simulations of wild-type beta 1 and beta 2 adrenergic receptors. *Biochemistry* 48(22): 4789–4797.

Vanni, S., M. Neri, I. Tavernelli, and U. Rothlisberger. 2010. A conserved protonation-induced switch can trigger "ionic-lock" formation in adrenergic receptors. *J. Mol. Biol.* 397(5): 1339–1349.

Vanni, S., M. Neri, I. Tavernelli, and U. Rothlisberger 2011. Predicting novel binding modes of agonists to beta adrenergic receptors using all-atom molecular dynamics simulations. *PLoS Comput. Biol.* 7(1): e1001053.

Venkatakrishnan, A. J., X. Deupi, G. Lebon, C. G. Tate, G. F. Schertler, and M. M. Babu. 2013. Molecular signatures of G-protein-coupled receptors. *Nature* 494(7436): 185–194.

Vilar, S., G. Ferino, S. S. Phatak, B. Berk, C. N. Cavasotto, and S. Costanzi. 2011. Docking-based virtual screening for ligands of G protein-coupled receptors: Not only crystal structures but also *in silico* models. *J. Mol. Graphics Modell.* 29(5): 614–623.

Wang, C., H. Wu, V. Katritch et al. 2013. Structure of the human smoothened receptor bound to an antitumour agent. *Nature* 497(7449): 338–343.

Yarnitzky, T., A. Levit, and M. Y. Niv. 2010. Homology modeling of G-protein-coupled receptors with x-ray structures on the rise. *Curr. Opin. Drug Discov. Devel.* 13(3): 317–325.

Yuan, S., H. Vogel, and S. Filipek. 2013. The role of water and sodium ions in the activation of the mu-opioid receptor. *Angew. Chem. Int. Ed. Engl.* 52(38): 10112–10115.

14

Fragment-Based Methods in Drug Design

Márton Vass, Gergely Makara, and György Miklós Keserű

CONTENTS

14.1 Fragment Design Principles

Drug discovery is a very complex and highly multidisciplinary process that requires constant reevaluation of best practices in order to improve the rather low success rate of the overall discovery workflow. Every decade or so a revolutionary new principle is introduced that slowly begins to transform key steps of the well-established drug development process, which includes target identification and validation, lead identification, lead optimization, and preclinical and clinical development. These true game-changers that have significantly enhanced the arsenal of tools available to biologists and medicinal chemists include computer-aided drug discovery, parallel and combinatorial chemistry, biologics, high-throughput screening (HTS), and in the early twenty-first century fragment-based drug discovery (FBDD).

In the 1990s, HTS became a paramount hit identification method via enabling the storage and screening of millions of small molecules by technology development and miniaturization. However, soon it became evident that an increase in the sheer number of molecules does not provide a satisfactory solution for the challenges mounted by the practically infinite chemical space (Fox et al. 2004, 2006; Parker and Bajorath 2006). HTS hit rates of truly novel leads for several important protein families have been low (Macarron 2006) while properties of HTS hits and consequentially leads developed starting from HTS hits have often been suboptimal leading to low clinical success rates and industrial productivity in terms of approved new chemical entities (Proudfoot 2002; Leeson and Springthorpe 2007; Keserű and Makara 2009). The notion of FBDD was brought about to approach the lead identification problem from an angle very different from that of HTS. The screening of smaller molecules rather than drug-like larger ones not only improves hit rates without the burden of screening ever-increasing number of small molecules (Hann et al. 2001) but also brings the promise of more balanced properties for candidates developed from fragments via the use of various efficiency indices (Hopkins et al. 2014). As with all novel hit finding screening strategies, the performance of fragment screening greatly depends on the design and selection of the screening library properly tailored to the screening method of choice.

14.1.1　Fragment-Screening Strategies and Their Influence on Library Design

Fragment screenings can be conducted via either biophysical or biochemical techniques. Biophysical methods including nuclear magnetic resonance (NMR), x-ray crystallography, and surface plasmon resonance (SPR) are predominant in the literature (Neumann et al. 2007; Congreve et al. 2008) and every day practice in FBDD, although biochemical fragment screens are on the rise. Combinations of the two have also been applied with success where usually biochemical screening is carried out first on a larger library in order to filter down the compound list for the lower throughput NMR or x-ray techniques (Card et al. 2005). Biochemical and SPR screens can easily process tens of thousands of compounds while typically NMR or x-ray methods employ a 1000–5000 member screening set. Due to anticipated weak affinity of fragments (0.5–5 mM range) from a small library, NMR and x-ray screens are usually conducted in the millimolar range requiring high solubility. Biochemical and SPR screens of larger fragment libraries might yield more potent hits, therefore screening can be conducted at a lower fragment concentration softening the solubility requirement. The highest possible solubility for the starting point of optimization programs is beneficial from a freedom of operation point of view, and it can also be managed via the judicious use of lipophilicity indices to avoid undesirable inflation of lipophilicity (Hopkins et al. 2014). Thus, it is important to avoid the needless inclusion of extremely hydrophilic and soluble fragments because of the negative effect of the desolvation penalty on the affinity of the hits. On the contrary, reaching the highest possible affinity is critical for fragment hit selection because generally only highly efficient ligands are considered for follow-up (Abad-Zapatero 2007). Thus, adjustment of the solubility range of the library members should be done with care to ensure good behavior in the assay without increasing the expected potency range of the hits. An additional impact of the screening technique on the library design might involve preferred atoms (such as halogens) for x-ray crystallography that can act as a beacon in the interpretation of the electron density (Wilcken et al. 2012; Tiefenbrunn et al. 2014). In summary, the fragment screening method will influence the library size, the desired solubility range, and in some cases it will bias the composition of the fragments toward the inclusion of preferred atoms.

14.1.2 Fragment Sources

A very important basic decision that shall be made at the very beginning of the library design process is where the fragments will be procured from. Tens of thousands of fragment-like chemicals can be purchased from fine chemical vendors, fragments can be obtained from the corporate database of intermediates, and internal compound collections or fragments can be synthesized. The decision on the source of the fragment compounds will also greatly influence novelty and exclusivity. It can readily be assumed that fragments purchased from commercial vendors could very well be part of screening collections of other companies or institutions while molecules selected out of internal intermediate collections could be proprietary especially if database searches confirm their novelty. Fragments designed for synthesis after database queries are also a good source of proprietary fragments, however, high-throughput and cost-effective synthesis of fragment molecules is not trivial as the small molecule size and high hydrophilic character make synthesis, purification, and drying (volatility) challenging using parallel chemistry, HPLC purification, and drying techniques that were developed for lead- and drug-like molecules. In the last few years, it has been recognized that there could be significant overlap among fragment collections strengthening the desire of several organizations to acquire proprietary fragments. Fragment hits will undergo significant modification, growth, or both during lead optimization potentially suggesting that even from the same fragment hit different and novel leads and candidates can be developed. On the contrary, high ligand efficiency (LE) is required for hits to be followed up. This ensures that the basic fragment core must have good interactions in the binding site making its replacement or modification a low priority in optimizations, which significantly raises the possibility of IP conflict between lead series developed at different organizations from the same fragment hit. Conversely, the same argument about a novel skeleton in the fragment hit will practically guarantee that the developed candidate has good freedom of operation and patentability. As a result several organizations—but not all—have put a considerable focus on enriching their fragment library with novel templates.

Novel scaffolds or ring systems can be the fruit of design by medicinal chemists or *de novo* computational algorithms. Additionally, ambitious initiatives by academic groups have made the possibility of systematic generation of all combinations of basic atoms a reality. A database of chemically tractable small molecules composed of up to 13 heavy atoms of C, N, O, S, and Cl has been created and made available to the chemical community for analysis (Venhorst et al. 2010; Blum et al. 2011). In this database called GDB-13, 12.8 million fragment-like molecules were identified indicating the vastness of chemical space even in the fragment universe. Another evaluation has shown that a large number of the almost 25,000 theoretically possible aromatic mono and bicyclic frameworks—adding up to a high percentage of the total—have not been published at all serving as an excellent and convenient source of novel fragments for synthesis (Pitt et al. 2009). Both of these studies make it rather obvious that while fragment libraries do a much better job at sampling fragment chemical space than HTS libraries sample drug-like chemical space, the small molecule universe <300 Da is still inconceivably vast, making it rather unlikely that a few thousand fragments can cover it sufficiently (Makara 2007). This sampling problem shall maintain focus on the identification of screening techniques that enable the meaningful and artifact-free evaluation of much larger fragment libraries.

Fragments can also be designed by retrosynthetic analysis (Lewell et al. 1998) and defragmentation of leads and drugs found in comprehensive databases (Bemis and Murcko 1996; Fejzo et al. 1999) providing the best likelihood of finding biologically active scaffolds, albeit the novelty of such fragments is likely to be minimal. Much higher novelty can be expected from the same deconstructive approach of natural products leading to "nature-inspired" fragments (Wetzel et al. 2009). It has been pointed out that 83% of the skeletons in natural products are absent in commercial databases of small molecules (Hert et al. 2009). A related interesting approach was conceived by Davies et al. (2009) claiming that fragments derived from metabolites could be a good source of fragments ("fragments of life"). However, it has been shown that when a known ligand is deconstructed into its fragments those small pieces do not necessarily bind in the same position as seen in the binding of the parent, somewhat questioning the underlying scientific rationale of deconstructive approaches (Babaoglu and Shoichet 2006). Preferred substructures that are enriched in candidate molecules (Bemis and Murcko 1996; Fejzo et al. 1999) or HTS frequent hitters have also been suggested to enhance success rates of fragment screenings. While hit rates would certainly benefit, novelty, IP position, and possibly selectivity would likely suffer from such preferred substructures.

14.1.3 Fragment Properties

The success of the fragment screening approach lies in better sampling of the smaller chemical space of molecules of low complexity (Hann et al. 2001). Very low complexity will, however, lead to hits with promiscuous or multiple binding modes that are difficult to interpret or meaningfully follow-up (Good et al. 2012). Thus, as it is with most properties, there is a desirable range to strive for and therefore it is paramount to keep a check on molecular complexity and have it efficiently controlled by a direct measure or via properties that are indirectly linked to it. Such properties are heavy atom count, number of H-bond donor atoms, number of H-bond acceptor atoms. As a guidance, the rule of three (RO3) was introduced early on to place an upper limit on certain properties that affect molecular complexity, solubility, and lead-likeness (Congreve et al. 2003). The rules (MW $\leq$ 300, logP $\leq$ 3, H-bond donors $\leq$ 3, H-bond acceptors $\leq$ 3, TPSA $\leq$ 60) say nothing about the lower limit values that shall be considered to maximize the hit-rate and detectability in screening as well as to minimize multiple binding modes. For instance, benzene or cyclopentane fully conforms to the RO3 but few people would consider them fragment-like. Siegal et al. (2007) suggested 150 Da as a lower MW limit for fragment libraries. Moreover, several groups have applied a lower limit to H-bond donors, H-bond acceptors, or some sort of combination of the two, although there are no guidance rules for H-bonding lower limit values. High-energy H-bonding requires directional precision; thus putting a requirement into the filters for a number of such interactions will certainly lower the likelihood of multiple high-affinity binding modes of fragment hits.

Influenced by the RO3 most researchers use MW to control the size component of complexity. Clearly, molecular weight and the number of heavy atoms are related, but it is important to keep in mind that the number of heavy atoms and complexity are more relevant than molecular weight. For instance, a methyl group and a chlorine atom fill approximately similar volumes and have similar hydrophobic properties but chlorine's molecular weight is 21.5 Da larger. Thus, controlling molecular weight will inherently penalize heavier elements such as halogens (F, Cl, or Br) or sulfur in favor of H and C needlessly disregarding the relevance of such heavier atoms to drug discovery. Fortunately, this issue can easily be avoided by employing heavy atom count in place of MW. Since the statistical average (Hopkins et al. 2004) for MW per heavy atom is around 13.2, a heavy atom count range of 11–22 is an adequate and preferable substitute for MW range of 150–300 Da without biasing against heavier elements (Tiefenbrunn et al. 2014). An additional consideration favoring the use of heavy atom count for size and complexity control is that LE indices that guide hit selection (Hopkins et al. 2004) also rely on heavy atom count for the normalization of binding contribution, therefore it would be prudent to apply the same for design of the very library the hits originate from.

Since solubility of fragments at the screening concentration is paramount, it can be advised to either compute or preferably measure the solubility of the selected library members in aqueous media. *In silico* prediction of solubility is still rather unreliable and the results should be taken with a grain of salt. It might be advisable to set a cutoff value an order of magnitude higher than the desired minimum solubility. On the contrary, the experimental determination of solubility via HPLC techniques is achievable for a few thousand samples of an NMR or x-ray fragment library, but it could be a daunting task to do so as an experimental filter for selection out of a larger set.

An emerging hot topic is the flatness or three-dimensional (3D) shape of drugs and leads and—as a consequence—fragments (Lovering et al. 2009; Ritchie and Macdonald 2009; Over et al. 2013). It has been suggested that historically available compound collections, screening libraries, and lead series in medicinal chemistry programs contain too many flat—usually aromatic or heteroaromatic—compounds that not only trigger significant solubility and ADMET challenges but also overpopulate certain areas of chemical space leaving the 3D-shaped molecule space unexplored. The latter has been suggested to potentially be one of the reasons for poor hit rates against certain therapeutic targets or protein classes. A popular description of flatness is the fsp3 value (fraction sp3) that is the ratio of sp3 versus sp2 hybridized heavy atoms in a given molecule. The higher the fsp3 value the less flat the molecule appears to be. As a result of the recognition that there is a need to enrich collections in nonflat compounds, it could be recommended to compute the fsp3 value and strive for a good distribution of flat and 3D-shaped molecules in the library.

Several groups have suggested that fragments possessing chemical handles for optimization should be abundant in screening libraries in order to provide a natural direction to grow the hit molecule (Siegal et al. 2007; Albert et al. 2007). While it would certainly be nice to have a built-in direction for optimization into the hits, in reality it is impossible to know *a priori* which part or moiety of the molecules would be amenable to modification. Chemical handles typically include H-bond donor or acceptor functionalities that are often part of a key interaction in the active site, rendering them unavailable for quick derivatization. Moreover, most fragment optimizations begin with the careful analysis of an x-ray or NMR structure by computational and medicinal chemists, when the most promising position and the nature of modification or substitution are identified and simulated. Thus, for the above reasons the prerequisite for chemical handles seems an overly restrictive and intuitively unnecessary filter that limits the available molecules without providing significant and consistent benefits.

14.1.4 Fragment Diversity

Following important decisions of the library screening method and library source filtrations, and filtrations to tailor the fragment pool to desirable ranges, diversity analysis might be applied to limit the final screening set to the size applicable for the screening method or the available resources. There is, however, an important consequence of ranking hits by LE as follows. Since only highly ligand efficient fragments are accepted for follow-up, most interactions made by the fragment hit with its target protein shall be reasonably energetically favorable making structural regio- or stereoisomers highly unlikely to be redundant. Standard 2D fingerprints typically score the presence or absence of moieties with more weight than their relative position within the molecular framework thereby often eliminating these isomers from representative most-diverse subsets. Therefore, it is recommended that as a final step a visual review of both included and excluded structures be conducted after diversity analysis in order to assure that important or preferred structural motifs are not discarded over molecules that do not feel fragment-like. A summary of the full fragment design process is indicated in Figure 14.1.

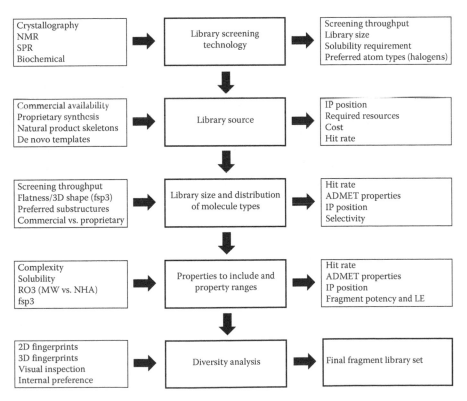

FIGURE 14.1
Decision graph and workflow of the fragment design process.

14.2 Virtual Fragment Screening

As described above, sampling efficiency of the fragment chemical space by experimental fragment screening is limited, since most of the biophysical screening technologies routinely applied in FBDD programs have limited throughput. As a result, experimental fragment screening is usually restricted to investigate several thousands of fragments. This approach still provides a more complete coverage of the chemical space than realized in HTS campaigns, but efficient sampling of the fragment chemical space requires combining experimental approaches with virtual screening. Virtual screening technologies consist of ligand-based and structure-based approaches. Since most of the FBDD programs use structure-guided optimization tools (Ferenczy and Keserű 2013), the preference of structure-based virtual screening in the hit discovery phase of FBDD programs is more than expected.

High-throughput docking is the ultimate choice of structure-based virtual screening, and it is used routinely for exploring the drug-like universe. Fragment docking, having specific challenges relative to docking of drug-like compounds, however, is much less studied. The challenges and the limited experience collected with fragments prompted a number of research groups to investigate the performance of industry standard docking programs. Due to the small size and limited complexity of fragments, docking represents a number of inherent challenges. First, considering the architecture of the protein-binding sites there are a large number of interaction sites available that would generate a number of false positives in virtual fragment screening. Docking programs discriminate between these sites by estimating energetic contribution of separate interactions to the binding free energy. Fragments, however, typically show low-to-moderate potency due to the limited number of interactions formed. Consequently, scoring functions used for estimating the binding free energy need to be extremely sensitive to the type and extent of interactions formed between the fragment and the binding site. Second, the small volume of fragments relative to the binding site complicates the identification of relevant binding modes. Increased translational and rotational freedom relative to larger molecules makes the conformational analysis of fragment-protein complexes more difficult. Given the limited sampling efficiency of high-throughput docking tools, this could result in incorrect fragment poses. Finally, the scoring functions used in most docking software are optimized for drug-like compounds. The development of adequate scoring functions is not an easy task even for drug-like molecules. Fragments, however, form significantly less interactions and therefore scoring and ranking fragments are expected to be even more problematic.

Here, we summarize the attempts published on the validation of commercially available docking programs in fragment settings and then review the most relevant applications of virtual fragment screening.

14.2.1 Validation Studies on Fragment Docking

One of the first investigative studies was published by an AstraZeneca team exploring various docking and scoring protocols for fragment docking using Glide (Kawatkar et al. 2009). In this work the authors tested Glide SP and Glide XP scoring with and without the expanded funnel (EF) option developed for the enhanced sampling of possible binding modes. The performance of fragment docking was evaluated on two targets, prostaglandin D2 synthase (PGDS) and DNA ligase in both self-docking and cross-docking paradigms. Results from PGDS docking were analyzed in detail. Considering the 2 Å limit in RMSD, the authors found that five out of the seven ligands (71%) were docked correctly by Glide SP in self-docking mode. Changing GlideScore (GS) to Emodel score had no effect. The enhanced sampling option was unable to improve this performance but decreased the success rate (57%). Interestingly Glide XP, that uses a more sophisticated scoring scheme, gave much inferior rate with (14%) and without (14%) the expanded funnel option. Although the overall docking performance is usually improved by postprocessing in the case of drug-like compounds, here MM-GBSA rescoring gave lower success rates (14–43% depending on the minimization protocol) relative to the simplest Glide SP approach. Glide SP outperformed Glide XP in cross-docking mode as well. Four out of the six fragments (67%) were docked with RMSD smaller than 2 Å that was further improved by the expanded funnel option to 83%. Again, changing Glide Score (GS) to Emodel had no effect while post-processing on average decreased the success rate (33–67%). In contrast, Glide XP found no fragments within the 2 Å RMSD limit while the success rate was somewhat improved using the expanded funnel option (33%). Focusing on the best-performing Glide SP-based protocols, average RMSDs were calculated in both self-docking and cross-docking modes (see Table 14.1).

It is interesting to see that Glide SP performed very similar in self-docking and cross-docking modes. Although the expanded funnel option was less useful in the self-docking mode, it improved the success rate significantly in cross-docking applications. Some improvement in the average RMSD was also observed. The most striking observations of these authors were that

TABLE 14.1

Docking Performance of Glide SP and Glide SP-EF on PGDS in Self-Docking and Cross-Docking Modes

	Glide SP		Glide SP-EF	
	Self-Docking	Cross-Docking	Self-Docking	Cross-Docking
Success rate (%)	71	67	57	83
Avg. RMSD (Å)	1.89	2.67	3.15	2.38

Success rate refers to the percentage of docking solutions within 2 Å RMSD relative to the experimental structure. Average RMSD was calculated for 7 and 6 fragments in self-docking and cross-docking modes, respectively.

Glide SP gave much better results than Glide XP. Considering the fact that XP is more resource intensive than SP, the better performance of the latter underlines its usefulness in virtual fragment screening applications. Since cross-docking mimics real-life screening applications better than self-docking, the use of expanded funnel option might be validated. On the contrary, neither Emodel scoring nor MM-GBSA rescoring or postdocking minimization seems beneficial.

Schrödinger, the developer of Glide also published a small-scale study on 12 targets (Loving et al. 2009). Since the objective of this study was developing a method for the elucidation of key features for fragment recognition rather than validation, the authors tested Glide XP only in self-docking mode. Glide XP docking was performed by default and in fragment-specific settings. In the latter, the number of poses per ligand was increased reflecting to the sampling problem of small volume fragments. Scoring difficulties prompted setting the scoring window wider and keeping the best 1000 poses for energy minimization, however, Glide XP scoring scheme was retained. Using the set of fragment-protein crystal structures described by Congreve et al. (2008), these authors found that Glide XP docked all of the fragments within 2 Å RMSD (success rate: 100%). The average RMSD value was calculated to be 0.49 and 0.53 Å for the default and fragment-specific settings, respectively. Consequently, it seems that fragment-specific settings have little effect on the docking accuracy.

Astex scientists have published a more complex study validating the docking program GOLD on 11 targets (Verdonk et al. 2011). In this work the authors investigated whether fragment docking is more difficult than docking drug-like compounds. To achieve this goal, they used an in-house set of protein–ligand complexes that included fragments and drug-like ligands. GOLD with four scoring functions was used to dock both subsets in self-docking, cross-docking, and ensemble-docking modes. Docking was combined with different rescoring protocols including energy minimization and scoring with the AMBER force field. Docking performance was evaluated by success rates calculated as the percentage of docking solutions within 1.5 and 2 Å RMSD relative to the experimental structure of fragments and drug-like compounds, respectively. Investigating the effect of different scoring functions (Goldscore, Chemscore, ChemPLP, and ASP), it was concluded that the performance dropped significantly (15–20%) from self-docking to cross-docking mode while results of the latter were somewhat improved in ensemble-docking mode. ChemPLP outperformed other scoring functions in both cases. Table 14.2 summarizes success rates obtained by GOLD-ChemPLP with and without AMBER rescoring for fragments and drug-like compounds in self-docking, cross-docking, and ensemble-docking modes.

The most important observation of these authors was that GOLD performs pretty equally well on fragments and drug-like compounds. Although rescoring with other scoring functions gave some minor improvements on the success rate, this was not always the case. Contrarily, however, AMBER

TABLE 14.2

Docking Performance (Success Rate %) of GOLD with ChemPLP Scoring in Self-Docking, Cross-Docking, and Ensemble Docking of Fragments and Druglike Molecules

Success Rate	GOLD-ChemPLP			GOLD-ChemPLP/AMBER		
	Self	Cross	Ensemble	Self	Cross	Ensemble
Fragments	63.5	35.6	41.2	69.2	41.2	53.1
Druglike	70.3	31.6	49.0	75.7	33.8	48.3

rescoring improved the success rate significantly. The authors related this beneficial effect to the more sophisticated description of interactions, particularly electrostatics and the structure relaxing effect of energy minimization. Investigating the outcome of docking in ensemble mode, it was interesting to see that the primary reason for fragment docking failures is scoring errors, while the contribution of scoring and sampling errors is more balanced for drug-like molecules. This finding was rationalized by the limited flexibility of fragments relative to drug-like compounds and the smaller energy gaps between fragment-binding modes. The greater sensitivity of fragment docking on scoring is in line with the more significant effect of AMBER rescoring on the docking performance.

Since fragments are typically less potent than drug-like compounds, it was logical to check the effect of potency on the performance of docking but it turned out that potency has no impact on success rates. However, splitting the full set of ligands into low- and high-LE subsets, the authors found significant differences between the success rates in each docking mode (see Table 14.3) favoring the highly ligand-efficient fragments.

This is the result of compounds with high LE forming higher number and better quality interactions within the binding site assisting discrimination between the different possible binding modes and identification of the best one. In summary, the most important findings of this study were that GOLD performed similar on fragments and drug-like compounds and fragment ranking could be improved by AMBER rescoring. The authors identified scoring as the major source of docking failure for fragments and suggested the development of new force field-based scoring protocols and also the use of more sophisticated methods for the calculation of ligand–protein interactions.

TABLE 14.3

Docking Performance (Success Rate %) of GOLD in Self-Docking, Cross-Docking, and Ensemble Docking of Ligands with Low and High LE

Success Rate	Self-Docking	Cross-Docking	Ensemble Docking
Low LE	55	26	35
High LE	73	45	57

TABLE 14.4

Docking Performance of Glide SP and XP with and without Expanded Sampling and Different Pre- and Postprocessing Options

Method	None	Pre	Post	Pre + Post
SP	72%	76%	76%	80%
SP-ES	69%	75%	73%	82%
XP	70%	71%	72%	77%
XP-ES	68%	71%	74%	76%

The most comprehensive evaluation of Glide in virtual fragment docking was published by our laboratory (Sándor et al. 2010). In this study, we investigated the performance of Glide on 78 targets represented by 190 fragment-protein complexes. In total we tested 16 different docking protocols involving two docking algorithms Glide SP and XP, two sampling options including default and expanded sampling (indicated by –ES suffix), and four processing options including both pre- and postprocessing minimizations (default), preprocessing only, postprocessing only, and lack of pre- and postprocessing. Results obtained in self-docking mode are summarized in Table 14.4.

In line with the early AstraZeneca results, we found that Glide SP outperformed XP. Expanded sampling had only minor effect on the docking performance, but pre- and postprocessing minimizations improved the success rates significantly. The effect of different protocols on docking accuracy is depicted in Figure 14.2. Comparative RMSD data demonstrates that similar

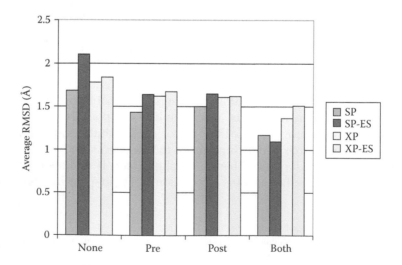

FIGURE 14.2
(See color insert.) Docking accuracy obtained by different protocols in self-docking mode. (Adapted with permission from Sándor, M. et al. 2010. *J. Chem. Inf. Model.* 50(6): 1165–1172. Copyright 2010, American Chemical Society.)

to the trend seen in success rates the average RMSD is the lowest for Glide SP used in combination with pre- and postprocessing minimizations.

Analyzing the possible source of docking failures, we found that the majority of docking errors are related to scoring problems, however, in some cases sampling errors also contributed. On Figure 14.3, we exemplify

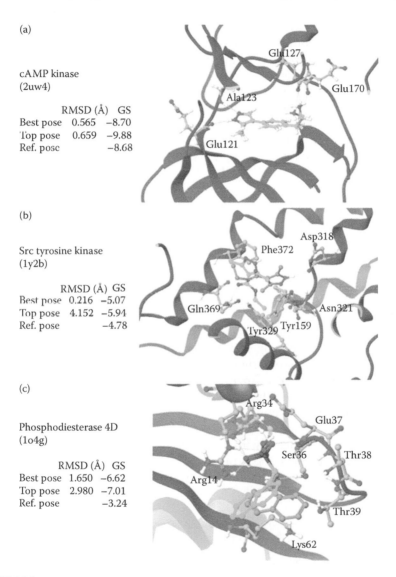

(a)

cAMP kinase
(2uw4)

	RMSD (Å)	GS
Best pose	0.565	−8.70
Top pose	0.659	−9.88
Ref. pose		−8.68

(b)

Src tyrosine kinase
(1y2b)

	RMSD (Å)	GS
Best pose	0.216	−5.07
Top pose	4.152	−5.94
Ref. pose		−4.78

(c)

Phosphodiesterase 4D
(1o4g)

	RMSD (Å)	GS
Best pose	1.650	−6.62
Top pose	2.980	−7.01
Ref. pose		−3.24

FIGURE 14.3
(**See color insert.**) Typical examples for accurate docking (a), scoring error (b), and sampling error (c) obtained by Glide SP docking with pre- and postprocessing in self-docking mode. (Adapted with permission from Sándor, M. et al. 2010. *J. Chem. Inf. Model.* 50(6): 1165–1172. Copyright 2010, American Chemical Society.)

accurate docking, scoring errors, and sampling errors. Figure 14.3a represents the best scenario seen in the case of cAMP kinase. The top scoring pose of the fragment inhibitor (green) has a reasonably low RMSD relative to the position observed in the crystal structure (reference pose colored orange) and its GS is pretty close to that of the reference pose. Interestingly, the best pose identified by the lowest RMSD has a score almost identical to that of the experimental reference pose. Figure 14.3b shows a docking failure related to scoring error as found in the case of SH2 domain of Src kinase. Although the score of the best pose with the lowest RMSD is close enough to that of the crystal structure (reference pose colored orange), unfortunately the top-ranked pose (green) with the lowest GS has a very high RMSD. In addition, the score of the top pose is much lower than that of the reference pose indicating that the docking failure is caused by a scoring error. Finally, Figure 14.3c exemplifies a sampling error on phosphodiesterase 4D. In this complex, the experimentally observed pose (reference pose colored orange) has an unusually high score. Both the top and the best pose have much lower GS but none of them have reasonably low RMSD. In these poses, the naphthyl ring of the fragment oriented in the opposite direction relative to the experimental binding mode that suggests a sampling problem.

Cross-docking experiments were performed with those eight targets that had more than five crystal structures available in the Protein Data Bank (PDB). Table 14.5 reports success rates and docking accuracy obtained by Glide SP with and without expanded sampling. Analyzing the results of cross-docking, we conclude that Glide SP and XP performed very similarly. Considering the resource point of view, SP is clearly a more reasonable choice. Similar to our previous experience, expanded sampling showed no significant effect on docking performance and accuracy.

Our comprehensive study showed that the docking performance and accuracy of Glide are similar for fragments and drug-like compounds. This is in line with the conclusion in the Astex paper investigating another docking code GOLD. Investigating the impact of scoring function, we showed that Glide SP outperforms XP. Expanded sampling option has virtually no impact on the results that is in accordance with the finding of the AstraZeneca team. In line with the beneficial effect of postprocessing with AMBER, we found that pre- and postprocessing minimization improve the performance of Glide SP.

TABLE 14.5

Docking Performance and Accuracy of Glide SP with and Without Expanded Sampling Found in Cross-Docking Experiments on Eight Targets

Method	Self-Docking		Cross-Docking	
	Avg. RMSD (Å)	Success Rate	Avg. RMSD(Å)	Success Rate
SP	1.08	83.1%	2.06	62.9%
SP-ES	1.13	82.9%	2.36	58.5%
XP	1.04	84.7%	1.98	63.8%

Summarizing the most important findings of these validation studies, there are at least three points to be carefully considered before designing a virtual fragment screening protocol: preparation of the protein and the fragment set to be docked, choice of scoring function, and treating protein flexibility. As the case with docking drug-like compounds, successful fragment docking requires the adequate preparation of both the proteins and the fragment sets. It is more or less obvious that the protonation state of the fragments as well as the protein must be carefully adjusted. In addition to protomers, all of the possible tautomers of the fragments should be taken into account. It is highly advisable to double check the protein structures used for virtual fragment screening. These structural investigations should deal with the crystallographic properties (resolution, B-factors, completeness, etc.) as well as with electron density maps ensuring that the shape and orientation of key components of the binding site are correct.

Validation studies reviewed here suggest that sampling is not the major issue associated with virtual fragments screening indicated by the fact that the expanded sampling option and other fragment-specific settings did not improve the performance of docking programs. Contrarily, however, scoring is one of the major challenges that is responsible for most of the docking failures found when docking fragments. Fortunately, there are several strategies that improve the scoring of fragments. First, there are protocols that employ the otherwise very successful MM-PBSA (Kawatkar et al. 2012) or MM-GBSA (Kawatkar et al. 2009) rescoring. Interestingly, this was not very promising on the targets investigated by the AstraZeneca team, however, more data are needed for a firm conclusion. Rescoring by QM/MM calculations represents another option for improving the scoring protocol (Gleeson and Gleeson 2009). Statistical methods such as the linear interaction energy approach (Huang et al. 2006) or grand canonical Monte Carlo methods (Moore 2005) have also been applied for minimizing scoring problems during virtual fragment screening. Development of fragment-specific scoring functions is also a viable alternative (Fukunishi et al. 2009). Since fragments have particular physicochemical and interaction profiles, these differentiating features could be considered to define a scoring scheme specifically tailored for fragments. Promising results of the Astex team with the AMBER force field suggests that scoring could be improved by force field-based protocols.

Combination of rescoring with fixed, constrained, or relaxed minimization could further benefit from taking the induced fit effects into account. Improved docking performance observed in ensemble-docking mode relative to that found in cross-docking using GOLD indicates the importance of protein flexibility also supported by improvements achieved by pre- and postprocessing minimizations. In addition to different crystal structures, ensembles can be generated from molecular dynamics (MD) frames. The conformational space of the target protein could be at least partially explored by MD that would provide a conformational ensemble for subsequent fragment docking (Ekonomiuk et al. 2009). Alternatively, a metadynamics-based approach would also help describing the dynamics of fragment recognition by protein binding sites (Limongelli et al. 2010).

14.2.2 Case Studies of Virtual Fragment Screening

Among the biophysical methods used frequently for fragment screening, the heaviest restriction on the number of compounds in a screening campaign is imposed by x-ray crystallography. Even when fragments are screened in cocktails and automated high-throughput detection is used, the number of fragments screened is in the several hundred–low thousand range. It is thus not surprising that virtual screening to enrich fragments with a higher chance of binding to the target was first reported in combination with x-ray crystallographic screening. Astex reported the use of focused libraries in their Pyramid screening campaigns against five enzyme targets in 2005 (Hartshorn et al. 2005). They used different methodologies to assemble fragment libraries of 500–1000 against the five targets. They acquired a general 327-member set from frequent ring systems and linkers found in drug molecules, and used GOLD docking to identify target-specific sets. The in-house commercial compound library was filtered using fragment physicochemical criteria and then docked to multiple crystal structures of the enzymes using pharmacophore constraints. Different scoring functions were analyzed and the ones best-reproducing known fragment binding modes for each target were used in fragment selection. The focused kinase set contained 116 fragments and the focused phosphatase set contained 264 compounds. Fragments were screened in cocktails of four and hit rates of 0.5–10% were reported. In another article by Astex, a screening campaign against thrombin was described in detail (Howard et al. 2006). A virtual screening protocol similar to the one in the previous article was used but additional pharmacophores were also designed to reward the placement of hydrophobic groups in the S1 pocket. Finally, 80 fragments were screened using x-ray crystallography and three of the hits were disclosed in the article, two of which were found in the S1 pocket but one surprisingly occupied the S2–S4 region while leaving the S1 pocket vacant. Two of the fragments were linked based on their binding mode to afford a 1.4 nM inhibitor. Similar fragment enrichment for crystallization was performed using the Glide docking software against the BRD4 bromodomain in a recent publication (Zhao et al. 2013). The ZINC database was filtered for fragment criteria, clustered and cherry picked by medicinal chemists to arrive at a 487-member library. These compounds were docked with the single precision protocol in Glide to the crystal structure with conserved water molecules retained using an additional H-bond constraint. After visual inspection of the results, 60 cocrystals with 41 fragments were obtained and nine showed clear electron density in the binding site.

Most virtual fragment screening studies that have been reported are against crystal structures of enzymes and specifically kinases. In some cases, homology models have also been used when the experimental structure was not available and more recently virtual screening has been applied also to new target classes such as G protein-coupled receptors (GPCRs) and protein–protein interface (PPI) targets. FlexX was used to dock fragments to the crystal structure of dipeptidyl peptidase IV (Rummey et al. 2006). Ten thousand small primary aliphatic amines originating from the Available Chemical Directory (ACD) were filtered by docking. Two of four selected acceptor points were required to be engaged in H-bond contact and in addition a spatial constraint within the S1 pocket was defined. After visual inspection of the results, 14 fragments were screened in a biochemical assay and seven produced greater than 50% inhibition at 100 µM. Teotico et al. (2009) and Chen and Shoichet (2009) from the Shoichet laboratory were the first to compare the performance of virtual fragment screening to drug-like molecule screening and HTS. They used AmpC and CTX-M β-lactamases as model systems in their studies. They used crystal structures with the catalytic waters retained for docking of 137,639 and 67,489 fragments filtered from the ZINC database, respectively (in the former, restrictions on H-bond donor and acceptor numbers were relaxed). DOCK 3.5.54 was used for docking and the top 500 and 1000 poses were visually inspected for contacts to key catalytic residues and chemical novelty. For the AmpC β-lactamase, 48 fragments were purchased and tested in both enzyme and SPR assays, of which 23 had K_i values lower than 10 mM. Also eight crystal structures were determined, four provided good agreement with the docking pose, two had a larger RMSD but retained key contacts, and finally for two docking failed to identify the experimental binding mode. In this article, 20 random fragments were also screened, of which none showed inhibitory activity. For the CTX-M β-lactamase, 69 fragments were purchased and out of the 10 validated hits in the enzyme assay, crystal structures for five were determined. Four showed good agreement with the docking pose and one had a larger RMSD but key contacts were recovered. In this latter article, also a lead-like library of 1.1 million compounds was docked and out of the 37 compounds tested none showed activity in the enzyme assay. The authors conclude that fragment docking generally provides reliable binding modes and that docking is able to prioritize fragments for screening. However, the head-to-head comparison of hit rates to random screening was very limited. DOCK 3.5.54 was also used to dock 26,084 commercially available fragments to the crystal structure of pteridine reductase 1 (Mpamhanga et al. 2009). Results were also filtered by a pharmacophore hypothesis and for chemical novelty and subsequently clustered by their H-bonding patterns. Clusters were visually inspected and finally 45 compounds were tested of which 10 showed higher than 30% inhibition at 100 µM. One crystal structure was obtained, which confirmed the predicted binding mode. The same group used DOCK 3.5.54 to dock 64,000 fragments from ACD to the crystal structure of 6-phosphogluconate dehydrogenase (Ruda et al. 2010). After a similar virtual screening methodology, 71 promising compounds were identified for purchase, of which 10 were true hits in the enzymatic assay at 200 μM but IC_{50} values were only determined for 3 providing higher than 50% inhibition at 50 μM. More recently, FlexX 3.1 was used in a virtual screening campaign against crystal structures of aldo-keto reductase 1C1 and 1C3 (Brožič et al. 2012). The ZINC database was filtered for trusted vendors and fragment likeness, which provided a library of 143,000 compounds to be docked to the two binding sites using an H-bonding constraint to the catalytic tyrosine. Thirty-seven available compounds for AKR1C1 and 33 available compounds for AKR1C3 were obtained and out of the 70 tested compounds 11 were insoluble at the assay conditions but 24 were discovered with low μM K_i values for AKR1C1, AKR1C3, or both, thus even selectivity could be pursued in this study, which is not always the case for fragments.

A homology model of phosphatidylinositide 3-kinase p110β was constructed at AstraZeneca for virtual fragment screening, since an experimental structure for this enzyme was not available at the time (Giordanetto et al. 2011). The homology model was based on two crystal structures of the p110γ isoform and constructed using MODELLER. A total of 183,330 unique fragments from the AstraZeneca compound collection were docked using Glide 5.0 single precision protocol. Binding modes were analyzed for hydrogen-bond interactions with 3 residues and hydrophobic contacts with 8 residues in the binding site, clustered and after visual inspection 210 compounds were selected for screening. Eighteen fragments belonging to 5 chemical families displayed measurable IC_{50s} but no high selectivity against other PI3K isoforms. Since only an apo crystal structure of mitogen-activated protein kinase-interacting kinase 1 was available, Oyarzabal et al. (2010) decided to use several complementary ligand-based virtual fragment screening methodologies to identify pharmacological tools for this enzyme. They used the CNIO in-house library and a commercial compound library to filter fragments matching the models. Two hundred and forty-nine structures were selected using a staurosporine-derived pharmacophore, 140 molecules from similarity searches against known MNK1 and MNK2 ligands, 124 compounds using FTrees similarity, 231 compounds using 3D similarity eMaps plus 400 diverse compounds representing the CNIO compound library. Out of the 1236 compounds finally selected by these methods, 26 were confirmed as hits with IC_{50} values less than 10 μM for MNK1. One was selective against MNK2, while another showed activity on MNK1 and MNK2 but was selective against 24 other kinases, thus it could be used as a pharmacological tool and a starting point for medicinal chemistry optimization.

The SAMPL3 challenge initiative by OpenEye provided opportunity for a head-to-head comparison of virtual fragment screening methodologies and experimental screening on a validated data set. The test data for SAMPL3 was provided by Newman et al. (2009), where 500 fragments from the Maybridge fragment library were soaked into crystals of bovine pancreatic trypsin and their structures were determined by x-ray crystallography.

Binding affinity data were also obtained by SPR, 20 of the 500 fragments were designated as actives with a $k_D < 1$ mM. Modelers could submit sorted lists of the 500 fragments and evaluate their results in the context of the full experimental data. One group used RosettaLigand for docking after selecting the best methodology on previously known trypsin ligand binding modes and affinities from the PDB (Kumar and Zhang 2012). They used multiple crystal structures for docking and rescoring by interaction fingerprints (IFPs), which methodology provided an area under the receiver operating characteristic curve (ROC AUC) of 0.843 (where 0.500 means random selection and 1.000 means perfect enrichment of actives). However, surprisingly for the prospective data set this method provided nearly random selection and an AUC of only 0.505 with no sign of early enrichment of actives in the sorted list of fragments. Analysis of the data showed that the use of a different scoring function and differently derived partial charges for the ligands might have provided better enrichment. Another group also used the data from the PDB for selecting the best retrospective methodology (Surpateanu and Iorga 2012). They used a single high-resolution structure of trypsin for docking and evaluated five different protocols with GOLD 5.0 and four protocols with Glide 5.5 and found that GOLD with GoldScore was more reliable in pose prediction and affinity ranking than Glide. Using their three top-ranked protocols, they obtained high AUC values of 0.776–0.787 for the prospective data set with substantial early enrichments. The four protocols using Glide showed inferior performance also on the prospective data set.

With the advances in crystal structure determination of membrane-embedded and transiently interacting proteins, recently virtual fragment screening has also been attempted on new target classes, namely GPCRs and PPI targets. de Graaf et al. (2011) and Sirci et al. (2012) performed virtual fragment screening against the crystal structure of the histamine H_1 receptor and a homology model of the histamine H_3 receptor based on the H_1R crystal structure. In the former article, 108,790 fragments from ZINC containing a basic moiety were docked into the H_1R crystal structure using a protocol optimized retrospectively on H_1R binding data from the ChEMBL database. The PLANTS software was used for docking, binding modes were filtered for ionic interaction with the conserved aspartate residue and interaction fingerprints were used for rescoring calculating the similarity to the crystallographic doxepin binding mode. Out of the 354 fragments passing these filters, 282 were chemically novel and after visual inspection 26 were screened in biochemical assay. Of these, 19 had affinities ranging from 10 μM to 6 nM for H_1R providing an unprecedented hit rate of 73%. In the virtual screening against H_3R both structure-based and ligand-based protocols were applied. Retrospective validation on in-house and ChEMBL data was carried out and Fingerprint for Ligands and Proteins (FLAP) methods were found superior to both ligand-based methods such as ECFP-4 fingerprint based similarity metrics and shape-based ROCS similarity and structure-based methods such as docking by GOLD or PLANTS software. The FLAP method uses four-point pharmacophores to align molecules with known biological activity. Linear discriminant analysis is then used to identify a reference ligand for the alignment of molecules and derive a linear combination of probe scores that is capable of discriminating molecules with different biological activity. FLAP is trained on a similar number of active and inactive molecules and is thus not biased toward any biological activity range. A total of 156,090 positively charged fragment-like compounds from ZINC were subjected to both structure-based and ligand-based FLAP models and 202 consensus hits and the top 200 molecules from the ligand-based model were visually inspected. Twenty-nine novel compounds were selected for testing, of which 18 were confirmed with affinities ranging from 0.5 to 10 μM for H_3R. A head-to-head comparison of target immobilized NMR screening (TINS) and virtual screening was carried out against the adenosine A_{2A} receptor by ZoBio (Chen et al. 2013). In that study an in-house library of 500 chemically diverse fragments was docked using DOCK3.6 to an antagonist-bound crystal structure of the $A_{2A}AR$ prior to experimental screening. The TINS screen resulted in 94 primary hits, but only five were confirmed in a radioligand displacement assay. Four of these hits were found in the top 25 fragments by docking. To test whether docking identified false negatives of the NMR screen, five compounds with reasonable binding modes were selected from the top 50 fragments of the ranked library and screened in the radioligand displacement assay, three of which turned out to be inhibitors with high LE. After these encouraging results 328,000 commercially available fragments from ZINC were docked using the same protocol to the $A_{2A}AR$ structure, the top 500 binding modes were visually inspected and 22 were ordered and screened. Fourteen molecules showed significant radioligand displacement and the K_i values ranged from 2 to 240 μM. Finally, an article by Rouhana et al. (2013) described virtual fragment screening against a protein–protein interaction target, the Arno Sec7 domain regulating GDP/GTP nucleotide exchange by the Arf1 ADP-ribosylation factor. They identified hot spots on the experimentally determined Arf1-Arno4M complex with a computational alanine scanning approach. Arno4M contains four mutations that allowed the crystallization of the complex. Surflex was used to dock the ~3000 fragments of the ChemBridge fragment library to four identified subsites at the computationally back-mutated wild-type Arno surface. After visual inspection of the top solutions to identify bad contacts, 33 fragments were purchased together with 40 randomly selected fragments. Four of these fragments were confirmed inhibitors that did not show aggregation-based effects. All four fragments were identified in the docking screen and none from the randomly selected set. Taken together, these results show that virtual fragment screening is a viable approach for enriching active fragments for experimental screening and hit rates as high as 73% can be achieved. It seems that workflows generally include docking with pharmacophore constraints or postprocessing with pharmacophore hypotheses or interaction fingerprints and visual inspection of the predicted contacts with the target and some medicinal chemistry expertise to maximize the outcome of virtual screening.

14.3 Fragment Optimization

Once validated and well-characterized fragment hits have emerged from a screening campaign the hit-to-lead optimization can begin. As opposed to lead optimization from an HTS hit where usually large and lipophilic compounds need to be converted into smaller and less lipophilic ones while moderately increasing potency, fragment optimization needs a qualitatively different mindset, as a larger increase in potency is needed accompanied by a moderate increase in molecule size and maintenance of good physicochemical parameters. For example, Astex has reported 50 Da lower molecular mass and 1 clogP unit lower lipophilicity for their leads compared to literature HTS leads (Murray et al. 2012), but it is at least as much the result of company culture as it is of the favorable properties of fragments. In FBDD, not only the library design and screening campaign have to be conducted in the most rigorous way, but control over the parameters needs to be maintained throughout the whole optimization process. While this is not a trivial task, the success and entering speed of fragment-originated candidates in clinical trials can be seen as a victory march of FBDD. In 2011 Vemurafenib, the first drug discovered using a fragment-based strategy was approved after only 6 years of going from concept to approval (Tsai et al. 2008). The structure-guided optimization of Vemurafenib is shown in Figure 14.4. In

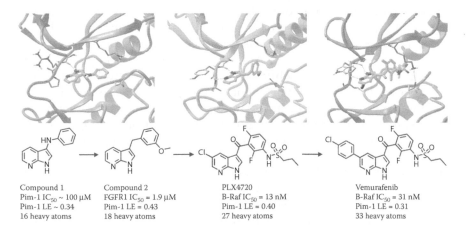

Compound 1	Compound 2	PLX4720	Vemurafenib
Pim-1 IC$_{50}$ ~ 100 µM	FGFR1 IC$_{50}$ = 1.9 µM	B-Raf IC$_{50}$ = 13 nM	B-Raf IC$_{50}$ = 31 nM
Pim-1 LE ~ 0.34	Pim-1 LE = 0.43	Pim-1 LE = 0.40	Pim-1 LE = 0.31
16 heavy atoms	18 heavy atoms	27 heavy atoms	33 heavy atoms

FIGURE 14.4
(**See color insert.**) Structure-guided optimization of Vemurafenib.

the beginning of 2013, there were 25 fragment-originated compounds in clinical trials. Fragments can tackle targets even formerly tagged as undruggable, like BACE-1, which is now a popular target of FBDD campaigns and all-known potent inhibitors are derived from fragments (Huang et al. 2006). While in its infancy FBDD was often only used as a last resort for targets where all other methods failed, now it has become a well-established alternative for HTS or analog-based lead identification.

14.3.1 Background of Fragment Optimization

The physical background of the superiority of fragment hits lies in their ability to form high-quality interactions with the protein targets. Fragments can be seen as the minimal interaction pattern needed for binding to the respective target. An analysis of 1297 high-resolution complex structures from the PDB revealed that fragments form on average two H-bonds with near optimal geometry while also experiencing favorable hydrophobic embedding in the so-called hot spot of the protein target. These characteristic H-bonds are well conserved among different small molecules bound to the same protein. It has also been shown that larger compounds feature only one extra optimal geometry H-bond on average compared to fragment-sized ligands (Ferenczy and Keserű 2012). The conserved H-bonding pattern can also be regarded as the foundation stone for fragment optimization. For structure-based optimization and understanding of the SAR to be possible, it is a prerequisite that initial fragment hits do not change their binding modes throughout the optimization process. Astex has indeed shown that for 39 of their fragment hit-lead pairs the average shift of the fragment binding pose was only 0.8 Å RMSD and for no individual pair the shift exceeded 1.5 Å RMSD (Murray et al. 2012). Orita et al. (2011) have found a similar 0.7 Å mean shift for 25 fragment hit-lead pairs from the literature with a maximum of 1.7 Å. During optimization not only the fragment binding mode but the protein structure might change as well. Astex has reported essentially no fragment-induced protein movements (maximal protein atom movement <1 Å) in the fragment screening against one-third of 25 protein targets while for half of the targets induced fit effects accompanied by a protein movement larger than 5 Å were found for specific fragments. Examples included amino acid side chain movements, helix collapse, movement of the flap region in kinases or other loop rearrangements (Murray et al. 2012). Figure 14.5 shows maximum ligand and protein movements found by Astex.

The conservation of the binding mode facilitates predictions based on the complex structure. In an ideal scenario, the optimization process is monitored by crystallography or structural information from NMR. Using this information from the complexes modifications of the ligand can be evaluated in an iterative manner using hypotheses derived from medicinal chemistry knowledge or computational models and testing these hypotheses

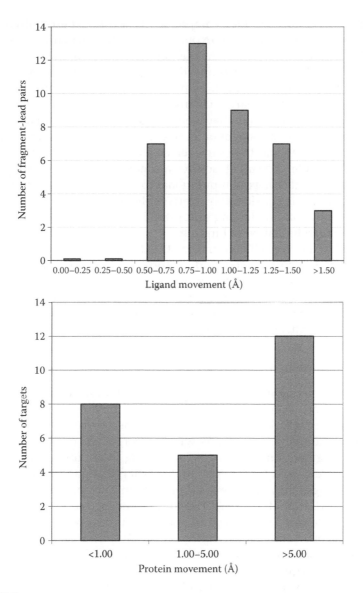

FIGURE 14.5
Maximum ligand and protein movement in fragment optimization at Astex.

experimentally. As seen in fragment library design and fragment screening, computational tools can be used in every aspect of fragment optimization as well and form an efficient combination together with experiment. Such a workflow, in general, includes the enumeration of the chemical space around the fragment hit and then filtering the enumerated structures using predictive models for various desired properties—the basic principles of *de novo* drug design. The top few idea compounds that fulfill the required criteria are then synthesized and tested experimentally, and structural information is used as a seed in the next round of iteration. The two basic steps in this workflow, namely enumeration and filtering, can be done using medicinal chemistry knowledge, however, computers have the advantage of being able to enumerate a much larger chemical space than humans. Also, models might suggest modifications that would otherwise elude human thinking, thus contributing to the navigation in free IP space. When models with good predictivity are available, they can even entirely guide the optimization process. When complex crystal structures are not available, homology modeling or ligand-based *de novo* computational tools can be of use. Optimization without structure is considerably more challenging and will require more synthesis for hypothesis testing and establishing SAR and heavier investments into characterization of binding.

In the following, we will summarize the different strategies for fragment optimization, structure-based and ligand-based computational methods applied in the process with focus on recent developments in techniques and methodologies. For further information, the reader is referred to recent reviews discussing computational techniques in FBDD (Loving et al. 2010; Rabal et al. 2011; Sheng and Zhang 2013).

14.3.2 Computational Tools Used in Fragment Optimization

The two main strategies to optimize fragments into novel chemical entities are growing and linking. In growing, a single protein-bound fragment is identified and new functional groups are attached to this core fragment one by one to exploit new interactions with the target. As outlined earlier, the anchoring fragment rarely changes its binding mode upon growing; however, the protein structure might undergo larger ligand-induced conformational changes and even new subpockets might open during fragment optimization (Edink et al. 2011). The initial binding mode of the fragment can be available from experiment or docking studies. When the x-ray structure of the protein-fragment complex is available, finding the best growing vectors and functional groups can be done automatically using computational *de novo* design tools.

In linking, two or more protein-bound fragments are identified and joined together synthetically by suitable linkers that allow all of the fragments to retain their binding modes and specific interactions. Fragments suitable for linking might come from cocrystallization of fragment cocktails with the target, second-site screening by SPR or NMR, particularly interligand Overhauser effect (ILOE) experiments, or virtual identification of simultaneously accommodated fragments in the binding site with tools such as multiple copy simultaneous search (MCSS) (Schubert and Stultz 2009), simultaneous docking of multiple fragments (Li, H. et al. 2011; Hoffer and Horvath 2013), or sequential docking (Vass and Keserű

2013). In theory, the linked compound should have binding free-energy greater than the sum of the binding free-energies of its constituting fragments because of the preorganization of binding elements. Although this approach might seem straightforward, it is often difficult to pursue synthetically, because of the high entropy loss of the linked fragments and the linker itself compared to the unlinked fragments (Ichihara et al. 2011). Thus, the selection of the ideal linker is not an easy task and computational tools can be of great help. de Kloe et al. (2009) collected a remarkable variety of fragment optimizations from the literature including both growing and linking examples.

De novo design tools have the same general workflow: enumeration of the possible chemical space using the fragment as a seed and scoring of the resulting virtual compounds using a suitable fitness function. They can differ in the implementation of these steps, namely the types of building blocks used in enumeration, the rules for attaching these building blocks to the core fragment, the algorithm used for optimization in the chemical space, and the fitness function with respect to which the optimization is pursued. Building blocks can be atoms, functional groups, or small fragments. Atom-based methods like LEGEND (Nishibata and Itai 1991) have the advantage that they can theoretically enumerate the whole chemical space and find truly novel structures, however, these approaches consider too many possible molecules, many of which are problematic in terms of chemical stability, synthetic accessibility, or drug-likeness. If small fragments are used as building blocks the number of molecules to be considered is much lower and they are more probably synthetically accessible and drug-like. Fragment building block libraries can be assembled by methods described in the first section: filtering of public databases or proprietary building blocks as in AutoGrow (Durrant et al. 2009), fragmentation of drug-like molecules as in COLIBREE (Hartenfeller et al. 2008), Flux (Fechner and Schneider 2006, 2007), MEGA (Nicolaou et al. 2009), PROTOBUILD (Bhurruth-Alcor et al. 2011), and using pharmacophore or bioisostere libraries as in Fragment hopping (Ji et al. 2008) and PhDD (Huang et al. 2010). Such libraries may be categorized into ring systems, linkers, and side chains if these specific subsets need to be used, for example, a linker library for fragment linking in CONFIRM (Thompson et al. 2008). Modern *de novo* tools mostly use fragment libraries instead of atom-based build-up.

The simplest way of fragment assembly is the brute-force method, when all fragments are attached to all growing or linking vectors and unwanted chemistry or compounds not fitting in the binding site are filtered out. However, there are various ways of getting rid of the enumeration overhead. It is possible to identify possible growing vectors based on the crystal structures as in AutoGrow and to use retrosynthetic assembly rules to ensure synthetic accessibility already in the enumeration phase as in FlexNovo (Degen and Rarey 2006) and Flux. PROTOBUILD uses both approaches to reduce the search space. It is also possible to enumerate only those compounds that fulfill predefined min–max criteria of specific molecular descriptors such as molecular weight, logP, rotatable bond count, and so on, further reducing enumeration and evaluation costs (Parn et al. 2007). Fragment assembly may also be biased toward drug-like compounds if the frequency of specific fragment linking is matched to the frequencies in a drug-like or natural product database as done in FOG (Kutchukian et al. 2009). Another method of fragment assembly is hybridization of molecules with known or predicted binding modes. The BREED algorithm identifies overlapping bond vectors in a set of compounds bound in the same binding site and swaps the fragments on the two ends of the bond (Pierce et al. 2004). If one of the bonded atoms is hydrogen, the method can be utilized as a fragment growing technique. A few novel methods inspired by the original BREED algorithm have been described: automatic tailoring and transplanting (AutoT&T) uses virtual screening hits for breeding taking into account synthetic accessibility (Li, Y. et al. 2011), while MED-Hybridise breeds multiple ligands in one iteration step using local similarity of protein surfaces from protein–ligand complexes from the whole PDB (Moriaud et al. 2009).

The choice of optimization algorithm is crucial in efficient sampling of the huge chemical space of drug-like molecules and in finding the appropriate regions, which correspond to compounds with optimal affinity, chemical, physicochemical, and ADMET properties. Nature-inspired algorithms such as genetic algorithms, evolutionary graph-theory, particle swarm optimization, and ant colony optimization turned out to be especially useful in navigating the huge chemical space and guiding the optimization against multiobjective constraints (Hiss et al. 2010). For example, AutoGrow, Flux, MEGA, PROTOBUILD, GANDI (Dey and Caflisch 2008), and LigBuilder 2.0 (Yuan et al. 2011) use evolutionary algorithms in the search, while COLIBREE and MLSD use particle swarm optimization.

Fitness functions may include structure- or ligand-based prediction of affinity using the previously presented scoring and rescoring methods or validated pharmacophore, QSAR and 3D-QSAR models in the lack of crystal structures. Synthetic accessibility is often assessed using the RECAP (Lewell et al. 1998), SYNOPSIS (Vinkers et al. 2003), SYLVIA (Boda et al. 2007), or DOGS (Hartenfeller et al. 2012) algorithms. Further fitness parameters include diversity and novelty, drug-likeness and ADMET properties, which all have a large number of models described in the literature.

Modern *de novo* tools have the advantage of integrating validated building block libraries, efficient enumeration algorithms, and multiobjective scoring schemes. For example, FlexNovo uses the incremental build-up strategy of the FlexX docking algorithm, large fragment libraries for enumeration and it includes spatial, physicochemical, and diversity filters. FlexNovo has been integrated into the NovoBench platform (Zaliani et al. 2009), which also includes synthetic accessibility prediction and ligand-based search algorithms in order to be used in projects with different amount of structural information. AutoGrow uses the free AutoDock software to enumerate and redock evolved fragments into the protein-binding site using an evolutionary algorithm. GANDI is a novel tool that is based on the linking strategy of predocked fragments from a user-defined fragment library. Its optimization scheme combines an evolutionary algorithm with taboo search simultaneously evaluating force field energy and similarity to known reference compounds. The relative weights of these can be tuned; thus the method may be used in a purely structure- or ligand-based mode or in a combination of the two. Fragment hopping uses minimal pharmacophoric elements to find fragments from five different fragment libraries and places them in the preferred spatial orientation proposed by LUDI (Böhm 1992), and MCSS then joins them together. Evaluation of the virtual compounds includes diversity, isozyme selectivity, redocking, and ADMET filters. LigBuilder 2.0 uses a genetic algorithm to grow or link fragments in an iterative scheme and uses the embedded SYLVIA tool for assessing synthetic accessibility. It also evaluates binding site complementarity, drug-likeness, and ADMET filters. MEGA is a new multiobjective optimization *de novo* design framework that combines evolutionary algorithms with graph-theory to design structurally diverse molecules satisfying one or more objectives. It uses ChillScore to score interactions with the target and also similarity to known reference compounds. MOEA (van der Horst et al. 2012) and LiGen (Beccari et al. 2013) are among the latest reported integrated *de novo* design tools. Both feature a highly customizable workflow with both structure- and ligand-based fitness functions, ADMET predictions, and efficient communication with external software. Synthetic accessibility prediction is part of LiGen but not of MOEA.

Ligand-based *de novo* design algorithms are useful when the structure of the protein-fragment complex is not available as is usually the case with membrane protein targets such as GPCRs and ion channels. COLIBREE, Flux, PhDD, NEWLEAD (Tschinke and Cohen 1993), SQUIRREL (Proschak et al. 2009), EA-Inventor (Tripos International, St. Louis, MO), and Qsearch (Lippert et al. 2011) are examples of pharmacophore-based *de novo* platforms. NEWLEAD was the first pharmacophore-based *de novo* design method; however, it can only process specific pharmacophoric functional groups rather than chemical features. Flux reassembles fragments obtained by the RECAP procedure using predefined assembly rules and an evolutionary algorithm evaluating the resulting compounds with topological atom-pair descriptors and similarity to reference molecules as fitness function. COLIBREE uses particle swarm optimization to vary linkers and side chains on a fixed scaffold evaluating topological pharmacophore similarity to reference ligands as the fitness function. This allows for positive and negative design to be performed simultaneously. SQUIRREL compares both molecular shape and potential pharmacophore features and can suggest bioisosteric replacement groups for a reference compound. PhDD is able to work with abstract pharmacophore models assessing also drug-likeness, bioactivity, and synthetic accessibility. Tripos's EA-Inventor works on connection tables of structure populations using an evolutionary algorithm. Any user-defined scoring function can be used as the fitness function. EAISFD combines the EA-Inventor algorithm for structure evolution with Surflex-Dock for scoring (Liu et al. 2007). EAISFD has later been developed into the commercial product Muse (Certara, L.P., St. Louis, MO). Another approach called NovoFLAP combines the EA-Inventor algorithm with a powerful ligand-based scoring function that uses both molecular shape and pharmacophore features in a multiconformational context (FLAP) (Damewood et al. 2010). Qsearch is a fast algorithm that stochastically constructs new molecules from fragment spaces considering a 3D pharmacophore including not only feature addition steps but also undecoration of the compounds. Finally, an interesting and surprising approach called the metastructure approach can provide an alternative route for lead identification when no structural information of the target is available (Henen et al. 2012). This method searches for protein targets with similar activity but possibly completely different fold based only on primary sequence and exploits structural information of known active ligands of the similar protein targets in *de novo* compound design.

14.3.3 Fragment Optimization for Targets with Little or No Structural Information

GPCRs constitute the largest target family in drug design, however, due to the complex nature of the membrane-embedded dynamics, their crystallization is not yet a routine task and it usually requires heavy protein engineering investments as well. Besides the undruggable rhodopsin, beta adrenergic and adenosine receptors are the only GPCRs with multiple reported x-ray structures; thus structure-based design efforts could only be successfully undertaken mainly in these receptor subfamilies so far. Altogether x-ray structures of 21 out of the 779 distinct GPCRs have been solved (May 2014), thus coverage is still small and for the majority of GPCR drug targets homology modeling with limited accuracy is the only possibility for structure-based studies. Fragment-based lead discovery on GPCRs has been reviewed by Visegrády and Keserű (2013). Virtual fragment screening has been reported on histamine H_1 (de Graaf et al. 2011) and H_3 (Sirci et al. 2012) and adenosine A_{2A} receptors (Chen et al. 2013). Limited expansion of fragment hits has been pursued in the absence of structural information, for example, on adenosine A_3 (Stoddart et al. 2012) and melanocortin MC_4 receptors (Albert et al. 2007). Structure-based optimization of several fragment-like adenosine A_{2A} receptor hits using Glide for docking has been reported by Heptares (Congreve et al. 2012; Langmead et al. 2012) and a complete *in silico*-assisted lead discovery project has also been reported for the A_{2A} receptor by ZoBio and academic groups (Chen et al. 2013). In this project, NMR and docking-based virtual screening were run parallel and showed fair agreement, while also a larger fragment library was screened virtually, which provided further hits. Altogether 14 validated hits were identified and three of them were subsequently expanded guided by MD simulations and free energy calculations (FEP) using the free GROMACS software.

Use of modern *de novo* design tools in the absence of structural information has been reported in the optimization of GnRH receptor, serotonin $5HT_{1B}$ receptor, and selective adenosine A_1 receptor ligands. EA-Inventor was used by Neurocrine to select optimal side-chain combinations for a core identified by virtual screening for GnRHR (Feher et al. 2008). Compounds were selected based on similarity to reference compounds, fitting to a 3D pharmacophore and property filters, but synthetic accessibility was checked by medicinal chemists. NovoFLAP was used by AstraZeneca to design the first nonbasic $5HT_{1B}$ antagonist (Damewood et al. 2010). The basic amine moiety from a reference dihydrochromene ligand was redesigned to afford compounds with no hERG or phospholipidosis liabilities. Finally, MOEA was developed and used by academic groups in the design of adenosine A_1 receptor ligands selective against adenosine A_{2A}, A_{2B}, and A_3 receptors (van der Horst et al. 2012). A 3D pharmacophore model for A_1 and three support vector machine (SVM) models for selectivity along with ADMET filters (Lipinski parameters, solubility, and mutagenicity) were used in compound selection, which in this case was also supported by synthetic accessibility check by medicinal chemists.

14.3.4 LE Metrics in Fragment Optimization

Fragment-based optimization, as any medicinal chemistry optimization, is a multiobjective task, where not only affinity to the target but also selectivity, antitarget activity, pharmacodynamic and pharmacokinetic properties all have to be balanced. Fragments have the advantage of possessing favorable binding and physicochemical properties from the start and the goal is to maintain these favorable properties during optimization. LE and lipophilic efficiency metrics provide an aid in navigating the complex multiparametric property space of compounds. The original LE metric as the binding free-energy per heavy atom of the ligand was introduced by Hopkins in 2004 with selection of HTS hits with better optimizability in mind (Hopkins et al. 2004). Ligands with LE values greater than 0.3 kcal/mol are generally considered efficient binders. Alternative metrics with molar mass (in BEI) or polar surface area (in SEI) instead of heavy atom count were proposed by Abad-Zapatero (2007). Since then it was shown that the LE metric is size dependent and overemphasizes the effectiveness of very small fragments. Thus, if fragments are prioritized solely based on LE, smaller ligands will stand a higher chance of good ranking. An LE metric scaled by an exponential factor of heavy atom count was proposed by Reynolds et al. (2007) and the percentage of the actual LE of the maximal achievable LE is called fit quality (FQ). Orita et al. (2009) used a similar approach with a different exponential scaling

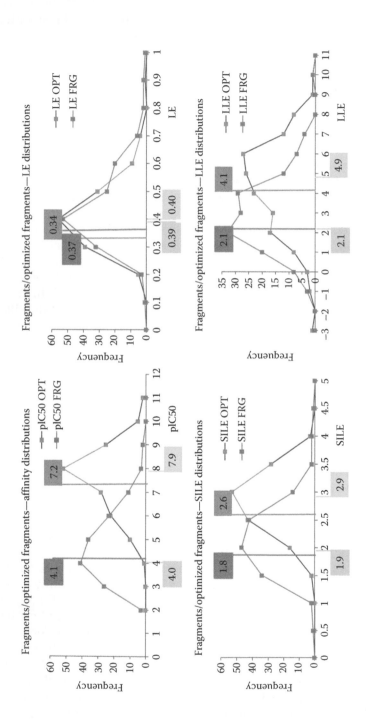

FIGURE 14.6
(See color insert.) Distribution of affinity, LE, SILE, and LLE of fragment hits and optimized compounds. (Adapted with permission from Ferenczy, G. G. and G. M. Keserü. 2013. *J. Med. Chem.* 56(6): 2478–2486. Copyright 2013, American Chemical Society.)

function based on the golden ratio. Nissink (2009) proposed an alternative solution for the problem, namely, instead of the heavy atom count, the cubic root of the heavy atom count was used in the formula of size-independent ligand efficiency (SILE). Though simpler than FQ, SILE has been debated to retain some size dependency.

Lipophilic efficiency metrics were introduced later in order to simultaneously consider binding efficiency and lipophilicity, which is known to have a great effect on compound quality and attrition by being more selective and having fewer ADMET and pharmacokinetics-related problems. Ligand-lipophilicity efficiency (LLE) (the difference between the negative logarithm of affinity and logp) was introduced by Leeson and Springthorpe (2007) to estimate the maximally accepted lipophilicity for a compound of given potency. They proposed a separation of at least 5 log units between potency and lipophilicity. LELP defined by the ratio of logp and LE was introduced by Keserű and Makara (2009). Though the LELP function behaves undesirably for compounds with logp ≤ 0, this is rarely a problem in lead discovery programs. It was shown that compounds with LELP values lower than 10 have higher chances to be free of ADME and safety issues in terms of permeability, clearance, efflux transport, CYP induction, hERG inhibition, and cell viability (Tarcsay et al. 2012). While LLE does not separate HTS and fragment hits, LELP has the advantage of discriminating preferred starting points effectively. The simultaneous application of the LLE > 5 and LELP < 10 cutoffs could select compounds advanced to phase II clinical trials and approved drugs from other compound types. Orita et al. (2011) and more recently Hopkins et al. (2014) reviewed the use of different efficiency indices.

Ferenczy and Keserű (2013) analyzed trends in 145 fragment optimization programs and found that accompanying a median affinity increase of 3 and logp increase of 1.5 log units LE is generally unchanged, while SILE is preferably increased during fragment optimization. LLE and LELP usually also increase but not in such a straightforward manner (see Figure 14.6). Hence the authors propose the monitoring of SILE and LELP in the course of optimization in order to arrive at efficient and safe compounds that have a higher chance of being successful.

References

Abad-Zapatero, C. 2007. Ligand efficiency indices for effective drug discovery. *Expert Opin. Drug Discov.* 2(4): 469–488.

Albert, J. S. et al. 2007. An integrated approach to fragment-based lead generation: Philosophy, strategy and case studies from AstraZeneca's drug discovery programmes. *Curr. Top. Med. Chem.* 7(16): 1600–1629.

Babaoglu, K. and B. K. Shoichet. 2006. Deconstructing fragment-based inhibitor discovery. *Nat. Chem. Biol.* 2(12): 720–723.

Beccari, A. R., Cavazzoni, C., Beato, C., and G. Costantino. 2013. LiGen: A high performance workflow for chemistry driven *de novo* design. *J. Chem. Inf. Model.* 53(6): 1518–1527.

Bemis, G. W. and M. A. Murcko. 1996. The properties of known drugs. 1. Molecular frameworks. *J. Med. Chem.* 39(15): 2887–2893.

Bhurruth-Alcor, Y. et al. 2011. Synthesis of novel PPARalpha/gamma dual agonists as potential drugs for the treatment of the metabolic syndrome and diabetes type II designed using a new *de novo* design program PROTOBUILD. *Org. Biomol. Chem.* 9(4): 1169–1188.

Blum, L. C., van Deursen, R., and J.-L. Reymond. 2011. Visualization and subsets of the chemical universe database GDB-13 for virtual screening. *J. Comput. Aided Mol. Des.* 25(7): 637–647.

Boda, K., Seidel, T., and J. Gasteiger. 2007. Structure and reaction based evaluation of synthetic accessibility. *J. Comput. Aided. Mol. Des.* 21(6): 311–325.

Böhm, H. J. 1992. The computer program LUDI: A new method for the *de novo* design of enzyme inhibitors. *J. Comput. Aided. Mol. Des.* 6(1): 61–78.

Brožič, P. et al. 2012. Selective inhibitors of aldo-keto reductases AKR1C1 and AKR1C3 discovered by virtual screening of a fragment library. *J. Med. Chem.* 55(17): 7417–7424.

Card, G. L. et al. 2005. A family of phosphodiesterase inhibitors discovered by cocrystallography and scaffold-based drug design. *Nature Biotechnology* 23(2): 201–207.

Chen, D. et al. 2013. Complementarity between *in silico* and biophysical screening approaches in fragment-based lead discovery against the A(2A) adenosine receptor. *J. Chem. Inf. Model.* 53(10): 2701–2714.

Chen, Y. and B. K. Shoichet. 2009. Molecular docking and ligand specificity in fragment-based inhibitor discovery. *Nat. Chem. Biol.* 5(5): 358–364.

Congreve, M., Carr, R., Murray, C., and H. Jhoti. 2003. A "Rule of Three" for fragment-based lead discovery? *Drug Discov. Today* 8(19): 876–877.

Congreve, M., Chessari, G., Tisi, D., and A. J. Woodhead. 2008. Recent developments in fragment-based drug discovery. *J. Med. Chem.* 51(13): 3661–3680.

Congreve, M. et al. 2012. Discovery of 1,2,4-triazine derivatives as adenosine A(2A) antagonists using structure based drug design. *J. Med. Chem.* 55(5): 1898–1903.

Damewood, J. R., Lerman, C. L., and B. B. Masek. 2010. NovoFLAP: A ligand-based *de novo* design approach for the generation of medicinally relevant ideas. *J. Chem. Inf. Model.* 50(7): 1296–1303.

Davies, D. et al. 2009. Discovery of leukotriene A4 hydrolase inhibitors using metabolomics biased fragment crystallography. *J. Med. Chem.* 52(15): 4694–4715.

de Graaf, C. et al. 2011. Crystal structure-based virtual screening for fragment-like ligands of the human histamine H(1) receptor. *J. Med. Chem.* 54(23): 8195–8206.

de Kloe, G. E., Bailey, D., Leurs, R., and I. J. de Esch. 2009. Transforming fragments into candidates: Small becomes big in medicinal chemistry. *Drug Discov. Today* 14(13–14): 630–646.

Degen, J. and M. Rarey. 2006. FlexNovo: Structure-based searching in large fragment spaces. *Chem. Med. Chem.* 1(8): 854–868.

Dey, F. and A. Caflisch. 2008. Fragment-based *de novo* ligand design by multiobjective evolutionary optimization. *J. Chem. Inf. Model.* 48(3): 679–690.

Durrant, J. D., Amaro, R. E., and J. A. McCammon. 2009. AutoGrow: A novel algorithm for protein inhibitor design. *Chem. Biol. Drug Des.* 73(2): 168–178.

EA-Inventor; Tripos International: St. Louis, MO. http://www.tripos.com

Edink, E. et al. 2011. Fragment growing induces conformational changes in acetylcholine-binding protein: A structural and thermodynamic analysis. *J. Am. Chem. Soc.* 133(14): 5363–5371.

Ekonomiuk, D. et al. 2009. Flaviviral protease inhibitors identified by fragment-based library docking into a structure generated by molecular dynamics. *J. Med. Chem.* 52(15): 4860–4868.

Fechner, U. and G. Schneider. 2006. Flux(1): A virtual synthesis scheme for fragment-based *de novo* design. *J. Chem. Inf. Model.* 46(2): 699–707.

Fechner, U. and G. Schneider. 2007. Flux(2): Comparison of molecular mutation and crossover operators for ligand-based *de novo* design. *J. Chem. Inf. Model.* 47(2): 656–667.

Feher, M. et al. 2008. The use of ligand-based *de novo* design for scaffold hopping and sidechain optimization: Two case studies. *Bioorg. Med. Chem.* 16(1): 422–427.

Fejzo, J. et al. 1999. The SHAPES strategy: An NMR-based approach for lead generation in drug discovery. *Chem. Biol.* 6(10): 755–769.

Ferenczy, G. G. and G. M. Keserű. 2012. Thermodynamics of fragment binding. *J. Chem. Inf. Model.* 52(4): 1039–1045.

Ferenczy, G. G. and G. M. Keserű. 2013. How are fragments optimized? A retrospective analysis of 145 fragment optimizations. *J. Med. Chem.* 56(6): 2478–2486.

Fox, S. et al. 2004. High throughput screening: Searching for higher productivity. *J. Biomol. Screen.* 9(4): 354–358.

Fox, S. et al. 2006. High throughput screening: Update on practices and success. *J. Biomol. Screen.* 11(7): 864–869.

Fukunishi, Y. et al. 2009. *In silico* fragment screening by replica generation (FSRG) method for fragment-based drug design. *J. Chem. Inf. Model.* 49(4): 925–933.

Giordanetto, F., Kull, B., and A. Dellsén. 2011. Discovery of novel class 1 phosphatidylinositide 3-kinases (PI3K) fragment inhibitors through structure-based virtual screening. *Bioorg. Med. Chem. Lett.* 21(2): 829–835.

Gleeson, M. P. and D. Gleeson. 2009. QM/MM as a tool in fragment based drug discovery. A cross-docking, rescoring study of kinase inhibitors. *J. Chem. Inf. Model.* 49(6): 1437–1448.

Good, A. C. et al. 2012. Implications of promiscuous Pim-1 kinase fragment inhibitor hydrophobic interactions for fragment-based drug design. *J. Med. Chem.* 55(6): 2641–2648.

Hann, M. M., Leach, A. R., and G. Harper. 2001. Molecular complexity and its impact on the probability of finding leads for drug discovery. *J. Chem. Inf. Comput. Sci.* 41(3): 856–864.

Hartenfeller, M., Proschak, E., Schuller, A., and G. Schneider. 2008. Concept of combinatorial *de novo* design of drug-like molecules by particle swarm optimization. *Chem. Biol. Drug Des.* 72(1): 16–26.

Hartenfeller, M. et al. 2012. DOGS: Reaction-driven *de novo* design of bioactive compounds. *PLoS Comput. Biol.* 8(2): e1002380.

Hartshorn, M. J. et al. 2005. Fragment-based lead discovery using x-ray crystallography. *J. Med. Chem.* 48(2): 403–413.

Henen, M. A., Coudevylle, N., Geist, L., and R. Konrat. 2012. Toward rational fragment-based lead design without 3D structures. *J. Med. Chem.* 55(17): 7909–7919.

Hert, J. et al. 2009. Quantifying biogenic bias in screening libraries. *Nat. Chem. Biol.* 5(7): 479–483.

Hiss, J. A., Hartenfeller, M., and G. Schneider. 2010. Concepts and applications of "natural computing" techniques in *de novo* drug and peptide design. *Curr. Pharm. Des.* 16(15): 1656–1665.

Hoffer, L. and D. Horvath. 2013. S4MPLE–sampler for multiple protein-ligand entities: Simultaneous docking of several entities. *J. Chem. Inf. Model.* 53(1): 88–102.

Hopkins, A. L., Groom, C. R., and A. Alex. 2004. Ligand efficiency: A useful metric for lead selection. *Drug Disc. Today* 9(10): 430–431.

Hopkins, A. L. et al. 2014. The role of ligand efficiency metrics in drug discovery. *Nature Rev. Drug Disc.* 13(2): 105–121.

Howard, N. et al. 2006. Application of fragment screening and fragment linking to the discovery of novel thrombin inhibitors. *J. Med. Chem.* 49(4): 1346–1355.

Huang, D. et al. 2006. *In silico* discovery of b-secretase inhibitors. *J. Am. Chem. Soc.* 128(16): 5436–5443.

Huang, Q., Li, L. L., and S. Y. Yang. 2010. PhDD: A new pharmacophore-based *de novo* design method of drug-like molecules combined with assessment of synthetic accessibility. *J. Mol. Graph. Model.* 28(8): 775–787.

Ichihara, O., Barker, J., Law, R. J., and M. Whittaker. 2011. Compound design by fragment-linking. *Mol. Inf.* 30: 298–306.

Ji, H. et al. 2008. Minimal pharmacophoric elements and fragment hopping, an approach directed at molecular diversity and isozyme selectivity. Design of selective neuronal nitric oxide synthase inhibitors. *J. Am. Chem. Soc.* 130(12): 3900–3914.

Kawatkar, S., Moustakas, D., Miller, M., and D. Joseph-McCarthy. 2012. Virtual fragment screening: Exploration of MM-PBSA re-scoring. *J. Comput. Aided Mol. Des.* 26(8): 921–934.

Kawatkar, S., Wang, H., Czerminski, R., and D. Joseph-McCarthy. 2009. Virtual fragment screening: An exploration of various docking and scoring protocols for fragments using Glide. *J. Comput. Aided Mol. Des.* 23(8): 527–539.

Keserű, G. M. and G. M. Makara. 2009. The influence of lead discovery strategies on the properties of drug candidates. *Nature Rev. Drug Disc.* 8(3): 203–212.

Kumar, A. and K. Y. Zhang. 2012. Computational fragment-based screening using RosettaLigand: The SAMPL3 challenge. *J. Comput. Aided. Mol. Des.* 26(5): 603–616.

Kutchukian, P. S., Lou, D., and E. I. Shakhnovich. 2009. FOG: Fragment optimized growth algorithm for the *de novo* generation of molecules occupying druglike chemical space. *J. Chem. Inf. Model.* 49(7): 1630–1642.

Langmead, C. J. et al. 2012. Identification of novel adenosine A(2A) receptor antagonists by virtual screening. *J. Med. Chem.* 55(5): 1904–1909.

Leeson, P. D. and B. Springthorpe. 2007. The influence of drug-like concepts on decision-making in medicinal chemistry. *Nature Rev. Drug Disc.* 6(11): 881–890.

Lewell, X. Q., Judd, D. B., Watson, S. P., and M. M. Hann. 1998. RECAP—Retrosynthetic combinatorial analysis procedure: A powerful new technique for identifying privileged molecular fragments with useful applications in combinatorial chemistry. *J. Chem. Inf. Comput. Sci.* 38(3): 511–522.

Li, H., Liu, A., and Z. Zhao. 2011. Fragment-based drug design and drug repositioning using multiple ligand simultaneous docking (MLSD): Identifying celecoxib and template compounds as novel inhibitors of signal transducer and activator of transcription 3 (STAT3). *J. Med. Chem.* 54(15): 5592–5596.

Li, Y., Zhao, Y., Liu, Z., and R. Wang. 2011. Automatic tailoring and transplanting: A practical method that makes virtual screening more useful. *J. Chem. Inf. Model.* 51(6): 1474–1491.

Limongelli, V. et al. 2010. Molecular basis of cyclooxygenase enzymes (COXs) selective inhibition. *Proc. Natl. Acad. Sci. USA* 107(12): 5411–5416.

Lippert, T. et al. 2011. *De novo* design by pharmacophore-based searches in fragment spaces. *J. Comput. Aided. Mol. Des.* 25(10): 931–945.

Liu, Q., Masek, B., Smith, K., and J. Smith. 2007. Tagged fragment method for evolutionary structure-based *de novo* lead generation and optimization. *J. Med. Chem.* 50(22): 5392–5402.

Lovering, F., Bikker, J., and C. Humblet. 2009. Escape from flatland: Increasing saturation as an approach to improve clinical success. *J. Med. Chem.* 52(21): 6752–6756.

Loving, K., Alberts, I., and W. Sherman. 2010. Computational approaches for fragment-based and *de novo* design. *Curr. Top. Med. Chem.* 10(1): 14–32.

Loving, K., Salam, N. K., and W. Sherman. 2009. Energetic analysis of fragment docking and application to structure-based pharmacophore hypothesis generation. *J. Comput. Aided Mol. Des.* 23(8): 541–554.

Macarron, R. 2006. Critical Review of the role of HTS in drug discovery. *Drug Discov. Today* 11(7–8): 277–279.

Makara, G. M. 2007. On sampling of fragment space. *J. Med. Chem.* 50(14): 3214–3221.

Moore, W. R. Jr. 2005. Maximizing discovery efficiency with a computationally driven fragment approach. *Curr. Opin. Drug Discov. Devel.* 8(3): 355–364.

Moriaud, F. et al. 2009. Computational fragment-based approach at PDB scale by protein local similarity. *J. Chem. Inf. Model.* 49(2): 280–294.

Mpamhanga, C. P. et al. 2009. One scaffold, three binding modes: Novel and selective pteridine reductase 1 inhibitors derived from fragment hits discovered by virtual screening. *J. Med. Chem.* 52(14): 4454–4465.

Murray, C. W., Verdonk, M. L., and D. C. Rees. 2012. Experiences in fragment-based drug discovery. *Trends Pharmacol. Sci.* 33(5): 224–232.

Muse, C., L.P., St. Louis, MO. http://www.certara.com/products/molmod/muse/

Neumann, T., Junker, H.-D., Schmidt, K., and R. Sekul. 2007. SPR-based fragment screening: Advantages and applications. *Curr. Top. Med. Chem.* 7(16): 1630–1642.

Newman, J. et al. 2009. Practical aspects of the SAMPL challenge: Providing an extensive experimental data set for the modeling community. *J. Biomol. Screen.* 14(10): 1245–1250.

Nicolaou, C. A., Apostolakis, J., and C. S. Pattichis. 2009. *De novo* drug design using multiobjective evolutionary graphs. *J. Chem. Inf. Model.* 49(2): 295–307.

Nishibata, Y. and A. Itai. 1991. Automatic creation of drug candidate structures based on receptor structure. Starting point for artificial lead generation. *Tetrahedron* 47(43): 8985–8990.

Nissink, J. W. 2009. Simple size-independent measure of ligand efficiency. *J. Chem. Inf. Model.* 49(6): 1617–1622.

Orita, M., Ohno, K., and T. Niimi. 2009. Two "Golden Ratio" indices in fragment-based drug discovery. *Drug Discov. Today* 14(5–6): 321–328.

Orita, M. et al. 2011. Lead generation and examples opinion regarding how to follow up hits. *Methods Enzymol.* 493: 383–419.

Over, B. et al. 2013. Natural-product-derived fragments for fragment-based ligand discovery. *Nat Chem.* 5(1): 21–28.

Oyarzabal, J. et al. 2010. Discovery of mitogen-activated protein kinase-interacting kinase 1 inhibitors by a comprehensive fragment-oriented virtual screening approach. *J. Med. Chem.* 53(18): 6618–6628.

Parker, C. N. and J. Bajorath. 2006. Towards unified compound screening strategies: A critical evaluation of error sources in experimental and virtual high-throughput screening. *QSAR Comb. Sci.* 25(12): 1153–1161.

Parn, J., Degen, J., and M. Rarey. 2007. Exploring fragment spaces under multiple physicochemical constraints. *J. Comput. Aided. Mol. Des.* 21(6): 327–340.

Pierce, A. C., Rao, G., and G. W. Bemis. 2004. BREED: Generating novel inhibitors through hybridization of known ligands. Application to CDK2, p38, and HIV protease. *J. Med. Chem.* 47(11): 2768–2775.

Pitt, W. R., Parry, D. M., Perry, B. G., and C. R. Groom. 2009. Heteroaromatic rings of the future. *J. Med. Chem.* 52(9): 2952–2963.

Proschak, E., Sander, K., and H. Zettl. 2009. From molecular shape to potent bioactive agents II: Fragment-based *de novo* design. *Chem. Med. Chem.* 4(1): 45–48.

Proschak, E. et al. 2009. From molecular shape to potent bioactive agents I: Bioisosteric replacement of molecular fragments. *Chem. Med. Chem.* 4(1): 41–44.

Proudfoot, J. R. 2002. Drugs, leads, and drug-likeness: An analysis of some recently launched drugs. *Bioorg. Med. Chem. Lett.* 12(12): 1647–1650.

Rabal, O., Urbano-Cuadrado, M., and J. Oyarzabal. 2011. Computational medicinal chemistry in fragment-based drug discovery: What, how and when. *Future Med. Chem.* 3(1): 95–134.

Reynolds, C. H., Bembenek, S. D., and B. A. Tounge. 2007. The role of molecular size in ligand efficiency. *Bioorg. Med. Chem. Lett.* 17(15): 4258–4261.

Ritchie, T. J. and S. J. F. Macdonald. 2009. The impact of aromatic ring count on compound developability—Are too many aromatic rings a liability in drug design? *Drug Discov. Today.* 14(21–22): 1011–1020.

Rouhana, J. et al. 2013. Fragment-based identification of a locus in the Sec7 domain of Arno for the design of protein-protein interaction inhibitors. *J. Med. Chem.* 56(21): 8497–8511.

Ruda, G. F. et al. 2010. Virtual fragment screening for novel inhibitors of 6-phosphogluconate dehydrogenase. *Bioorg. Med. Chem.* 18(14): 5056–5062.

Rummey, C., Nordhoff, S., Thiemann, M., and G. Metz. 2006. *In silico* fragment-based discovery of DPP-IV S1 pocket binders. *Bioorg. Med. Chem. Lett.* 16(5): 1405–1409.

Sándor, M., Kiss, R., and G. M. Keserű. 2010. Virtual fragment docking by glide: A validation study on 190 protein–fragment complexes. *J. Chem. Inf. Model.* 50(6): 1165–1172.

Schubert, C. R. and C. M. Stultz. 2009. The multi-copy simultaneous search methodology: A fundamental tool for structure-based drug design. *J. Comput. Aided. Mol. Des.* 23(8): 475–489.

Sheng, C. and W. Zhang. 2013. Fragment informatics and computational fragment-based drug design: An overview and update. *Med. Res. Rev.* 33(3): 554–598.

Siegal, G., Ab, E., and J. Schultz. 2007. Intergration of fragment screening and library design. *Drug Discov. Today.* 12(23–24): 1032–1039.

Sirci, F. et al. 2012. Virtual fragment screening: Discovery of histamine H3 receptor ligands using ligand-based and protein-based molecular fingerprints. *J. Chem. Inf. Model.* 52(12): 3308–3324.

Stoddart, L. A. et al. 2012. Fragment screening at adenosine-A(3) receptors in living cells using a fluorescence-based binding assay. *Chem. Biol.* 19(9): 1105–1115.

Surpateanu, G. and B. I. Iorga. 2012. Evaluation of docking performance in a blinded virtual screening of fragment-like trypsin inhibitors. *J. Comput.-Aided. Mol. Des.* 26(5): 595–601.

Tarcsay, A., Nyíri, K., and G. M. Keserű. 2012. Impact of lipophilic efficiency on compound quality. *J. Med. Chem.* 55(3): 1252–1260.

Teotico, D. G. et al. 2009. Docking for fragment inhibitors of AmpC beta-lactamase. *Proc. Natl. Acad. Sci. USA* 106(18): 7455–7460.

Thompson, D. C. et al. 2008. CONFIRM: Connecting fragments found in receptor molecules. *J. Comput. Aided. Mol. Des.* 22(10): 761–772.

Tiefenbrunn, T. et al. 2014. Crystallographic fragment-based drug discovery: Use of a brominated fragment library targeting HIV protease. *Chem. Biol. Drug Des.* 83(2): 141–148.

Tsai, J. et al. 2008. Discovery of a selective inhibitor of oncogenic B-Raf kinase with potent antimelanoma activity. *Proc. Natl. Acad. Sci. USA* 105(8): 3041–3046.

Tschinke, V. and N. C. Cohen. 1993. The NEWLEAD program: A new method for the design of candidate structures from pharmacophoric hypotheses. *J. Med. Chem.* 36(24): 3863–3870.

van der Horst, E., Marqués-Gallego, P., and T. Mulder-Krieger. 2012. Multi-objective evolutionary design of adenosine receptor ligands. *J. Chem. Inf. Model.* 52(7): 1713–1721.

Vass, M. and G. M. Keserű. 2013. Fragments to link. A multiple docking strategy for second site binders. *Med. Chem. Commun.* 4(3): 510–514.

Venhorst, J., Nunez, S., and C. G. Kruse. 2010. Design of a high fragment efficiency library by molecular graph theory. *ACS Med. Chem. Lett.* 1(9): 499–503.

Verdonk, M. L. et al. 2011. Docking performance of fragments and druglike compounds. *J. Med. Chem.* 54(15): 5422–5431.

Vinkers, H. M. et al. 2003. SYNOPSIS: SYNthesize and OPtimize System *in Silico*. *J. Med. Chem.* 46(13): 2765–2773.

Visegrády, A. and G. M. Keserű. 2013. Fragment-based lead discovery on G-protein-coupled receptors. *Expert. Opin. Drug. Discov.* 8(7): 811–820.

Wetzel, S. et al. 2009. Interactive exploration of chemical space with Scaffold Hunter. *Nat. Chem. Biol.* 5(8): 581–583.

Wilcken, R. et al. 2012. Halogen-enriched fragment libraries as leads for drug rescue of mutant p53. *J. Am. Chem. Soc.* 134(15): 6810–6818.

Yuan, Y., Pei, J., and L. Lai. 2011. LigBuilder 2: A practical *de novo* drug design approach. *J. Chem. Inf. Model.* 51(5): 1083–1091.

Zaliani, A. et al. 2009. Second-generation *de novo* design: A view from a medicinal chemist perspective. *J. Comput. Aided. Mol. Des.* 23(8): 593–602.

Zhao, L. et al. 2013. Fragment-based drug discovery of 2-thiazolidinones as inhibitors of the histone reader BRD4 bromodomain. *J. Med. Chem.* 56(10): 3833–3851.

Section III

Challenges

15

Role of Water Molecules and Hydration Properties in Modeling Ligand–Protein Interaction and Drug Design

Alfonso T. García-Sosa

CONTENTS

15.1 Introduction

Recent findings are changing the view of water molecules in binding events from that of a passive role to a fundamental and driving one. Water molecules can bridge protein–ligand interactions and guide their specificity, energetics both enthalpically and entropically, and kinetics, and all these outcomes depend on the shape, size, chemical, and dynamical nature of protein-binding sites and ligands.

Water molecules may be replaced upon ligand binding, or they can be conserved, or even join concurrent with ligand binding, and in all of these events, binding affinity may be maintained, reduced, or even increased (García-Sosa et al. 2003; Barelier et al. 2013; García-Sosa 2013). Ligands with more water molecules can in some cases actually be stronger than ligands with fewer waters, or no waters (Barelier et al. 2013; García-Sosa 2013).

The polar character and molecular topography of molecular surfaces (shape and physicochemistry of cavities) are determinant for networks of hydrogen-bonded waters, and for the thermodynamics of the hydrophobic effect or the different types of hydrophobic effect, both entropic and enthalpically driven (Snyder et al. 2013).

Water molecules should thus not be disregarded, but considered an integral part of all biomolecular interactions (García-Sosa 2013). Appropriate consideration of these effects can lead molecular design in protein-water-ligand binding systems (García-Sosa and Mancera 2010).

15.2 Water in Biological Systems

Water is essential to living organisms as we know them. It was a likely component of the primordial soup that gave rise to life on earth, and has distinct physicochemical properties that afford it a unique role as solvent, media, support, chemical reaction and energy intermediate, among many others. Indeed, proteins require water to function, and these coordinated functions and equilibria define life (Ball 2003, 2013). Water, in particular the liquid state, is searched for in astronomical environments as a possible location for extraterrestrial life.

15.3 Hydration Effects for Biomolecules and Small Molecules

Water molecules occupy the space between molecules, but they also dictate the structure of biomolecules. Proteins orient their polar amino acids to the outer surface, burying nonpolar groups in their interior. Given that the structure of biomolecules is a major determinant of their function, the role of water is multipronged. Individual water molecules occupy hydration sites on the surface of biomolecules. A first or primary solvation shell can be detected, peaking in radial distribution functions at around 3.5–4 Å, followed by second- and higher-order solvation shells surrounding a biomolecule. This first hydration shell or layer is fundamental to the protein's activity, and has longer duration of contacts than the bulk solvent: from sub-nanosecond, to femto- or picoseconds, respectively (Zhang et al. 2007). They also form networks that can be regular in pentagons and other geometries, surrounding hydrophobic groups in patches (Poornima and Dean 1995a,b,c), and involve cooperative networks of hydrogen bonding. The change in the energy of these water molecule networks can easily determine the energetics of the whole biomolecular system (Baron et al. 2010). Protein folding and protein denaturing, as well as transport, can also be influenced by water molecules. Water also has a direct role in enthalpy–entropy compensation events.

15.4 Explicit Water Molecules in Biomolecular Interfaces

Different methods and tools exist to deal with explicit water molecules in biomolecular interfaces. Consolv uses a k-nearest neighbor algorithm to classify water molecules and their propensity to hydrate polar groups in proteins (Sanschagrin and Kuhn 1998).

15.4.1 WaterScore

WaterScore was developed using a multivariate logistic regression in order to distinguish those explicit water molecules in a protein binding site that were more likely to remain tightly bound to the protein atoms, and which water molecules were likely to be easily displaceable (García-Sosa et al. 2003). Sets of high-resolution x-ray crystal protein structure pairs were compared, to establish which water molecule hydration sites were conserved, that is, an explicit water molecule was observed in the exact same site in another crystal structure of the same protein, versus those displaced (loosely bound). A major feature of the method is the availability to fast score water molecules, using functions that are clearly interpretable and related to observable physicochemical parameters. These parameters are crystallographic B-factor (also called isotropic temperature factor, a measure of the mobility of atoms in a crystal structure determination), number of protein contacts within 3.5 Å (a measure of the degree of association between water molecule and protein surface), and solvent accessible contact surface area (a measure of the degree of exposure of an explicit water molecule to the bulk solvent). The outcome is a probability of an explicitly observed water molecule in a protein-binding site to be classified as conserved or tightly bound, versus displaceable. The probability outcome lies between 0 and 1, and follows a smooth sigmoidal distribution with positive contributions by number of protein contacts, and negative coefficients for B-factor and solvent accessible contact surface area. That is, those water molecules with lower mobility or higher degree of confidence in their crystallographic structure determination, those with higher association to the protein surface, and those less exposed to bulk solvent were shown to be the most likely to reappear in the same position in other crystal structures of the same protein.

15.4.2 Distributions of Protein–Ligand Complexes' Energies and Properties According to the Presence or Absence of Tightly Bound Water Bridges

Experimentally determined inhibition, K_i, or dissociation, K_d, constants for 2332 high-resolution x-ray crystal structures show that there is no statistically significant difference in binding energy between binding sites with tightly bound water molecules and those without (García-Sosa 2013). Other physicochemical properties and ligand efficiencies (Hetényi et al. 2007; García-Sosa et al. 2008, 2009, 2010, 2011, 2012a,b,c; García-Sosa 2013; García-Sosa and Maran 2013) such as molecular mass (MW), number of heavy atoms (NHA), number of carbons (NoC), (García-Sosa et al. 2008), number of atoms, number of hydrogens, number of bonds, number of rings, aliphatic rings, aromatic rings, aromatic atoms, hydrogen bond donors, hydrogen bond acceptors, rotatable bonds, molecular surface area (MSA), polar surface area (PSA), molecular polarizability, Wiener index, Balaban index, Harary index, hyper-Wiener index, Platt index, Randic index, Szeged index, Wiener polarity, the logarithm of the octanol/water partition coefficient ($logP_{octanol/water}$), ΔGbind/MW, ΔGbind/NHA, ΔGbind/NoC, ΔGbind/MSA, ΔGbind/PSA, ΔGbind/Wiener, as well as a lipophilic efficiency index: $log(-\Delta Gbind/P)$ (García-Sosa et al. 2010) and their distributions were also compared between both groups. Lower $logP$ and better developability for tightly hydrated compounds were also beneficial. During ligand optimization, stronger potency is not always required or beneficial. These results also held for drugs/nondrugs comparisons.

The results showed that both agonist and antagonist compounds that use tightly bound water bridges were smaller, less lipophilic, and less planar; had deeper ligand efficiency indices, and in general, possessed better physicochemical properties for further development than agonists and antagonists that did not use tightly bound water bridges (García-Sosa 2013). Tightly bound, bridging water molecules may therefore, in some cases, be replaced and targeted as a strategy, though sometimes keeping them as bridges may be better from a pharmacodynamic point of view. The receptor may have many structure conformations available with the hydrated binding site being one of them. Also, different ligands will have a different ability to select either tightly hydrated or nontightly hydrated or nonhydrated receptor binding site conformations (García-Sosa 2013). Figure 15.1 shows the strong coupling and important mediation that tightly bound water molecules can have in the interior of a protein–ligand binding site.

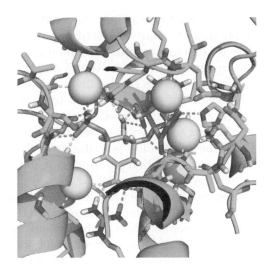

FIGURE 15.1
(**See color insert.**) Strong and important mediation of tightly bound waters in protein–ligand binding shown by a cyclohexene ligand in cocrystal with a phosphate synthase protein.

15.5 Theoretical and Computational Approaches to Hydration Modeling

Water and hydration can be used in biomolecular simulation and computational techniques in several different ways. The most elaborate, though thorough, approach considers waters as explicit, dynamic, flexible, and polarizable molecules. Implicit solvation methods, in contrast, consider a homogeneous region of space surrounding a solute molecule (itself modeled with molecular mechanics force fields), and calculate energies based on electrostatic contributions and nonpolar surface areas. Such methods are used in molecular mechanics/Poisson-Boltzmann-Surface Area (MM/PBSA) and molecular mechanics/Generalized-Born-Surface Area (MM/GBSA) methods for calculating the solvation free energy components of binding, apart from so-called gas-phase energies and entropy components.

Docking is a method of searching for geometries of ligands inside receptor binding sites, and they judge their fit based on structural and energetic scores using a scoring function, usually additive over interaction atom pairs (*i* and *j*). The scoring function for the program Autodock is of the form (Huey et al. 2007):

$$V_{tot} = W_{elec} \sum_{i,j} \frac{q_j q_i}{\varepsilon(r_{ij}) r_{ij}} + W_{vdw} \sum_{i,j} \left(\frac{A_{ij}}{r_{ij}^{12}} - \frac{B_{ij}}{r_{ij}^{6}} \right) + W_{hbond} \sum_{i,j} E(t) \left(\frac{C_{ij}}{r_{ij}^{12}} - \frac{D_{ij}}{r_{ij}^{10}} \right)$$

$$+ W_{sol} \sum_{i,j} (S_i V_j + S_j V_i) e^{(-r_{ij}^2 / 2\sigma^2)} \tag{15.1}$$

where V_{tot} is the total calculated interaction energy, W terms represent different weight constants that are adjusted based on experimental data. The electrostatic term uses a Coulomb potential based on charges and distances between atoms. The van der Waals term calculates dispersion and repulsion interactions using a Lennard-Jones 6/12 potential using A and B parameters from the Amber force field. The hydrogen bond term is a 10/12 potential moderated by the directionality of the possible hydrogen bonds formed, with constants C and D providing well depths at certain distances for O–H and N–H (C), and S–H (D). The desolvation potential uses the volume V of the atoms around another atom, a solvation parameter (S), the distance between them, r, and a distance weighting factor, σ, of 3.5 Å.

FlexX is a docking program that uses a particle concept to precompute favorable discrete water position on the protein surface and to turn off or on these discrete water molecules in specific places of the protein–ligand binding site during docking if they can make additional hydrogen bonds with the ligand (Rarey et al. 1999). A similar option to turn on or off explicit, discrete water molecules are available in the docking software GOLD (Verdonk et al. 2005).

Docking scoring functions can also add explicit water molecules as extensions of ligand structures, to be evaluated during the docking program's search algorithm, and using predetermined water-probe grid maps in the case of AutoDock (Forli and Olson 2012). Only water in grid hotspots and contributing to the enthalpy of the protein–ligand interaction are kept, otherwise, they are "released" to solvent, that is, the docking pose displacing them is favored in the docking pose and ranking search iteration. If they are exposed to solvent, they are discarded with no energy effect, if they are involved a steric clash with protein, then their release provides an entropic reward to the score.

Autodock Vina was used to develop WaterDock, a tool that enables predicting the binding site of water molecules (Ross et al. 2012). Data-mining, heuristic, and machine learning were applied to identify conserved and displaced water molecules in the Astex Diverse Set of protein–ligand complexes. Free energy calculations of different types of explicit water molecules in protein-binding sites, coupled to Bayesian classifiers, have been carried out to compare the different classes of water molecules (Barillari et al. 2007).

Loosely bound water molecules that appear in x-ray crystal protein structures in ligand-binding sites are typically in unstable or imperfect interactions. Their replacement by a well-placed and chemically suited group can be beneficial, and that has been observed repeatedly (Young et al. 2007; Abel et al. 2008, 2011; Guimaraes and Mathiowetz 2010; Nguyen et al. 2014). WaterMap uses the knowledge of these loose sites in order to drive ligand interactions (Young et al. 2007; Abel et al. 2008, 2011; Guimaraes and Mathiowetz 2010). Those water molecules that have less local enthalpy and energy (calculated through molecular dynamics calculations) compared to bulk are used to position ligand atoms. Tightly bound water molecules, on the contrary, will be harder to displace correctly.

Grid-based (Nguyen et al. 2014) and inhomogeneous fluid (Lazaridis 1998) analysis of hydration sites can also provide information on water molecules, and different from implicit solvation models. The transition from loose to tightly ordered in a binding site can even be the driving force in enthalpy and energy changes in a biomolecular association (Timson et al. 2013).

Explicit, tightly bound water molecules on the protein surface do not have the same physicochemical and thermodynamic properties as those in the bulk, that is, bulk or solution waters, and therefore, they should be considered an integral part of the protein. This means that they should not be part of desolvation areas or energy calculations because they can be more ordered than bulk water, that is, their hydrogen bonds and their cooperative intermolecular interactions between them and protein and ligand are stronger than those they would make in solution.

In the double-decoupling method, the standard free energy of water molecules can be calculated and used in connection with thermodynamics integration methods (Hamelberg and McCammon 2004).

15.6 Applications of Explicit Water in Drug Design

Once a water molecule, a group of water molecules or a hydration site has been identified as important for a protein–ligand interaction, and that binding site has been validated for a possible therapeutic effect due to ligand or substrate binding occurring and inhibition or agonist/antagonist activity following, then the following step is how to include those explicit water molecules in drug design.

Biomolecule–water–ligand systems display a delicate interplay of effects that include differences in bulk solvent and in the binding site, as well as conformational states. Compound design may take into account these effects and their change due to modification of a ligand with chemically relevant series of functional groups (García-Sosa and Mancera 2010). In the classical example case of cyclical urea inhibitors of HIV-1 protease, a tightly bound water molecule was targeted with ligand functional groups (a cyclic urea), where a larger hydrophobic effect and lower ligand entropy helped to increase binding (Lam et al. 1994). However, waters may be included in docking (García-Sosa et al. 2011), *de novo* design (García-Sosa et al. 2005; García-Sosa and Mancera 2006), and pharmacophores, (Lloyd et al. 2004) among others (Mikol et al. 1995; Helms and Wade 1998; Ekstrom et al. 2002; Branson and Smith 2004; Hattotuwagama et al. 2006; Monecke et al. 2006; Calderon-Kawasaki et al. 2007; Geroult et al. 2007; Graneto et al. 2007; Kroemer 2007; Seo et al. 2007; Amadasi et al. 2008; Bottcher et al. 2008; Clark 2008; Huang and Shoichet 2008; Huang et al. 2008; Raub et al. 2008; Ellermann et al. 2009; Villacanas et al. 2009; de Beer et al. 2010; de Courcy et al. 2010; Kutchukian and Shakhanovich 2010; Loving et al. 2010; Michel et al. 2010; Andaloussi et al. 2011; Gresh et al. 2011; Huggins and Tidor 2011; Knegtel and Robinson 2011; Meanwell 2011; Rechfeld et al. 2011; Rossato et al. 2011; Waszkowycz et al. 2011; Wong and Lightstone 2011; Trujillo et al. 2012; Zheng et al. 2013).

15.6.1 GRID (Goodford)

The program GRID allows calculating binding sites on molecules that can have favorable energies (Goodford 1985). A GRID map can be run to search for water molecules that the ligand does not displace. If those water molecules are not making hydrogen bonds, then they could be trapped in hydrophobic regions, and as such, would be destabilizing to ligand binding and be unfavorable. Ligand molecules can also be designed to displace these loose, trapped waters.

15.6.2 Cyclin-Dependent Kinase 2, CDK2

One strategy to employ is to use two or more running scenarios, one including an explicit tightly bound water molecule, and another excluding it. The result of each ligand–protein and ligand–water–protein calculation can be compared and the deepest energy (or best score) case kept for further analysis. The inclusion or exclusion of an explicit water molecule will affect the volume, shape, flexibility, dynamics, polarity, and binding partners available to protein and ligand.

As an example, inhibitors of cyclin-dependent kinase 2 (CDK2) were designed (García-Sosa and Mancera 2006). CDK2 is an important enzyme in the cell–lifecycle and is well placed as a target for cancer treatment. The inclusion of an explicit water molecule affected (constrained) the chemical diversity of the fragments produced in the computational *de novo* structure generation.

Also, the inclusion of the tightly bound water molecule HOH100 in *de novo* structure generation runs changed the orientation and binding modes of the ligands, as well as their interaction scores. The change in diversity comes from the position of the explicit, tightly bound water molecule since it is close to the hinge region groups that are recognized to be critical for interaction in CDK2. These groups are the glutamate 81 backbone C=O, and leucine 83 backbone NH and C=O. Given the shape and volume of the binding site in this region, the inclusion of water HOH100 favors those fragments that can connect the critically important groups for binding and the water molecule. It guided the generated ligands to the more favorable section of the binding site. Ideally placed groups for connecting water molecule and hinge region atoms were heterocyclic, moderately small ligands. Each run strategy: (a) including water molecule HOH100; (b) neglecting the water molecule HOH100; or (c) targeting the hydration site of water molecule100, gave different scaffolds and binding motifs. Some of the binding motifs obtained confirmed those for known inhibitors, such as compound BMS-387032 (also called SNS-032) that displaces water molecule HOH100, as well as roscovitine and isopentenyladenine that use water molecule HOH100 in the binding site.

15.6.3 Poly-ADP Ribose Polymerase, PARP

Another example is the search for inhibitors of poly-ADP ribose polymerase (PARP). This is another enzyme that is an important target in cancer treatment, since it repairs damage to DNA previously achieved by chemo- or radiotherapy. It undoes the work, so to speak, of these treatments, so inhibiting it with small molecules would allow those treatments to be more effective. There are two explicit, tightly bound water molecules in the PARP binding site, specifically the nicotinamide binding subsite, HOH 52 and HOH 107 (PDB 1efy). Running structure generation or virtual screening with these two water molecules required nine runs, where each water molecule is included or neglected and the protein interaction groups they shield are considered or not (García-Sosa et al. 2005). The best scoring ligands were produced with two runs: (a) one that included all compulsory groups (atoms shown to interact with several active ligands: Gly 863 O + Gly 863 N + Ser 904 Oγ) + HOH 52+ Ser 864 Oγ; or (b) the three compulsory groups+ Glu 988 Oε1 (the protein group shielded by HOH 52).

Using structure generation or ligand screening runs with both waters reduces chemical diversity the most, but using one specific water molecule or its associated protein groups gave the best scoring ligands. Ignoring all waters does give the highest diversity, but not the best scores. In this case, all nine runs gave clues as to the best size of the binding site, and the best water molecule to include. This knowledge is not straightforward, and requires running the calculations to derive the information that allows improving computational strategies for ligand generation and design.

The scores of the ligands between runs with water and without water were comparable, so these results indicate that although displacing or using tightly bound water molecules can enhance the ligand chemical diversity, there are small differences when comparing the binding energies of ligands computed with docking scoring functions.

15.6.4 Explicit Water Molecules in Pharmacophores

Sets of features present in a protein–ligand-binding site can be used to generate pharmacophores, that is, the smallest possible number of groups assembled in three-dimensional (3D) space that represent the spatial arrangement of chemical groups responsible for the binding of a compound to its receptor. For herpes target thymidine kinase, analysis of the groups in the protein-binding site did not reveal ligand or protein groups in positions that were linking both. Closer analysis of the x-ray crystal structures revealed that these partner groups were explicit water molecules, scored as tightly bound (Lloyd et al. 2004).

It is an often overlooked feature of protein-ligand binding that empty spaces will almost invariably be filled by water molecules at some point in time. Some hydration sites will have higher occupancies than others but an ever present competition unfolds between chemical groups in ligands and protein and water molecules, for binding interactions. When these are of an appropriate nature, such as polar–polar or hydrophobic interactions, hydrogen bonds, *etc.*, then there will be a favorable contribution to binding. When polar groups of any of these three participants are enclosed in hydrophobic spaces, the binding energy usually suffers as a result.

15.6.5 Explicit Water Molecules in HCV, ITK, and Other Targets

Barreca et al. (2014) also showed that including explicit water molecules improved the outcome of virtual screening for inhibitors of the hepatitis C virus enzyme NS5B polymerase. This improvement was found for those compounds that used those explicit waters in the binding site in their complexes to the protein. The reverse effect was shown for those compounds lacking water. The work represents a way forward for treatments that may sidestep the need to use interferon in hepatitis C treatment, as well as showing the importance of including explicit water molecules in protein structures in addition to the influence of the flexibility of the protein on virtual screening results. The described *in silico* procedure was confirmed by the synthesis and evaluation of pyrazolobenzothiazine inhibitors (Manfroni et al. 2014).

Water molecules are also critical for the thermodynamics of proline-rich systems such as the Abl-SH3 domain (Palencia et al. 2004). Thermodynamically unfavorable waters were also used to explain selectivity and design more selective ligands for the interleukin-2 inducible T-cell kinase (Knegtel and Robinson 2011).

Tightly bound waters helped predict and construct an algorithm for protein solvation, called AcquaAlta (Rossato et al. 2011). The algorithm was based on the geometric arrangements of water molecules in crystal structures in the Cambridge Structural Database. *Ab initio* calculations were also performed to judge the propensity of ligand hydration. Considering loosely bound waters decreased the effectiveness of the method for predicting water molecule binding to polar groups and bridging protein and ligand groups.

Even the calculation of nonpolar solvation free energies, usually conducted solely using continuum methods including protein surface areas or volumes, requires explicit water molecules to describe the process and accurately predict them (Genheden et al. 2011). Even in a solvent-exposed binding site, water molecules in the binding site were thus found to have distinct properties from bulk water.

15.6.6 Rigorous Free Energy/Thermodynamic Integration Methods Using Explicit, Tightly Bound Water

A way of including explicit water molecules in designing ligands and bio-molecules would require a correct consideration and calculation of all the effects: energetic, both enthalpic and entropic, as well as dynamic such as conformational, and standard free energy, of the water molecule and its pos-sible chemical group substitutions. This has been precisely achieved (García-Sosa and Mancera 2010) by a study extending the double-decoupling method. Different chemical groups substituted a tightly bound, explicit water mol-ecule bridging protein and ligand by mutation of this water through modifi-cation of the ligand chemical structure. The biological system is the Abl-SH3 domain tyrosine kinase in complex with a peptide ligand and the chemi-cal functional groups included methyl, ethyl, hydroxyl, amine, and amide groups. This responds to a chemically intuitive optimization procedure, where the designer is faced with different chemical routes to modify the ligand. These different chemical functional groups include different sizes, hydrogen bonding capabilities, desolvation energies, flexibilities, polarities, and so on that can have an effect on binding, as well as on solvation, crys-tallization, side-effects, administration, distribution, metabolism, excretion, and toxicity properties, among many others.

The calculations include the energy required to substitute the replaced tightly bound water molecule back into the bulk solvent, which requires energy in the way of cavity formation, hydrogen-bond breaking and form-ing, and can have different hydrogen bonding abilities in the bulk compared to the binding site. It is because of this that each tightly bound, explicit water molecule replacement with a different chemical functional group depends on an exquisite balance of factors in the binding site as compared to the bulk.

The way to calculate the energy of placing a water molecule (solvation energy of a single water molecule) into the bulk solvent is to delete (mutate) a water molecule from the solvent and reverse the sign of the energy change (see Figure 15.2), since it has the same magnitude but opposite direction of the equilibrium reaction. The result of 6.6 kcal/mol for this calculation was in excellent agreement with 6.32 kcal/mol determined experimentally.

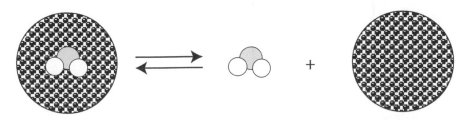

FIGURE 15.2
The free energy of inserting a water molecule into the bulk of water molecules in solution has the same magnitude but reverse sign of extracting a water molecule from bulk solution.

Also required is the energy of removing the tightly bound water molecule bridge from the protein–ligand complex. The calculations also include the correction for the standard free energy of a water molecule (Hamelberg and McCammon 2004). The total energy for removing the tightly bound water molecule and solvating it (introducing it) in bulk solvent was 1.8 kcal/mol. This is a considerable amount of energy required for its removal, or alternatively, the amount of energy neglected when the water molecule is just overlooked in computer modeling calculations. Given that water molecules are commonly overlooked in modeling practices, the finding shows the importance of their inclusion or consideration of the energy required to remove them. The positive value for the transformation shows that it is unfavorable for the system to lose the water molecule, that is, it is more stable as a tightly bound water molecule bridge.

Calculations were performed using molecular dynamics techniques for free energy determination, called thermodynamic integration, where the reaction coordinates are gradually modified in windows during a simulation run, so as to approximate equilibrium. Each window involves a change in the partial charges of the atoms and includes equilibration runs between each window. The number of windows varied, up to over 300 windows per transformation. Initial and final partial charges correspond to the initial and final states of chemical transformation. The annihilation of the tightly bound, bridging water molecule was calculated using absolute energies, while the differences in energy between the ligands were calculated relative to each other, and relative to the wild-type, tightly hydrated state. Transformations were conducted in a thermodynamic cycle, calculating the changes required in the binding site (ΔG_{compl}), as well as the changes in solution (ΔG_{aq}), to compute the overall relative free energy of binding associated with a chemical transformation. This is shown in cycle B in Figure 15.3, where L1 and L2 are ligands differing in a functional group, and P denotes a protein or nucleic acid receptor.

All modifications were made in the *ortho* position of the phenol ring of a tyrosine amino acid on the peptide ligand. The crystal structure and

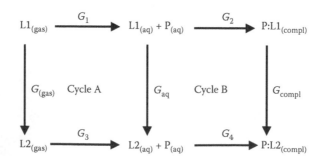

FIGURE 15.3
Closed and complete cycle for calculating the free energy of binding of a ligand mutation with a receptor.

molecular dynamics simulations show that there is a highly present (95% of the time) hydrogen bond between the tightly bound water molecule bridge and the hydroxyl group on serine 12 of the protein.

Hysteresis and other error measures showed errors smaller than 1 kcal/mol for all cases. A full cycle of transformation gave a value of 0.5 kcal/mol, close to the ideal value of zero. The calculated relative free energies of solvation of the ligands were in agreement with experimental values.

The only ligand modifications that were predicted to be favorable in energy were the replacement of the tightly bound water molecule with a hydroxyl, an ethyl, or a formamide group. The hydroxyl group has the best features of the functional groups used to mimic and replace the hydrogen bound interactions that the tightly bound water molecule was forming both with the protein serine and the ligand phenolic OH. The ethyl group does not replace the water molecules' hydrogen bonds but increases the nonpolar interactions through van der Waals contacts even if it has to pay a larger penalty through a higher desolvation free energy (3.2 kcal/mol). For formamide, the overall balance between changes in binding site and in solution gives a free energy change that is nearly zero, but slightly favorable by −0.4 kcal/mol. Formamide is a large group that introduces steric challenges, but is also able to form hydrogen bonds with protein and ligand.

The amino and methyl group substitutions were unfavorable due to the combined energy changes in the complex as well as in solution being smaller than the energy required to replace the tightly bound water molecule.

No new water molecule was observed to occupy the same hydration site as the one that was occupied by the tightly bound water molecule. The study is the first to consider rigorously all energetic and dynamic effects as well as ground state corrections on tightly bound, protein–ligand-bridging water molecule substitution by a series of different chemical functional groups. The transformations indicate that there is an initial energy barrier to overcome, that of replacing the tightly bound water molecule and that not any chemical group is suited for this task. The changes in the interactions involved in the protein–ligand binding, as well as the changes of these species in solvent, indicate that very precise, specific, and delicately balanced changes occur. The overall energy outcome can depend on any of these substeps, as well as on the size, electronic properties, and geometric suitability of a group for the hydration site.

15.7 Concluding Remarks

During drug design if a bridging water molecule is observed in a biomolecular structure in a protein–ligand binding site, it can be replaced if it is not strongly bound to the surface. If it is tightly bound to the protein and/or ligand, then its replacement must be done with full analysis of all outcomes of subsequent ligand modification, since the balance between replacement and conservation will be more refined. These options result in different ligands for either hydrated or nonhydrated binding cases.

References

Abel, R., N. K. Salam, J. Shelley, R. Farid, R. A. Friesner, and W. Sherman. 2011. Contribution of explicit solvent effects to the binding affinity of small-molecule inhibitors in blood coagulation factor serine proteases. *Chem. Med. Chem.* 6(6):1049–1066.

Abel, R., T. Young, R. Farid, B. J. Berne, and R. A. Friesner. 2008. Role of the active-site solvent in the thermodynamics of factor Xa ligand binding. *J. Am. Chem. Soc.* 130(9):2817–2831.

Amadasi, A., J. A. Surface, F. Spyrakis, P. Cozzini, A. Mozzarelli, and G. E. Kellogg. 2008. Robust classification of "relevant" water molecules in putative protein binding sites. *J. Med. Chem.* 51(4):1063–1067.

Andaloussi, M., L. M. Henriksson, A. Wieckowska, A. et al. 2011. Design, synthesis, and x-ray crystallographic studies of alpha-aryl substituted fosmidomycin analogues as inhibitors of mycobacterium tuberculosis 1-deoxy-D-xylulose 5-phosphate reductoisomerase. *J. Med. Chem.* 54(14):4964–4976.

Ball, P. 2003. How to keep dry in water. *Nature* 423(6935):25–26.

Ball, P. 2013. Water in biology. A forum for discussing the behaviour of water in the living cell. http://waterinbiology.blogspot.com/ Accessed 17 December 2013.

Barelier, S., S. E. Boyce, I. Fish, M. Fischer, D. B. Goodin, and B. K. Shoichet. 2013. Roles for ordered and bulk solvent in ligand recognition and docking in two related cavities. *PLoS ONE* 7(8):e69153.

Barillari, C., J. Taylor, R. Viner, and J. W. Essex. 2007. Classification of water molecules in protein binding suites. *J. Am. Chem. Soc.* 129(9):2577–2587.

Baron, R., P. Setny, and J. A. McCammon. 2010. Water in cavity-ligand recognition. *J. Am. Chem. Soc.* 132(34):12091–12097.

Barreca, M. L., N. Iraci, G. Manfroni, R. Gaetani, C. Guercini, S. Sabatini, O. Tabarrini, and V. Cecchetti. 2014. Accounting for target flexibility and water molecules by docking to ensembles of target structures: The HCV NS5B palm site I inhibitors case study. *J. Chem. Inf. Model.* 54(2):481–497.

Bottcher, J., A. Blum, A. Heine, W. E. Diederich, and G. Klebe. 2008. Structural and kinetic analysis of pyrrolidine-based inhibitors of the drug-resistant Ile84Val mutant of HIV-1 protease. *J. Mol. Biol.* 383(2):347–357.

Branson, K. M. and B. J. Smith. 2004. The role of virtual screening in computer-aided structure-based drug design. *Aust. J. Chem.* 57:1029–1037.

Calderon-Kawasaki, K., S. Kularatne, Y. H. Li, B. C. Noll, W. R. Scheidt, and D. H. Burns. 2007. Synthesis of urea picket porphyrins and their use in the education of the role buried solvent plays in the selectivity and stoichiometry of anion binding receptors. *J. Org. Chem.* 72(24):9081–9087.

Clark, D. E. 2008. What has virtual screening ever done for drug discovery? *Expert Opin. Drug Discovery* 3(8):841–851.

de Beer, S. B. A., N. P. E. Vermeulen, and C. Oostenbrink. 2010. The role of water molecules in computational drug design. *Curr. Top. Med. Chem.* 10(1):55–66.

de Courcy, B., J.-P. Piquemal, C. Garbay, and N. Gresh. 2010. Polarizable water molecules in ligand-macromolecule recognition. Impact on the relative affinities of competing pyrrolopyrimidine inhibitors for FAK kinase. *J. Am. Chem. Soc.* 132(10):3312–3320.

Ekstrom, J. L., T. A. Pauly, M. D. Carty et al. 2002. Structure-activity analysis of the purine binding site of human liver glycogen phosphorylase. *Chem. Biol.* 9(8):915–924.

Ellermann, M., R. Jakob-Roetne, C. Lerner et al. 2009. Molecular recognition at the active site of the catechol-o-methyl-transferase: Energetically favorable replacement of a water molecule imported by a bisubstrate inhibitor. *Angew. Chem. Int. Ed.* 48(48):9092–9096.

Forli, S. and A.J. Olson. 2012. A force field with discrete displaceable waters and desolvation entropy for hydrated ligand docking. *J. Med. Chem.* 55(2):623–638.

García-Sosa, A. T. 2013. Hydration properties of ligands and drugs in protein binding sites: Tightly-bound, bridging water molecules and their effects and consequences on molecular design strategies. *J. Chem. Inf. Model.* 53(6):1388–1405.

García-Sosa, A. T., S. Firth-Clark, and R. L. Mancera. 2005. Including tightly-bound water molecules in *de novo* drug design. Exemplification through the *in silico* generation of poly(ADP-ribose)polymerase ligands. *J. Chem. Inf. Model.* 45(3):624–633.

García-Sosa, A. T., C. Hetényi, and U. Maran. 2010. Drug efficiency indices for improvement of molecular docking scoring functions. *J. Comput. Chem.* 31(1):174–184.

García-Sosa, A. T. and R. L. Mancera. 2006. The effect of a tightly bound water molecule on saffold diversity in the computer-aided *de novo* ligand design of CDK2 inhibitors. *J. Mol. Model.* 12:422–431.

García-Sosa, A. T. and R. L. Mancera. 2010. Free energy calculations of mutations involving a tightly bound water molecule and ligand substitutions in a ligand-protein complex. *Mol. Inf.* 29(8–9):589–600. "Hot Article in Biochemistry 2011", named by Wiley.

García-Sosa, A. T., R. L. Mancera, and P. M. Dean. 2003. WaterScore: A novel method for distinguishing between bound and displaceable water molecules in the crystal structure of the binding site of protein-ligand complexes. *J. Mol. Mod.* 9(3):172–182.

García-Sosa, A. T. and U. Maran. 2013. Drugs, non-drugs, and disease category specificity: Organ effects by ligand pharmacology. *SAR QSAR Environ. Res.* 24(4):585–597.

García-Sosa, A. T., U. Maran, and C. Hetényi. 2012a. Molecular property filters describing pharmacokinetics and drug binding. *Curr. Med. Chem.* 19(11):1646–1662.

García-Sosa, A. T., M. Oja, C. Hetényi, and U. Maran. 2012b. Disease-specific differentiation between drugs and non-drugs using principal component analysis of their molecular descriptor space. *Mol. Inf.* 31(5):369–383.

García-Sosa, A. T., M. Oja, C. Hetényi, and U. Maran. 2012c. DrugLogit: Logistic discrimination between drugs and non-drugs including disease-specificity by assigning probabilities based on molecular properties. *J. Chem. Inf. Model.* 52(8):2165–2180.

García-Sosa, A. T., S. Sild, and U. Maran. 2008. Design of multi-binding-site inhibitors, ligand efficiency, and consensus screening of avian influenza H5N1 wild-type neuraminidase and of the oseltamivir-resistant H274Y variant. *J. Chem. Inf. Model.* 48(10):2074–2080.

García-Sosa, A. T., S. Sild, and U. Maran. 2009. Docking and virtual screening using distributed grid technology. *QSAR Comb. Sci.* 28(8):815–821.

García-Sosa, A. T., S. Sild, K. Takkis, and U. Maran. 2011. Combined approach using ligand efficiency, cross-docking, and anti-target hits for wild-type and drug-resistant Y181C HIV-1 reverse transcriptase. *J. Chem. Inf. Model.* 51(10):2595–2611.

Genheden, S., P. Mikulskis, L. H. Hu, J. Kongsted, P. Soderhjelm, and U. Ryde. 2011. Accurate predictions of nonpolar solvation free energies require explicit consideration of binding-site hydration. *J. Am. Chem. Soc.* 133(33):13081–13092.

Geroult, S., M. Hooda, S. Virdee, and G. Waksman. 2007. Prediction of solvation sites at the interface of src SH2 domain complexes using molecular dynamics simulations. *Chem. Biol. Drug Des.* 70:87–99.

Goodford, P. J. 1985. A computational procedure for determining energetically favorable binding sites on biologically important macromolecules. *J. Med. Chem.* 28(7):849–857.

Graneto, M. J., R. G. Kurumbail, M. L. Vazquez et al. 2007. Synthesis, crystal structure, and activity of pyrazole-based inhibitors of p38 kinase. *J. Med. Chem.* 50(23):5712–5719.

Gresh, N., B. de Courcy, J.-P. Piquemal, J. Foret, S. Courtiol-Legourd, and L. Salmon. 2011. Polarizable water networks in ligand-metalloprotein recognition. Impact on the relative complexation energies of Zn-dependent phosphomannose isomerase with D-mannose 6-phosphate surrogates. *J. Phys. Chem. B* 115(25):8304–8316.

Guimaraes, C. R. and A. M. Mathiowetz. 2010. Addressing limitations with the MM-GB/SA scoring procedure using the WaterMap method and free energy perturbation calculations. *J. Chem. Inf. Model* 50(4):547–559.

Hamelberg, D. and J. A. McCammon. 2004. Standard free energy of releasing a localized water molecule from the binding pockets of protein: Double-decoupling method. *J. Am. Chem. Soc.* 126(24):7683–7689.

Hattotuwagama, C. K., M. N. Davies, and D. R. Flower. 2006. Receptor-ligand binding sites and virtual screening. *Curr. Med. Chem.* 13(11):1283–1304.

Helms, V. and R. C. Wade. 1998. Computational alchemy to calculate absolute protein-ligand binding free energy. *J. Am. Chem. Soc.* 120:2710–2713.

Hetényi, C., U. Maran, A.T. García-Sosa, and M. Karelson. 2007. Structure-based calculation of drug efficiency indices. *Bioinformatics* 23(20):2678–2685.

Huang, H. C., D. Jupiter, M. Qiu, J. M. Briggs, and V. VanBuren. 2008. Cluster analysis of hydration waters around the active sites of bacterial alanine racemase using a 2-ns MD simulation. *Biopolymers* 89(3):210–219.

Huang, N. and B. K. Shoichet. 2008. Exploiting ordered waters in molecular docking. *J. Med. Chem.* 51(16):4862–4865.

Huey, R., G.M. Morris, A.J. Olson, and D.S. Goodsell. 2007. A semiempirical free energy force field with charge-based desolvation. *J. Comput. Chem.* 28(6):1145–1152.

Huggins, D. J. and B. Tidor. 2011. Systematic placement of structural water molecules for improved scoring of protein-ligand interactions. *Protein Eng., Des. Sel.* 24(10):777–789.

Knegtel, R. M. A. and D. D. Robinson. 2011. A role for hydration in interleukin-2 inducible T cell kinase (ltk) selectivity. *Mol. Inf.* 30(11–12):950–959.

Kroemer, R. T. 2007. Structure-based drug design: Docking and scoring. *Curr. Protein Pept. Sci.* 50:5712–5719.

Kutchukian, P. S. and E. I. Shakhnovich. 2010. *De novo* design: Balancing novelty and continued chemical space. *Expert Opin. Drug Discov.* 5(8):789–812.

Lam, P. Y. S., P. K. Jadhav, C. J. Eyermann et al. 1994. Rational design of potent, bioavailable, nonpeptide cyclic ureas as HIV protease inhibitors. *Science* 263(5145):380–384.

Lazaridis, T. 1998. Inhomogeneous fluid approach to solvation thermodynamics. 1. Theory. *J. Phys. Chem. B* 102(18):3531–3541.

Lloyd, D. G., A. T. García-Sosa, I. L. Alberts, N. P. Todorov, and R. L. Mancera, R. L. 2004. The effect of tightly bound water molecules on the structural interpretation of ligand-derived pharmacophore models. *J. Comput.-Aided Mol. Des.* 18(2):89–100.

Loving, K., I. Alberts, and W. Sherman. 2010. Computational approaches for fragment-based and *de novo* design. *Curr. Top. Med. Chem.* 10(1):14–32.

Manfroni, G., D. Manvar, M. L. Barreca, N. Kaushik-Basu, P. Leyssen, J. Paeshuyse, R. Cannalire et al. 2014. New pyrazolobenzothiazine derivatives as hepatitis C virus NS5B polymerase palm site I inhibitors. *J. Med. Chem.* 57(8):3247–3262.

Meanwell, N. A. 2011. Synopsis of some recent tactical applications of bioisosteres in drug design. *J. Med. Chem.* 54(8):2529–2591.

Michel, J., J. Tirado-Rives, and W. L. Jorgensen. 2010. Prediction of the water content in protein binding sites. *J. Phys. Chem. B* 113(40):13337–13346.

Mikol, V., C. Papageorgiou, and X. Borer. 1995. The role of water molecules in the structure-based design of (5-hydroxynorvaline)-2-cyclosporin: Synthesis, biological activity, and crystallographic analysis with cyclophilin A. *J. Med. Chem.* 38(17):3361–3367.

Monecke, P., T. Borosch, R. Brickmann, and S. M. Kast. 2006. Determination of the interfacial water content in protein-protein complexes from free energy simulations. *Biophys. J.* 90(3):841–850.

Nguyen, C. N., A. Cruz-Balberdy, M. K. Gilson, and T. Kurtzman. 2014. Thermodynamics of water in an enzyme active site: Grid-based hydration analysis of coagulation faxtor Xa. *J. Chem. Theory Comput.* 10(7):2769–2780.

Palencia, A., E. S. Cobos, P. L. Mateo, J. C. Martinez, and I. Luque. 2004. Thermodynamic dissection of the binding energetics of proline-rich peptides to the Abl-SH3 domain: Implications for rational ligand design. *J. Mol. Biol.* 336(2):527–537.

Poornima, C. S. and P. M. Dean. 1995a. Hydration in drug design. 2. Influence of local site surface shape on water binding. *J. Comput.-Aided Mol. Des.* 9:513–520.

Poornima, C. S. and P. M. Dean. 1995b. Hydration in drug design. 3. Conserved water molecules at the ligand-binding sites of homologous proteins. *J. Comput.-Aided Mol. Des.* 9:521–531.

Poornima, C.S. and P. M. Dean. 1995c. Hydration in drug design. 1. Multiple hydrogen-bonding features of water molecules in mediating protein-ligand interactions. *J. Comput.-Aided Mol. Des.* 9:500–512.

Rarey, M., B. Kramer, and T. Lengauer. 1999. The particle concept: Placing discrete water molecules during protein-ligand docking predictions. *Proteins* 34(1):17–28.

Raub, S., A. Steffen, A. Kamper, and C. M. Marian. 2008. AIScore—Chemically diverse empirical scoring function employing quantum chemical binding energies of hydrogen-bonded complexes. *J. Chem. Inf. Model.* 48(7):1492–1510.

Rechfeld, F., P. Gruber, J. Hofmann, and J. Kirchmair. 2011. Modulators of protein-protein interactions—Novel approaches in targeting protein kinases and other pharmaceutically relevant biomolecules. *Curr. Top. Med. Chem.* 11(11):1305–1319.

Ross, G. A., G. M. Morris, and P. C. Biggin. 2012. Rapid and accurate prediction and scoring of water molecules in protein binding sites. *PLoS One* 7:e32036.

Rossato, G., B. Ernst, A. Vedani, and M. Smiesko. 2011. AcquaAlta: A directional approach to the solvation of ligand-protein complexes. *J. Chem. Inf. Model.* 51(8):1867–1881.

Sanschagrin, P. C. and L. A. Kuhn. 1998. Cluster analysis of consensus water sites in thrombin and trypsin shows conservation between serine proteases and contributions to ligand specificity. *Prot. Sci.* 7(10):2054–2064.

Seo, J., J. Igarashi, H. Li et al. 2007. Structure-based design and synthesis of Nw-nitro-L arginine-containing peptidomimetics as selective inhibitors of neuronal nitric oxide synthase. Displacement of the heme structural water. *J. Med. Chem.* 50(9):2089–2099.

Snyder, P. W., M. R. Lockett, D. T. Moustakas, and G. M. Whitesides. 2013. Is it the shape of the cavity, or the shape of the water in the cavity? *Eur. Phys. J. Special Topics* 223(5):853–891.

Timson, M. J., M. R. Duff, G. Dickey, A. M. Saxton, J. I. Reyes-De-Corcuera, and E. E. Howell. 2013. Further studies on the role of water in R67 dihydrofolate reductase. *Biochemistry* 52(12):2118–2127.

Trujillo, J. I., J. R. Kiefer, W. Huang et al. 2012. Investigation of the binding pocket of human hematopoietic prostaglandin (PG) D2 synthase (hH-PGDS): A tale of two waters. *Bioorg. Med. Chem. Lett.* 22 (11):3795–3799.

Verdonk, M. L., G. Chessari, J. C. Cole et al. 2005. Modeling water molecules in protein-ligand docking using GOLD. *J. Med. Chem.* 48(20):6504–6515.

Villacanas, O., S. Madurga, E. Giralt, and I. Belda. 2009. Explicit treatment of water molecules in protein-ligand docking. *Curr. Comput.-Aided Drug Des.* 5(3):145–154.

Waszkowycz, B., D. E. Clark, and E. Gancia. 2011. Outstanding challenges in protein-ligand docking and structure-based virtual screening. *Wiley Interdiscip. Rev.: Comput. Mol. Sci.* 1(2):229–259.

Wong, S. E. and F. C. Lightstone. 2011. Accounting for water molecules in drug design. *Expert Opin. Drug Discov.* 6(1):65–74.

Young, T., R. Abel, B. Kim, B. J. Berne, and R. A. Friesner. 2007. Motifs for molecular recognition exploiting hydrophobic enclosure in protein-ligand binding. *Proc. Natl. Acad. Sci. USA* 104(3):808–813.

Zhang, L., L. Wang, Y.-T. Kao, W. Qiu, Y. Yang, O. Okobiah, and D. Zhong. 2007. Mapping hydration dynamics around a protein surface. *Proc. Nat. Acad. Sci. USA* 104(47):18461–18466. Bibcode:2007PNAS.10418461Z.

Zheng, M., Y. Li, B. Xiong, H. Jiang, and J. Shen. 2013. Water PMF for predicting the properties of water molecules in protein binding site. *J. Comput. Chem.* 34(7):583–592.

16

How Protein Flexibility Can Influence Docking/Scoring Simulations

Pietro Cozzini, Luca Dellafiora, Tiziana Ginex, and Francesca Spyrakis

CONTENTS

16.1 Introduction

Flexibility has always represented a fundamental issue for *in silico* chemistry, especially for docking. In many cases, a limited simulation of proteins intrinsic flexibility can, in fact, result in meaningless binding scores, even if a reliable and possibly correct binding pose is obtained (Cozzini et al. 2008).

The old and too simple "lock and key" model does not represent the real behavior of biological system (e.g., protein-ligand-water): we need a locksmith, that is, an appropriate modeling tool, to make the key fit the lock (Kellogg and Abraham 1992).

The fundamental basis for computational simulations is represented by structural data, which might come from x-ray or neutron diffraction, nuclear magnetic resonance (NMR) analyses, or homology modeling simulations.

We always used to consider x-ray information as more reliable and more representative of the possible "real structure" of our target protein or protein–ligand complex (Ischima and Torchia 2000). Nevertheless, we have to keep in mind that x-ray solved structures generally represent frozen models of our systems, not accounting for the real and intrinsic protein dynamics. Fortunately, some diffraction parameters could help us in considering and simulating flexibility, as the resolution, the R factor, the thermal motions encoded into the B factors, the occupancy, and so on.

The resolution of the structure is a measure of the quality of the original crystal, and it refers to the amount of information obtained from a crystal in a protein crystallography experiment. We generally consider a resolution value lower than 2.0 Å a marker for "good" structures.

The standard crystallographic R factor is a measure of how well the refined structure predicts the observed data and a reasonable model should give an R not greater than Resolution/10.

The occupancy defines the degree of occupancy of a volume by a specific atom or group of atoms. It is again a measure for the mobility of a group of atoms. In some cases an oxygen atom, belonging to a water molecule (hydrogens are not recognized by x-ray), can show an occupancy of 50% in two distinct positions. It means this water moves between two position centers, and it is not reliable for a good model especially if this water is decisive as bridge between ligand and protein.

The B factors, also known as temperature factors, are parameters accounting for the mobility of each protein atom around a center point, and modeling the static and dynamic disorder. Pdb files retrieved from the Protein Data Bank (PDB) (Bernstein et al. 1977) constitute the main source for protein structural data, and contain information related to the "total" B factor or "mean" B factor, representing the general mobility of the whole protein, and related to specific B "local" factors for each atom. We have to consider that if the B factor of a residue or of a group of atoms is greater than the total protein B factor, it means that that specific region is more mobile than the whole protein, which could be extremely relevant if that particular region falls within the binding site.

B factors are defined as $B = 8\pi^2 U$, where U is a measure of the movements of an atom along three axis due to the isotropic (or anisotropic) thermal motion; for example, in case of isotropic approximation, a B factor value equal to 20 corresponds to an indetermination of 0.25 Å for that specific atom around its equilibrium position. Thermal motions are depicted as ellipsoid where the size along three axes represents the motion along the specific axis (Farrugia 2012).

More structural information about protein mobility could be obtained from NMR studies that are able to distinguish among several conformation states, supplying more structure models for docking. Obviously, if the protein is very flexible in solution, NMR could be unable to determine few stable average models.

A good example of a flexible protein is represented by the Estrogen Receptor (ER). The ER (in the alpha or beta form) is a nuclear receptor (NR) involved in several pathologies, as breast cancer or bone osteoporosis. It belongs to the NRs superfamily, a set of proteins that plays major functions in eukaryotic cell development, reproduction, differentiation, and metabolic homeostasis (Sladek 2011). This huge family counts more than 150 members, steroidal and nonsteroidal receptors and a high number of orphan receptors for which no relevant ligands have been identified.

Even if a significant fraction of family members have been used as drug targets, NRs could also be considered as "nutraceutical" targets since they can interact with food metabolites, xenobiotics, and toxins as well as with drugs.

Endocrine Disrupting Chemicals (EDCs) or simple Endocrine Disruptors (EDs) are compounds in the environment or diet that interfere with normal hormone biosynthesis, signaling, and metabolism (Diamanti-Kandarakis et al. 2009). Many EDCs are able to interfere with the physiological activation of NRs and many of them act through direct interaction with ERs and Androgen Receptors (ARs), causing a wide array of developmental, reproductive, or metabolic diseases (Luccio-Camelo and Prins 2011; Shanle and Xu 2011).

In particular, it has been widely reported that the ER is able to bind different classes of chemicals, food additives, mycotoxins, plasticizers, PCBs, polyphenols, and the like (Fisher 2004).

ER is a ligand-activated receptor, containing six functional domains (A–F): a transcription activation domain (A/B. AF-1), a DNA binding domain (C or DBD), a hinge domain (D), and the second transcription activation domain (E/F, AF-2) also known as the Ligand Binding Domain (LBD) and representing the most important region for docking simulations.

ER shows two different level of flexibility, a "macro" flexibility mainly involving helix 12 (H12), and a "micro" flexibility given by the local arrangements of some residues (His524, Asp353, Arg394), lining the binding site and adjusting according to ligands binding.

Many crystal structures of ER-ligand complexes have been solved and deposited in PDB. Based on these data, we might think that ER can assume only a "close" or "agonist" (e.g., PDB code 2YJA) or an "open" or "antagonist" conformation (e.g., PDB code 1XPC) (see Figure 16.1). Nevertheless, the absence of the crystal structure of the ER apo form and of the intermediate conformations between the close and open models give important clues about the high level of protein dynamics and about the limit of working with crystallographic structures, often able to consider only a few static representation of the real protein conformational space.

In the perspective of providing a more complete description of ER motions, Dal Palu et al. (2012) looked for open/closed intermediate conformations using an innovative *in silico* technique based on constraint logic programming.

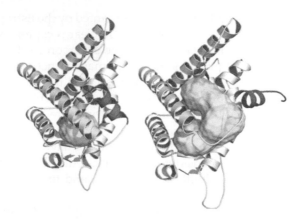

FIGURE 16.1
(See color insert.) The close and open ER α conformations. H12 is colored in red, while the binding site volume is shown in yellow.

Choosing the right conformation for docking experiments still represents a challenging task, in particular when the available models significantly differ one from each other. In the ER case, the close/agonist conformation is generally chosen for simulating the binding of ligands similar to the endogenous substrate 17-β estradiol, while the open/antagonist conformation is used for ligands more similar to the known antagonists Raloxifene or Tamoxifen (Tsai et al. 1999).

A possible solution to avoid the *a priori* choice of a specific conformation could be given by docking each possible ligand in both the open and closed structures. Nevertheless this strategy could lead to a number of false positive given by the ability of smaller molecules to fit the larger open form binding site in many different, and not reliable, forms. A more promising solution could be represented by docking the ligands of interest in a set of intermediate conformations, generated by classical or enhanced molecular dynamics (MD) simulations, and then by selecting the highest scored complexes, possibly corresponding to the more reliable states.

Thus, till now we are forced to assume the close conformation to dock molecules with the same scaffold of 17β estradiol and with some of the three attachment points well known in ER LBD cavity: two polar interactions at the ends of the molecule and a Π–Π interaction between the hydrophobic scaffold of the ligand and the hydrophobic amino acids of the cavity.

In the following paragraphs, we provide (i) an overview of the methodologies and the algorithms used to model protein flexibility in docking, (ii) a description of the MD techniques used to describe limited and extended dynamics, and of the pros and cons related to MD simulations, and (iii) a real case study, that is, the AR, describing how docking and scoring techniques can take into account the intrinsic protein flexibility and when it is really worth to do it.

16.2 Docking Softwares: Methods and Fexibility

The tight structural complementarity between protein and ligand in a host–guest complex is due to mutual conformational changes, as a consequence of the binding event, commonly referred to as "induced-fit." Ligands undergo some conformational motions in order to satisfy spatial requirements of the target ligand-binding pocket. It is to be noted that in some cases small molecules conformation within protein–ligand complex may not correspond to the lower energy state of the molecule in solution (Perola and Charifson 2004). In the meanwhile, proteins may be subjected to several ligand-induced conformational changes comprised between small side-chain adjustments and massive reorganization of entire domains. Since molecular docking is a computational method mostly aimed to compute the binding event between a given host (typically a protein) and guests (typically small molecules), docking procedures need to consider, at least in some extent, mutual conformational reorganizations arising from protein–ligand interaction. However, in order to deal with the effects of protein flexibility on docking simulations, it should be kept in mind how flexibility is treated in docking studies. Some of the most valuable approaches for taking into account intrinsic protein and ligand flexibility in docking simulations are reported below.

16.2.1 Ligand Flexibility

Albeit ligand flexibility still represents a challenging task, it is a common practice to simulate it in docking techniques. The strategies handling ligand motions can be classified depending on how they treat molecule body. We can distinguish between whole-molecule approaches and fragment-based techniques (Sotriffer 2011) or, according to the algorithm used to generate poses, among systematic, random, or stochastic methods, and simulation methods. According to the latter categorization, the systematic search algorithms attempt to explore all the degrees of freedom in a molecule by using conformational search methods (namely, all rotatable bonds are systematically rotated until all possible combinations have been generated and evaluated), or fragmentation methods (where ligand is split into fragments and then reconstructed in the ligand pocket), or database methods (which use libraries of pregenerated conformations). Random search algorithms sample the conformational space by performing random changes to a single ligand or a population of ligands and each change is accepted or rejected on the basis of predefined probability functions. Such approaches mainly use Monte Carlo methods, where the acceptance criteria for obtained poses are based on a Boltzmann probability function, genetic algorithms, which represent the ligand conformations in a modular fashion by using operations similar to mutations and crosses, and Tabu search methods, where the investigation of already explored areas is prevented.

In the most straightforward whole-molecule approaches, the ligand conformational space and orientation search are performed separately. Thus, ensembles of conformers are first generated and then docked into the target pocket (Wang et al. 1999). The multiconformer docking may be effective in the case of molecules sharing a limited number of low-energy conformations, but for highly flexible molecules it becomes less suitable since the number of possible conformers drastically increases. Alternatively, a more rigorous treatment of whole-molecule ligand flexibility is performed by sampling the ligand conformational space during docking simulations (Sotriffer 2011). GOLD (Genetic Optimisation for Ligand Docking; [Verdonk et al. 2003]), Autodock (Morris et al. 2009), and Autodock Vina (Trott and Olson 2010), for instance, exploit genetic algorithms to generate and sample poses. In such cases, the quality of results is affected by the starting genes, the number of evolutionary events, and the scoring function used to identify the more favorable conformers. The main drawback of these approaches is that they may be too slow when the ligands are markedly flexible and the number of consistent conformers increases substantially (Halperin et al. 2002). Another popular example is given by ICM method, which generates conformational ensembles operating on internal coordinates and employs multiple stochastic runs to sample poses (Neves et al. 2012). Conversely, in fragment-based techniques the ligand is dissected into molecular fragments, which can be individually docked and reconnected (typically used in *de novo* design programs) or built incrementally according to a given fragmentation scheme. A popular example of these approaches is represented by FlexX (Kramer et al. 1999; Rarey et al. 1996), based on a robust incremental construction algorithm by which ligands are deconstructed into fragments and then rebuilt into the active site using different placement strategies. Another example is given by the Surflex software (Jain 2003), a fully automatic flexible molecular docking algorithm based on incremental strategies combining the scoring function from the Hammerhead docking system (Welch et al. 1996) with a search engine that relies on a surface-based molecular similarity method. The more recent Surflex-Dock presents some methodological enhancements for search process such as ring flexibility, ligand energetic modeling, and knowledge-based docking (Jain 2007). A different strategy is adopted by the Electronic High Throughput Screening program (eHiTS; Zsoldos et al. 2006) as it attempts to find a global optimum based on individually docked fragments, instead of using the incremental model.

16.2.2 Protein Flexibility

While ligand flexibility is commonly considered in docking simulations, handling protein motions still remains a challenge, mainly because of the dynamic complexity and the computational time required for running the simulations. Ideally, since the proteins are inherently dynamic and flexible systems (Kamerzell and Middaugh 2008; Spyrakis et al. 2011), the perfect tool should be able to treat proteins as full-flexible bodies in order to simulate any ligand-induced conformational rearrangement. In practice, such a tool cannot be implemented. The exhaustive calculation of protein motions and the simultaneous docking of ensemble of ligand conformers (pregenerated or generated and sampled during docking simulations) are still unfeasible mainly due to the high cost in terms of computing time needed to sufficiently explore protein conformational space. However, over the years several strategies have been developed to compute the most important degrees of protein flexibility. According to the categorization proposed by Teodoro and Kavraki (Teodoro and Kavraki 2003), five main approaches have been reported: (i) Soft-docking methods. These methods typically allow some degree of atom–atom overlapping depenalizing intermolecular clashes. The conformational adjustments are not explicitly calculated since protein flexibility is implicitly considered by reducing van der Waals contributions to the total energy evaluation. In this way, docking simulations are usually fast but the extension and the magnitude of the "soft" region is not easily *a priori* determined. Also, these methodologies are not usable in case of particularly flexible proteins where ligand-induced conformations substantially different from the input structure are difficult to obtain. (ii) Methods based on the selection of a limited number of degree of freedom within the ligand-binding pocket (e.g., rotations around single bonds). Only subsets of movable atoms are explicitly computed, thus reducing the complexity of computation. Typically, these subsets contain atoms of the side-chains lining the binding site and the conformers are modeled by using continuous torsional degrees of freedom or rotamers libraries. Alternatively, flexibility of pocket side-chains may be modeled replacing with alanine a given set of residues, which are then reconstructed after ligand placement. This approach is adopted, for instance, by the software Glide (Sherman et al. 2006) that uses soft docking for the preliminary placement of ligand, applies pocket minimization after side-chains reconstruction (which includes backbone and ligand) and finally re-docked the ligand without using any soft potential. (iii) Multistructures docking approaches. In these methods protein flexibility is considered by using ensembles of target structures experimentally determined (i.e., NMR or crystallographic data) or computed (e.g., MD simulations). The possibility of considering the entire target flexibility represents the main advantage, even if these methodologies are strictly dependent on the nature of the experimental data. The protein conformational space portrayed by structural studies (i.e., the quantity and quality of different structures of a given target) obviously affects computations based on ensembles of structures experimentally determined but, at some extent, also on computed ensembles since simulations typically use as starting point structures determined by NMR or x-ray analyses. A popular example is represented by the FlexX variant FlexE (Claussen et al. 2001), where the algorithm superimposes target conformations, merges similar parts and handles dissimilar moieties as independent alternatives. Then, according to the scoring function used, the program selects the substructures combination that better complements the ligand under analysis. (iv) Techniques based on molecular simulations, that is, Monte Carlo or MD simulations. The former are based on the random sampling of the conformational space, whereas the latter apply the laws of classical mechanic. The main advantage is given by the possibility of computing high degree of flexibility, otherwise unreachable, even if, on the other hand, the computational costs grow proportionally. (v) Methods based on the employment of collective degree of freedom. Collective degrees of freedom are not native degrees of freedom of molecules, rather they consist of global protein motions resulting from a simultaneous change of all or part of the native degrees of freedom. For instance, in methods based on the calculation of normal modes, the dynamics of protein structure can be described as a superposition of harmonic high-frequency motions and coupled anharmonic low-frequency motions of collective variables corresponding to the normal modes of vibration (Go et al. 1983). By assuming that the protein is at an energy minimum, its flexibility can be represented by using the low-frequency normal modes as degrees of freedom for the system (Teodoro and Kavraki 2003).

As reported above, during the binding event protein and ligand undergo several mutual and simultaneous conformational changes aimed at reaching a minimum energetic state. According to this, the categorization proposed by Wong (2008) acquires relevance, who distinguishes docking strategies on the basis of the coupling of ligand and protein flexibility. Respect to decoupling strategies, which typically generate protein and ligand conformations independently, partially coupled and, even more, fully coupled ligand-protein motion methods represent the most promising techniques. Often these strategies are multistep processes that may involve adaptation and integration of already existing tools. For instance, the actual version of RosettaLigand (Davis and Baker 2009; Meiler and Baker 2006) considers ligand and protein flexibility simultaneously, including all residue side-chains of binding pocket and backbone. The new method extends the RosettaLigand algorithm, which uses Monte Carlo sampling and the Rosetta full-atom energy function. The authors clearly showed how including protein backbone flexibility was useful for correctly docking ligands of Meiler and Baker test set (Meiler and Baker 2006). Another example worthy of mention is given by the docking program GalaxyDock2 (Shin et al. 2013), in which both ligand and receptor conformational degrees of freedom are simultaneously optimized. The program performs conformational space annealing global optimization to find the optimal binding pose of a ligand both in the rigid-receptor mode and in the flexible-receptor mode. Respect to the previous version, GalaxyDock2 uses a more effective method for the generation of initial conformations. Specifically, it uses a fast geometry-based docking method based on the beta-complex (Kim et al. 2010, 2011) that is a structure derived from the Voronoi diagram of receptor atoms. This new feature could enhance both the computational speed and binding mode prediction accuracy.

16.3 Molecular Dynamics Approaches for Modeling Flexibility

It is widely known that motion is essential for proteins' function (Cozzini et al. 2008; Spyrakis et al. 2011). Catalysis, chaperone-assisted folding, protein–protein interactions, protein–nucleic acids interactions, and allosteric regulations, are only some of the biological events requiring proteins breathing and movement.

The presence of multiple structures in the PDB for a single protein in slightly or highly different conformations supports the necessary breathing and dynamics of biological molecules. Since the conformational adjustment of many proteins is often related to the interaction with substrates or ligands, the availability of both known and unknown conformational states is obviously fundamental when trying to discover or design new potential drugs (Nichols et al. 2012). The strategy of using more conformations in computer-aided drug design approaches has been widely applied since it was demonstrated that including protein flexibility improves the quality of the predictions (Sinko et al. 2013). Conformations can be obtained through x-ray and NMR experiments, as reported in the introduction or, alternatively, through Monte Carlo, MD, or enhanced sampling calculations.

If MD applications have always been disadvantaged because of their time-consuming and expensive character, in terms of hardware architecture and time needed for system setting up and simulations running, recent software and hardware advances have made these techniques much more feasible and easy to apply (Amaro and Li 2010; Henzler and Rarey 2010; Kokh et al. 2011; Lill 2011).

The most important and advanced hardware improvements have been represented by the development of the special purpose supercomputer Anton for long MD simulations and by the use of graphics processing units (GPU) for accelerated computing, which also represents a less expensive solution, in comparison to CPU-based high-performance computing (HPC). Some of the most popular softwares as Amber, NAMD, and Gromacs have released specific codes for running simulations on GPU (Stone et al. 2007), and benchmark studies have revealed an impressive improvement in the calculation time (http://www.nvidia.com/object/molecular_dynamics. html). The same DHFR test case was performed at 38.49 ns/day with Amber 12 on 32 Intel E5-2670 2.60 GHz processors and at 54.46 ns/day on a single NVIDIA GTX580 GPU. Also, GPU performances could be improved when running calculations in parallel (http://ambermd.org/gpus/benchmarks. htm). The Anton machine has extended MD simulations into the millisecond scale (Shaw et al. 2008), thus allowing the investigation of drugs binding to their protein target (Shan et al. 2011) and of small protein folding processes (Lindorff-Larsen et al. 2011). An interesting review on the development of molecular modeling algorithms that leverage GPU computing, and on the continuing evolution of GPU technology has been provided by Stone and coworkers (2010). At the same time, softwares and algorithms for enabling large-scale samplings have been developed and will be reported later.

16.3.1 The Dynamic Pharmacophore Model

The first MD application for drug design was performed more than 30 years ago (McCammon et al. 1977), but the first experimental confirmation of the utility of using multiple computationally generated structures in an ensemble-based approach arrived 23 years later, when Carlson et al. simulated the dynamics of the apo HIV-1 integrase catalytic domain (Carlson et al. 2000; Lins et al. 1999). Eleven conformations were selected and used to define a dynamic pharmacophore model (DPM), subsequently used to screen the Available Chemical Database, looking for new potential inhibitors. More than 30% of the identified compounds were able to inhibit the target and the DPM re-ranking outperformed any single static pharmacophore model. A similar approach was later applied to HIV-1 protease. Better performances in terms of discrimination between binders and nonbinders were achieved when the MD simulation length was increased (Meagher and Carlson 2004). These results interestingly pointed out how longer simulations length might lead to improved results for CADD applications. A few years later, Carlson's group used the DPM strategy to simulate the flexibility of MDM2-p53 binding site and to search for new inhibitors. Starting from a library of 35,000 compounds, four molecules were found to inhibit the target at 50 µM concentration, after being screened against a 6-site pharmacophore model of the active site (Bowman et al. 2007).

In the last years, more and more experimental evidences have supported the capability of MD-generated ensembles to closely replicate the structural dynamics of proteins in solution (Salmon et al. 2009).

16.3.2 The Relaxed Complex Scheme

An alternative strategy for using multiple MD-generated structures in drug discovery is the relaxed complex scheme (RCS) (Amaro et al. 2008a; Lin et al. 2003). Different from the construction of an average pharmacophore, RCS approaches use snapshots extracted from MD simulation for screening ligand libraries, thus taking into account both protein and ligand flexibility. These approaches normally combine MD calculations to docking algorithms and scoring functions, used for the identification of the lower energy, and thus more probable, complexes.

RCS techniques have been applied by Lin et al. (2002) to the FKBP binding protein, demonstrating that docking results are extremely sensitive to receptor conformations. Improved rescoring functions based on MM-PBSA models was adopted. Schames et al. (2004) performed 2 ns MD simulation onto HIV-1 integrase, identifying a new possible pocket adjacent to the known binding site. Docking of ligands into the alternative pocket gave better results than docking into the active site, thus opening the unexpected possibility for the design of new inhibitors. Further experiments demonstrated the reliability of the simulations and supported again the necessity of taking into account receptor flexibility in CADD (Summa et al. 2008). RCS techniques have also been successfully applied by Durrant et al. (2010) when looking for inhibitors of *Tripanosoma brucei* uridine diphosphate galactose 4′-epimerase, (Durrant et al. 2010) and by Sinko et al. (2011) for targeting the antibacterial target undecaprenyl pyrophosphate synthase and looking for rarely sampled ligand-bound conformational states. New compounds have also been identified through RCS methodologies by Cheng and coworkers (2008), for inhibiting neuraminidase in avian influenza.

16.3.3 Clustering

Given the constant improvement of hardware and software performances, and the increasing feasibility of running increasingly longer simulations, methods for clustering and selecting representative conformations have become more and more necessary. The advantage is mainly associated with the reduction of the data quantity and the calculation time required for the following docking and scoring analyses, since some properly selected structures may cover a large conformational space without redundant information. More represented structures should, in principle, correspond to more favorable energetic states and might, thus, be overscored in order to account more than rarely sampled conformations. Unfortunately, this does not represent a universal solution since, sometimes, very rare structure could be the most important in compound binding.

First, clustering methodologies used as discriminating factor the root mean square deviation (RMSD), which should extract the most diverse and dominant conformations generated during MD simulations. Also, more populated clusters should correspond to more energetically favorable, and thus more representative and reliable, conformations.

RMSD-based clustering has been applied to both DPM and RCS approaches. Again looking for HIV-1 integrase inhibitors Deng et al. refined a DPM procedure via RMSD-based clustering. The final conformational ensemble comprised 10 different conformations, collectively representing 50% of the trajectory, that were used to screen an in-house database of about 400 compounds. Of these, 23 compounds were selected and nine proved to be active at a concentration equal or less than 100 μM (Deng et al. 2005). An RMSD clustering example was also provided by Chen et al., who applied it to RCS-based simulations. The authors run a 40 ns-long simulation of avian influenza N1 neuraminidase in both apo and complex forms. Interestingly, the MD was run onto the whole tetramer, while clustering was performed onto individual monomers, thus increasing to 160 ns the global simulation time (Cheng et al. 2008). Multicopy MD approaches have proved to enhance sampling, in comparison with standard single long trajectories (Caves et al.

1998). Members of the three most representative clusters were used for screening the NCIDS1 dataset with AutoDock finding, among 25 selected compounds, 10 with K_i lower than 500 µM. Of these, seven compounds were identified thanks to the presence of conformations characterized by large structural rearrangements.

An alternative and more recent technique for clustering snapshots extracted from MD simulations is represented by QR-factorization. This approach, proposed by O'Donoghue and Luthey-Schulten, is aimed at removing the redundancy from a multiple structural alignment by choosing those structures that better preserve the phylogenetic tree topology of the homologous groups (O'Donoghue and Luthey-Schulten 2005). Application of the QR-factorization approach by Amaro et al. on the RNA editing ligase 1 enzyme in *Tripanosoma brucei* demonstrated its capability of drastically reducing the number of representative conformations and of selecting active compounds which, through standard screening procedure, would not have been identified. The authors concluded that redocking into the QR-reduced set was an efficient way of describing and capturing the intrinsic protein flexibility, without loosing energetic information (Amaro et al. 2008b).

Even if good results have been widely obtained and new inhibitors found in a number of different cases, some simulated conformations may sometimes perform worse than crystallographic structures and, unfortunately, trustworthy protocols for choosing most predictive and reliable models from a simulation are not yet available (Nichols et al. 2011). Thus, if x-ray structures providing a sufficiently large sampling of the conformational space of a specific protein are available, they should represent the best choice rather than using computationally generated conformations (Osguthorpe et al. 2012).

It is, in fact, a general opinion that ensemble-based screening is superior to single-structure screening, in particular when extensive crystallographic data are not available.

This failure can also be attributed to the difficulty of sampling large conformational adjustments with standard MD simulations, thus pointing out the necessity of implementing methods able to provide wider conformational sampling. The timescale of biological motion covers a wide range, from femtosecond required for simple bond vibrations to seconds for more complex collective motions (Henzler-Wildman and Kern 2007), clearly impossible to be reproduced through standard MD simulation.

16.3.4 Enhanced Sampling Techniques

Although microsecond all-atom simulations of entire proteins were performed on dedicated heavily parallel systems (Dror et al. 2009), the simulation of macromolecular aggregates on the microsecond time scale requires further simplifications (Tozzini 2010).

In this perspective, a number of nonconventional MD methodologies able to explore large domain motions and significant active site rearrangements in a computational efficient way have been developed. The rapid progress in computational power and algorithm development is providing the scientific community the necessary tools for shedding light onto complex large-scale conformational transitions and their functional implications, thus opening new possibility for drug design and discovery (Spyrakis et al. 2011).

Coarse-grained techniques enhance the sampling of slow and large-scale motions via simplified descriptions of the degrees of freedom, which are integrated into a few (i.e., coarse graining). Very different levels of coarse-grained techniques can be considered ranging from the "united atoms" approach, where only the hydrogen atoms are eliminated, to mesoscale models with interacting sites representing whole proteins. Overall, the system is modeled as a bead ensemble: lower is the number of the beads, less expensive is the simulation and faster the time required to perform it.

Coarse-grained MD approaches, where some of the fine atomistic details of the system are smoothed over or averaged out, are suggested for analyzing large-scale structural changes. The combination of coarse-grained methods with enhanced computer power easily allows the simulation of submicrometric systems in a timescale ranging from microseconds to milliseconds, thus coinciding with those that can be reached with the most advanced spectroscopic techniques. The use of more rigorous parameterization methods and novel algorithms for sampling the configurational space improved the value of the simulations even if they still cannot be considered as predictive as all-atom simulations (Tozzini 2005). Nevertheless, the absence of atomistic details seriously limits the reliability of the sampled conformations for docking experiments. Hybrid methods combining coarse-grained models of proteins with an atomistic description of the active site have been recently developed, to enhance the potential of these approaches in examining molecular recognition processes (Neri et al. 2005).

Enhanced sampling can also be achieved through techniques that rely on the modification of the conventional MD sampling. Thus, the system can be forced to explore the conformational space by facilitating the escape from local energy minimum wells by using non-Boltzmann sampling, as in the locally enhanced sampling (LES) methods. In LES, a given number of non-interacting copies of the fragment to be explored (i.e., a residue side chain or a ligand is considered, whereas the interaction of each fragment with the rest of the system is reduced by a suitable factor from their original magnitudes (Czerminski and Elber 1991). Other examples of valuable methods for enhancing sampling are provided by Replica Exchange (RE), umbrella sampling, metadynamics, or accelerated MD simulations (AMD). Most of these methodologies require the *a priori* definition of the reaction coordinate, which will guide the energetic evolution of the system and allow the calculation of the free energy variation between known conformational states. Unfortunately, when looking for new conformations, these might not result as the most suitable tools (Sinko et al. 2013).

16.3.4.1 Replica Exchange Molecular Dynamics

One of the simplest artificial biases for speeding the conformational sampling is raising the system temperature, which increases fluctuations through increasing the average velocity of the atoms (Sugita and Okamoto 1999). RE were first reported by Swendens and Wang and are based on running a number of simulations at different temperatures, exchanging temperature and coordinates every fixed number of steps based on Metropolis criteria (Swendens and Wang 1986). The temperature set should be chosen in order to ensure that no replica is trapped in local minima and the number of replicas should be sufficiently large to ensure the swapping of adjacent replicas.

Even if RE technique has been widely used to study folding processes (Garcia and Onuchic 2003), in the last years, several applications to drug design have been reported (Kokubo et al. 2013; Okamoto et al. 2013).

Extensions of the REMD include multidimensional replica-exchange methods (MREM) (Sugita et al. 2000), also referred to as Hamiltonian REM (Fukunishi et al. 2002), and replica-exchange umbrella sampling (REUS), which combines the conventional umbrella sampling methodology (REF) (Torrie and Valleau 1997) with REM and revealed to be particularly appropriate for free-energy calculations (Sugita et al. 2000).

16.3.4.2 Umbrella Sampling

Different from other accelerated methods, focusing on energy minima, umbrella sampling is capable of sampling the conformational space also in high-energy regions and, consequently, of giving reliable estimations of the free energy difference (Patey and Valleau 1975; Torrie and Valleau 1974, 1997). To reach this aim, an additional term is added to the potential energy, in order to ensure an efficient sampling all along the entire reaction coordinate. Umbrella sampling often uses harmonic biasing potentials in a series of windows along the reaction coordinate, or a single window in combination with an adaptive biasing potential aimed to match the whole free energy profile. In each window, the sampling is performed through conventional MD or Hamiltonian RE. Again, the choice of the reaction coordinate is crucial for having predictive results (Sinko et al. 2013).

16.3.4.3 Metadynamics

Metadynamics approaches (Laio and Parrinello 2002) have been used as valuable tools for reconstructing the free energy surface and for simulating rare conformational events in different fields as biophysics (Biarnes et al. 2007; Domene et al. 2008; Fiorin et al. 2006; Petraglio et al. 2008; Rohrig et al. 2006), material science (Behler et al. 2008; Di Pietro et al. 2006; Donadio et al. 2001; Prestipino and Giaquinta 2008), crystal structure prediction (Karamertzanis et al. 2008; Martonak et al. 2006; Oganov et al. 2005), and chemistry (Blumberger et al. 2006; Ensing et al. 2006, 2004; Schreiner et al.

2008). The capability of crossing high-energy barriers is enhanced by adding to the Hamiltonian of the system a history-dependent potential energy function of a determined set of collective variables (CVs). In particular, the bias potential is added by dropping Gaussians along the sampled trajectory, discouraging the system from generating already experienced conformations.

The most difficult part of running metadynamics is related to the selection and definition of CVs, which can greatly affect the simulation results and become more complicated as the system dimension increases. Criteria for picking the best CVs have been reported in literature (Barducci et al. 2011; Laio and Gervasio 2008), as well as examples of failure in case of not proper CVs selection (Branduardi et al. 2005). Unfortunately, a "trial and error" procedure is often the best choice. In general, CVs should clearly differentiate among the initial, final, and intermediate states, describe the most relevant slow conformational events, and their number should be as much as possible limited, to avoid long simulations necessary for filling the whole free energy surface (Spyrakis et al. 2011). CVs are always function of the system coordinates. They can be as simple as interatomic distances, angles and torsions, or much more complicated as the potential energy, normal modes, and essential coordinates derived from essential dynamics (Spiwok et al. 2007) or more specific as the helicity of the backbone or the dihedral correlation (Piana and Laio 2007).

Despite these drawbacks, a number of applications of metadynamics to protein–ligand interaction, also accounting for full receptor flexibility, have been reported (Gervasio et al. 2005; Limongelli et al. 2010; Masetti et al. 2009; Pietrucci et al. 2009; Provasi et al. 2009). The enhanced sampling allows, in fact, the identification of bottlenecks or unfavorable interactions occurring during the ligand-binding pathway. A good description of ligand migration has been reported by Ceccarelli et al. (2004) for the translocation of ampicillin through OmpF in *Escherichia coli* (Ceccarelli et al. 2004) and by Branduardi et al. (2005) for trimethylamonium migration through the acetylcholinesterase gorge.

16.3.4.4 Accelerated MD Simulations

AMD were developed by McCammon and coworkers (Hamelberg et al. 2004; Hamelberg and McCammon 2006), starting from the work of Voter (1997), for improving the exploration of large biological systems energy landscape. Different from other aforementioned methods, AMD do not need the *a priori* definition of a coordinate reaction and are ideally suited for an efficient exploration of the configurational space.

These methodologies are able to increase the transition of high-energy barriers, without having any knowledge or taking into account the underling energy landscape (Hamelberg et al. 2004). In particular, a biased potential is added to the real one, in order to reduce the energy barriers between the minima states through an increase of the corresponding potential energies.

The addition of the bias potential significantly increases the probability of escaping from minima regions, according to the boost energy value and the form of the bias potential.

AMD methods have been applied for exploring the intrinsic conformational flexibility of GB3 protein (Markwick et al. 2007), and for investigating the conformational switching in Ras protein (Grant et al. 2009). Yang and coworkers (2009) used AMD for studying the folding mechanism of the trpzip2 β-hairpin and obtaining multiple folding and unfolding trajectories in relatively short amount of simulation time.

16.4 Androgen Receptor: A Case Study

Androgen Receptor belongs to the great family of ligand-inducible transcriptional factors, identified as NRs, with four main structural and functional domains. The binding of the endogenous ligand testosterone or the more potent 5α-reductase-derived metabolite Dihydrotestosterone (DHT) induces protein homo-dimerization and translocation into the nucleus, where the recruitment of cofactorial proteins and activation of transcriptional machinery take place (Claessens et al. 2001; Li and Al-Azzawi 2009).

From a physiological point of view, androgenic/anabolic activity is responsible of the development of male features during embryogenesis, bone and muscles maintenance, and sexual maturation. AR is also a crucial biological target for hormone-related prostate cancer treatment (Lamb et al. 2014; Shafi et al. 2013). In the last 10 years, several studies showed that AR can bind different molecular chemotypes as exogenous ligands. In particular, *in silico* (Vuorinen et al. 2013) and *in vitro* approaches predicted and confirmed the potential toxicological effects of pesticides (Kojima et al. 2003), environmental chemicals as phthalates (Araki et al. 2005) and organochlorine food contaminants (Schrader and Cooke 2000) able to interact with AR.

In an effort to split anabolic (side effects as osteoanabolism for treatment of sarcopenia and myoanabolism for treatment of osteoporosis) to androgenic (virilizing and feminizing side effects caused by an excess of 5α-reductase or aromatase substrates) effects, the testosterone scaffold has been deeply investigated and optimized for improving its binding affinity and reducing the related hepatotoxic effects. As a result, nonsteroidal Selective Androgen Receptors Modulators (SARMs) and "pure" antiandrogens have been developed, in order to modulate androgenic activity without interfering with endogenous testosterone levels and related metabolic biochemical pathways.

Nonsteroidal AR antagonists can be divided into three main categories: first-generation monoaryl-propionamidic derivatives as Flutamide, hydantoin derivatives as Nilutamide, and second-generation diaryl-propionamidic derivatives as R-Bicalutamide.

As shown in Figure 16.2, ligands able to interact with ARs are characterized by a wide structural heterogeneity. In the case of the pro-drug Flutamide, or of its active metabolite Hydroxyflutamide, the substitution of the Cα methyl with a 4-Fluorophenylsulphonyl group leads to the more active derivative R-Bicalutamide. The increased affinity has been mainly attributed to the π–π interaction made between the Trp741 indole moiety and the ligand aromatic B-ring. This is a result of a wide local conformational plasticity of AR-LBP.

As shown in Figure 16.3, the comparison of all currently available PDB structures for human AR has revealed two main crystallographic model of protein–ligand interaction. These models can be summarized by the full agonist form of AR cocrystallized with its endogenous ligand testosterone, and by the partial agonist model of AR complexed with EM-5744 and SARM S22, respectively, steroidal and nonsteroidal selective modulators. In the full agonist model, the testosterone makes H-bond interactions with Arg745, Asn705, and Thr877. The nonsteroidal partial agonist model differs from the former for the implication of Leu704 as well as for the lack of Thr877 in H-bonding the ligand. CoMFA analysis reveals that a planar region close to Arg745 is important for ligand activity. Moreover, the following displacement

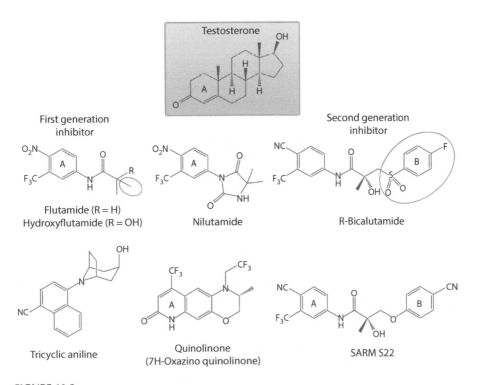

FIGURE 16.2
Principal classes of synthetic ligands for AR compared to the natural ligand testosterone. (As described in Mohler, M. L., C. E. Bohl, A. Jones et al. 2009. *J. Med. Chem.* 52(12):3597–3617.)

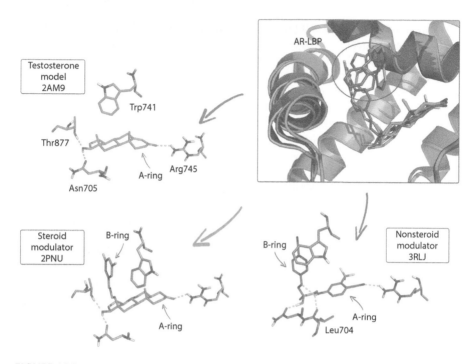

FIGURE 16.3

(See color insert.) Model of ligand–protein interaction for testosterone (green, PDB code 2AM9), steroidal modulator EM-5744 (yellow, PDB code 2PNU), nonsteroidal modulator SARM-S22 (violet, PDB code 3RLJ). The presence of a bulky protruding B-ring induces conformational rearrangement of Trp741 side chain and of other two methionine residues (not showed).

of Trp741 indole ring and the close methionines in H6 allows the accommodation of an accessory perpendicular B-ring near the region delimited by Thr877 and Asn705 (Hong et al. 2003). The concerted H12 partial displacement and the Trp741 flipping lead to the opening of a B-ring tunnel, which allows the accommodation of the propionamidic SARMs derivatives. The presence of such bulkier moieties and the following displacement of Trp741, Met895, and of the whole N-terminal portion of H12 negatively influence the ligands affinity and activity, resulting in agonist-to-antagonist switching as shown by SARM-S1 (an R-Bicalutamide derivative) or by the pure antagonists R-Bicalutamide. It is interesting to note that the replacement of Trp741 with Leu741 causes the gain of agonist activity of SARM-S1 in the W741L AR mutant (Bohl et al. 2005), whereas mutation at codon 895 (from Methionine to Threonine) gives a antagonism-to-agonism switching for R-Bicalutamide, thus suggesting that the antagonist effect of S1 and R-Bicalutamide could be related to steric clashes with Met895 and Trp741 side chains. The superimposition of the crystallographic structures reveals how a local flexibility is distributed among the 20 residues of AR-LBP: AR-T877A mutant (PDB code 2OZ7) cocrystallized with Cyproterone Acetate (CPA; [Bohl et al. 2007]) reveals that conformational changes for Met895, Trp741, Leu701, Leu880, Met780, Phe876 allows the accommodation of 17α-acetyl/17β-methyl-keto groups of CPA with a local unfolding of H11 C-terminal region. The area delimited by Arg745, Gln711, and Phe764 is quite "stable" and selectively accommodates planar A-ring of ligand through an *edge-to-face* aromatic interaction with Phe764 and H-bonds with Arg745 and/or Asn711 (see Figure 16.4).

Starting from crystallographic available data, it is possible to define three main levels of local flexibility into the AR-LBP: the most flexible (green-circled) area that includes residues of H6, the medium flexible (blue-circled) area that includes residues of H3, H8, H11, L11-12, and the "stable" (red-circled) area that includes residues of H3, H6, and β-sheet1. Considering that the conformational plasticity of AR-LBP amino acids side chains allows the accommodation of different structural chemotypes, the local side chains flexibility could be of pivotal importance. In this perspective, the *inactive* and *active* antagonism on AR could be associated, respectively, to a great degree of local conformational instability produced by accommodation of small ligand as HF or Nilutamide, and to an important *pseudo-local* conformational instability produced by bulkier ligands as R-Bicalutamide.

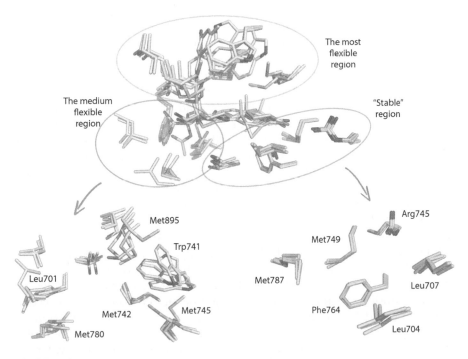

FIGURE 16.4
(See color insert.) Superimposition of different AR structure: the most flexible (green-circled), medium flexible (blue-circled), and "stable" (red-circled) regions are shown. All different ligands are represented in gray. Backbone atoms are not reported for clarity. (PDB codes 2AM9, 3RLJ, 2PNU, and 2OZ7.)

Up to now, the structural instability of AR in the presence of pure antagonists as R-Bicalutamide has made impossible the acquisition of a crystallographic wild-type structure of any antagonism-like form. So, if for ERs we can talk about local, related to side chains, and global, mainly attributed to H12, flexibility, for AR we can just refer to local adjustments. A similar conformational macroflexibility can be neither confirmed nor excluded.

From a computational point of view, the absence of a crystallographic model of antagonism has not precluded the possibility to find new antagonists. For instance, Li and coworkers (2013) discovered novel antiandrogens by using the crystallographic agonist model 2PNU and hypothesizing that, if a compound is more affine than testosterone to AR-LBP, it could work as competitive antagonist.

In such an ambiguous scenario, what can we do with a molecular mechanic approach? *In silico* approaches allow to predict guest–host interactions, assessing a free energy value to the obtained complex as an index of effectiveness of interaction (Vuorinen et al. 2013). This allows to hypothesize binding affinity and, in some cases, toxicological potencies of lead molecules. Regardless of the approach adopted, the focus is to build a model with a high predictive power, measured as "sensitivity" (percentage of actives found) and "specificity" (percentage of inactive discarded). In many cases, high specificity causes loss of sensitivity. Moreover, the choice of the scoring/ranking function as well as the algorithm of poses generation can drastically affect the results. From a crystallographic point of view, we can consider a semiflexible docking approach giving flexibility to more instable aminoacid side chains and full conformational freedom to each putative ligand. A set up docking study has revealed to give good predictions in preliminary evaluations of toxicity, with a significant economic and time gain (Ginex et al. 2014). It could allow to do binding affinities evaluations and hypothesize putative mechanism of action, even if we have to take into account the risk of finding false positives when allowing a high degree of local flexibility. Interestingly, a cross-docking study performed on the same system in rigid conditions (full conformational freedom only for ligand) has allowed to distinguish between testosterone-like full agonist and SARMs-like partial agonist model. Docking with GOLD demonstrated that the lack of flexibility for Trp741, Met742, Met745, and Met895 side chains can dramatically affect a good and energetically favorable positioning of SARM and pure antagonist propionamides, as R-Bicalutamide into the steroid-binding pocket. We chose testosterone, SARM S22, and R-Bicalutamide as examples of, respectively, full agonist, partial agonist, and antagonist whereas the respective crystallographic structures 2AM9, 3RLJ, and 1Z95 as structural models of activity. Cross-docking was performed with GOLD suite v. 5.1 (CCDC, Cambridge, UK). The default GOLDScore fitness function was applied for performing the energetic evaluations (Jones et al. 1997). Despite the enthalpic contribution

TABLE 16.1

HINT Scores for Cross-Docking of the Full Agonist (Testosterone), a Partial Agonist (SARM S-22) and a Pure Antagonist (R-Bicalutamide) in Their Three Crystallographic Structures (PDB code 2AM9, 3RLJ, and 1Z95)

Compound	2AM9 Model	3RLJ Model	1Z95 Model
R-Bicalutamide	Negative	133	282
SARM S-22	Negative	224	117
Testosterone	242	Negative	Negative

to the free-energy calculation of protein–ligand interactions already considered by GOLD, HINT scoring function (Cozzini et al. 2002) was applied to the entire GOLD output or a more exhaustive computing of the entropic term of *in silico* free energy calculation.

The cross-docking results (Table 16.1) revealed that in all rigid conditions testosterone can be accommodate only in 2AM9, whereas both SARM S22 and R-Bicalutamide can only fit in 3RLJ and 1Z95 (SARM-like/"antagonists" models).

Obviously, rigid docking is more selective and less permissive than the flexible one. It could allow a proper modeling of the activity of known ligands, but enhance the risk of false-negative predictions. Moreover, in the AR case, a good and energetically favored accommodation of a putative ligand into the steroid binding pocket could not necessarily mean that compound acts as an agonist! Recent studies suggested that the transcriptional activity in AR is also related to allosteric interaction between cofactorial proteins on AF-2 site (Grosdidier et al. 2012), small molecules on BF-3 site (Lack et al. 2011; Munuganti et al. 2013), and hormone binding pocket in AR-LBD. In these conditions, a docking approach can, clearly, only allow to estimate binding affinity but not activity. On the contrary, a ligand-based virtual screening did not give better results in terms of selectivity because of the high-ligand promiscuity into the 3-ketosteroid class of NRs. AR, GR, MR, and PR activity are endogenously modulated by closely related ligands that possess a steroid nucleus and a 3-keto function. The substantial absence of molecular diversity between natural steroid ligands as well as the high heterogeneity of synthetic active and not active compounds (SARM S22 instead of R-Bicalutamide, see Figure 16.2) significantly affects the predictive power of a ligand-based global model, making very difficult the discrimination of an agonist from an antagonist without experimental data. At the same time, a local model drastically limits the field of action. It could be suitable to evaluate compounds closely related to those used to build the model, but it fails to evaluate chemicals with different scaffolds. In this perspective, the use of complementary models, in other words, computational models specialized in the analysis of different properties and/or phenomena of guest–host interactions, could allow to overcome the problem.

16.5 Conclusions

We are conscious that in this chapter not all the problems regarding flexibility and docking/scoring simulations are exhaustively depicted, but we tried to address the reader to the most evident and important problems to be considered in order to achieve the best possible model for simulation. We describe the problems using two well-known biological systems belonging to NR family, ER, and AR. It is obvious that a sum of small inaccuracies can produce a bad model and lead to much more false-positive or false-negative solutions. We do not take care of some false negatives in medicinal chemistry because the aim is to define one or more lead compounds as base for a further "possible" drug development. In case of *in silico* food safety, where we screen a set of molecules to predict if they can interact with selected targets, we cannot afford to neglect some false negatives that can act as endocrine disruptors or toxins, then a right model able to allow good prediction is mandatory for best results. Thus, we have to take into account all kinds of movements of our molecules.

References

Amaro, R. E., R. Baron, and J. A. McCammon. 2008a. An improved relaxed complex scheme for receptor flexibility in computer-aided drug design. *J. Comput. Aided Mol. Des.* 22(9):693–705.

Amaro, R. E. and W. W. Li. 2010. Emerging methods for ensemble-based virtual screening. *Curr. Top. Med. Chem.* 10(1):3–13.

Amaro, R. E., A. Schnaufer, H. Interthal, W. Hol, K. D. Stuart, and J. A. McCammon. 2008b. Discovery of drug-like inhibitors of an essential RNA-editing ligase in *Trypanosoma brucei*. *Proc. Natl. Acad. Sci. U S A* 105(45):17278–17283.

Araki, N., K. Ohno, M. Nakai, M. Takeyoshi, and M. Iida. 2005. Screening for androgen receptor activities in 253 industrial chemicals by *in vitro* reporter gene assays using AR-EcoScreen cells. *Toxicol. In Vitro* 19(6):831–842.

Barducci, A., M. Bonomi, and M. Parrinello. 2011. Metadynamics. *WIRES Comput. Mol. Sci.* 1:826–843.

Behler, J., R. Martonak, D. Donadio, and M. Parrinello. 2008. Metadynamics simulations of the high-pressure phases of silicon employing a high-dimensional neural network potential. *Phys. Rev. Lett.* 100(18):185501.

Bernstein, F. C., T. F. Koetzle, G. J. Williams et al. 1977. The Protein Data Bank: A computer-based archival file for macromolecular structures. *J. Mol. Biol.* 112(3): 535–542.

Biarnes, X., A. Ardevol, A. Planas, C. Rovira, A. Laio, and M. Parrinello. 2007. The conformational free energy landscape of beta-D-glucopyranose. Implications for substrate preactivation in beta-glucoside hydrolases. *J. Am. Chem. Soc.* 129(35):10686–10693.

Blumberger, J., B. Ensing, and M. L. Klein. 2006. Formamide hydrolysis in alkaline aqueous solution: Insight from ab initio metadynamics calculations. *Angew. Chem. Int. Ed. Engl.* 45(18):2893–2897.

Bohl, C. E., D. D. Miller, J. Chen, C. E. Bell, and J. T. Dalton. 2005. Structural basis for accommodation of nonsteroidal ligands in the androgen receptor. *J. Biol. Chem.* 280(45):37747–37754.

Bohl, C. E., Z. Wu, D. D. Miller, C. E. Bell, and J. T. Dalton. 2007. Crystal structure of the T877A human androgen receptor ligand-binding domain complexed to cyproterone acetate provides insight for ligand-induced conformational changes and structure-based drug design. *J. Biol. Chem.* 282(18):13648–13655.

Bowman, A. L., Z. Nikolovska-Coleska, H. Zhong, S. Wang, and H. A. Carlson. 2007. Small molecule inhibitors of the MDM2-p53 interaction discovered by ensemble-based receptor models. *J. Am. Chem. Soc.* 129(42):12809–12814.

Branduardi, D., F. L. Gervasio, A. Cavalli, M. Recanatini, and M. Parrinello. 2005. The role of the peripheral anionic site and cation-pi interactions in the ligand penetration of the human AChE gorge. *J. Am. Chem. Soc.* 127(25):9147–9155.

Carlson, H. A., K. M. Masukawa, K. Rubins et al. 2000. Developing a dynamic pharmacophore model for HIV-1 integrase. *J. Med. Chem.* 43(11):2100–2114.

Caves, L. S., J. D. Evanseck, and M. Karplus. 1998. Locally accessible conformations of proteins: Multiple molecular dynamics simulations of crambin. *Protein Sci.* 7(3):649–666.

Ceccarelli, M., C. Danelon, A. Laio, and M. Parrinello. 2004. Microscopic mechanism of antibiotics translocation through a porin. *Biophys. J.* 87(1):58–64.

Cheng, L. S., R. E. Amaro, D. Xu, W. W. Li, P. W. Arzberger, and J. A. McCammon. 2008. Ensemble-based virtual screening reveals potential novel antiviral compounds for avian influenza neuraminidase. *J. Med. Chem.* 51(13):3878–3894.

Claessens, F., G. Verrijdt, E. Schoenmakers et al. 2001. Selective DNA binding by the androgen receptor as a mechanism for hormone-specific gene regulation. *J. Steroid. Biochem. Mol. Biol.* 76(1–5):23–30.

Claussen, H., C. Buning, M. Rarey, and T. Lengauer. 2001. FlexE: efficient molecular docking considering protein structure variations. *J. Mol. Biol.* 308(2):377–395.

Cozzini, P., M. Fornabaio, A. Marabotti, D. J. Abraham, G. E. Kellogg, and A. Mozzarelli. 2002. Simple, intuitive calculations of free energy of binding for protein-ligand complexes. 1. Models without explicit constrained water. *J. Med. Chem.* 45(12):2469–2483.

Cozzini, P. and G. E. Kellogg. (eds.). 2012. *Computational Approaches to Nuclear Receptors*. Cambridge, UK: RSC Publishing, 176 p.

Cozzini, P., G. E. Kellogg, F. Spyrakis et al. 2008. Target flexibility: An emerging consideration in drug discovery and design. *J. Med. Chem.* 51 (20):6237–6255.

Czerminski, R. and R. Elber. 1991. Computational studies of ligand diffusion in globins: I. Leghemoglobin. *Proteins* 10(1):70–80.

Dal Palu, A., F. Spyrakis, and P. Cozzini. 2012. A new approach for investigating protein flexibility based on Constraint Logic Programming. The first application in the case of the estrogen receptor. *Eur. J. Med. Chem.* 49:127–140.

Davis, I. W. and D. Baker. 2009. RosettaLigand docking with full ligand and receptor flexibility. *J. Mol. Biol.* 385(2):381–392.

Deng, J., K. W. Lee, T. Sanchez, M. Cui, N. Neamati, and J. M. Briggs. 2005. Dynamic receptor-based pharmacophore model development and its application in designing novel HIV-1 integrase inhibitors. *J. Med. Chem.* 48(5):1496–1505.

Di Pietro, E., M. Pagliai, G. Cardini, and V. Schettino. 2006. Solid-state phase transition induced by pressure in LiOH x H_2O. *J. Phys. Chem. B* 110(27):13539–13546.

Diamanti-Kandarakis, E., J. P. Bourguignon, L. C. Giudice et al. 2009. Endocrine-disrupting chemicals: An Endocrine Society scientific statement. *Endocr. Rev.* 30(4):293–342.

Domene, C., M. L. Klein, D. Branduardi, F. L. Gervasio, and M. Parrinello. 2008. Conformational changes and gating at the selectivity filter of potassium channels. *J. Am. Chem. Soc.* 130(29):9474–9480.

Donadio, D., M. Bernasconi, and M. Boero. 2001. Ab initio simulations of photoinduced interconversions of oxygen deficient centers in amorphous silica. *Phys. Rev. Lett.* 87(19):195504.

Dror, R. O., D. H. Arlow, D. W. Borhani, M. O. Jensen, S. Piana, and D. E. Shaw. 2009. Identification of two distinct inactive conformations of the beta2-adrenergic receptor reconciles structural and biochemical observations. *Proc. Natl. Acad. Sci. USA* 106(12):4689–4694.

Durrant, J. D., M. D. Urbaniak, M. A. Ferguson, and J. A. McCammon. 2010. Computer-aided identification of *Trypanosoma brucei* uridine diphosphate galactose 4'-epimerase inhibitors: Toward the development of novel therapies for African sleeping sickness. *J. Med. Chem.* 53(13):5025–5032.

Ensing, B., M. De Vivo, Z. Liu, P. Moore, and M. L. Klein. 2006. Metadynamics as a tool for exploring free energy landscapes of chemical reactions. *Acc. Chem. Res.* 39(2):73–81.

Ensing, B., A. Laio, F. L. Gervasio, M. Parrinello, and M. L. Klein. 2004. A minimum free energy reaction path for the E2 reaction between fluoro ethane and a fluoride ion. *J. Am. Chem. Soc.* 126(31):9492–9493.

Farrugia, L. J. 2012. WinGX and ORTEP for Windows: An update. *J. Appl. Cryst.* 45:849–854.

Fiorin, G., A. Pastore, P. Carloni, and M. Parrinello. 2006. Using metadynamics to understand the mechanism of calmodulin/target recognition at atomic detail. *Biophys. J.* 91(8):2768–2777.

Fisher, J. S. 2004. Are all EDC effects mediated via steroid hormone receptors? *Toxicology* 205(1–2):33–41.

Fukunishi, F., O. Watanabe, and S. Takada. 2002. On the Hamiltonian replica exchange method for efficient sampling of biomolecular systems: Application to protein structure prediction. *J. Chem. Phys.* 116:9058–9067.

Garcia, A. E. and J. N. Onuchic. 2003. Folding a protein in a computer: An atomic description of the folding/unfolding of protein A. *Proc. Natl. Acad. Sci. USA* 100(24):13898–13903.

Gervasio, F. L., A. Laio, and M. Parrinello. 2005. Flexible docking in solution using metadynamics. *J. Am. Chem. Soc.* 127(8):2600–2607.

Ginex, T., C. Dall'Asta, and P. Cozzini. 2014. Preliminary hazard evaluation of androgen receptor-mediated endocrine-disrupting effects of thioxanthone metabolites through structure-based molecular docking. *Chem. Res. Toxicol.* 27(2):279–289.

Go, N., T. Noguti, and T. Nishikawa. 1983. Dynamics of a small globular protein in terms of low-frequency vibrational modes. *Proc. Natl. Acad. Sci. USA* 80(12):3696–3700.

Grant, B. J., A. A. Gorfe, and J. A. McCammon. 2009. Ras conformational switching: Simulating nucleotide-dependent conformational transitions with accelerated molecular dynamics. *PLoS Comput. Biol.* 5(3):e1000325.

Grosdidier, S., L. R. Carbo, V. Buzon et al. 2012. Allosteric conversation in the androgen receptor ligand-binding domain surfaces. *Mol. Endocrinol.* 26(7):1078–1090.

Halperin, I., B. Ma, H. Wolfson, and R. Nussinov. 2002. Principles of docking: An overview of search algorithms and a guide to scoring functions. *Proteins* 47(4):409–443.

Hamelberg, D. and J. A. McCammon. 2006. Accelerating conormational transitions in biomolecular systems. *Ann. Rep. Comp. Chem.* 2:221–232.

Hamelberg, D., J. Mongan, and J. A. McCammon. 2004. Accelerated molecular dynamics: A promising and efficient simulation method for biomolecules. *J. Chem. Phys.* 120(24):11919–11929.

Henzler, A. M. and M. Rarey. 2010. In pursuit of fully flexible protein-ligand docking: Modeling the bilateral mechanism of binding. *Mol. Inform.* 29(3):164–173.

Henzler-Wildman, K. and D. Kern. 2007. Dynamic personalities of proteins. *Nature* 450(7172):964–972.

Hong, H., H. Fang, Q. Xie, R. Perkins, D. M. Sheehan, and W. Tong. 2003. Comparative molecular field analysis (CoMFA) model using a large diverse set of natural, synthetic and environmental chemicals for binding to the androgen receptor. *SAR QSAR Environ. Res.* 14(5–6):373–388.

http://ambermd.org/gpus/benchmarks.htm

http://www.nvidia.com/object/molecular_dynamics.html

Ishima, R. and D. A. Torchia. 2000. Protein dynamics from NMR. *Nat. Struct. Biol.* 7(9):740–743.

Jain, A. 2007. Surflex-Dock 2.1: Robust performance from ligand energetic modeling, ring flexibility, and knowledge-based search. *J. Comput. Aided Mol. Des.* 21(5):281–306.

Jain, A. N. 2003. Surflex: Fully automatic flexible molecular docking using a molecular similarity-based search engine. *J. Med. Chem.* 46(4):499–511.

Jones, G., P. Willett, R. C. Glen, A. R. Leach, and R. Taylor. 1997. Development and validation of a genetic algorithm for flexible docking. *J. Mol. Biol.* 267(3):727–748.

Kamerzell, T. J. and C. R. Middaugh. 2008. The complex inter-relationships between protein flexibility and stability. *J. Pharm. Sci.* 97(9):3494–3517.

Karamertzanis, P. G., P. Raiteri, M. Parrinello, M. Leslie, and S. L. Price. 2008. The thermal stability of lattice-energy minima of 5-fluorouracil: Metadynamics as an aid to polymorph prediction. *J. Phys. Chem. B* 112(14):4298–4308.

Kellogg, G. E. and D. J. Abraham. 1992. KEY, LOCK, and LOCKSMITH: Complementary hydropathic map predictions of drug structure from a known receptor-receptor structure from known drugs. *J. Mol. Graph.* 10(4):212–217, 226.

Kim, D. S., Y. Cho, K. Sugihara, D. Ryu, and D. Kim. 2010. Three-dimensional beta-shapes and beta-complexes via quasi-triangulation. *Comput. Aided Des.* 42:911–929.

Kim, D. S., C. M. Kim, C. I. Won et al. 2011. BetaDock: Shape-priority docking method based on beta-complex. *J. Biomol. Struct. Dyn.* 29(1):219–242.

Kojima, H., M. Iida, E. Katsura, A. Kanetoshi, Y. Hori, and K. Kobayashi. 2003. Effects of a diphenyl ether-type herbicide, chlornitrofen, and its amino derivative on androgen and estrogen receptor activities. *Environ. Health Perspect.* 111(4):497–502.

Kokh, D. B., R. C. Wade, and W. Wenzel. 2011. Receptor flexibility in small-molecule docking calculations. *Comput. Mol. Sci.* 1(2):298–314.

Kokubo, H., T. Tanaka, and Y. Okamoto. 2013. Two-dimensional replica-exchange method for predicting protein-ligand binding structures. *J. Comput. Chem.* 34(30):2601–2614.

Kramer, B., M. Rarey, and T. Lengauer. 1999. Evaluation of the FLEXX incremental construction algorithm for protein-ligand docking. *Proteins* 37(2):228–241.

Lack, N. A., P. Axerio-Cilies, P. Tavassoli et al. 2011. Targeting the binding function 3 (BF3) site of the human androgen receptor through virtual screening. *J. Med. Chem.* 54(24):8563–8573.

Laio, A. and F. L. Gervasio. 2008. Metadynamics: A method to simulate rare events and reconstruct the free energy of biophysics, chemistry and material sicence. *Rep. Prog. Phys.* 71:126601.

Laio, A. and M. Parrinello. 2002. Escaping free-energy minima. *Proc. Natl. Acad. Sci. USA* 99(20):12562–12566.

Lamb, A. D., C. E. Massie, and D. E. Neal. 2014. The transcriptional programme of the androgen receptor (AR) in prostate cancer. *BJU Int.* 113(3):358–366.

Li, H., M. D. Hassona, N. A. Lack et al. 2013. Characterization of a new class of androgen receptor antagonists with potential therapeutic application in advanced prostate cancer. *Mol. Cancer Ther.* 12(11):2425–2435.

Li, J. and F. Al-Azzawi. 2009. Mechanism of androgen receptor action. *Maturitas* 63(2):142–148.

Lill, M. A. 2011. Efficient incorporation of protein flexibility and dynamics into molecular docking simulations. *Biochemistry* 50(28):6157–6169.

Limongelli, V., M. Bonomi, L. Marinelli et al. 2010. Molecular basis of cyclooxygenase enzymes (COXs) selective inhibition. *Proc. Natl. Acad. Sci. USA* 107(12):5411–5416.

Lin, J. H., A. L. Perryman, J. R. Schames, and J. A. McCammon. 2002. Computational drug design accommodating receptor flexibility: The relaxed complex scheme. *J. Am. Chem. Soc.* 124(20):5632–5633.

Lin, J. H., A. L. Perryman, J. R. Schames, and J. A. McCammon. 2003. The relaxed complex method: Accommodating receptor flexibility for drug design with an improved scoring scheme. *Biopolymers* 68(1):47–62.

Lindorff-Larsen, K., S. Piana, R. O. Dror, and D. E. Shaw. 2011. How fast-folding proteins fold. *Science* 334(6055):517–520.

Lins, R. D., J. M. Briggs, T. P. Straatsma et al. 1999. Molecular dynamics studies on the HIV-1 integrase catalytic domain. *Biophys. J.* 76(6):2999–3011.

Luccio-Camelo, D. C. and G. S. Prins. 2011. Disruption of androgen receptor signaling in males by environmental chemicals. *J. Steroid. Biochem. Mol. Biol.* 127(1–2):74–82.

Markwick, P. R., G. Bouvignies, and M. Blackledge. 2007. Exploring multiple timescale motions in protein GB3 using accelerated molecular dynamics and NMR spectroscopy. *J. Am. Chem. Soc.* 129(15):4724–4730.

Martonak, R., D. Donadio, A. R. Oganov, and M. Parrinello. 2006. Crystal structure transformations in SiO_2 from classical and ab initio metadynamics. *Nat. Mater.* 5(8):623–626.

Masetti, M., A. Cavalli, M. Recanatini, and F. L. Gervasio. 2009. Exploring complex protein-ligand recognition mechanisms with coarse metadynamics. *J. Phys. Chem. B* 113(14):4807–4816.

McCammon, J. A., B. R. Gelin, and M. Karplus. 1977. Dynamics of folded proteins. *Nature* 267(5612):585–590.

Meagher, K. L. and H. A. Carlson. 2004. Incorporating protein flexibility in structure-based drug discovery: Using HIV-1 protease as a test case. *J. Am. Chem. Soc.* 126(41):13276–13281.

Meiler, J. and D. Baker. 2006. ROSETTALIGAND: Protein-small molecule docking with full side-chain flexibility. *Proteins* 65(3):538–548.

Mohler, M. L., C. E. Bohl, A. Jones et al. 2009. Nonsteroidal selective androgen receptor modulators (SARMs): Dissociating the anabolic and androgenic activities of the androgen receptor for therapeutic benefit. *J. Med. Chem.* 52(12):3597–3617.

Morris, G. M., R. Huey, W. Lindstrom et al. 2009. AutoDock4 and AutoDockTools4: Automated docking with selective receptor flexibility. *J. Comput. Chem.* 30(16):2785–2791.

Munuganti, R. S., E. Leblanc, P. Axerio-Cilies et al. 2013. Targeting the binding function 3 (BF3) site of the androgen receptor through virtual screening. 2. Development of 2-((2-phenoxyethyl) thio)-1H-benzimidazole derivatives. *J. Med. Chem.* 56(3):1136–1148.

Neri, M., C. Anselmi, M. Cascella, A. Maritan, and P. Carloni. 2005. Coarse-grained model of proteins incorporating atomistic detail of the active site. *Phys. Rev. Lett.* 95(21):218102.

Neves, M. A., M. Totrov, and R. Abagyan. 2012. Docking and scoring with ICM: The benchmarking results and strategies for improvement. *J. Comput. Aided Mol. Des.* 26(6):675–686.

Nichols, S. E., R. Baron, A. Ivetac, and J. A. McCammon. 2011. Predictive power of molecular dynamics receptor structures in virtual screening. *J. Chem. Inf. Model.* 51(6):1439–1446.

Nichols, S. E., R. V. Swift, and R. E. Amaro. 2012. Rational prediction with molecular dynamics for hit identification. *Curr. Top. Med. Chem.* 12(18):2002–2012.

O'Donoghue, P. and Z. Luthey-Schulten. 2005. Evolutionary profiles derived from the QR factorization of multiple structural alignments gives an economy of information. *J. Mol. Biol.* 346(3):875–894.

Oganov, A. R., R. Martonak, A. Laio, P. Raiteri, and M. Parrinello. 2005. Anisotropy of Earth's D″ layer and stacking faults in the $MgSiO_3$ post-perovskite phase. *Nature* 438(7071):1142–1144.

Okamoto, Y., H. Kokubo, and T. Tanaka. 2013. Ligand docking simulations by generalized-ensemble algorithms. *Adv. Protein Chem. Struct. Biol.* 92:63–91.

Osguthorpe, D. J., W. Sherman, and A. T. Hagler. 2012. Exploring protein flexibility: incorporating structural ensembles from crystal structures and simulation into virtual screening protocols. *J. Phys. Chem. B* 116(23):6952–6959.

Patey, G. N. and J. P. Valleau. 1975. Monte-Carlo method for obtaining interionic potential of mean force in ionic solution. *J. Chem. Phys.* 64:2334–2339.

Perola, E. and P. S. Charifson. 2004. Conformational analysis of drug-like molecules bound to proteins: An extensive study of ligand reorganization upon binding. *J. Med. Chem.* 47(10):2499–2510.

Petraglio, G., M. Bartolini, D. Branduardi et al. 2008. The role of Li+, Na+, and K+ in the ligand binding inside the human acetylcholinesterase gorge. *Proteins* 70(3):779–785.

Piana, S. and A. Laio. 2007. A bias-exchange approach to protein folding. *J. Phys. Chem. B* 111(17):4553–4559.

Pietrucci, F., F. Marinelli, P. Carloni, and A. Laio. 2009. Substrate binding mechanism of HIV-1 protease from explicit-solvent atomistic simulations. *J. Am. Chem. Soc.* 131(33):11811–11818.

Prestipino, S. and P. V. Giaquinta. 2008. Liquid-solid coexistence via the metadynamics approach. *J. Chem. Phys.* 128(11):114707.

Provasi, D., A. Bortolato, and M. Filizola. 2009. Exploring molecular mechanisms of ligand recognition by opioid receptors with metadynamics. *Biochemistry* 48(42):10020–10029.

Rarey, M., B. Kramer, T. Lengauer, and G. Klebe. 1996. A fast flexible docking method using an incremental construction algorithm. *J. Mol. Biol.* 261(3):470–489.

Rohrig, U. F., A. Laio, N. Tantalo, M. Parrinello, and R. Petronzio. 2006. Stability and structure of oligomers of the Alzheimer peptide Abeta16-22: From the dimer to the 32-mer. *Biophys. J.* 91(9):3217–3229.

Salmon, L., G. Bouvignies, P. Markwick et al. 2009. Protein conformational flexibility from structure-free analysis of NMR dipolar couplings: Quantitative and absolute determination of backbone motion in ubiquitin. *Angew. Chem. Int. Ed. Engl.* 48(23):4154–4157.

Schames, J. R., R. H. Henchman, J. S. Siegel, C. A. Sotriffer, H. Ni, and J. A. McCammon. 2004. Discovery of a novel binding trench in HIV integrase. *J. Med. Chem.* 47(8):1879–1881.

Schrader, T. J. and G. M. Cooke. 2000. Examination of selected food additives and organochlorine food contaminants for androgenic activity in vitro. *Toxicol. Sci.* 53(2):278–288.

Schreiner, E., N. N. Nair, and D. Marx. 2008. Influence of extreme thermodynamic conditions and pyrite surfaces on peptide synthesis in aqueous media. *J. Am. Chem. Soc.* 130(9):2768–2770.

Shafi, A. A., A. E. Yen, and N. L. Weigel. 2013. Androgen receptors in hormone-dependent and castration-resistant prostate cancer. *Pharmacol. Ther.* 140(3):223–238.

Shan, Y., E. T. Kim, M. P. Eastwood, R. O. Dror, M. A. Seeliger, and D. E. Shaw. 2011. How does a drug molecule find its target binding site? *J. Am. Chem. Soc.* 133(24):9181–9183.

Shanle, E. K. and W. Xu. 2011. Endocrine disrupting chemicals targeting estrogen receptor signaling: Identification and mechanisms of action. *Chem. Res. Toxicol.* 24(1):6–19.

Shaw, D. E., M. M. Deneroff, R. O. Dror et al. 2008. Anton, a special-purpose machine for molecular dynamics simulation *Commun. ACM* 51:91–97.

Sherman, W., T. Day, M. P. Jacobson, R. A. Friesner, and R. Farid. 2006. Novel procedure for modeling ligand/receptor induced fit effects. *J. Med. Chem.* 49(2):534–553.

Shin, W. H., J. K. Kim, D. S. Kim, and C. Seok. 2013. GalaxyDock2: Protein-ligand docking using beta-complex and global optimization. *J. Comput. Chem.* 34(30): 2647–2656.

Sinko, W., C. de Oliveira, S. Williams et al. 2011. Applying molecular dynamics simulations to identify rarely sampled ligand-bound conformational states of undecaprenyl pyrophosphate synthase, an antibacterial target. *Chem. Biol. Drug Des.* 77(6):412–420.

Sinko, W., S. Lindert, and J. A. McCammon. 2013. Accounting for receptor flexibility and enhanced sampling methods in computer-aided drug design. *Chem. Biol. Drug Des.* 81(1):41–49.

Sladek, F. M. 2011. What are nuclear receptor ligands? *Mol. Cell Endocrinol.* 334(1–2):3–13.

Sotriffer, C. A. 2011. Accounting for induced-fit effects in docking: What is possible and what is not? *Curr. Top. Med. Chem.* 11(2):179–191.

Spiwok, V., P. Lipovova, and B. Kralova. 2007. Metadynamics in essential coordinates: Free energy simulation of conformational changes. *J. Phys. Chem. B* 111(12):3073–3076.

Spyrakis, F., A. BidonChanal, X. Barril, and F. J. Luque. 2011. Protein flexibility and ligand recognition: Challenges for molecular modeling. *Curr. Top. Med. Chem.* 11(2):192–210.

Stone, J. E., D. J. Hardy, I. S. Ufimtsev, and K. Schulten. 2010. GPU-accelerated molecular modeling coming of age. *J. Mol. Graph. Model.* 29(2):116–125.

Stone, J. E., J. C. Phillips, P. L. Freddolino, D. J. Hardy, L. G. Trabuco, and K. Schulten. 2007. Accelerating molecular modeling applications with graphics processors. *J. Comput. Chem.* 28(16):2618–2640.

Sugita, Y., A. Kitao, and Y. Okamoto. 2000. Multidimensional replica-exchange method for free-energy calculations. *J. Chem. Phys.* 113:6042–6051.

Sugita, Y. and Y. Okamoto. 1999. Replica-exchange molecular dynamics method for protein folding. *Chem. Phys. Lett.* 314:141–151.

Summa, V., A. Petrocchi, F. Bonelli et al. 2008. Discovery of raltegravir, a potent, selective orally bioavailable HIV-integrase inhibitor for the treatment of HIV-AIDS infection. *J. Med. Chem.* 51(18):5843–5855.

Swendens, R. H. and J. S. Wang. 1986. Replica Monte Carlo simulation of spin glasses. *Phys. Rev. Lett.* 57:2607–2609.

Teodoro, M. L. and L. E. Kavraki. 2003. Conformational flexibility models for the receptor in structure based drug design. *Curr. Pharm. Des.* 9(20):1635–1648.

Torrie, G. M. and J. P. Valleau. 1974. Monte-Carlo free energy estimates using non-Boltzmann sampling—Application to subcritical Lennard-Jones fluid. *Chem. Phys. Lett.* 28:578–581.

Torrie, G. M. and J. P. Valleau. 1997. Non-physical sampling distributions in Monte-Carlo free-energy estimation—Umbrella sampling. *J. Comput. Phys.* 23:187–199.

Tozzini, V. 2005. Coarse-grained models for proteins. *Curr. Opin. Struct. Biol.* 15(2):144–150.

Tozzini, V. 2010. Multiscale modeling of proteins. *Acc. Chem. Res.* 43(2):220–230.

Trott, O. and A. J. Olson. 2010. AutoDock Vina: Improving the speed and accuracy of docking with a new scoring function, efficient optimization, and multithreading. *J. Comput. Chem.* 31(2):455–461.

Tsai, C. J., S. Kumar, B. Ma, and R. Nussinov. 1999. Folding funnels, binding funnels, and protein function. *Protein Sci* 8(6):1181–1190.

Verdonk, M. L., J. C. Cole, M. J. Hartshorn, C. W. Murray, and R. D. Taylor. 2003. Improved protein-ligand docking using GOLD. *Proteins* 52(4):609–623.

Voter, A. 1997. A method for accelerating the molecular dynamics simulation of infrequent events. *J. Chem. Phys.* 106:4665–4677.

Vuorinen, A., A. Odermatt, and D. Schuster. 2013. *In silico* methods in the discovery of endocrine disrupting chemicals. *J. Steroid. Biochem. Mol. Biol.* 137:18–26.

Wang, J., P. A. Kollman, and I. D. Kuntz. 1999. Flexible ligand docking: A multistep strategy approach. *Proteins* 36(1):1–19.

Welch, W., J. Ruppert, and A. N. Jain. 1996. Hammerhead: Fast, fully automated docking of flexible ligands to protein binding sites. *Chem. Biol.* 3(6):449–462.

Wong, C. F. 2008. Flexible ligand-flexible protein docking in protein kinase systems. *Biochim. Biophys. Acta* 1784(1):244–51.

Yang, L., Q. Shao, and Y. Q. Gao. 2009. Thermodynamics and folding pathways of trpzip2: An accelerated molecular dynamics simulation study. *J. Phys. Chem. B* 113(3):803–808.

Zsoldos, Z., D. Reid, A. Simon, B. S. Sadjad, and A. P. Johnson. 2006. eHiTS: An innovative approach to the docking and scoring function problems. *Curr. Protein Pept. Sci.* 7(5):421–435.

17

In Silico *Approaches Assisting the Rational Design of Low Molecular Weight Protein–Protein Interaction Modulators*

Bruno O. Villoutreix, Melaine A. Kuenemann, David Lagorce, Olivier Sperandio, and Maria A. Miteva

CONTENTS

17.1 Introduction

Proteins associate to create macromolecular machines of various complexities (e.g., dimers or large multiprotein complexes). The subunits creating these various complexes can be identical or heterogeneous and the interaction can be transient (nonobligate) or permanent (obligatory) (Keskin et al. 2008; Jubb et al. 2012; Metz et al. 2012a; Surade and Blundell 2012; Kastritis and Bonvin 2013). In basically all situations, the formation of permanent or transient complexes is critical to carry out biological functions necessary for life (e.g., illustration of such statements can be easily found just by looking at relatively well-studied biological system like blood coagulation [Villoutreix and Sperandio 2010], or at recent discoveries in the field of cancer [White et al. 2008; Garner and Janda 2011; Ivanov et al. 2013], infectious diseases [Franzosa and Xia 2011; Palu and Loregian 2013; Zoraghi and Reiner 2013], or CNS diseases [Blazer and Neubig 2009], among others). In fact, recent advances in genomics and proteomics have brought to light vast networks of protein–protein interactions (PPIs) often referred to as the interactome (Vidal et al. 2011; Jaeger and Aloy 2012). As a result, we are gaining a far greater understanding about the disease state as the characterization of individual genes/proteins potentially involved in the disease process has been shifting to investigations taking into account the dynamic nature of gene's/protein's networks (Schadt et al. 2009; Penrod et al. 2011; Bultinck et al. 2012; Jaeger and Aloy 2012; Csermely et al. 2013; Furlong 2013; Medina-Franco et al. 2013). In the coming years, high-throughput interactomics data should allow the scientific community to draw a complete map of all the interactions taking place in the cells and tissues (Jaeger and Aloy 2012). Already at present, even if the picture is not complete, hundreds of thousands of interactions have been identified and stored in public databases and the rate is growing exponentially (Mosca et al. 2013) (see Box 17.1).

BOX 17.1   SHORT INTRODUCTION TO PPI NETWORK

Mapping PPIs has not only provided insights into protein function but has facilitated the modeling of functional pathways. One of the most common approaches for the detection of pairs of interacting proteins is the yeast two-hybrid (Y2H) system. The interaction of two proteins transcriptionally activates a reporter gene, and a color reaction can then be seen. Another approach to PPI detection is to use quantitative mass spectrometry to analyze the composition of a partially purified protein complex. Microarray-based analysis can also be used and is relatively high-throughput (simultaneous analysis of thousands of parameters within a single experiment). Experimental methods aimed at investigating PPI have generated a substantial amount of information usually stored in databases. However, the data generated are prone to errors and many information are still missing. In order to propose a more complete picture of potential interactions including those not detected by the experimental methods, several *in silico* tools have been developed. A number of PPI prediction tools are based on the use of genomic data. Some approaches also make use of data-mining techniques to extract useful information from large data sources. A PPI network can then be built, this one has several properties. In general, the process begins with the representation of the PPI network structure (Figure 17.1). The simplest representation

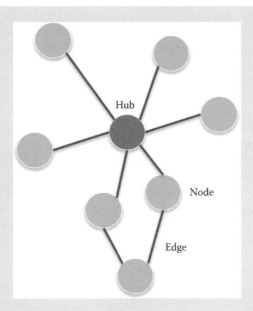

FIGURE 17.1
PPI network representation.

takes the form of a mathematical graph consisting of nodes and edges
(or links). Proteins are then usually represented as nodes; two proteins that interact physically are represented as adjacent nodes connected by an edge. Proteins with many interaction partners (hubs)
are often divided into date and party hubs, depending on whether
their interactions can occur simultaneously or discretely. A party hub
has multiple interfaces on its surface, meaning it can interact with
multiple partners at once. A date hub, on the other hand, tends to
have multiple partners that share the same or overlapping interfaces,
meaning only one partner can be bound at a single time. Essential
proteins tend to be more interconnected than nonessential ones and
human disease-associated proteins tend also to be more interconnected than nondisease proteins. One example is p53 (a critical tumor
suppressor), a highly interconnected protein, or thrombin, a key protein of the blood coagulation system. Of interest, viral, bacterial, or
fungal pathogens tend to target hub proteins. Warning, there are still
many ongoing debates about protein networks or the importance of
party and date hubs, and readers should thus pay attention to different views about these concepts.

Despite their therapeutic relevance, most small molecule drugs do not in general hit PPIs but rather enzymes, ion channels, nuclear hormone receptors, and G-protein coupled receptors (Chene 2006; Villoutreix et al. 2008). The modulation (inhibition or stabilization) of PPIs by drug-like molecules was for many years thought to be impossible or far too risky as compared to conventional targets (Wells and McClendon 2007; Thiel et al. 2012). In fact, these last 50 years, PPIs have been essentially modulated by therapeutic antibodies, and therapeutic proteins and peptides (or modified peptides or more recently stapled peptides) (Loregian and Palu 2005; White et al. 2008; Wilson 2009; Cummings and Hamilton 2010; Raj et al. 2012; Azzarito et al. 2013). However, while biologics can possess outstanding qualities and be valuable in some pathological conditions (Craik et al. 2013), some of these molecules tend to be problematic for at least three reasons (Lu et al. 2012; Meunier 2012): (a) most of them are difficult or impossible to administrate orally with our present knowledge, (b) adverse immune reactions can occur, and (c) biologics are usually expensive to develop, and/or produce, and/or store with treatment for one patient easily reaching over $100,000 per year (CML 2013) (a cost that most healthcare systems are not able to afford, and the associated problem of aligning the cost of small chemical compounds to the cost of biologics). Although significant advances have been made and will take place in the coming years (Teague 2011), several obstacles will have to be overcome, from cost to delivery issues (Wanner et al. 2011). Yet, some biologics are clearly on the rise (Robinson et al. 2008; Kaspar and Reichert 2013; London et al. 2013a,b), they have interesting potentials for PPIs and can obviously be used as chemical probes (e.g., peptides). We will not discuss biologics in the present chapter but interested readers can find relevant information in several recent reviews (see e.g., Leader et al. 2008; Craik et al. 2013; Kaspar and Reichert 2013). Along the same line, due to space limitation, we will only slightly comment on the use of fragments for PPI modulation and readers can find numerous recent reviews on the topic including the recent review article of Winter et al. (2012b). It is here interesting to note that small molecules and biologics can be combined (e.g., a small molecule can be given with a monoclonal antibody [mAb], or the grafting of a small molecule to a protein including mAb can be valuable in some cases). Along the same line, small molecules could be given together with biologics, not to gain a synergistic effect but rather to allow proper functioning of the biologics like for instance to avoid aggregation of an mAb by using a small molecule PPI inhibitor (e.g., proof of concept study with the mAb bevacizumab or Avastin) (Westermaier et al. 2013).

There are many reasons that have led to the widespread perception that modulation of PPIs could not be addressed by small drug-like molecules such as PPI interfaces are usually described as large, flat, lacking a well-defined ligand-binding cavity characteristic of conventional targets (Wells and McClendon 2007; Higueruelo et al. 2009; Morelli et al. 2011; Bienstock 2012; Surade and Blundell 2012); the lack of appropriate high-throughput screening (HTS) technologies and/or the low hit rates observed upon running HTS experiments (Makley and Gestwicki 2013; Ngounou Wetie et al. 2014); the paucity of small molecules in traditional screening libraries dedicated to PPIs reinforced by the observations that small PPI hit molecules often have physicochemical characteristics slightly outside of what would be expected for a typical oral drug starting point (Pagliaro et al. 2004; Villoutreix et al. 2008; Sperandio et al. 2010b; Wanner et al. 2011; Taboureau et al. 2011). In the recent years however, several research articles have challenged the dogma, new strategies have emerged and interesting modulators of PPIs have been reported. In this chapter, we introduce the field and discuss some key challenges and then comment several *in silico* tools and databases that can assist the rational design of PPI modulators. Then, we illustrate PPI hit discovery on three selected systems, the modulation of VEGF-VEGFR (Gautier et al. 2011), of the calmodulin-edema factor (Laine et al. 2010), and of the interferon-α (IFN-α) with its receptor (Geppert et al. 2012).

17.2 Key Challenges Associated with the Modulation of PPIs by Low Molecular Weight Molecules

The traditional target-based small molecule drug discovery workflow (Wyatt et al. 2011; Duffy et al. 2012) begins with target identification (most drug targets are proteins, historically drawn from a few families, such as enzymes, receptors, and ion channels). This step involves analysis of the disease mechanism, genomics to rank genes with respect to physiological functions and proteomics to identify candidate proteins and protein interactions that could be inhibited or enhanced by a drug (Schenone et al. 2013). In a second step, the target is validated, at least to some extent, using genetic engineering, transgenic animal models, antisense DNA/RNA, or chemical probes among others (one generally knows that a target is a good target at the end of the process once the drug is on the market!). Once a target is expected to be important in a disease process, it is necessary to find and optimize small molecules that can act on it. This step usually requires experimental screening of a large compound collection but cost can be lowered and hit rates improved in many cases by using appropriate combination of *in silico* and *in vitro* screening (Villoutreix et al. 2009, 2013; Taboureau et al. 2011). Clearly, drug discovery is much more complicated than finding a binder but still, identification of relevant hits is an essential step (Wanner et al. 2011). These initial hits have then to be optimized in terms of potency/efficacy, selectivity, ADME-Tox (absorption, distribution, metabolism, excretion, and toxicity), and pharmacokinetics (PK) properties to achieve relevant therapeutic effects. Along all these steps, it is important to align the target, clinical goals, and chemical properties in such a way that a target product profile gets defined (i.e., a listing of the essential attributes required for a specific drug to be a clinically successful product and to be of substantial benefit over existing therapies) (Wyatt et al. 2011). After years of research (e.g., 5–7 years), if the molecules are deemed appropriate, clinical trials start. This final step can be followed by postmarket research to discover new applications of the newly reported drug. From this short overview of the process, it is clear that developing a new drug from the original idea to the launch of the final product is a very complex endeavor, the entire process can take 12–15 years and cost around $1 billion. It should be borne in mind that in general, this journey is characterized by very high attrition rates (Hughes et al. 2011; Duffy et al. 2012).

From these observations, it is clear that each and every step represents a challenge and for many years, the modulation of PPIs by low molecular weight compounds was considered impossible. In fact, many of the known difficulties pertaining to drug discovery are even more acute when it comes to the design of PPI modulators (this is also true for all the so-called challenging targets) while some difficulties tend to be specific to these untapped target opportunities (Domling 2008). A nonexhaustive list of challenges (real or perceived) is introduced below:

1. *Number of PPI and PPI selection*: Considering about half million possible PPIs in human (i.e., about 300,000) (Zhang et al. 2012) (so far only about 10% of pairwise interactions have been charted [Ruffner et al. 2007]) that could take place within and between cells, a first difficulty involves the selection of the right PPI target (selecting a target is always challenging but in the case of PPI, it can be even more difficult). Some *in vitro* and bioinformatics studies suggest that targeting protein nodes that possess a higher number of functional connections in a PPI network (hub proteins, see Box 17.1) could be beneficial in some disease conditions such as cancer and infectious diseases while in other cases, it would be beneficial to target bridges or edges instead of hubs (Jaeger and Aloy 2012; Furlong 2013). Although many progresses have been made in the area of target selection, much effort is needed and the present research on network and systems pharmacology should definitely shed new light and greatly assist the selection of the right target or of the right pathway (Rask-Andersen et al. 2011).

2. *PPI assays*: In general, a high-throughput assay has to be developed. This is a difficult task and it is important to dedicate enough time and funding to this step in order to avoid accumulating artifact compounds as much as possible (Wanner et al. 2011; Makley and Gestwicki 2013). It has been our experience that such assays tend to be developed too late in the project or too early, in some cases against the wrong protein partner, thereby slowing down the initial screening phase.

3. *Interface druggability and flexibility, docking, and scoring*: Also, still related to the selection of targets, comes the notion of druggability, here defined as the likelihood of finding high-affinity low-molecular weight binders (i.e., also called ligandability [Surade and Blundell 2012]). There are here many concepts and tools that can be applied depending on the available knowledge, but often, computational tools in the area of druggability prediction require the three-dimensional (3D) structure of the targets (see below). Traditionally, target-based drug discovery (with low-molecular weight compounds) has relied on designing or finding molecules that fit in a relatively well-defined concave binding pocket. However, PPIs have in general not evolved to bind a low-molecular weight chemical compound; interfaces tend to be flat, relatively large, often lacking a clear ligand-binding cavity (see below) (Fuller et al. 2009). Also, protein–protein interfaces tend to dynamically adapt to upcoming ligands (small- or large macro-molecules), and transient cavities not visible in some experimental structures can appear on the molecular surface during (or prior to) the binding event (Eyrisch and Helms 2007). In such cases, while the flexibility at the interface poses a significant challenge for structure-based drug design approaches, molecular simulation tools can assist and complement x-ray or nuclear magnetic resonance (NMR) studies (Rueda et al. 2010; Sperandio et al. 2010a; Ulucan et al. 2012). In fact, such flexibility features at the interface can turn out to be valuable for PPI drug designers. An important discovery critical to the notion of PPI druggability that gave hope to the rational design of small-molecule modulators was the finding that within a protein–protein binding interface only a small number of amino acids is crucial for the interaction (hotspots, residues that make a major contribution to the binding free energy) (Clackson and Wells 1995; Bogan and Thorn 1998). More recently, thanks to the availability of experimental 3D structures and innovative computational approaches, it has been shown that when a main hotspot region at a protein–protein interface has a concave topology, with one or two additional hotspots close enough to be reached from the first main hotspot site by a drug-sized molecule, then the region is likely to be druggable (Kozakov et al. 2011; Zerbe et al. 2012). Interestingly and as described below, identification of hotspots, binding pockets, and prediction of druggable regions is possible in many cases using theoretical means with a relatively high likelihood of success. Another point to make in this section is that currently available docking scoring tools for small molecules were not developed to target relatively flat PPI subpockets, suggesting that it will be important to design new *in silico* methods/protocols specific of PPIs.

4. *3D structures of PPIs*: Some additional complications in the field of PPI modulation have been the lack of structural knowledge about the

individual proteins forming the complex or about the macromolecular complex and the fact that some PPIs involve at least one partner (or one region) that is intrinsically disordered (Eyrisch and Helms 2007; Baker and Best 2014). Second-generation structural genomics initiatives together with advances in *in silico* PPI predictions should improve the situation in the coming years (Leis et al. 2010; Grosdidier and Fernandez-Recio 2012; Taboureau et al. 2011; Mosca et al. 2013). In this context, *in silico* simulation algorithms are important to identify transient binding pockets in the interface area and it is in some cases possible to fold a small protein (or part of a protein) in the context of another macromolecule (Eyrisch and Helms 2007; Sperandio et al. 2010a; Bowman and Geissler 2012; Baker and Best 2014; Johnson and Karanicolas 2013; Khan et al. 2013). Still about the notion of flexibility, some studies suggest that allosteric modulation could be a good strategy to act on PPIs (Gonzalez-Ruiz and Gohlke 2006; Schon et al. 2011; Ma and Nussinov 2013) but, while it is interesting from many points including the energetic of the interaction and possibly selectivity, the underlying complexity in terms of computational simulations and experimental approaches is such that further research is needed before the rational design of PPI allosteric modulators becomes mainstream. Fortunately, with tools able to identify possible binding pockets and hotspot residues or patches only with the structure of one partner, the design of a PPI modulator can still be initiated even if the 3D structure of the complex is not yet known.

5. *PPI compound collections*: Most often, PPI are screened with traditional compound collections and the hit rate is then usually very low (Barker et al. 2013). This often lead research groups to develop relatively expensive biologics, or to use low-throughput (yet efficient in many cases) fragment-based approaches while it could be that only redesigning the compound collection would be sufficient to improve the chance of finding interesting binders. Several studies have indeed shown that it should be possible to design a compound collection enriched in PPI modulators and much progress is expected in this area in a near future (Reynes et al. 2010; Sperandio et al. 2010b; Morelli et al. 2011; Fry et al. 2013). The reasoning behind is simple: most screening collections contain scaffolds and molecules specific or related to previously screened enzymes or membrane receptors, however, as mentioned above, the binding pockets of orthosteric PPI modulators at the protein–protein interfaces are in general different from those found in traditional protein targets (Fuller et al. 2009; Gautier et al. 2011) suggesting that it is important to expand the screening collections and explore new areas of the chemical space (Pagliaro et al. 2004; Sperandio et al. 2010b).

6. *ADME-Tox properties of PPI small-molecule modulators*: Another issue involves the ADME-Tox properties of the small molecules supposed to be modulating PPIs. Investigation of known PPI binders showed that the presently known molecules tend to have a larger molecular weight (average MW of 421 Da for protein–protein inhibitors versus 341 Da for regular drugs), higher log P (a mean value of ~5.1 for protein–protein inhibitors was found while it is around 3.5 for enzyme inhibitors) and have a more complex 3D structure than typical drugs, underlining further the need of rationally designing the screening collection. Of course, this general view does not apply to all PPI modulators (Bologa et al. 2006; Higueruelo et al. 2009; Sperandio et al. 2010b; Morelli et al. 2011; Villoutreix et al. 2012; Labbe et al. 2013). For example, many compounds that are known to inhibit PPIs (because of some of the physicochemical properties listed above, e.g., high lipophilicity) tend to violate several rules of thumb commonly used to select compounds after screening, or to prepare a compound collection or to predict bioavailability or toxicity (Gleeson 2008; Leeson and St-Gallay 2011; Hann and Keseru 2012; Taboureau et al. 2011; Bohnert and Gan 2013). Such rules can be, for instance, the Lipinski rule of five (Lipinski et al. 2001) or the 3/75 rule (computed log P < 3 and topological polar surface area (TPSA) > 75) as compounds with high-log P and low TPSA are approximately six times more likely to be toxic compared to low-log P/high TPSA compounds (Hughes et al. 2008) (see Box 17.2). In fact, because of some of these physicochemical

---

BOX 17.2   SHORT COMMENTS ABOUT ADME-TOX PROPERTIES AND RELATED RULES OF THUMB

Several rules of thumb have been reported these last years to assist the design of a compound collection or to help select the best compounds for further optimizations. There are many misapplications of these guidelines leading to much debates and eventually conflicts. A very well-known example is the rule of five by Lipinski, Lombardo, Dominy, and Feeney reported in 1997. These authors analyzed a set of orally delivered drugs and clinical candidates, and defined cutoffs that were separately chosen to capture about 90% of the ranges for four calculated properties:

Molecular mass ≤ 500
Calculated log P ≤ 5
Number of hydrogen bond donors ≤ 5
Number of hydrogen bond acceptors ≤ 10

These guidelines meant that a molecule whose properties fell outside these boundaries would be less likely orally absorbed. It was stated at that time that a compound with two parameters out of range would be subject to an alert but that the molecule should not be rejected without further investigation. Some drugs do not follow these rules and are yet orally available but this does not prevent considering the rules as they have to be understood: guidelines not rigid dogma. Then this set of rules went on and now tend to be misused as considered as a mean to define drug-likeness. These four properties are important (particularly log P and hydrogen bond donors) and are fundamentally interrelated. These rules certainly impact beyond oral bioavailability as it is known, for instance, that a high log P can be linked to hydrophobicity-associated toxicity. What many of these guidelines really formalize is that it is better to start with a smaller and less lipophilic molecule if the compound is intended to be orally bioavailable. Such a molecule should be easier to optimize and could be less toxic as less promiscuous (reduced risk of interacting with antitargets). While less than perfect, these rules still provide an efficient means of filtering compounds, they do not hinder research teams to learn from outliers but rather stimulate the design of new rules tuned to new and challenging targets underrepresented at the time they were drawn.

properties, some PPI modulators may fit the so-called class II (low solubility, high permeability) or class IV (low solubility, low permeability) category of the Biopharmaceutics Classification System (see for review [Dahan et al. 2009]). Along the physicochemical properties line of reasoning and rules of thumb, a GSK team showed that increasing lipophilicity usually contributes to lower drug efficiency and consequently such molecules tend to require higher doses, which in turn can increase the risk of adverse drug reactions (e.g., increased promiscuity leading to increase binding to antitargets) (Valko et al. 2012). Further, knowing that starting hits usually have to grow in size during the compound optimization phase with, in general, a further increase in log P (in fact, compounds that have more chance to succeed tend to preserve a relatively low lipophilicity during the optimization program) (Perola 2010), a clever design of PPI screening collection is required such as to obtain compounds with balanced ADME-Tox properties still compatible with the binding site features present at or near the protein–protein interfaces. This difficulty is reinforced by the usually low-hit rate observed when screening PPIs (in our hand often between 0.01% and 0.1% on various biological systems), underlining further the need of designing PPI-specific compound collections containing diverse molecules, exploring new areas of the chemical space and yet being compatible with oral and/or animal/human administration. Other difficulties could occur if a PPI compound has to hit a CNS target since the CNS physicochemical property ranges for molecular weight (around 300) and log P (around 2.8) (among others) are very stringent (Wager et al. 2010). However, although the ADME-Tox properties of PPI modulators are a legitimate concern, we have recently reviewed several PPI interfaces that can be modulated by hits that match the generally accepted rule of five-like guidelines (Villoutreix et al. 2012; Labbe et al. 2013). For the remaining molecules, it is true that some PPI modulators have a higher log P and molecular weight than many drug candidates that hit traditional targets, yet for the PPI modulators that have reached clinical trials, several seem to be orally available (Hann 2011). In addition, many studies highlight that some of these physical chemistry rules might be too restrictive (e.g., Faller et al. 2011; Zhao 2011) as, for instance, larger compounds could reduce their effective size and lipophilicity through hydrophobic collapse or by forming internal hydrogen bonds, thereby enhancing membrane permeability and possibly impacting the overall bioavailability (Bruncko et al. 2010; Alex et al. 2011; Ettorre et al. 2011; Zhao 2011). Furthermore, it has been stated that small PPI inhibitors tend to use more aromatic interactions than the corresponding protein partners that utilize also several charged residues, suggesting that new PPI modulators could possess more charged groups (this could improve some ADME-Tox properties while deteriorate others like permeability, but this information is important to explore) (Higueruelo et al. 2012). Tremendous amount of work is needed in this area while inspiration from natural compounds could help understand how to rationally go beyond several ADME-Tox rules of thumb (Ganesan 2008; Bauer et al. 2010). Overall, it is likely that such obstacles will be overcome in the coming years (Zinzalla and Thurston 2009; Villoutreix et al. 2012). *In silico* approaches that make use of multiparameter optimization protocols should indeed facilitate the design of molecules with balanced ADME-Tox properties, adequate potency and relevant selectivity tuned to the disease type (Segall 2012). Definitively, gain in knowledge will come from the analysis of compounds that are in advanced preclinical stages and in clinical trials. At present only around 30–50 compounds (Labbe et al. 2013) are at these stages but the increased research activity in this area should rapidly bring new insights that will favor rational and quality by design approaches.

17.3 Selected Databases and *In Silico* Tools to Assist the Design

In silico tools and associated databases are well established in the field of drug discovery, and we will discuss in this section some recently reported approaches that can assist the process (Zhong et al. 2007; Shublaq et al. 2013). First, databases, as they are at the heart of many research projects (i.e., data have to be collected and translated into knowledge). We will then focus on protein–protein interfaces and virtual screening. The URLs of hundreds of freely available tools and databases can be found at http://www.vls3d.com (Villoutreix et al. 2013), and we here mention only some very recent studies while we provide to the readers reviews that reference previously reported tools. These *in silico* methods/databases should ultimately help to answer some questions such as what is an appropriate interface for small molecule drug design, which regions of the chemical space should be explored, how to design a good starting collection or which screening protocols should be applied?

17.3.1 Some Selected and/or Recently Reported PPI-Related Databases

Several databases containing experimentally identified protein–protein complexes as well as predicted ones have been published these last years including protein interface databases (please see also Fernandez-Recio 2011; Orchard 2012; Winter et al. 2012a; Mosca et al. 2013). Often these databases do not contain information about the location of the interface but rather collate interactions from literature search and large-scale experiments. Other databases contain molecules cocrystallized at the PPI interfaces while yet others propose to visualize interacting networks or propose a comprehensive list of annotated small-molecule PPI modulators. For instance, databases containing information about possible PPIs include the Database of Interacting Proteins (DIP) (Salwinski et al. 2004), the Biomolecular Interaction Network (BIND) (Isserlin et al. 2011), the Molecular Interaction (MINT) (Licata et al. 2012), the Mammalian Protein–Protein Interaction (MIPS) (Pagel et al. 2005), the host–pathogen interaction database (HPIDB) (Kumar and Nanduri 2010), IntAct (Kerrien et al. 2012), BioGRID (Stark et al. 2011), STRING (Franceschini et al. 2013), among others. Obviously, errors and duplicates can be found in these databases and, in order to improve the quality of the data, the IMEx consortium was for instance created with the goal of sharing curation efforts (http://www.imexconsortium.org/about-imex). Structural information can be found at the Protein Data Bank (PDB) and for instance PISite collects interface data from the PDB (Higurashi et al. 2009). Structures of domain–domain interactions are available from 3did (Stein et al. 2011) and iPfam (Finn et al. 2005). Homology models can also be used to study further PPIs and increase coverage. The Interactome3D database (Mosca et al. 2013) provides 12,000 structurally resolved PPIs in eight organisms while Instruct contains over 6500 human PPIs (Meyer et al. 2013). Some other databases published in 2013 are reported in Table 17.1. One note for instance, the Protein Interaction and Molecule Search (PRIMOS) platform which represents a novel web portal that unifies six primary PPI databases (BIND; DIP; HPRD [Human Protein Reference Database]; IntAct; MINT and MIPS, Munich Information Center for Protein Sequences) into a

TABLE 17.1

Some PPI and Protein–Ligand Interaction-Related Databases Reported in 2013–2014

Name	Comments	Links	References
HippDB	The database catalogs every PPI whose structure is available in the PDB and which exhibits one or more helices at the interface	http://www.nyu.edu/ projects/arora/hippdb/	Bergey et al. (2012)
iRefWeb	iRefWeb is a bioinformatics resource that offers access to a large collection of data on PPIs in over a thousand organisms	http://wodaklab.org/ iRefWeb	Turinsky et al. (2014)
PRIMOS	PRIMOS: an integrated database of reassessed PPIs providing web-based access to *in silico* validation of experimentally derived data	http://primos. fh-hagenberg.at	Rid et al. (2013)
2P2Idb	A hand-curated structural database dedicated to PPIs with known orthosteric modulators	http://2p2idb.cnrs-mrs. fr	Basse et al. (2013)
TissueNet database	Database of human tissue PPIs	http://netbio.bgu.ac.il/ tissuenet/	Barshir et al. (2013)
PrePPI	A database that combines predicted and experimentally determined PPIs using a Bayesian framework	http://bhapp.c2b2. columbia.edu/PrePPI)	Zhang et al. (2012, 2013a)
TIMBAL	A database holding small-molecules modulating PPIs	http://www-cryst.bioc. cam.ac.uk/timbal	Higgueruelo et al. (2013)
SynSysNet	Integration of experimental data on synaptic PPIs with drug-target relations	http://bioinformatics. charite.de/synsysnet	von Eichborn et al. (2013)
iPPI-DB	A manually curated and interactive database of small nonpeptide inhibitors of PPIs	http://www.ippidb. cdithem.fr/	Labbe et al. (2013)
INstruct	A database of high-quality 3D structurally resolved protein interactome networks	http://instruct.yulab.org	Meyer et al. (2013)
STRING	A database of known and predicted PPIs	http://string-db.org/	Franceschini et al. (2013)

Note: More data can be found at www.vls3d.com.

single consistent repository (Rid et al. 2013). Along the same line, iRefWeb is a bioinformatics resource that offers access to a large collection of data on PPIs in over a thousand organisms. This collection is consolidated from 14 major public databases (Turinsky et al. 2014). Databases dedicated to small molecule modulators of PPIs are for instance 2P2Idb (manually curated) (Basse et al. 2013), TIMBAL (Higueruelo et al. 2013), and iPPI-DB (manually curated) (Labbe et al. 2013). Exploring and navigating these collections should help gain insights into privileged scaffolds or substructures particularly well suited to bind at the PPI interface and can help to derive new rules to design ADMET-friendly collections dedicated to PPIs.

17.3.2 Protein–Protein Interfaces, Hot Spots, and Ligand Binding Pockets

A first set of tools is dedicated to the prediction of protein–protein binding sites, which is technically very different from the prediction of ligand-binding sites (Fernandez-Recio 2011) (NB: it is also important to note that some tools could be flagged as binding site predictors while they also evaluate hotspots). Information about protein–protein binding sites is important for drug discovery as it helps to select a target and to design experiments to probe the interface. Diverse protein–protein binding site prediction methods have been reported, mostly based on sequence conservation, residue propensities, surface topology (planarity and protrusion), electrostatics, hydrophobicity, and solvent accessibility (Tuncbag et al. 2009; Leis et al. 2010; Fernandez-Recio 2011; Wanner et al. 2011; Bienstock 2012; Grosdidier and Fernandez-Recio 2012) (numerous online tools can be found here [Villoutreix et al. 2013], see also Table 17.2). Some protein–protein binding site prediction approaches are based on the protein sequence like the interaction sites identified from sequence (ISIS) approach (Ofran and Rost 2007) and PPIcons (even if the tool used some structural information during training) (Sriwastava et al. 2013) or SPPIDER (it runs with or without information about the 3D structure) (Porollo and Meller 2007). It has been noted that methods that use structural information tend to be more accurate than sequence-based approaches (see, for instance, Mosca et al. 2013). Some recently published tools or databases are the latest version of protein interactions by structural matching (PRISM) (Tuncbag et al. 2011), PrePPI (a database of predicted and experimentally determined protein–protein interactions) (Zhang et al. 2012) or BIPS (Biana Interolog Prediction Server) (Garcia-Garcia et al. 2012). A related concept involves the investigation of overlaps between small molecules and protein-binding sites within families of protein structures (i.e., bifunctional sites, so far about 8000 proteins from the human proteome have been annotated with bifunctional residues [Davis 2011]). Davis and Sali (Davis and Sali 2010) reported the HOMOLOBIND software (Davis 2011), a tool that identifies residues in protein sequences with significant similarity to structurally characterized binding sites. Yet, it should be mentioned

TABLE 17.2

Some Standalone and Online Tools Reported in 2013–2014 Dealing with PPI Prediction, Hotspots, and Binding Pockets

Name	Comments	Links	References
PPIcons	PPIcons: identification of PPI sites in selected organisms (standalone)	http://code.google.com/p/cmater-bioinfo/	Sriwastava et al. (2013)
iLoops	A PPI prediction server based on structural features	http://sbi.imim.es/iLoopsServer/index.php	Planas-Iglesias et al. (2013)
PPIevo	PPI prediction from PSSM-based evolutionary information (standalone)	http://lbb.ut.ac.ir/Download/LBBsoft/PPIevo/	Zahiri et al. (2013)
DockTrina	Docking triangular protein trimers (standalone)	http://nano-d.inrialpes.fr/software/docktrina/	Popov et al. (2014)
pyDockWEB	A web server for rigid-body protein–protein docking using electrostatics and desolvation scoring	http://life.bsc.es/servlet/pydock/home/	Jimenez-Garcia et al. (2013)
F(2)Dock 2.0 and GB-rerank	A rigid-body protein–protein docking software (standalone)	http://www.cs.utexas.edu/~bajaj/cvc/software/f2dock.shtml	Chowdhury et al. (2013)
SwarmDock	A server for flexible protein–protein docking	http://bmm.cancerresearchuk.org/~SwarmDock/	Torchala et al. (2013)
ATTRACT	Docking program (standalone)	http://www.t38.ph.tum.de/index.php?id = 88	de Vries and Zacharias (2013)
MEGADOCK	An all-to-all PPI prediction system using tertiary structure data (standalone)	http://www.bi.cs.titech.ac.jp/megadock/	Matsuzaki et al. (2013)
AlloSite	Predict allosteric binding site	http://202.120.138.35/AST/Allosite/index.jsp	Huang et al. (2013)
Frustratometer	An Energy Landscape Theory inspired algorithm that aims at quantifying the degree of local frustration manifested in protein molecules	http://lfp.qb.fcen.uba.ar/embnet/index.php	Jenik et al. (2012)
FTFLEX extension of FTMAP	Flexible protein mapping	http://ftflex.bu.edu/	Grove et al. (2013)

(Continued)

TABLE 17.2 (*Continued*)

Some Standalone and Online Tools Reported in 2013–2014 Dealing with PPI Prediction, Hotspots, and Binding Pockets

Name	Comments	Links	References
FTProd	Binding site comparison across multiple structures (standalone)	https://amarolab.ucsd.edu/ftprod/	Votapka and Amaro (2013)
2P2I scoring function	A scoring function to predict the druggability of protein–protein interfaces	http://2p2idb.cnrs-mrs.fr/2p2i_score.html	Basse et al. (2013)
DrosteP	Tool to evaluate the conservation of pockets detected on the protein surface by CastP (standalone)	http://www.icb.cnr.it/project/drosteppy/	Cammisa et al. (2013)
TRAPP	A tool for analysis of transient binding pockets in proteins	http://www.mcm.h-its.org/trapp/	Kokh et al. (2013)
eFindSite	Improved prediction of ligand binding sites in protein models using meta-threading, machine learning, and auxiliary ligands	http://brylinski.cct.lsu.edu/efindsite	Brylinski and Feinstein (2013)
PocketAnnotate	Functional annotation of proteins	http://proline.biochem.iisc.ernet.in/pocketannotate/index.php	Anand et al. (2012)
APoc	Large-scale identification of similar protein pockets (standalone)	http://cssb.biology.gatech.edu/APoc	Gao and Skolnick (2013)
SKEMPI	Structural kinetic and energetic database of mutant protein interactions and its use in empirical models	http://life.bsc.es/pid/mutation_database/	Moal and Fernandez-Recio (2012)

Note: More data can be found at www.vls3d.com.

that some studies suggest that PPIs appear to be rarely conserved unless a very high sequence similarity is observed. Consequently, some research groups suggest that approaches applying inferred interactions should be used with care (see, for instance, Lewis et al. 2012). Protein–protein docking approaches and template-based structure modeling of PPI tools can also be used to propose interaction regions (Hwang et al. 2014; Szilagyi and Zhang 2014). These tools usually benefit from the knowledge of predicted interacting residues, site-directed mutagenesis, and other experimental information such as SAXS, electron microscopy, or NMR. Many protein–protein docking engines have been reviewed like, for instance, in Taboureau et al. (2011) and Bienstock (2012) while some protein–protein docking tools released (or optimized) in 2013 include DockTrina (for docking triangular protein trimers) (Popov et al. 2014), ATTRACT (de Vries and Zacharias 2013), MEGADOCK (Matsuzaki et al. 2013), pyDockWEB (Jimenez-Garcia et al. 2013), F(2)Dock 2.0 and GB-rerank (Chowdhury et al. 2013), and SwarmDock (incorporating flexibility) (Torchala et al. 2013). These approaches can benefit from new scoring functions as illustrated by the combination of DockRank and the protein–protein docking tool ClusPro (Xue et al. 2014).

After locating the overall interacting regions or the specific residues involved in the interaction, small-molecule drug discovery projects dedicated to PPI requires the identification of a compound that should in principle bind to or near the PPI interface region (Isvoran et al. 2013). Modulation of a selected PPI could also be achieved, for example, with an allosteric modulator that binds away from the interface. While this is possible using HTS screening, this is very challenging via structure-based rational approaches. To identify an allosteric binding pocket (possible but difficult [Panjkovich and Daura 2012]) tools such as AlloSite (Huang et al. 2013) or the Frustratometer (Jenik et al. 2012) have been reported. Yet, to predict that the propagation of the structural changes (some allosteric signals may only alter the dynamics of the protein and not induce conformational changes [Duran-Frigola et al. 2013]) resulting from such protein-small ligand contact will act at the interface and that the function of such a small molecule could stabilize or impede the interaction are essentially impossible with the presently available experimental and *in silico* approaches. As a result, while allosteric modulators are definitively interesting, the rational design of such molecules is still very difficult. As such, in general *in silico* drug designer teams tend to focus on small molecules that are expected to bind at or near the interface (the molecule can however act through allosteric mechanism or by a combination of allostery and direct competition or by direct competition alone) rather than to sites that are far away from the main contact area.

To continue the project once a target has been identified and an overall interaction area has been found and in the case one has some structural information about the proteins involved in the complex, it is possible to use the concept of hotspots (residues that are responsible for the stabilization of the complex) (Clackson and Wells 1995) to rationally design PPI modulators.

These hotspots can be identified experimentally but a number of computational approaches can also be used (Thangudu et al. 2012). It should be remembered that hotspot residues are not so easy to identify experimentally (e.g., by alanine-scanning experiments that show that the binding energy is not equally distributed among all amino acids participating in the interaction) or *in silico* (see for instance discussions about possible misconceptions of alanine-scanning results [Metz et al. 2012a; Zerbe et al. 2012]). Hotspot residues (among the most conserved amino acids) are generally located around the center of the interface, and protected from bulk solvent by energetically less-important residues forming a hydrophobic O-ring. Tryptophan, arginine, and tyrosine are often hotspot residues whereas leucine, serine, threonine, and valine tend to be disfavored (Fernandez-Recio 2011). The surface area of a region containing some hotspot residues is around 600 $Å^2$, a size that is compatible with a small molecule (NB: traditional protein-small ligand interaction ~300–1000 $Å^2$), and much smaller than a typical protein–protein interface (e.g., 1200–2000 to well over 3000 $Å^2$) (Janin et al. 2008). *In silico* tools that help to predict hotspots can be the ISIS (interaction sites identified from sequence) approach mentioned above, and if structural data are available, *in silico* alanine-scanning can be carried out with, for example, FoldX (Schymkowitz et al. 2005), Robetta (Kim et al. 2004), HotPoint (Tuncbag et al. 2010), or DSPPI (Kruger and Gohlke 2010). Alternate methods have been developed that are based on probing a protein surface with organic fragments and predicting the locations of hot spots based on where fragments interact with high affinity. Tools like FTMAP (Kozakov et al. 2011) (computational mapping with 16 different chemical probes) and the FTFLEX extension of FTMAP (which takes into account side-chain flexibility on the fly) (Grove et al. 2013) can be used for hot-spot prediction while if multiple structures are available (or obtained via molecular dynamics [MD]), FTProd (Votapka and Amaro 2013) could be applied. Other methods for hotspot prediction can be based on protein–protein docking simulations, like for instance with the module pyDockNIP of the pyDock software package (Grosdidier and Fernandez-Recio 2008; Fernandez-Recio 2011). Hotspots can also be investigated by MD in water and in isopropanol/water cosolvent environment (see, for instance, Yang and Wang 2011). Related to hotspots is the concept of "anchor" sites, which contrary to hotspots have explicit concave/convex geometries appealing for pharmaceutical intervention (i.e., anchors can also be hotspots). The online tool ANCHOR was developed along this concept to assist the design of small molecule modulators of PPIs (Meireles et al. 2010). Another related concept is the notion of druggable interface. The 2P2I scoring function has been specifically designed to investigate such a feature (Basse et al. 2013). A question associated with the prediction of hotspots is to try to predict where a small molecule could bind at a PPI interface (i.e., one may want to touch a hotspot residue present in a binding pocket). Some of the tools mentioned above can do both, like for instance ANCHOR or FTMAP. These tools tend to work on a static structure (although one can generate alternative conformations prior to the computations) while some others combine identification of hotspots by MM-PBSA free energy decomposition on the basis of the structural ensemble generated by MD and generation of transient pockets using MD and FRODA simulations (Metz et al. 2012b). Another tool dedicated to PPI described by Koes and Camacho identifies and ranks clusters of interface residues in a PPI that are most suitable as starting points for rational small-molecule design. These clusters are called Small-Molecule Inhibitor Starting Points (SMISPs) and the approach is complementary to methods that identify binding sites through an analysis of the receptor surface (either through shape descriptors or chemical probes). The PocketQuery web service has been developed around this concept to predict hotspots, anchor residues, and hot regions (Koes and Camacho 2012). These authors expect, after a PDB-wide analysis, that about 48% of the protein complexes could be modulated with a low molecular weight molecule. A recent study aiming at characterizing the nature of protein residues at overlapping protein–protein and protein–ligand binding interfaces with the goal of predicting where a small molecule could bind was recently reported. The dataset used is available at the ABC2 database and the resulting prediction algorithm was applied on 10,000 protein–protein interfaces reported by Walter et al. (2013).

Although tools predicting binding pockets and the druggability of pockets have been essentially developed for regular targets, such methods can still be used (with cautions) prior to for instance structure-based virtual screening computations for PPIs. Binding pocket detection algorithms are essentially subdivided into two major classes, geometry-based and energy-based tools (Perot et al. 2010). In addition to predict binding pockets, some tools also provide a druggability score. In general, methods work on a static protein structure but some also take into account protein flexibility. There are in addition about 20 methods that evaluate pocket similarity. Several recent articles or reviews describe these tools and the underlying concepts (Perot et al. 2010; Fauman et al. 2011; Kufareva et al. 2012; Zheng et al. 2012; Dessailly et al. 2013; Trosset and Vodovar 2013; Wirth et al. 2013). Some recently reported approaches to predict pockets and/or pocket druggability (see Villoutreix et al. 2013) are Provar (Ashford et al. 2012), MetaPocket (Zhang et al. 2011), DrosteP (Cammisa et al. 2013), DoGSiteScorer (Volkamer et al. 2012), TRAPP (Kokh et al. 2013), or eFindSite (Brylinski and Feinstein 2013) while recent pocket comparisons tools include PocketAnnotate (Anand et al. 2012), APoc (Gao and Skolnick 2013), and SiteComp (Lin et al. 2012).

Additional information on PPI druggability could come from nonsynonymous single nucleotide polymorphisms (nsSNPs) (i.e., single base changes leading to a change to the amino acid sequence of the encoded protein) data because many of these variants are associated with disease. Clearly, the development of affordable techniques for sequencing genomes and the application of these approaches will generate vast amount of new data, including SNPs. Thus far, studies looking at the effects of nsSNPs were performed on individual proteins but now, the impact of nsSNPs on PPIs starts to be investigated (Yates and Sternberg 2013; Zhang et al. 2013b). It seems that when a disease-causing nsSNPs do not occur in a protein core region, they are preferentially located at a protein–protein interface rather than on noninterface regions (David et al. 2012). These studies could help find rules that assist the selection of a target. Along this line, the manually curated SKEMPI database has been developed and contains the effects of mutation on binding energies for about 2792 mutations across 85 protein–protein complexes (Moal and Fernandez-Recio 2012). New insights should definitively come from the analysis of such repository.

Further, it is important to note that many protein complexes seem to be dominated by a hot segment where the interaction is dominated by a continuous epitope and as such hot segments are good predictors of PPI druggability (London et al. 2013a). Still along this line of attempting to predict druggability, a recently reported study attempts to define classes of PPIs that could be more easily modulated by small molecules and suggests that the "tight and narrow" and "weak and narrow" protein–protein complex categories are good candidates (Smith and Gestwicki 2012). One does note the many different and yet related concepts in this section and definitively *in silico* methods have been instrumental to investigate PPIs.

17.3.3 Virtual Screening

The term "virtual screening" (or *in silico* screening) was first reported in the scientific literature in 1997 (Horvath 1997); it can be defined as a set of computer methods that analyzes large databases or collections of compounds in order to identify and prioritize likely hit candidates (Phatak et al. 2009). *In silico* screening search can be performed on libraries that contain physically existing compounds or on virtual libraries, and thus on compounds that are not yet synthesized. Noteworthy is the fact that virtual screening can be used on very large databases that no experimental approaches can tackle. It is important to remember that the easily accessible drug-like space contains about 10^{33} molecules (Polishchuk et al. 2013) and that with 17 atoms and simple chemistry rules, it is already possible to generate 166 billion compounds (Ruddigkeit et al. 2012). Yet, it should be noted that *in silico* screening goes much beyond number crunching, it helps to generate ideas, to reduce the cost and to gain knowledge. *In silico* screening experiments can be performed to complement HTS (and are indeed often integrated in screening campaigns), prior to experimental screening, or after HTS to rescue some compounds potentially missed by the *in vitro* readouts (see latent hits by Varin et al. (2012) (Tanrikulu et al. 2011). Furthermore, diverse *in silico* screening experiments can be applied after phenotypic screening or on complex formulations in an attempt to explain the mode of actions of the molecules (see, e.g., a chemoinformatics study performed on traditional Chinese and Ayurvedic medicines [Mohd Fauzi et al. 2013]) or for drug repurposing

(Liu et al. 2013). The complementarity between HTS and virtual screening has been shown in many studies, like for instance by screening both *in silico* and experimentally the same 198,000-compound collection against cruzain, a cysteine protease target for Chagas disease (Ferreira et al. 2010). Along the same line, a computer screening experiment performed on a subset of the ChemBridge compound collection (about 500,000 molecules) and a study making use of HTS (50,000 molecules using also molecules from ChemBridge) found quasi-identical hit molecules for the proteasome cancer target (Marechal et al. 2013; Ozcan et al. 2013).

Virtual screening approaches have been traditionally subdivided into two main approaches (Figure 17.2): first, ligand-based screening, in which 2D

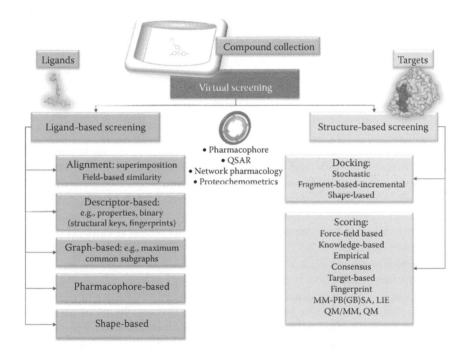

FIGURE 17.2
Main virtual screening methods. Some approaches can be considered to be at the interface between the two main screening concepts, ligand-based and structure-based, such as some types of pharmacophore modeling that use information derived from cocrystallized target-ligand complexes or in the case of proteochemometric modeling, QSAR, and systems pharmacology. Abbreviations: LIE: linear energy interaction; MM-PB(GB)SA, molecular mechanics-Poisson Boltzmann (Generalized Born) Solvent accessibility; QM/MM, quantum mechanics/molecular mechanics; QM, molecular mechanics. Additional information can be found in some recent reviews about virtual screening (From Stumpfe, D., P. Ripphausen, and J. Bajorath. 2012. *Future Med. Chem.* 4(5):593–602), fragment-based approaches (From Zoete, V., A. Grosdidier, and O. Michielin. 2009. *J. Cell Mol. Med.* 13(2):238–248.), structure-based tools for screening and compound optimization (From Joseph-McCarthy, D. et al. 2007. *Curr. Opin. Drug Discov. Devel.* 10(3):264–274.) or systems pharmacology (Taboureau et al. 2011), or pharmacophore. (From Voet, A. et al. 2013. *Curr. Top. Med. Chem.* 13(9):989–1001.)

or 3D chemical structures or molecular descriptors of known actives (and sometimes inactive molecules) are used to retrieve other compounds of interest from a database using some types of similarity measure or by seeking a common substructure or pharmacophore between the query molecule and the compounds in the database; and second, structure-based (or 3D receptor-based) screening in which compounds from the database are docked into a binding site (or over the entire surface) and are ranked using one or several scoring functions. Structure-based virtual screening also includes tools to perform binding site-derived pharmacophore search. There are some slight differences on how the methods are classified but the nomenclature used here is generally well accepted (Stumpfe et al. 2012). Of importance for PPIs is that structure-based screening can be carried out on homology models or on low-resolution structures (Cavasotto and Phatak 2009; Fan et al. 2009; Skolnick et al. 2013).

The structure-based virtual screening process can then be continued if deemed appropriate using different types of postprocessing approaches (see, for instance, Pencheva et al. 2008, 2013; Yuriev and Ramsland 2013). Ligand- and structure-based methods can be combined if the necessary information is available (Sperandio et al. 2008). Virtual screening methods are relatively well established, and numerous success stories in terms of hit identification, contribution to the development of drug candidates, or marketed products have been recently reviewed (Clark 2008; Villoutreix et al. 2009). This does not mean that the methods have no flaws but yet they contribute significantly to the identification of interesting molecules (Scior et al. 2012). Over 100 commercial and free tools are available to carry out virtual screening, many of these approaches have been discussed in several recent reviews (Liao et al. 2011; Ripphausen et al. 2012; Taboureau et al. 2011; Villoutreix et al. 2013; Yuriev and Ramsland 2013; Voet et al. 2013).

A compound collection is required to perform virtual screening and its preparation is obviously as mentioned above critical in the case of PPI screening (Sperandio et al. 2010b; Morelli et al. 2011). Physicochemical properties, structural alerts, and flags for promiscuity should in general be considered. This is also important because molecules have to be optimized (Zhu et al. 2013), and it has been noticed that artifact compounds (e.g., pan assay interference compounds [PAINS]) are reported at a growing rate (Baell and Holloway 2010; Whitty 2011; Taboureau et al. 2011) (warning, some authors do not find that some PAINS molecules are that problematic [Mok et al. 2013]). *In silico* tools such as the FAF-Drugs online server (Lagorce et al. 2011) can assist in the preparation of a compound collection and, for instance, evaluate physicochemical properties, search for the presence of PAINS and toxicophores as well as assess the potential of a compound (the molecule has to be in 3D) to be a PPI inhibitor according to the rules defined in Reynes et al. (2010). It is important to note that when searching for PPI modulators it might be necessary to apply soft *in silico* ADME-Tox filters to prepare the collection. For example, chemical groups that could react with a protein to form a covalent bond are usually not welcome in a drug discovery program, yet this could be useful when probing a PPI like in the case of inhibitors of the thyroid hormone receptor and coregulator proteins (Arnold et al. 2005). As mentioned above, traditional compound collections available in a screening center were usually not prepared to screen PPIs and as such, it could be valuable to generate focused collections enriched in potential PPI modulators. In order to do that, two available tools have been recently reported (if the 3D structure of the target is known obviously other approaches can also be applied). Using known PPI inhibitors and machine learning, the PPI-HitProfiler engine was developed and is the first freely available application ever reported (Reynes et al. 2010) (standalone application via the CDithem website http://www.cdithem. fr/). This tool is now available online via the FAF-Drugs-2 server (Lagorce et al. 2011). Another method to prepare compound collection enriched in PPI inhibitors is 2P2IHUNTER that filters orthosteric PPI modulators via a dedicated support vector machine developed using a set of PPI inhibitor cocrystallized at protein–protein interface (Hamon et al. 2013). While all virtual screening approaches can be used, some like pharmacophore derived from protein–protein interfaces (Voet et al. 2013) seem well suited to identify hits once a PPI target has been selected. Other tools like docking-scoring can be used although they have not been designed to target PPI pockets (the docking step can be affected by the lack of well-defined binding cavity and the scoring step is always sensitive). Yet, in a recent study performed over several ligand-docking engines, it was found that good docking solutions could be obtained using conventional docking-scoring tools (yet a drop of about 10% has been noticed as compared to regular pockets [Kruger et al. 2012]), suggesting that structure-based screening can already assist the design of PPI modulators although additional methodological developments are required.

17.4 Recent PPI Success Stories

Modulating PPI with a small molecule could be beneficial in many cases, even more so if the small molecule can be administered orally (Wells and McClendon 2007; Thiel et al. 2012). First, this could open new avenue for therapeutic intervention (Falchi et al. 2014). Further, designing catalytic site inhibitors can be limited by high structural similarity among enzymes of the same family, whereas the greater structural variability of protein–protein interfaces may provide a real opportunity for selectivity. Also, PPI modulators could be less prone to drug resistance than catalytic site inhibitors. In addition, even if two proteins bind with high affinity, they could be successfully out-competed by a weakly small molecule binder. Indeed, in some cases, the mere alteration of a binding equilibrium will be sufficient to produce a significant biological effect without the need to completely inhibit the selected PPI. In this paragraph, we will show that interesting hits could be found by combining *in silico* and *in vitro* screening approaches.

17.4.1 Inhibition of the VEGF-VEGFR Interaction

Vascular endothelial growth factor (VEGF) plays a key role in angiogenesis, one of the hallmarks of cancer (Ferrara and Kerbel 2005). VEGF binds to two major tyrosine kinase receptors (TKR), VEGFR-1 and VEGFR-2, on the surface of endothelial cells, thereby activating signal transduction and regulating both physiological and pathological angiogenesis. Whereas VEGFR-1 has been shown to stimulate endothelial cells migration (Kanno et al. 2000), VEGFR-2 is known to be the main mediator of signaling pathway in endothelial cells (Holmes et al. 2007). The VEGF-VEGFR system is a validated and promising target for anti-angiogenic treatments. Although the VEGF-VEGFR interface was found to be one of the flattest protein–protein interfaces available in the investigated dataset (with a planarity value of 1.7 Å [Gautier et al. 2011]), well below those of most transient protein–protein complexes (mean planarity value = 2.7 Å [Reynolds et al. 2009], successful structure-based *in silico* screening was performed by targeting the VEGF-binding zone of the extracellular domain D2 of VEGFR-1. As flexibility is known to be important at protein–protein interfaces, the DFprot server was used to investigate the possible plasticity of the D2 domain of VEGFR-1 (Garzon et al. 2007). Analysis of the x-ray structure and of the simulation suggested that this region of the D2 domain was essentially rigid and as such, the authors performed docking experiments on only one 3D structure of the D2 domain. Then, 8000 proprietary drug-like molecules were docked with Surflex (Jain 2003) onto the predicted binding pockets of the target (Figure 17.3). After the *in silico* analysis, 206 compounds were selected for *in vitro* assays. Twenty compounds inhibiting the formation of the VEGF-VEGFR complex in the micromolar range were identified. The bioactive molecules contained a (3-carboxy-2-ureido) thiophen unit and the best IC_{50} was ~10 µM. Moreover, the most potent compound 4321 (shown in Figure 17.4) decreased the auto-phosphorylation of VEGFR-1 induced by VEGF, inhibited HUVE cells capillary formation and disrupted the actin and tubulin networks. These findings suggest that the best hit could be a promising scaffold to probe this macromolecular complex and used as a starting point to develop new treatments of diseases linked to VEGFR-1.

17.4.2 Inhibition of the Calmodulin-Edema Factor Interaction

Edema factor (EF) is a calmodulin (CaM)-activated adenylyl cyclase (AC) toxin from *Bacillus anthracis* that contributes to anthrax pathogenesis. Anthrax is an important medical problem and the treatment of *B. anthracis* infections is still unsatisfying. It has been suggested that selective EF inhibitors could be valuable drugs for such infection. However, a key challenge is

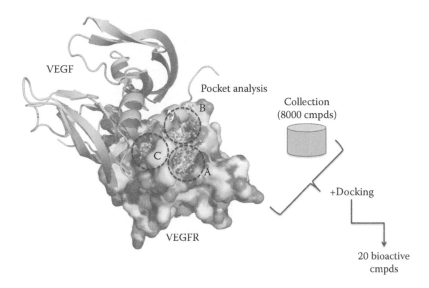

FIGURE 17.3
(**See color insert.**) VEGF-VEGFR binding pockets. The crystal structure of residues 8–109 of VEGF (cartoon diagram) in complex with VEGFR-1 D2 domain (shown here in solid surface representation; yellow, hydrophobic/aromatic; red, oxygen atom and/or negatively charged; blue, nitrogen atom and/or positively charged) is shown. A probe-mapping algorithm was used to analyze the interface area (green sphere highlights regions where carbon atoms can bind with reasonable affinity, blue spheres represent nitrogen atoms and red spheres, carbonyl groups). Three subpockets, A, B, and C, could be identified and are shown as dashed circles. Structure-based virtual screening was carried out over this entire zone and 20 molecules were identified. The best compound binds directly to the VEGFR-1 D2 domain and inhibits PPI.

to obtain compounds with high selectivity for AC toxins relative to mammalian membranious ACs and thus some efforts have been directed toward the development of EF inhibitors targeting directly the EF-CaM interaction. To this end, Blondel and coworkers (Laine et al. 2010) developed an *in silico* protocol combining simulation and docking-scoring methods (Figure 17.5). They modeled the putative conformational pathway of EF based on the known initial inactive (apo) and final active (CaM-bound) conformations. In fact, the binding of CaM to EF induces a major transition from a closed to an open form of EF. The transition path conformations were generated by using steered MD simulations and conjugate peak refinement approach. The path conformations were systematically analyzed with the PocketFinder module of ICM (www.molsoft.com). A druggable site that could block the conformational transition of EF when occupied with a small ligand was identified. This site involves amino acid residues from the so-called switches A, B, and C of the CaM-binding zone of EF, also called SABC pocket. Then, virtual screening of 28,000 molecules from the French National Chemical Library was performed on several different conformations selected from the conformational path using the software FlexX. The authors tested 18 compounds in

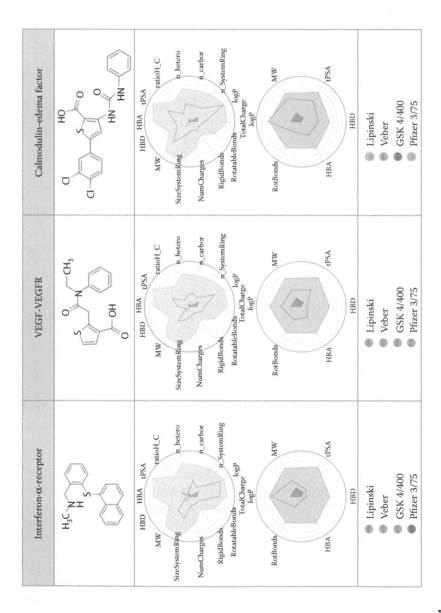

FIGURE 17.4

(See color insert.) Analysis of three PPI inhibitors. 2D structures and ADME-Tox properties evaluation (computed with FAF-Drugs) for the three best PPI inhibitors discussed in the success story section (see text for further explanations about the rules).

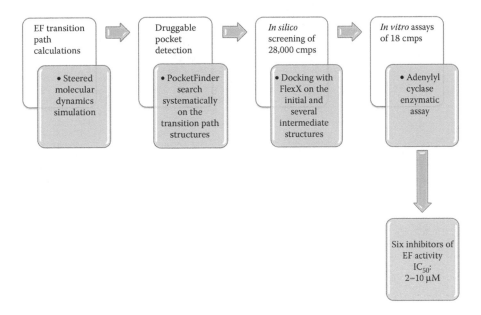

FIGURE 17.5
New inhibitors of CaM-EF complex formation. A workflow of the modeling and *in silico* screening protocol employed for the identification of new inhibitors of CaM-EF complex formation.

an *in vitro* assay and identified six compounds with a 5-phenyl-3-(3-phenylureido)thiophene-2-carboxylic acid scaffold that inhibit EF catalysis. The most potent compound (shown in Figure 17.4) inhibits the activity of EF with an IC_{50} of 2 µM. The scaffold offers ample opportunities for optimization. The compounds also inhibited the related AC toxin from Bordetella pertussis. The specific homology between the putative binding sites of both toxins supports that these pockets are the actual binding sites of the selected inhibitors.

17.4.3 Modulation of the Interferon-α (IFN-α) with Its Receptor

Interferons (IFNα and β) are proinflammatory cytokines that confer cellular resistance to vital infections. They constitute a first line of defense against pathogens. All type I IFNs bind to one specific cell surface receptor often named IFNAR. This PPI initiates a positive feedback loop leading to elevated IFN levels. Previous studies have shown that a high number of IFNα could contribute to the pathogenesis of a severe autoimmune disorder called lupus erythematosus (Swiecki and Colonna 2010). Geppert et al. (2012) were interested to search drug-like low molecular weight inhibitors of the PPI involving IFNα and its receptor IFNAR with the ultimate goal of reducing IFNα levels. Using a combination of PocketPicker (cavity extraction) and iPred hotspot detection performed on the IFNα interface, they identified a binding cavity of about 155 Å^3 surrounded by four predicted hotspot residues (Phe27, Leu30, Lys31, and Arg149) (Figure 17.6), confirming the results of a

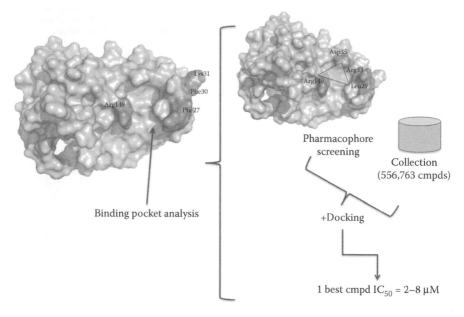

FIGURE 17.6
Modulation of the interferon-α (IFN-α) with its receptor. Using a combination of pocket detection and hotspot prediction tools, a binding cavity was found surrounded by four predicted hotspot residues (Phe27, Leu30, Lys31, and Arg149, dark gray, left side of the figure), confirming the results of a mutation study that highlighted the importance of this area for the interaction. Then, based on four important residues (Arg149, Asp35, Arg33, and Leu29, dark gray, right side of the figure), a permissive pharmacophore model was used for the screening of 556,763 commercially available compounds. Six compounds were manually extracted and docked and one best compound was identified.

mutation study that highlighted these residues as critical for the interaction. The authors also identified four residues (Arg149, Asp35, Arg33, and Leu29) in or next to the small putative binding pocket found with PocketPicker that were near this hotspot region and that could possibly bind part of a small molecule. Using these four residues surrounding the pocket, they generated a permissive pharmacophore model using the VirtualLigand tool. This pharmacophore was then used for the screening of 556,763 commercially available compounds. From the top-ranking 100 molecules, six compounds were selected interactively and docked using the Gold software into the IFNα pocket. The ability of inhibiting IFNα response was tested experimentally for these six compounds. Only the best scoring compound obtained by Gold was able to completely inhibit the investigated biological reaction ($IC_{50} = 2$–$8\ \mu M$). SPR measurements were also carried out during this analysis to validate direct binding and the authors determined a dissociation constant of about $4\ \mu M$ for the interaction between the best molecule and IFNα. An x-ray structure of the (IFN)–(IFNAR2-EC) complex (PDB ID: 3s9d) was published after completion of the Geppert et al. study and confirmed the importance of the identified hotspot residues. Thus, in that study, these authors were able to find a nonpeptidic low molecular weight molecule that inhibited the interaction between IFNα and its receptor using a combined *in silico–in vitro* approach.

17.5 Conclusion

Most disease-modifying proteins exert their functions through interactions with other proteins. Although PPIs are essential for cellular functions, targeting such interactions with small molecules (and if possible orally available compounds) has been a challenge thus far. Yet, as we gain knowledge about these macromolecular systems, we expect to see more and more modulators of PPIs entering clinical trials and most likely new drugs will become approved for this target class in the coming years. Drug repositioning could also be applied as illustrated by the discovery of raloxifene and bazedoxifene as novel inhibitors of the IL-6-GP130 interface (Li et al. 2014). Clearly, some biological systems are going to be easier to address with low molecular weight compounds than others just like in the case of enzymes. We have seen in this chapter that several *in silico* methods can be used in combination with *in vitro* experiments to assist the process. The many ongoing *in silico* developments worldwide should definitively contribute to a more efficient and rational discovery of new types of PPI modulators against an ever-increasing number and diversity of protein–protein complexes.

References

Alex, A., D. S. Millan, M. Perez, F. Wakenhut, and G. A. Whitlock. 2011. Intramolecular hydrogen bonding to improve membrane permeability and absorption in beyond rule of five chemical space. *Med. Chem. Commun.* 2(7):669–674.

Anand, P., K. Yeturu, and N. Chandra. 2012. PocketAnnotate: Towards site-based function annotation. *Nucleic Acids Res.* 40 Web Server issue:W400–W408.

Arnold, L. A., E. Estebanez-Perpina, M. Togashi et al. 2005. Discovery of small molecule inhibitors of the interaction of the thyroid hormone receptor with transcriptional coregulators. *J. Biol. Chem.* 280(52):43048–43055.

Ashford, P., D. S. Moss, A. Alex et al. 2012. Visualisation of variable binding pockets on protein surfaces by probabilistic analysis of related structure sets. *BMC Bioinformatics.* 13:39.

Azzarito, V., K. Long, N. S. Murphy, and A. J. Wilson. 2013. Inhibition of alpha-helix-mediated protein-protein interactions using designed molecules. *Nat. Chem.* 5(3):161–173.

Baell, J. B. and G. A. Holloway. 2010. New substructure filters for removal of pan assay interference compounds (PAINS) from screening libraries and for their exclusion in bioassays. *J. Med. Chem.* 53(7):2719–2740.

Baker, C. M. and R. B. Best. 2014. Insights into the binding of intrinsically disordered proteins from molecular dynamics simulation. *WIREs Comput. Mol. Sci.* 4:182–198.

Barker, A., J. G. Kettle, T. Nowak, and J. E. Pease. 2013. Expanding medicinal chemistry space. *Drug Discov. Today* 18(5–6):298–304.

Barshir, R., O. Basha, A. Eluk, I. Y. Smoly, A. Lan, and E. Yeger-Lotem. 2013. The TissueNet database of human tissue protein-protein interactions. *Nucleic Acids Res.* 41 Database issue:D841–D844.

Basse, M. J., S. Betzi, R. Bourgeas et al. 2013. 2P2Idb: A structural database dedicated to orthosteric modulation of protein-protein interactions. *Nucleic Acids Res.* 41 Database issue:D824–D827.

Bauer, R. A., J. M. Wurst, and D. S. Tan. 2010. Expanding the range of "druggable" targets with natural product-based libraries: An academic perspective. *Curr. Opin. Chem. Biol.* 14(3):308–314.

Bergey, C. M., A. M. Watkins, and P. S. Arora. 2012. HippDB: A database of readily targeted helical protein-protein interactions. *Bioinformatics* 29(21):2806–2807.

Bienstock, R. J. 2012. Computational drug design targeting protein-protein interactions. *Curr. Pharm. Des.* 18(9):1240–254.

Blazer, L. L. and R. R. Neubig. 2009. Small molecule protein-protein interaction inhibitors as CNS therapeutic agents: Current progress and future hurdles. *Neuropsychopharmacology* 34(1):126–141.

Bogan, A. A. and K. S. Thorn. 1998. Anatomy of hot spots in protein interfaces. *J. Mol. Biol.* 280(1):1–9.

Bohnert, T. and L. S. Gan. 2013. Plasma protein binding: From discovery to development. *J. Pharm. Sci.* 102(9):2953–2994.

Bologa, C. G., M. M. Olah, and T. I. Oprea. 2006. Chemical database preparation for compound acquisition or virtual screening. *Methods Mol. Biol.* 316(6):375–388.

Bowman, G. R. and P. L. Geissler. 2012. Equilibrium fluctuations of a single folded protein reveal a multitude of potential cryptic allosteric sites. *Proc. Natl. Acad. Sci. U.S.A.* 109(29):11681–11686.

Bruncko, M., S. K. Tahir, X. Song et al. 2010. N-aryl-benzimidazolones as novel small molecule HSP90 inhibitors. *Bioorg. Med. Chem. Lett.* 20(24):7503–7506.

Brylinski, M. and W. P. Feinstein. 2013. eFindSite: Improved prediction of ligand binding sites in protein models using meta-threading, machine learning and auxiliary ligands. *J. Comput. Aided. Mol. Des.* 27(6):551–567.

Bultinck, J., S. Lievens, and J. Tavernier. 2012. Protein-protein interactions: Network analysis and applications in drug discovery. *Curr. Pharm. Des.* 18(30):4619–4629.

Cammisa, M., A. Correra, G. Andreotti, and M. V. Cubellis. 2013. Identification and analysis of conserved pockets on protein surfaces. *BMC Bioinformatics* 14 Suppl 7:S9.

Cavasotto, C. N. and S. S. Phatak. 2009. Homology modeling in drug discovery: Current trends and applications. *Drug Discov. Today* 14(13–14):676–683.

Chene, P. 2006. Drugs targeting protein-protein interactions. *ChemMedChem.* 1(4):400–411.

Chowdhury, R., M. Rasheed, D. Keidel et al. 2013. Protein-protein docking with F(2) Dock 2.0 and GB-rerank. *PLoS One* 8(3):e51307.

Clackson, T. and J. A. Wells. 1995. A hot spot of binding energy in a hormone-receptor interface. *Science* 267(5196):383–386.

Clark, D. E. 2008. What has virtual screening ever done for drug discovery? *Expert. Opin. Drug Discov.* 3(8):841–851.

CML, Experts in. 2013. The price of drugs for chronic myeloid leukemia (CML) is a reflection of the unsustainable prices of cancer drugs: From the perspective of a large group of CML experts. *Blood* 121(22):4439–4442.

Craik, D. J., D. P. Fairlie, S. Liras, and D. Price. 2013. The future of peptide-based drugs. *Chem. Biol. Drug. Des.* 81(1):136–147.

Csermely, P., T. Korcsmaros, H. J. Kiss, G. London, and R. Nussinov. 2013. Structure and dynamics of molecular networks: A novel paradigm of drug discovery: A comprehensive review. *Pharmacol. Ther.* 138(3):333–408.

Cummings, C. G. and A. D. Hamilton. 2010. Disrupting protein-protein interactions with non-peptidic, small molecule alpha-helix mimetics. *Curr. Opin. Chem. Biol.* 14(3):341–346.

Dahan, A., J. M. Miller, and G. L. Amidon. 2009. Prediction of solubility and permeability class membership: Provisional BCS classification of the world's top oral drugs. *AAPS J.* 11(4):740–746.

David, A., R. Razali, M. N. Wass, and M. J. Sternberg. 2012. Protein-protein interaction sites are hot spots for disease-associated nonsynonymous SNPs. *Hum. Mutat.* 33(2):359–363.

Davis, F. P. 2011. Proteome-wide prediction of overlapping small molecule and protein binding sites using structure. *Mol. Biosyst.* 7(2):545–557.

Davis, F. P. and A. Sali. 2010. The overlap of small molecule and protein binding sites within families of protein structures. *PLoS Comput. Biol.* 6(2):e1000668.

de Vries, S. and M. Zacharias. 2013. Flexible docking and refinement with a coarse-grained protein model using ATTRACT. *Proteins* 81(3):2167–2174.

Dessailly, B. H., N. L. Dawson, K. Mizuguchi, and C. A. Orengo. 2013. Functional site plasticity in domain superfamilies. *Biochim. Biophys. Acta.* 1834(5):874–889.

Domling, A. 2008. Small molecular weight protein-protein interaction antagonists: An insurmountable challenge? *Curr. Opin. Chem. Biol.* 12(3):281–291.

Duffy, B. C., L. Zhu, H. Decornez, and D. B. Kitchen. 2012. Early phase drug discovery: Cheminformatics and computational techniques in identifying lead series. *Bioorg. Med. Chem.* 20(18):5324–5342.

Duran-Frigola, M., R. Mosca, and P. Aloy. 2013. Structural systems pharmacology: The role of 3D structures in next-generation drug development. *Chem. Biol.* 20(5):674–684.

Ettorre, A., P. D'Andrea, S. Mauro et al. 2011. hNK2 receptor antagonists. The use of intramolecular hydrogen bonding to increase solubility and membrane permeability. *Bioorg. Med. Chem. Lett.* 21(6):1807–1809.

Eyrisch, S. and V. Helms. 2007. Transient pockets on protein surfaces involved in protein-protein interaction. *J. Med. Chem.* 50(15):3457–3464.

Falchi, F., F. Caporuscio, and M. Recanatini. 2014. Structure-based design of small-molecule protein-protein interaction modulators: The story so far. *Future Med. Chem.* 6(3):343–357.

Faller, B., G. Ottaviani, P. Ertl, G. Berellini, and A. Collis. 2011. Evolution of the physicochemical properties of marketed drugs: Can history foretell the future? *Drug Discov. Today* 16(21–22):976–984.

Fan, H., J. J. Irwin, B. M. Webb, G. Klebe, B. K. Shoichet, and A. Sali. 2009. Molecular docking screens using comparative models of proteins. *J. Chem. Inf. Model.* 49(11):2512–2527.

Fauman, E. B., B. K. Rai, and E. S. Huang. 2011. Structure-based druggability assessment—Identifying suitable targets for small molecule therapeutics. *Curr. Opin. Chem. Biol.* 15(4):463–468.

Fernandez-Recio, J. 2011 Prediction of protein binding sites and hot spots. *WIREs Comp. Mol. Sci.* 1(5):680–698.

Ferrara, N. and R. S. Kerbel. 2005. Angiogenesis as a therapeutic target. *Nature* 438(7070):967–974.

Ferreira, R. S., A. Simeonov, A. Jadhav et al. 2010. Complementarity between a docking and a high-throughput screen in discovering new cruzain inhibitors. *J. Med. Chem.* 53(13):4891–4905.

Finn, R. D., M. Marshall, and A. Bateman. 2005. iPfam: Visualization of protein-protein interactions in PDB at domain and amino acid resolutions. *Bioinformatics* 21(3):410–412.

Franceschini, A., D. Szklarczyk, S. Frankild et al. 2013. STRING v9.1: Protein-protein interaction networks, with increased coverage and integration. *Nucleic Acids Res.* 41 Database issue:D808–D815.

Franzosa, E. A. and Y. Xia. 2011. Structural principles within the human-virus protein-protein interaction network. *Proc. Natl. Acad. Sci. U. S. A.* 108(26):10538–10543.

Fry, D., K. S. Huang, P. Di Lello et al. 2013. Design of libraries targeting protein-protein interfaces. *ChemMedChem.* 8(5):726–732.

Fuller, J. C., N. J. Burgoyne, and R. M. Jackson. 2009. Predicting druggable binding sites at the protein-protein interface. *Drug Discov. Today* 14(3–4):155–161.

Furlong, L. I. 2013. Human diseases through the lens of network biology. *Trends Genet.* 29(3):150–159.

Ganesan, A. 2008. The impact of natural products upon modern drug discovery. *Curr. Opin. Chem. Biol.* 12(3):306–317.

Gao, M. and J. Skolnick. 2013. APoc: Large-scale identification of similar protein pockets. *Bioinformatics* 29(5):597–604.

Garcia-Garcia, J., S. Schleker, J. Klein-Seetharaman, and B. Oliva. 2012. BIPS: BIANA Interolog Prediction Server. A tool for protein-protein interaction inference. *Nucleic Acids Res.* 40 Web Server issue:W147–W151.

Garner, A. L. and K. D. Janda. 2011. Protein-protein interactions and cancer: Targeting the central dogma. *Curr. Top. Med. Chem.* 11(3):258–280.

Garzon, J. I., J. Kovacs, R. Abagyan, and P. Chacon. 2007. DFprot: A webtool for predicting local chain deformability. *Bioinformatics* 23(7):901–902.

Gautier, B., M. A. Miteva, V. Goncalves et al. 2011. Targeting the proangiogenic VEGF-VEGFR protein-protein interface with drug-like compounds by *in silico* and *in vitro* screening. *Chem. Biol.* 18(12):1631–1639.

Geppert, T., S. Bauer, J. A. Hiss et al. 2012. Immunosuppressive small molecule discovered by structure-based virtual screening for inhibitors of protein-protein interactions. *Angew. Chem. Int. Ed. Engl.* 51(1):258–261.

Gleeson, M. P. 2008. Generation of a set of simple, interpretable ADMET rules of thumb. *J. Med. Chem.* 51(4):817–834.

Gonzalez-Ruiz, D. and H. Gohlke. 2006. Targeting protein-protein interactions with small molecules: Challenges and perspectives for computational binding epitope detection and ligand finding. *Curr. Med. Chem.* 13(22):2607–2625.

Grosdidier, S. and J. Fernandez-Recio. 2008. Identification of hot-spot residues in protein-protein interactions by computational docking. *BMC Bioinformatics* 9:447.

Grosdidier, S. and J. Fernandez-Recio. 2012. Protein-protein docking and hot-spot prediction for drug discovery. *Curr. Pharm. Des.* 18(30):4607–4618.

Grove, L. E., D. R. Hall, D. Beglov, S. Vajda, and D. Kozakov. 2013. FTFlex: Accounting for binding site flexibility to improve fragment-based identification of druggable hot spots. *Bioinformatics* 29(9):1218–1219.

Hamon, V., R. Bourgeas, P. Ducrot et al. 2013. 2P2I HUNTER: A tool for filtering orthosteric protein-protein interaction modulators via a dedicated support vector machine. *J. R. Soc. Interface* 11(90):20130860.

Hann, M. M. 2011. Molecular obesity, potency and other addictions in drug discovery. *MedChemComm.* 2:349–355.

Hann, M. M. and G. M. Keseru. 2012. Finding the sweet spot: The role of nature and nurture in medicinal chemistry. *Nat. Rev. Drug Discov.* 11(5):355–365.

Higueruelo, A. P., H. Jubb, and T. L. Blundell. 2013. TIMBAL v2: Update of a database holding small molecules modulating protein-protein interactions. *Database (Oxford)* 2013:39.

Higueruelo, A. P., A. Schreyer, G. R. Bickerton, T. L. Blundell, and W. R. Pitt. 2012. What can we learn from the evolution of protein-ligand interactions to aid the design of new therapeutics? *PLoS One* 7(12):e51742.

Higueruelo, A. P., A. Schreyer, G. R. Bickerton, W. R. Pitt, C. R. Groom, and T. L. Blundell. 2009. Atomic interactions and profile of small molecules disrupting protein-protein interfaces: The TIMBAL database. *Chem. Biol. Drug. Des.* 74(5):457–467.

Higurashi, M., T. Ishida, and K. Kinoshita. 2009. PiSite: A database of protein interaction sites using multiple binding states in the PDB. *Nucleic Acids Res.* 37 Database issue:D360–D364.

Holmes, K., O. L. Roberts, A. M. Thomas, and M. J. Cross. 2007. Vascular endothelial growth factor receptor-2: Structure, function, intracellular signalling and therapeutic inhibition. *Cell Signal.* 19(10):2003–2012.

Horvath, D. 1997. A virtual screening approach applied to the search for trypanothione reductase inhibitors. *J. Med. Chem.* 40(15):2412–2423.

Huang, W., S. Lu, Z. Huang et al. 2013. Allosite: A method for predicting allosteric sites. *Bioinformatics* 29(18):2357–2359.

Hughes, J. D., J. Blagg, D. A. Price et al. 2008. Physiochemical drug properties associated with *in vivo* toxicological outcomes. *Bioorg. Med. Chem. Lett.* 18(17):4872–4875.

Hughes, J. P., S. Rees, S. B. Kalindjian, and K. L. Philpott. 2011. Principles of early drug discovery. *Br. J. Pharmacol.* 162(6):1239–1249.

Hwang, H., T. Vreven, and Z. Weng. 2014. Binding interface prediction by combining protein-protein docking results. *Proteins* 82(1):57–66.

Isserlin, R., R. A. El-Badrawi, and G. D. Bader. 2011 The biomolecular interaction network database in PSI-MI 2.5. *Database (Oxford)*:baq037.

Isvoran, A., D. Craciun, V. Martiny, O. Sperandio, and M. A. Miteva. 2013. Computational analysis of protein-protein interfaces involving an alpha helix: Insights for terphenyl-like molecules binding. *BMC Pharmacol. Toxicol.* 14:31.

Ivanov, A. A., F. R. Khuri, and H. Fu. 2013. Targeting protein-protein interactions as an anticancer strategy. *Trends Pharmacol. Sci.* 34(7):393–400.

Jaeger, S. and P. Aloy. 2012. From protein interaction networks to novel therapeutic strategies. *IUBMB Life* 64(6):529–537.

Jain, A. N. 2003. Surflex: Fully automatic flexible molecular docking using a molecular similarity-based search engine. *J. Med. Chem.* 46(4):499–511.

Janin, J., R. P. Bahadur, and P. Chakrabarti. 2008. Protein-protein interaction and quaternary structure. *Q. Rev. Biophys.* 41(2):133–180.

Jenik, M., R. G. Parra, L. G. Radusky, A. Turjanski, P. G. Wolynes, and D. U. Ferreiro. 2012. Protein frustratometer: A tool to localize energetic frustration in protein molecules. *Nucleic Acids Res.* 40 Web Server issue:W348–W351.

Jimenez-Garcia, B., C. Pons, and J. Fernandez-Recio. 2013. pyDockWEB: A web server for rigid-body protein-protein docking using electrostatics and desolvation scoring. *Bioinformatics* 29(13):1698–1699.

Johnson, D. K. and J. Karanicolas. 2013. Druggable protein interaction sites are more predisposed to surface pocket formation than the rest of the protein surface. *PLoS Comput. Biol.* 9(3):e1002951.

Joseph-McCarthy, D., J. C. Baber, E. Feyfant, D. C. Thompson, and C. Humblet. 2007. Lead optimization via high-throughput molecular docking. *Curr. Opin. Drug Discov. Devel.* 10(3):264–274.

Jubb, H., A. P. Higueruelo, A. Winter, and T. L. Blundell. 2012. Structural biology and drug discovery for protein-protein interactions. *Trends Pharmacol. Sci.* 33(5):241–248.

Kanno, S., N. Oda, M. Abe et al. 2000. Roles of two VEGF receptors, Flt-1 and KDR, in the signal transduction of VEGF effects in human vascular endothelial cells. *Oncogene* 19(17):2138–2146.

Kaspar, A. A. and J. M. Reichert. 2013. Future directions for peptide therapeutics development. *Drug Discov. Today* 18(17–18):807–817.

Kastritis, P. L. and A. M. Bonvin. 2013. On the binding affinity of macromolecular interactions: Daring to ask why proteins interact. *J. R. Soc. Interface* 10(79):20120835.

Kerrien, S., B. Aranda, L. Breuza et al. 2012. The IntAct molecular interaction database in 2012. *Nucleic Acids Res.* 40 Database issue:D841–D846.

Keskin, O., A. Gursoy, B. Ma, and R. Nussinov. 2008. Principles of protein-protein interactions: What are the preferred ways for proteins to interact? *Chem. Rev.* 108(4):1225–1244.

Khan, W., F. Duffy, G. Pollastri, D. C. Shields, and C. Mooney. 2013. Predicting binding within disordered protein regions to structurally characterised peptide-binding domains. *PLoS One* 8(9):e72838.

Kim, D. E., D. Chivian, and D. Baker. 2004. Protein structure prediction and analysis using the Robetta server. *Nucleic Acids Res.* 32 Web Server issue:W526–W531.

Koes, D. R. and C. J. Camacho. 2012. Small-molecule inhibitor starting points learned from protein-protein interaction inhibitor structure. *Bioinformatics* 28(6):784–791.

Kokh, D. B., S. Richter, S. Henrich, P. Czodrowski, F. Rippmann, and R. C. Wade. 2013. TRAPP: A tool for analysis of transient binding pockets in proteins. *J. Chem. Inf. Model.* 53(5):1235–1252.

Kozakov, D., D. R. Hall, G. Y. Chuang et al. 2011. Structural conservation of druggable hot spots in protein-protein interfaces. *Proc. Natl. Acad. Sci. U. S. A.* 108(33):13528–13533.

Kruger, D. M. and H. Gohlke. 2010. DrugScorePPI webserver: Fast and accurate *in silico* alanine scanning for scoring protein-protein interactions. *Nucleic Acids Res.* 38:W480–W486.

Kruger, D. M., G. Jessen, and H. Gohlke. 2012. How good are state-of-the-art docking tools in predicting ligand binding modes in protein-protein interfaces? *J. Chem. Inf. Model.* 52(11):2807–2811.

Kufareva, I., Y. C. Chen, A. V. Ilatovskiy, and R. Abagyan. 2012. Compound activity prediction using models of binding pockets or ligand properties in 3D. *Curr. Top. Med. Chem.* 12(17):1869–1882.

Kumar, R. and B. Nanduri. 2010. HPIDB—A unified resource for host-pathogen interactions. *BMC Bioinformatics* 11 Suppl 6:S16.

Labbe, C. M., G. Laconde, M. A. Kuenemann, B. O. Villoutreix, and O. Sperandio. 2013. iPPI-DB: A manually curated and interactive database of small non-peptide inhibitors of protein-protein interactions. *Drug Discov. Today* 18(19–20):958–968.

Lagorce, D., J. Maupetit, J. Baell et al. 2011. The FAF-Drugs2 server: A multistep engine to prepare electronic chemical compound collections. *Bioinformatics* 27(14):2018–2020.

Laine, E., C. Goncalves, J. C. Karst et al. 2010. Use of allostery to identify inhibitors of calmodulin-induced activation of *Bacillus anthracis* edema factor. *Proc. Natl. Acad. Sci. U.S.A.* 107(25):11277–11282.

Leader, B., Q. J. Baca, and D. E. Golan. 2008. Protein therapeutics: A summary and pharmacological classification. *Nat. Rev. Drug Discov.* 7(1):21–39.

Leeson, P. D. and S. A. St-Gallay. 2011. The influence of the "organizational factor" on compound quality in drug discovery. *Nat. Rev. Drug Discov.* 10(10):749–765.

Leis, S., S. Schneider, and M. Zacharias. 2010. *In silico* prediction of binding sites on proteins. *Curr. Med. Chem.* 17(15):1550–1562.

Lewis, A. C., N. S. Jones, M. A. Porter, and C. M. Deane. 2012. What evidence is there for the homology of protein-protein interactions? *PLoS Comput Biol* 8(9):e1002645.

Li, H., H. Xiao, L. Lin et al. 2014. Drug design targeting protein-protein interactions (PPIs) using multiple ligand simultaneous docking (MLSD) and drug repositioning: Discovery of raloxifene and bazedoxifene as novel Inhibitors of IL-6/ GP130 interface. *J. Med. Chem.* 57(3):632–641.

Liao, C., M. Sitzmann, A. Pugliese, and M. C. Nicklaus. 2011. Software and resources for computational medicinal chemistry. *Future Med. Chem.* 3(8):1057–1085.

Licata, L., L. Briganti, D. Peluso et al. 2012. MINT, the molecular interaction database: 2012 update. *Nucleic Acids Res.* 40 Database issue:D857–D861.

Lin, Y., S. Yoo, and R. Sanchez. 2012. SiteComp: A server for ligand binding site analysis in protein structures. *Bioinformatics* 28(8):1172–1173.

Lipinski, C. A., F. Lombardo, B. W. Dominy, and P. J. Feeney. 2001. Experimental and computational approaches to estimate solubility and permeability in drug discovery and development settings. *Adv. Drug Deliv. Rev.* 46(1–3):3–26.

Liu, Z., H. Fang, K. Reagan et al. 2013. *In silico* drug repositioning: What we need to know. *Drug Discov. Today* 18(3–4):110–115.

London, N., B. Raveh, and O. Schueler-Furman. 2013a. Druggable protein-protein interactions—From hot spots to hot segments. *Curr. Opin. Chem. Biol.* 17(6):952–959.

London, N., B. Raveh, and O. Schueler-Furman. 2013b. Peptide docking and structure-based characterization of peptide binding: From knowledge to know-how. *Curr. Opin. Struct. Biol.* 23(6):894–902.

Loregian, A. and G. Palu. 2005. Disruption of protein-protein interactions: Towards new targets for chemotherapy. *J. Cell Physiol.* 204(3):750–762.

Lu, Z. J., S. J. Deng, D. G. Huang et al. 2012. Frontier of therapeutic antibody discovery: The challenges and how to face them. *World J. Biol. Chem.* 3(12):187–196.

Ma, B. and R. Nussinov. 2013. Druggable orthosteric and allosteric hot spots to target protein-protein interactions. *Curr. Pharm. Des.* 20(8): 1293–1301.

Makley, L. N. and J. E. Gestwicki. 2013. Expanding the number of "druggable" targets: Non-enzymes and protein-protein interactions. *Chem. Biol. Drug Des.* 81(1):22–32.

Marechal, X., E. Genin, L. Qin et al. 2013. 1,2,4-Oxadiazoles identified by virtual screening and their non-covalent inhibition of the human 20S proteasome. *Curr. Med. Chem.* 20(18):2351–2362.

Matsuzaki, Y., N. Uchikoga, M. Ohue et al. 2013. MEGADOCK 3.0: A high-performance protein-protein interaction prediction software using hybrid parallel computing for petascale supercomputing environments. *Source Code Biol. Med.* 8(1):18.

Medina-Franco, J. L., M. A. Giulianotti, G. S. Welmaker, and R. A. Houghten. 2013. Shifting from the single to the multitarget paradigm in drug discovery. *Drug Discov. Today* 18(9–10):495–501.

Meireles, L. M., A. S. Domling, and C. J. Camacho. 2010. ANCHOR: A web server and database for analysis of protein-protein interaction binding pockets for drug discovery. *Nucleic Acids Res.* 38 Web Server issue:W407–W411.

Metz, A., E. Ciglia, and H. Gohlke. 2012a. Modulating protein-protein interactions: From structural determinants of binding to druggability prediction to application. *Curr. Pharm. Des.* 18(30):4630–4647.

Metz, A., C. Pfleger, H. Kopitz, S. Pfeiffer-Marek, K. H. Baringhaus, and H. Gohlke. 2012b. Hot spots and transient pockets: Predicting the determinants of small-molecule binding to a protein-protein interface. *J. Chem. Inf. Model.* 52(1):120–33.

Meunier, B. 2012. Does chemistry have a future in therapeutic innovations? *Angew. Chem. Int. Ed. Engl.* 51(35):8702–8706.

Meyer, M. J., J. Das, X. Wang, and H. Yu. 2013. INstruct: A database of high-quality 3D structurally resolved protein interactome networks. *Bioinformatics* 29(12):1577–1579.

Moal, I. H. and J. Fernandez-Recio. 2012. SKEMPI: A structural kinetic and energetic database of mutant protein interactions and its use in empirical models. *Bioinformatics* 28(20):2600–2607.

Mohd Fauzi, F., A. Koutsoukas, R. Lowe et al. 2013. Chemogenomics approaches to rationalizing the mode-of-action of traditional Chinese and Ayurvedic Medicines. *J. Chem. Inf. Model.* 53:661–673.

Mok, N. Y., S. Maxe, and R. Brenk. 2013. Locating sweet spots for screening hits and evaluating pan-assay interference filters from the performance analysis of two lead-like libraries. *J. Chem. Inf. Model.* 53(3):534–544.

Morelli, X., R. Bourgeas, and P. Roche. 2011. Chemical and structural lessons from recent successes in protein-protein interaction inhibition (2P2I). *Curr. Opin. Chem. Biol.* 15(4):475–481.

Mosca, R., T. Pons, A. Ceol, A. Valencia, and P. Aloy. 2013. Towards a detailed atlas of protein-protein interactions. *Curr. Opin. Struct. Biol.* 23(6):929–940.

Ngounou Wetie, A. G., I. Sokolowska, A. G. Woods, U. Roy, K. Deinhardt, and C. C. Darie. 2014. Protein-protein interactions: Switch from classical methods to proteomics and bioinformatics-based approaches. *Cell Mol. Life Sci.* 71(2):205–228.

Ofran, Y. and B. Rost. 2007. ISIS: Interaction sites identified from sequence. *Bioinformatics* 23(2):e13–e16.

Orchard, S. 2012. Molecular interaction databases. *Proteomics* 12(10):1656–1662.

Ozcan, S., A. Kazi, F. Marsilio et al. 2013. Oxadiazole-isopropylamides as potent and noncovalent proteasome inhibitors. *J. Med. Chem.* 56(10):3783–3805.

Pagel, P., S. Kovac, M. Oesterheld et al. 2005. The MIPS mammalian protein-protein interaction database. *Bioinformatics* 21(6):832–834.

Pagliaro, L., J. Felding, K. Audouze et al. 2004. Emerging classes of protein-protein interaction inhibitors and new tools for their development. *Curr. Opin. Chem. Biol.* 8(4):442–449.

Palu, G. and A. Loregian. 2013. Inhibition of herpesvirus and influenza virus replication by blocking polymerase subunit interactions. *Antiviral Res.* 99(3):318–327.

Panjkovich, A. and X. Daura. 2012. Exploiting protein flexibility to predict the location of allosteric sites. *BMC Bioinformatics* 13:273.

Pencheva, T., D. Jereva, M. A. Miteva, and I. Pajeva. 2013. Post-docking optimization and analysis of protein-ligand interactions of estrogen receptor alpha using AMMOS software. *Curr. Comput. Aided Drug. Des.* 9(1):83–94.

Pencheva, T., D. Lagorce, I. Pajeva, B. O. Villoutreix, and M. A. Miteva. 2008. AMMOS: Automated molecular mechanics optimization tool for *in silico* screening. *BMC Bioinformatics* 9:438.

Penrod, N. M., R. Cowper-Sal-lari, and J. H. Moore. 2011. Systems genetics for drug target discovery. *Trends Pharmacol. Sci.* 32(10):623–630.

Perola, E. 2010. An analysis of the binding efficiencies of drugs and their leads in successful drug discovery programs. *J. Med. Chem.* 53(7):2986–2997.

Perot, S., O. Sperandio, M. A. Miteva, A. C. Camproux, and B. O. Villoutreix. 2010. Druggable pockets and binding site centric chemical space: A paradigm shift in drug discovery. *Drug Discov. Today* 15(15–16):656–667.

Phatak, S. S., C. C. Stephan, and C. N. Cavasotto. 2009. High-throughput and *in silico* screenings in drug discovery. *Expert Opin. Drug. Discov.* 4(9):947–959.

Planas-Iglesias, J., M. A. Marin-Lopez, J. Bonet, J. Garcia-Garcia, and B. Oliva. 2013. iLoops: A protein-protein interaction prediction server based on structural features. *Bioinformatics* 29(18):2360–2362.

Polishchuk, P. G., T. I. Madzhidov, and A. Varnek. 2013. Estimation of the size of drug-like chemical space based on GDB-17 data. *J Comput Aided Mol Des* 27(8):675–679.

Popov, P., D. W. Ritchie, and S. Grudinin. 2014. DockTrina: Docking triangular protein trimers. *Proteins* 82:34–44.

Porollo, A. and J. Meller. 2007. Prediction-based fingerprints of protein-protein interactions. *Proteins* 66(3):630–645.

Raj, M., B. N. Bullock, and P. S. Arora. 2012. Plucking the high hanging fruit: A systematic approach for targeting protein-protein interactions. *Bioorg. Med. Chem.* 21(14):4051–4057.

Rask-Andersen, M., M. S. Almen, and H. B. Schioth. 2011. Trends in the exploitation of novel drug targets. *Nat. Rev. Drug Discov.* 10(8):579–590.

Reynes, C., H. Host, A. C. Camproux et al. 2010. Designing focused chemical libraries enriched in protein-protein interaction inhibitors using machine-learning methods. *PLoS Comput. Biol.* 6(3):e1000695.

Reynolds, C., D. Damerell, and S. Jones. 2009. ProtorP: A protein-protein interaction analysis server. *Bioinformatics* 25(3):413–414.

Rid, R., W. Strasser, D. Siegl et al. 2013. PRIMOS: An integrated database of reassessed protein-protein interactions providing web-based access to *in silico* validation of experimentally derived data. *Assay Drug Dev. Technol.* 11(5):333–346.

Ripphausen, P., D. Stumpfe, and J. Bajorath. 2012. Analysis of structure-based virtual screening studies and characterization of identified active compounds. *Future Med. Chem.* 4(5):603–613.

Robinson, J. A., S. Demarco, F. Gombert, K. Moehle, and D. Obrecht. 2008. The design, structures and therapeutic potential of protein epitope mimetics. *Drug Discov. Today* 13(21–22):944–951.

Ruddigkeit, L., R. van Deursen, L. C. Blum, and J. L. Reymond. 2012. Enumeration of 166 billion organic small molecules in the chemical universe database GDB-17. *J. Chem. Inf. Model.* 52(11):2864–2875.

Rueda, M., G. Bottegoni, and R. Abagyan. 2010. Recipes for the selection of experimental protein conformations for virtual screening. *J. Chem. Inf. Model.* 50(1):186–193.

Ruffner, H., A. Bauer, and T. Bouwmeester. 2007. Human protein-protein interaction networks and the value for drug discovery. *Drug Discov. Today* 12(17–18):709–716.

Salwinski, L., C. S. Miller, A. J. Smith, F. K. Pettit, J. U. Bowie, and D. Eisenberg. 2004. The database of interacting proteins: 2004 update. *Nucleic Acids Res.* 32 Database issue:D449–D451.

Schadt, E. E., S. H. Friend, and D. A. Shaywitz. 2009. A network view of disease and compound screening. *Nat. Rev. Drug Discov.* 8(4):286–295.

Schenone, M., V. Dancik, B. K. Wagner, and P. A. Clemons. 2013. Target identification and mechanism of action in chemical biology and drug discovery. *Nat. Chem. Biol.* 9(4):232–240.

Schon, A., S. Y. Lam, and E. Freire. 2011. Thermodynamics-based drug design: Strategies for inhibiting protein-protein interactions. *Future Med. Chem.* 3(9):1129–1137.

Schymkowitz, J., J. Borg, F. Stricher, R. Nys, F. Rousseau, and L. Serrano. 2005. The FoldX web server: An online force field. *Nucleic Acids Res.* 33 Web Server issue:W382–W388.

Scior, T., A. Bender, G. Tresadern et al. 2012. Recognizing pitfalls in virtual screening: A critical review. *J. Chem. Inf. Model.* 52(4):867–881.

Segall, M. D. 2012. Multi-parameter optimization: Identifying high quality compounds with a balance of properties. *Curr. Pharm. Des.* 18(9):1292–1310.

Shublaq, N., C. Sansom, and P. V. Coveney. 2013. Patient-specific modelling in drug design, development and selection including its role in clinical decision-making. *Chem. Biol. Drug Des.* 81(1):5–12.

Skolnick, J., H. Zhou, and M. Gao. 2013. Are predicted protein structures of any value for binding site prediction and virtual ligand screening? *Curr. Opin. Struct. Biol.* 23(2):191–197.

Smith, M. C. and J. E. Gestwicki. 2012. Features of protein-protein interactions that translate into potent inhibitors: Topology, surface area and affinity. *Expert Rev. Mol. Med.* 14:e16.

Sperandio, O., M. A. Miteva, and B. O. Villoutreix. 2008. Combining structure-based and ligand-based virtual ligand screening. *Curr. Comput. Aided Drug. Des.* 4:250–258.

Sperandio, O., L. Mouawad, E. Pinto, B. O. Villoutreix, D. Perahia, and M. A. Miteva. 2010a. How to choose relevant multiple receptor conformations for virtual screening: A test case of Cdk2 and normal mode analysis. *Eur. Biophys. J.* 39(9):1365–1372.

Sperandio, O., C. H. Reynes, A. C. Camproux, and B. O. Villoutreix. 2010b. Rationalizing the chemical space of protein-protein interaction inhibitors. *Drug Discov. Today* 15(5–6):220–229.

Sriwastava, B. K., S. Basu, U. Maulik, and D. Plewczynski. 2013. PPIcons: Identification of protein-protein interaction sites in selected organisms. *J. Mol. Model.* 19(9):4059–4070.

Stark, C., B. J. Breitkreutz, A. Chatr-Aryamontri et al. 2011. The BioGRID interaction database: 2011 update. *Nucleic Acids Res.* 39 Database issue:D698–D704.

Stein, A., A. Ceol, and P. Aloy. 2011. 3did: Identification and classification of domain-based interactions of known three-dimensional structure. *Nucleic Acids Res.* 39 Database issue:D718–D723.

Stumpfe, D., P. Ripphausen, and J. Bajorath. 2012. Virtual compound screening in drug discovery. *Future Med. Chem.* 4(5):593–602.

Surade, S. and T. L. Blundell. 2012. Structural biology and drug discovery of difficult targets: The limits of ligandability. *Chem. Biol.* 19(1):42–50.

Swiecki, M. and M. Colonna. 2010. Unraveling the functions of plasmacytoid dendritic cells during viral infections, autoimmunity, and tolerance. *Immunol Rev.* 234(1):142–162.

Szilagyi, A. and Y. Zhang. 2014. Template-based structure modeling of protein-protein interactions. *Curr. Opin. Struct. Biol.* 24:10–23.

Taboureau, O., J. B. Baell, J. Fernandez-Recio, and B. O. Villoutreix. 2011 Established and emerging trends in computational drug discovery in the structural genomics era. *Chem. Biol.* 19(1):29–41.

Tanrikulu, Y., B. Kruger, and E. Proschak. 2011. The holistic integration of virtual screening in drug discovery. *Drug Discov. Today* 18(7–8):358–364.

Teague, S. J. 2011. Learning lessons from drugs that have recently entered the market. *Drug Discov. Today* 16(9–10):398–411.

Thangudu, R. R., S. H. Bryant, A. R. Panchenko, and T. Madej. 2012. Modulating protein-protein interactions with small molecules: The importance of binding hotspots. *J. Mol. Biol.* 415(2):443–453.

Thiel, P., M. Kaiser, and C. Ottmann. 2012. Small-molecule stabilization of protein-protein interactions: An underestimated concept in drug discovery? *Angew. Chem. Int. Ed. Engl.* 51(9):2012–2018.

Torchala, M., I. H. Moal, R. A. Chaleil, J. Fernandez-Recio, and P. A. Bates. 2013. SwarmDock: A server for flexible protein-protein docking. *Bioinformatics* 29(6):807–809.

Trosset, J. Y. and N. Vodovar. 2013. Structure-based target druggability assessment. *Methods Mol. Biol.* 986:141–164.

Tuncbag, N., A. Gursoy, R. Nussinov, and O. Keskin. 2011. Predicting protein-protein interactions on a proteome scale by matching evolutionary and structural similarities at interfaces using PRISM. *Nat. Protoc.* 6(9):1341–1354.

Tuncbag, N., G. Kar, O. Keskin, A. Gursoy, and R. Nussinov. 2009. A survey of available tools and web servers for analysis of protein-protein interactions and interfaces. *Brief Bioinform.* 10(3):217–232.

Tuncbag, N., O. Keskin, and A. Gursoy. 2010. HotPoint: Hot spot prediction server for protein interfaces. *Nucleic Acids Res* 38 Web Server issue:W402–W406.

Turinsky, A. L., S. Razick, B. Turner, I. M. Donaldson, and S. J. Wodak. 2014. Navigating the global protein-protein interaction landscape using iRefWeb. *Methods Mol. Biol.* 1091:315–331.

Ulucan, O., S. Eyrisch, and V. Helms. 2012. Druggability of dynamic protein-protein interfaces. *Curr. Pharm. Des.* 18(30):4599–4606.

Valko, K., E. Chiarparin, S. Nunhuck, and D. Montanari. 2012. *In vitro* measurement of drug efficiency index to aid early lead optimization. *J. Pharm. Sci.* 101(11):4155–4169.

Varin, T., M. C. Didiot, C. N. Parker, and A. Schuffenhauer. 2012. Latent hit series hidden in high-throughput screening data. *J. Med. Chem.* 55(3):1161–1170.

Vidal, M., M. E. Cusick, and A. L. Barabasi. 2011. Interactome networks and human disease. *Cell* 144(6):986–998.

Villoutreix, B. O., K. Bastard, O. Sperandio et al. 2008. *In silico–in vitro* screening of protein-protein interactions: Towards the next generation of therapeutics. *Curr. Pharm. Biotechnol.* 9(2):103–122.

Villoutreix, B. O., R. Eudes, and M. A. Miteva. 2009. Structure-based virtual ligand screening: Recent success stories. *Comb. Chem. High Throughput Screen.* 12(10):1000–1016.

Villoutreix, B. O., C. M. Labbe, D. Lagorce, G. Laconde, and O. Sperandio. 2012. A leap into the chemical space of protein-protein interaction inhibitors. *Curr. Pharm. Des.* 18(30):4648–4667.

Villoutreix, B. O., D. Lagorce, C. M. Labbe, O. Sperandio, and M. A. Miteva. 2013. One hundred thousand mouse clicks down the road: Selected online resources supporting drug discovery collected over a decade. *Drug Discov. Today* 18:1081–1089.

Villoutreix, B. O. and O. Sperandio. 2010. *In silico* studies of blood coagulation proteins: From mosaic proteases to nonenzymatic cofactor inhibitors. *Curr. Opin. Struct. Biol.* 20(2):168–179.

Voet, A., E. F. Banwell, K. K. Sahu, J. G. Heddle, and K. Y. Zhang. 2013. Protein interface pharmacophore mapping tools for small molecule protein: Protein interaction inhibitor discovery. *Curr. Top. Med. Chem.* 13(9):989–1001.

Volkamer, A., D. Kuhn, F. Rippmann, and M. Rarey. 2012. DoGSiteScorer: A web server for automatic binding site prediction, analysis and druggability assessment. *Bioinformatics* 28(15):2074–2075.

von Eichborn, J., M. Dunkel, B. O. Gohlke et al. 2013. SynSysNet: Integration of experimental data on synaptic protein-protein interactions with drug-target relations. *Nucleic Acids Res.* 41 Database issue:D834–D840.

Votapka, L. and R. E. Amaro. 2013. Multistructural hot spot characterization with FTProd. *Bioinformatics* 29(3):393–394.

Wager, T. T., R. Y. Chandrasekaran, X. Hou et al. 2010. Defining desirable central nervous system drug space through the alignment of molecular properties, *in vitro* ADME, and safety attributes. *ACS Chem. Neurosci.* 1(6):420–434.

Walter, P., J. Metzger, C. Thiel, and V. Helms. 2013. Predicting where small molecules bind at protein-protein interfaces. *PLoS One* 8:1–12.

Wanner, J., D. C. Fry, Z. Peng, and J. Roberts. 2011. Druggability assessment of protein-protein interfaces. *Future Med. Chem.* 3(16):2021–2038.

Wells, J. A. and C. L. McClendon. 2007. Reaching for high-hanging fruit in drug discovery at protein-protein interfaces. *Nature* 450(7172):1001–1009.

Westermaier, Y., M. Veurink, T. Riis-Johannessen, S. Guinchard, R. Gurny, and L. Scapozza. 2013. Identification of aggregation breakers for bevacizumab (Avastin(R)) self-association through similarity searching and interaction studies. *Eur. J. Pharm. Biopharm.* 85:773–780.

White, A. W., A. D. Westwell, and G. Brahemi. 2008. Protein-protein interactions as targets for small-molecule therapeutics in cancer. *Expert Rev. Mol. Med.* 10:e8.

Whitty, A. 2011. Growing PAINS in academic drug discovery. *Future Med. Chem.* 3(7):797–801.

Wilson, A. J. 2009. Inhibition of protein-protein interactions using designed molecules. *Chem. Soc. Rev.* 38(12):3289–3300.

Winter, C., A. Henschel, A. Tuukkanen, and M. Schroeder. 2012a. Protein interactions in 3D: From interface evolution to drug discovery. *J. Struct. Biol.* 179(3):347–358.

Winter, A., A. P. Higueruelo, M. Marsh, A. Sigurdardottir, W. R. Pitt, and T. L. Blundell. 2012b. Biophysical and computational fragment-based approaches to targeting protein-protein interactions: Applications in structure-guided drug discovery. *Q. Rev. Biophys.* 45(4):383–426.

Wirth, M., A. Volkamer, V. Zoete et al. 2013. Protein pocket and ligand shape comparison and its application in virtual screening. *J. Comput. Aided Mol. Des.* 27(6):511–524.

Wyatt, P. G., I. H. Gilbert, K. D. Read, and A. H. Fairlamb. 2011. Target validation: Linking target and chemical properties to desired product profile. *Curr. Top. Med. Chem.* 11(10):1275–1283.

Xue, L. C., R. A. Jordan, Y. El-Manzalawy, D. Dobbs, and V. Honavar. 2014. DockRank: Ranking docked conformations using partner-specific sequence homology based protein interface prediction. *Proteins* 82:250–267.

Yang, C-Y. and S. Wang. 2011. Hydrophobic binding hot spots of Bcl-xL protein–protein interfaces by cosolvent molecular dynamics simulation. *ACS Med. Chem. Lett.* 2:280–284.

Yates, C. M. and M. J. Sternberg. 2013. The effects of non-synonymous single nucleotide polymorphisms (nsSNPs) on protein-protein interactions. *J. Mol. Biol.* 425:3949–3963.

Yuriev, E. and P. A. Ramsland. 2013. Latest developments in molecular docking: 2010–2011 in review. *J. Mol. Recognit.* 26(5):215–239.

Zahiri, J., O. Yaghoubi, M. Mohammad-Noori, R. Ebrahimpour, and A. Masoudi-Nejad. 2013. PPIevo: Protein-protein interaction prediction from PSSM based evolutionary information. *Genomics* 102:237–242.

Zerbe, B. S., D. R. Hall, S. Vajda, A. Whitty, and D. Kozakov. 2012. Relationship between hot spot residues and ligand binding hot spots in protein-protein interfaces. *J. Chem. Inf. Model.* 52(8):2236–2244.

Zhang, Q. C., D. Petrey, L. Deng et al. 2012. Structure-based prediction of protein-protein interactions on a genome-wide scale. *Nature* 490(7421):556–560.

Zhang, Q. C., D. Petrey, J. I. Garzon, L. Deng, and B. Honig. 2013a. PrePPI: A structure-informed database of protein-protein interactions. *Nucleic Acids Res.* 41 Database issue: D828–D833.

Zhang, Z., Y. Li, B. Lin, M. Schroeder, and B. Huang. 2011. Identification of cavities on protein surface using multiple computational approaches for drug binding site prediction. *Bioinformatics* 27(15):2083–2088.

Zhang, Z., S. Witham, M. Petukh et al. 2013b. A rational free energy-based approach to understanding and targeting disease-causing missense mutations. *J. Am. Med. Inform. Assoc.* 20(4):643–651.

Zhao, H. 2011. Lead optimization in the nondrug-like space. *Drug Discov. Today* 16(3–4):158–163.

Zheng, X., L. Gan, E. Wang, and J. Wang. 2012. Pocket-based drug design: Exploring pocket space. *AAPS J.* 15(1):228–41.

Zhong, S., A. T. Macias, and A. D. MacKerell, Jr. 2007. Computational identification of inhibitors of protein-protein interactions. *Curr. Top. Med. Chem.* 7(1):63–82.

Zhu, T., S. Cao, P. C. Su et al. 2013. Hit identification and optimization in virtual screening: Practical recommendations based on a critical literature analysis. *J. Med. Chem.* 56(17):6560–6572.

Zinzalla, G. and D. E. Thurston. 2009. Targeting protein-protein interactions for therapeutic intervention: A challenge for the future. *Future Med. Chem.* 1(1):65–93.

Zoete, V., A. Grosdidier, and O. Michielin. 2009. Docking, virtual high through-put screening and *in silico* fragment-based drug design. *J. Cell Mol. Med.* 13(2):238–248.

Zoraghi, R. and N. E. Reiner. 2013. Protein interaction networks as starting points to identify novel antimicrobial drug targets. *Curr. Opin. Microbiol.* 16(5):566–572.

18

Incorporating Binding Kinetics in Drug Design

Chung F. Wong

CONTENTS

18.1 Introduction

Despite the introduction of many new technologies such as high-throughput screening, combinatorial chemistry, and various -omics, the number of new drugs approved per year remains constant over several decades. At the same time, productivity, measured by number of drugs approved per year per billion dollars spent, inflation adjusted, has trended down by more than a factor of 10 from 1950 to 2010 (Group 2011). Although multiple factors could cause this unwelcomed trend, overlooking important factors in early stage drug discovery, resulting in high attrition rates in different phases of clinical trials after substantial resources have already been spent, could be one contributor. Drug-binding kinetics could be one of these hidden factors.

Accumulating evidences support the notion that drug-binding kinetics could play an important role in determining whether a molecule can be a useful drug. Long residence time is one concept that has become popular.

A number of publications advocated that good drugs should have long residence time in their biological receptors so that they could produce long-lasting therapeutic effects (Swinney 2004, 2006a,b, 2009; Copeland et al. 2006; Tummino and Copeland 2008; Zhang and Monsma 2009; Lu and Tonge 2010). And scientists often define residence time as the inverse of the dissociation constant, k_{off}, of a drug candidate from its receptor.

Evidences supporting this proposal include the study by Berezov et al. (2001), who designed peptide mimics to bind to the extracellular domain of the receptor tyrosine kinase HER2. They found that the desired cellular interference correlated better with the dissociation constant than with the binding affinity of the peptide mimics. Another example came from studies correlating the response of T cells with the types of MHC/peptide complexes that they interacted. Whether the presented peptide by MHC was an agonist, partial agonist, antagonist, or one that did not trigger any T-cell response correlated with the duration of interaction between T cells and MHC/peptide complexes (Matsui et al. 1994; Lyons et al. 1996; Davis et al. 1998; Germain and Stefanova 1999; Savage et al. 1999; van der Merwe and Davis 2003). In another study, Lu and Tonge found the *in vivo* activity of alkyl diphenyl ethers to correlate better with residence time than with inhibition constant K_I (Lu and Tonge 2008; Lu et al. 2009).

However literature search and simulations using pathway models of cell signaling (Goyal et al. 2009; Bairy and Wong 2011; Wong and Bairy 2013) have found drug-binding kinetics to influence drug efficacy in more ways than requiring long-residence time. For example, fast off rate, or short residence time, is sometimes important to make a molecule a useful drug. The drug memantine for treating Alzheimer patients provides one example. Fast off rate plays a role in reducing its toxicity (Lipton 2006). Memantine functions by blocking the N-methyl D aspartate receptor. This synaptic receptor mediates signaling by the neurotransmitter glutamate. Alzheimer patients produce overly activated glutamate signals that overexcite several pathways leading to apoptosis. Memantine suppresses such unwanted trigger of cell death. However, it reduces toxic effects by not suppressing neurotransmission by the N-methyl D aspartate receptor completely because the receptor is also required for normal functions such as memory and learning. Memantine achieves this by having fast off rate so that neurotransmitters can still access the receptor when needed. In another study, Kapur and Seeman hypothesized that atypical antipsychotics acting on the 5-HT$_2$ receptor-reduced extrapyramidal side effects and undesirable sustained prolactin elevation by dissociating rapidly from the off target dopamine D$_2$ receptors (Kapur and Seeman 2001). By moving in and out of the dopamine D$_2$ receptors often, atypical antipsychotics let dopamine enter the receptors during dopamine surges. In contrast, the older generation typical antipsychotics bind to the dopamine D$_2$ receptors with long residence time, leaving few ligand-free receptors available for dopamine binding.

A literature search also found residence time, or k_{off}, alone could not provide the whole story. For example, Wu et al. (2005) provided an example in which k_{on}, rather than k_{off}, of engineered antibodies linked better with the ability of the antibodies to neutralize the respiratory syncytial virus. Simulation studies applying drugs to different protein kinase targets in quantitative cell signaling models have also suggested biological targets that transmit signals quickly to downstream molecules soon after they are activated require fast-binding drugs to block them (Goyal et al. 2009; Bairy and Wong 2011; Wong and Bairy 2013).

Therefore, to take full advantage of drug-binding kinetics in drug discovery, drug developers need to consider not only long residence time (or small k_{off}), but also short residence time (or large k_{off}), and association rate. And association rate, not k_{on} alone, is emphasized here, as our simulations have found it feasible to have a drug candidate entering the binding pocket of a drug target via more than one entrance (Huang and Wong 2007, 2012b). Under such conditions, association rate rather than association rate constant is required to compare the effectiveness of different compounds in blocking a drug target, as discussed further below.

18.2 Guiding Principles for Designing Drugs with Favorable Binding Kinetics Are Still Lacking

Unlike drug-binding thermodynamics, scientists still lack good guiding principles for designing drugs with kinetic parameters that could improve drug efficacy. To develop drugs with binding kinetics that could improve drug efficacy, drug developers need to first find out what binding kinetics produce better drugs and then to design drug candidates with the needed kinetics. Although not done much yet, scientists could use various experimental and computational techniques to address the first issue. For example, scientists could use various existing techniques to measure drug-binding kinetics in the "test tube" and correlate the results with *in vitro* and *in vivo* assays to identify kinetic parameters that favorable drug candidates should have. On the computational side, models of systems biology (e.g., Goyal et al. 2009; Bairy and Wong 2011; Wong and Bairy 2013) could eventually become realistic enough to inform what kinetics a drug need to have to produce useful therapeutic effects to treat a specific ailment. However, this introductory chapter focuses on addressing the second issue: how can one go about designing drugs once one knows what binding kinetics they need to have. To do this effectively requires a better molecular understanding of drug-binding kinetics and quantitative models that can aid rational design to avoid spending resources on trying many things randomly. Unfortunately, at this time, scientists still lack such understanding and models. In a recent article, Copeland made the point for the specific case of designing drugs with long residence time that "we have not been able to address the question of residence time structure–activity relationships in any systemic fashion" (Copeland 2011). Nevertheless, several published computational studies have provided some preliminary glimpses.

For example, Huang and Wong (2007) described the application of a mining-minima approach to facilitate the construction of the docking pathways between para-nitrocatechol sulfate (pNCS) and the protein tyrosine phosphatase YopH of *Yersinia pestis*, and analyzed the interaction patterns between the ligand and the protein along the pathways to gain insight into the design of molecules with certain desired drug-binding kinetics. Table 18.1 gives an example (Wong 2014) that shows that some amino acid residues interacted with the ligand only when the ligand was in the binding pocket, some participated only when the ligand was at the protein surface near the entrance to the docking pathway, but some interacted with the ligand almost all through the docking pathway inside the protein. Such analysis suggested some ways that a lead compound could be modified to achieve certain preferred binding kinetics. For example, if one wishes to find compounds with longer residence time, one might want to modify the portion of the compound that interacts with the residues that stabilize the bound form but not the transition state, because this would increase the activation barrier for dissociation. Note that to generate insights like this, it is insufficient to analyze the bound form alone.

The same article also found four, rather than one, major protein–ligand association pathways once the ligand reached the surface of the protein, as illustrated by the four energy profiles associated with the four paths within ~4 Å in Figure 18.1. In another article on docking a hexapeptide to the insulin receptor tyrosine kinase (Huang and Wong 2012a,b), two major entrance/exit sites were found (Figure 18.2). The possibility of multiple-docking pathways with multiple entry/exit sites significantly complicates the understanding of drug-binding kinetics and the rational design of drugs. For example, it is possible for different compounds to take different pathways, or they can use multiple pathways simultaneously but the flux through each pathway is different and dependent on compound and its concentration. These more complicated scenarios require quantitative models to give reliable insights. Some developments of such models are introduced below.

In another study, Colizzi et al. (2010) performed single-molecule force-pulling simulation on the binding of flavonoid inhibitors to β-hydroxyacyl-ACP dehydratase of *Plasmodium falciparum* and found active compounds to be harder to pull out than inactive ones. They also found that plots of force versus time clearly separated into two groups: one for active compounds, one for inactives. Thus, it is possible to use such plots to discern active inhibitors from inactive ones for some systems. In addition, by analyzing how the molecules interacted with the proteins along the undocking pathways, they found the 7-hydroxyl group of these compounds to not interact with the protein but the two hydroxyl groups on the phenyl ring gave the active compounds better resistance to be pulled out than the inactive compounds containing only one or no hydroxyl groups. Therefore, they added two

TABLE 18.1

Change of Protein–Ligand Interactions Along One Docking Pathway between pNCS and the Protein Tyrosine Phosphatase YopH in *Yersinia pestis*

Residue-Ligand Interaction Pairs	Distance Bins in Which the Interactions Were Found
C403-SG:OS2; C403-SG:OS4	0.7 Å, 2.7 Å
R409-NH2:OS2; R409-NE:OS2; R409-NE:OS4; R409-NH2:OS4; R409-NE:OS2	0.7 Å
R404-NH1:OH; R404-NH:OS2; R404-NH2:OS1; R404-NH2:OS3; R404-NE:OS4; R404-NH2:OS4; R404-NH2:OH; R404-NE:OS3; R404-NH2:OS2; R404-NH1:OS2;	0.7 Å, 2.7 Å, 3.5 Å, 4.3 Å, 5.5 Å
A405-NH:OS2; A405-NH:OS1; A405-NH:OS3	0.7 Å, 2.7 Å, 4.3 Å
V407-NH:OS3	0.7 Å
G406-NH:OS3;	0.7 Å
G408-NH:OS3; G408-NH:OS4;	0.7 Å
R230-NH2:OS2; R230-NH2:OS3	6.7 Å
Q446-NE2:OS2; Q446-OE1:OS2: Q446-NE2:OS1	4.3 Å, 5.5 Å, 6.7 Å
D356-OD2:OS4: D356-OD1:OS4; D356-OD2:OS1; D356-OD1:OS3; D356-OD2:OS3; D356-OD1:OH; D356-OD2:OH;	2.7 Å, 3.5 Å, 4.3 Å
Q357-NE2:OH; Q357-NE2:OS2; Q357-NE2:OS4; Q357-OE1:OH	3.5 Å, 4.3 Å, 5.5 Å, 6.7 Å
Q446-NE2:OS4; Q446-OE1:OS4; Q446-NE2:ON2; Q446-OE1:OS1; Q446-NE2:OH	4.3 Å, 5.5 Å, 6.7 Å
D356-OD1:OS2; D356-OD1:OS3	2.7 Å, 3.5 Å, 4.3 Å
R205-NH2:ON2; R205-NH2:ON1; R205-NH1:ON2; R205-NH1:ON1;	5.5 Å, 6.7 Å

Source: Modified from Huang, Z. and C. F. Wong. 2007. *Biophys. J.* 93(12):4141–4150.

Note: The table shows how different amino acids came into play at different values of the progress coordinate in one docking pathway as the ligand pNCS moved in and out of the protein. In moving from the smallest distance bin centered at 0.7 Å to that centered at 6.7 Å, the ligand moved from the bound pose to the surface of the protein near the entrance to the docking channel. The first column shows the atom pairs forming interactions between the protein and the ligand. OS2, OS3, and OS4 are the nonbridging oxygens of the sulfate group of pNCS. OS1 is the bridging oxygen. OH is the hydroxyl group of pNCS. ON1 and ON2 are the oxygens of the nitro group of pNCS. Residue and atom names are those used in the CHARMM force field (MacKerell Jr. et al. 1998). The second column shows the distance bins in which these interactions are found. Some amino acids only came into play when the ligand was bound (e.g., R409 only found in the innermost bin); some only interacted with the ligand when it was at the entrance of the channel leading from the protein surface to the binding site (e.g., R205 only found in the two outermost bins near the surface of the protein); some interacted with the ligand throughout most of the binding process (e.g., R404 found in most of the distance bins).

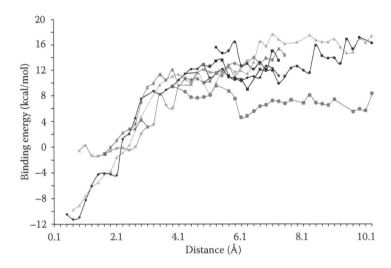

FIGURE 18.1
Four docking pathways of pNCS with the tyrosine phosphatase YopH in *Yersinia pestis.*
(Reproduced from Huang, Z. and C. F. Wong. 2007. *Biophys. J.* 93(12):4141–4150.)

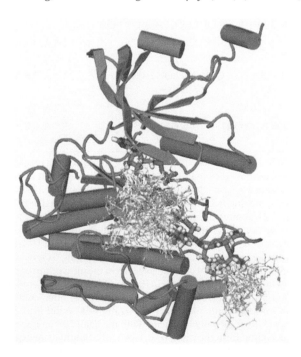

FIGURE 18.2
(See color insert.) The hexapeptide GDYMNM (shown in line model) utilizes two distinct sites
to enter or exit the catalytic domain of the insulin receptor tyrosine kinase (shown in cartoon).
(Reproduced from Huang, Z. and C. F. Wong. 2012b. *Proteins Struct. Funct. and Bioinformat.*
80(9):2275–2286.)

hydroxyl groups to the phenyl ring of the inactive compound kaempferol to form rhamnetin and the profile obtained from steered molecular dynamics simulation became similar to those of the active compounds. Rhamnetin was later confirmed experimentally to be active. This analysis resembles the examination of interaction patterns along docking pathways described above. Colizzi et al.'s successful application of such ideas to a drug-design problem encourages more similar analyses to be performed in the future. For example, could the patterns of interactions along a docking pathway also distinguish compounds with certain desired drug-binding kinetics from those without?

Despite these useful insights, such qualitative analyses of docking pathways are less effective in general cases such as when many pathways contribute to drug binding and unbinding. Quantitative models are indispensable in such cases. And there are special considerations in developing quantitative models for practical drug discovery.

18.3 In Practical Drug Discovery, Fast Quantitative Models for Studying Drug-Binding Kinetics Are Indispensable to Allow a Large Number of Compounds To Be Evaluated

Many methods (e.g., Fischer and Karplus 1992; Sugita and Okamoto 1999; Bolhuis et al. 2000; Henkelman et al. 2000; Cardenas and Elber 2003a,b; Chu et al. 2003; Peters et al. 2004; Ren et al. 2005; Hu et al. 2006; Elber 2007; Maragliano and Vanden-Eijnden 2007; Pan et al. 2008; Bowman et al. 2009a,b; Adelman and Grabe 2013; Donovan et al. 2013) that have been developed for studying large structural changes can potentially be used to study drug-binding kinetics. Researchers have already applied these methods to study different problems such as protein folding (e.g., Andrec et al. 2005; Deng et al. 2013; Han and Schulten 2013; Jimenez-Cruz and Garcia 2013), RNA polymerase II translocation (Da et al. 2014), rotary motion of F_1-ATPase (Okazaki and Hummer 2013), molecular motor (Elber and West 2010), and ATP movement across mitochondrial membrane (Adelman et al. 2011).

However, to be effective in practical drug discovery, one also needs to consider resources required for performing simulations because usually many molecules need to be evaluated before some are suggested for experimental synthesis and biological screening. To this end, fast approximate but inexpensive computational methods for trimming down a large number of molecules to a manageable number for pricier follow-up calculations will be useful. Therefore, instead of reviewing the methods mentioned above, this chapter introduces some recent ideas on developing quicker approximate methods for rapid evaluation of drug-binding kinetics.

18.4 Mining-Minima Approach for Studying Drug-Binding Kinetics

A mining-minima approach was previously employed to find approximate association and dissociation pathways and estimate the associated activation barriers (Huang and Wong 2007, 2012a,b; Wong 2008). This method employs suitable approximations to allow quick calculations.

The mining-mining approach first surveys the energy landscape of a protein–ligand system thoroughly via mining minima to identify a subspace from which docking/undocking pathways can be constructed. By first defining a small subspace to construct pathways, time can be saved by not constructing pathways that pass through configurational space with low transition probabilities.

To survey the energy landscape efficiently, this approach uses a simulated annealing cycling protocol to mine many local minima, characteristics of the complex energy landscape of a protein-ligand system (Elber and Karplus 1987; Frauenfelder et al. 1991). The large number of local minima spans not only energy wells but also energy tops. Thus, pathways connecting the unbound and bound states through some "transition states" can be constructed by suitably linking the minima.

The simulated annealing cycling protocol has been demonstrated to work well in molecular docking in protein kinase and phosphatase systems (Huang et al. 2008; Wong 2008; Huang and Wong 2009a,b, 2012). In this protocol, each molecular dynamics simulation contains a sequence of many short simulated annealing cycles. In each cycle, a system is heated up to a high temperature such as 1000 K and then cooled down to 0 K in ~10 ps. The heating encourages a system to move away from a local energy well to sample another region of the configurational space. The subsequent rapid cooling prevents the unfolding of the protein and traps the system into a new local minimum. One usually runs many such simulated annealing trajectories, starting with different initial atomic velocities, different placements of the ligand inside the protein, or/and different starting conformations of the protein. Because the trajectories are independent, many trajectories with different starting conditions can be run in parallel to reduce turn-around time.

Table 18.2 taken from reference (Huang and Wong 2007) illustrates one scheme to use the mining-minima approach to construct docking pathways (Huang and Wong 2007, 2012a,b; Wong and Bairy 2013). Huang and Wong (2007) had used this approach to study the docking between pNCS and the tyrosine phosphatase YopH in *Yersinia pestis* and that between the hexapeptide GDYMNM and the insulin receptor tyrosine kinase (Huang and Wong 2012a,b) as introduced briefly above.

18.5 Improving the Mining-Minima Approach by the Feynman Path Integral Formalism

The mining-minima approach provides quick estimates of the association and dissociation pathways of drug candidates in biomolecular targets. However, several approximations limit its reliability and it will be useful to add rigor to this approach without significantly increasing computational costs.

Approximations introduced in the mining-minima approach described above include neglecting energetic effects in deciding whether two structures or clusters of structures should be connected to form part of a pathway—only structural similarity is considered, using averaged energies of the clusters along a pathway to estimate association and dissociation activation barriers, and assuming different pathways contributed equally to the total transition probability. Here, we use the Feynman path integral formalism

TABLE 18.2

One Variation of the Mining-Minima Approach for Constructing Docking Pathways

(1) Perform simulated annealing cycling simulations to mine many energy minima.	(2) Cluster structures in energy minima according to structural similarity

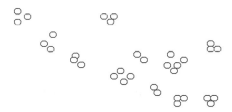 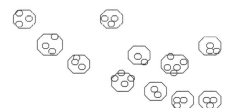

(3) Calculate the averaged energy of each cluster of structures	(4) Connect pairs of clusters to form portions of docking pathways, assuming transition probability proportional to structural similarity between clusters

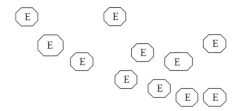

(5) Find continuous paths that can connect the docking structure with structures on the protein surface	(6) Construct energy profile along each path using the averaged energy of the clusters along the path

to relax these approximations, but without performing additional expensive simulations to control computational costs.

To reduce computational costs, one can first assume the collective motion of protein dynamics coupled with ligand docking follows a diffusive, or Brownian, process. Researchers often use this approximation to study configurational transitions in condensed and biomolecular systems (Johnson and Hummer 2012).

The Ermak-McCammon algorithm (Ermak and McCammon 1978) provides one way to simulate the Brownian motion of molecular systems:

$$\frac{d\vec{x}_i(t)}{dt} = -\left(\frac{D}{k_BT}\right)\left(\frac{\partial V(\vec{x})}{\partial \vec{x}}\right) + \vec{R}_i(t) \tag{18.1}$$

where $\vec{x}_i(t)$ represents the coordinates of the system at time t, $V(\vec{x})$ the interaction potential, D the diffusion tensor that is approximated by a scalar and a constant here, $\vec{R}_i(t)$ a random number having zero mean and a variance dependent on the diffusion coefficient, and k_BT the Boltzmann constant times the absolute temperature. Within this approximation, the Fokker–Planck form reads

$$\frac{\partial\rho(\vec{x},t)}{\partial t} = \left(\frac{D}{k_BT}\right)(\nabla^2 V\rho(\vec{x},t)) + \left(\frac{D}{k_BT}\right)(\nabla V \cdot \nabla\rho(\vec{x},t)) + D\nabla^2\rho(\vec{x},t) \tag{18.2}$$

where $\rho(\vec{x},t)$ is the probability density for finding the coordinate vector $\vec{x}$, which defines the structure of a protein–ligand system, at time t.

The transition probability $T(\vec{x}_t,t;\vec{x}_0,t_0)$ from structure $\vec{x}_0$ to $\vec{x}_t$ from time $t_0 = 0$ to time t can be expressed in the Feynman path integral form as

$$T(\vec{x}_t,t;\vec{x}_0,t_0)$$

$$= \int \prod_{\tau=0}^{t} \frac{dx_i}{\sqrt{4D\pi d\tau}} \cdots \prod_{\tau=0}^{t} \frac{dx_{3N_{atom}}}{\sqrt{4D\pi d\tau}} \cdot \exp\left\{-\frac{1}{4D}\sum_{i=1}^{3N_{atom}}\int_{0}^{t} d\tau\left(\dot{x}_i + \frac{D}{k_BT}\frac{\partial V}{\partial x_i}\right)^2\right\}$$

$$\exp\left\{\frac{1}{2}\sum_{i=1}^{3N_{atom}}\int_{0}^{t} d\tau\left(\frac{D}{k_BT}\frac{\partial^2 V}{\partial x_i^2}\right)\right\} \tag{18.3}$$

where N_{atom} is the number of atoms in the system.

For an initial probability density $\rho(\vec{x}_0,t_0=0)$ of a protein–ligand structure $\vec{x}_0$ at time $t_0 = 0$, the probability density $\rho(\vec{x},t)$ of finding the structure $\vec{x}_t$ at time t becomes

$$\rho(\vec{x}_t,t) = T(\vec{x}_t,t;\vec{x}_0,t_0)\rho(\vec{x}_0,t_0) = \int \prod_{\tau=0}^{t} \frac{dx_i}{\sqrt{4D\pi d\tau}} \cdots \prod_{\tau=0}^{t} \frac{dx_{3N_{atom}}}{\sqrt{4D\pi d\tau}}.$$

$$\exp\left\{ -\frac{1}{4D} \sum_{i=1}^{3N_{atom}} \int_0^t d\tau \left(\dot{x}_i + \frac{D}{k_B T} \frac{\partial V}{\partial x_i} \right)^2 \right\}$$

$$\exp\left\{ \frac{1}{2} \sum_{i=1}^{3N_{atom}} \int_0^t d\tau \left(\frac{D}{k_B T} \frac{\partial^2 V}{\partial x_i^2} \right) \right\} \rho(\vec{x}_0,t_0) \tag{18.4}$$

so that the ratio $\rho(\vec{x}_t,t)/\rho(\vec{x}_0,t_0)$ reads

$$\frac{\rho(\vec{x}_t,t)}{\rho(\vec{x}_0,t_0)} = T(\vec{x}_t,t;\vec{x}_0,t_0) = \int \prod_{\tau=0}^{t} \frac{dx_i}{\sqrt{4D\pi d\tau}} \cdots \prod_{\tau=0}^{t} \frac{dx_{3N_{atom}}}{\sqrt{4D\pi d\tau}}.$$

$$\exp\left\{ -\frac{1}{4D} \sum_{i=1}^{3N_{atom}} \int_0^t d\tau \left(\dot{x}_i + \frac{D}{k_B T} \frac{\partial V}{\partial x_i} \right)^2 \right\}$$

$$\exp\left\{ \frac{1}{2} \sum_{i=1}^{3N_{atom}} \int_0^t d\tau \left(\frac{D}{k_B T} \frac{\partial^2 V}{\partial x_i^2} \right) \right\} \tag{18.5}$$

This ratio provides an estimate of the rate constant k, assuming first-order kinetics, by

$$k(t) = \left(\frac{\rho(\vec{x}_t,t) - \rho(\vec{x}_t,0)}{t\rho(\vec{x}_0,t_0)} \right) = \frac{T(\vec{x}_t,t;\vec{x}_0,t_0=0)}{t} \tag{18.6}$$

Thus, a plot of $\langle T(\vec{x}_t,t;\vec{x}_0,t_0=0) \rangle$ versus t will allow a rate constant to be determined from its slope.

To estimate $k(t)$ using structures obtained from the mining-minima approach without running additional simulation, one can first discretize the path integral and obtain the contribution of each path to $T(\vec{x}_t,t;\vec{x}_0,t_0=0)$ by

$$T(\vec{x}_t,t;\vec{x}_0,t_0)_{path} = C_{path} \exp\left\{ -\frac{1}{4D} \sum_{i=1}^{3N_{atom}} \sum_{j=1}^{N} \Delta t_j \left(\frac{x_i(j+1) - x_i(j)}{\Delta t_j} + \frac{D}{k_B T} \frac{\partial V}{\partial x_i} \right)^2 \right\}$$

$$\exp\left\{ \frac{1}{2} \sum_{i=1}^{3N_{atom}} \sum_{j=1}^{N} \left(\frac{D}{k_B T} \frac{\partial^2 V}{\partial x_i^2} \right) \Delta t_j \right\} \tag{18.7}$$

where N is the number of discretized time slices between the two end states used to represent a path, C_{path} is a normalization constant, and x_i's are coordinates defined by the cluster structures obtained from mining-minima simulations.

Unlike the mining-minima approach described above, in which the probability of connecting two structural clusters is based on structural similarity alone, this Feynman path integral treatment incorporates energetic and dynamics effects as well.

To calculate $T(\vec{x}_t, t; \vec{x}_0, t_0)_{path}$ for all possible paths for each t can be expensive. If one uses $N_{cluster}$ to span the coordinate space for each time slice, the number of possible paths grows as $N_{cluster}{}^N$ for N time slices. Figure 18.3 schematically depicts the formation of pathways from the initial state to the final state through several time slices using four clusters ($N_{cluster} = 4$) to span the coordinate space. For the peptide-docking example given above, about 2000 clusters were obtained using 3 Å as the cutoff distance for forming clusters. Thus, even with only five time slices, $\sim 2000^5 = \sim 10^{16}$ paths are possible. One way to reduce the size of the problem is to employ the dominant path approximation in which one assumes the total transition probability to be given by that of the dominant path, the one that gives the largest transition probability. If one uses dynamic programming (Bellman 1957) to find the optimal path, the computational time grows only as $N_{cluster}^2 \times N$.

To illustrate the dominant path approximation, consider first a simple example of barrier crossing through the Eckart potential described by

$$V(x) = V_0 \sec h^2\left(\frac{\pi x}{a}\right) \tag{18.8}$$

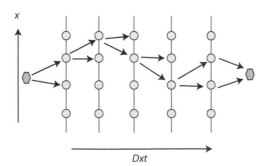

FIGURE 18.3
Schematic representation of paths formed between the initial state from the left to the final state at the right in the discretized representation of the Feynman path integral formalism in calculating the transition probability between the two states. In this example, four clusters are used to span the coordinate space (x) and five time slices are included. D is the diffusion constant in the Feynman path integral formalism and t represents the time. The figure shows only two of the 4^5 possible paths that can form between the two states.

where V_0 and a determine the height and width of the barrier, respectively. Figure 18.4 illustrates what an Eckart barrier looks like when $V_0 = 1$ kcal/mol and $a - 0.5$ Å.

Figure 18.5 uses the example of including one time slice to illustrate that the dominant path approximation works well for this test case. The transition probability of the most probable path was higher than those from the other paths by at least two orders of magnitude. In this calculation, a time step between time slices, Δt was determined by $2D\Delta t = \Delta x$ in which Δx was the distance between two adjacent points in this simple model. Thirteen equally spaced points were distributed along the x axis starting from $-1.5a$ to $1.5a$ to define the space for constructing pathways. The first state on the left at $-1.5a$ was taken as the initial state and the last state at $-1.5a$ was taken as the final state. The points in between gave the intermediate states that the pathways could go through, either one or multiple times.

Figure 18.6 plots the transition probability versus time using the dominant path approximation. One can see a linear region from which the rate constant can be determined from its slope. As the time increased, the transition probability deviated from linearity and decreased rapidly. To examine the origin of this behavior, one can look at the pathway of transitions. For example, the dominant pathway obtained by using 20 time slices between the two end states could be represented by $13 < -11 < -10 < -9 < -8 < -8 < -8 < -8 < -8 < -8 < -8 < -7 < -6 < -5 < -4 < -4 < -4 < -4 < -3 < -2 < -1 < -1$ in which the path moved from the initial state 1 quickly through state 2 and 3

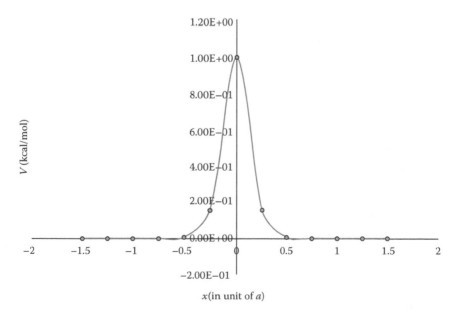

FIGURE 18.4
Eckart potential with $V_0 = 1$ kcal/mol and $a = 1$ Å in Equation 18.8.

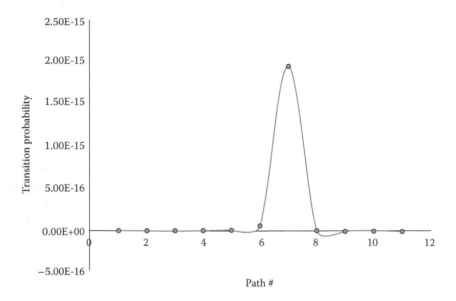

FIGURE 18.5

For the Eckart potential depicted in Figure 18.4, at a temperature of 300 K, and using only one time slice, the transition probability of the dominant path is significantly larger than the other paths so that the total transition probability can be approximated well by that of the dominant path.

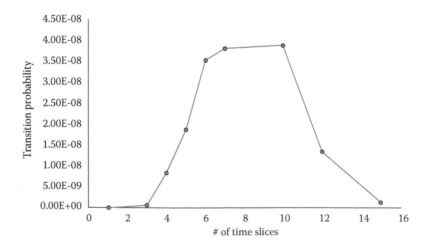

FIGURE 18.6

Dependence of the transition probability on transversal time for the Eckart potential depicted in Figure 18.4 and at a temperature of 300 K.

to state 4 at which it spent a long time before crossing the barrier (state 7). Afterwards, the system spent a long time at state 8 before reaching the final state 13. This was not a path that the system preferred to take and it gave negligible transition probability. The linear region represented pathways that the system favored to take. For these pathways, the distribution of residence times among the intermediate states was comparable. For example, using five time slices between the two end states gave the following pathway: $13 < -10 < -8 < -6 < -4 < -2 < -1$.

If multiple configurations form "predissociation/association states" at the surface of the protein, one can generalize the above treatment to include multiple configurations. For simplicity, one can first consider the following two-step mechanism for dissociation (and association for the reverse process):

$$P{:}L \underset{k_{-1}}{\overset{k_1}{\rightleftharpoons}} P{::}L \underset{k_{-2}}{\overset{k_2}{\rightleftharpoons}} P + L$$

where P denotes a protein, L a ligand, : a bound complex, and :: the collection of predissociation complexes. In many drug-binding processes, the first step represents activated process and the second represents the faster diffusional encounter between the protein and the ligand. If one treats the first part of the above two-step docking/undocking process as rate limiting, the rate law for ligand dissociation becomes

$$\frac{-d[P{:}L]}{dt} = k[P{:}L] \tag{18.9}$$

For the reverse process of ligand association, the rate law reads

$$\frac{d[P{:}L]}{dt} = k_{-1}[P{::}L] = k_{-1}(k_{-2}/k_2)[P][L] \tag{18.10}$$

To obtain the expression after the second equal sign, one assumes an equilibrium to be established between $P{::}L$ and $P + L$ based on the assumption that the interconversion between $P{::}L$ and $P{:}L$ is slow and rate-limiting, common for drug-binding.

18.6 Model to Facilitate the Calculation of Association Rate When a Ligand Enters Its Receptor through Multiple Sites

As discussed above, our previous studies of protein–ligand docking pathways with the mining-minima method have found multiple possible sites of ligand entry (Huang and Wong 2007, 2012a,b). Under these circumstances, it is inadequate to use rate constants $k_{association}$'s alone to compare the association rates among different drug candidates. The associate rates are needed. To further elaborate this requirement, consider a simple kinetic model of protein–ligand association described by

$$\frac{d[P{:}L]}{dt} = k[P][L] \tag{18.11}$$

If the protein and ligand concentrations, $[P]$ and $[L]$ respectively, are the same, it suffices to compare k for different ligands to rank their relative rate in association. However, multiple paths of association make this inadequate even for the same $[P]$ and $[L]$. Suppose one can still describe the kinetics going through each pathway by simple rate laws such that the overall rate of association involving m pathways now becomes

$$\frac{d[P{:}L]}{dt} = k_1 K_1 [P][L]_1 + \cdots + k_i K_i [P][L]_i + \cdots + k_m K_m [P][L]_m \tag{18.12}$$

In this general expression, the local ligand concentrations $[L]_i$ at all entrance sites, rather than the bulk ligand concentration, are required (K_i represents an equilibrium constant between the unbound states and the pre-association complex at site i, as in Equation 18.10). As previous Brownian dynamics simulation showed (Yu et al. 1996; Cerutti et al. 2003), the local ligand concentration could vary from site to site on a protein surface, could depend on the bulk concentration, and could depend on the conformation of the protein. Therefore, even for the same protein and ligand bulk concentrations, it is inadequate to use rate constants alone to compare the association rates between two ligands; it is essential to compare the rate, $d[P{:}L]/dt$, which depends on all the rate constants and the local ligand concentrations. This notion is supported indirectly by a recent experimental study by Hammes et al. (2009), who stressed the difference between comparing rate constants and comparing rates.

To speed up the estimation of local ligand concentrations, one can first perform implicit-solvent Brownian, rather than explicit-solvent molecular dynamics simulation. Using explicit-solvent molecular dynamics simulation to determine local ligand concentrations is expensive because the number density of a drug candidate is low. Short molecular dynamics simulations leave many space unvisited by the drug candidate, making it difficult to construct the probability distribution of a ligand on the surface of a biomolecule. However, even with computers many orders of magnitude slower long ago, Brownian dynamics simulation were performed to the microsecond time scale to allow the construction of the probability distribution of a ligand on a biomolecular surface to 1 Å resolution (Yu et al. 1996; Cerutti et al. 2003). Such Brownian dynamics simulation can be extended to study more complex drug candidates on the surface of biomolecules. If needed, the inhomogeneous concentration of a ligand surrounding the surface of a biomolecule can be further refined by explicit-solvent molecular dynamics simulation starting from the ligand distribution estimated from Brownian dynamics simulation.

18.7 Conclusions

This chapter summarizes and expands some discussions from a recent review (Wong 2014) on exploring how drug-binding kinetics could influence the design of efficacious drug candidates, and on employing simulation techniques to provide a molecular basis on understanding drug-binding kinetics and to aid drug design.

Although long residence time is an important concept in developing efficacious drugs, this chapter also emphasizes that drug-binding kinetics can come into play in other ways. Examples are given in which short residence time or association rate could be beneficial.

As it is still difficult to study drug-binding kinetics at the atomic level by any existing experimental technique, this chapter discusses the use of molecular simulation to gain insights into this problem. Although many methods have already been developed for studying large conformational or structural changes and they can be used to study drug-binding kinetics, practical considerations in drug discovery call for faster methods to evaluate a large number of potential drug candidates before subjecting a small subset to further evaluation by pricier computational or/and experimental methods. To this end, this chapter introduces a fast mining-minima approach that has already been used to study the docking/undocking pathways in protein-ligand systems, and examines how the Feynman path integral formalism can add rigor to this approach.

Although not many molecular simulations on studying drug-binding kinetics have appeared in the literature yet, the increasing awareness of the importance of considering binding kinetics in drug discovery should fuel more simulation work in the future—both in method development and in applications.

Acknowledgments

This chapter, which is expanded from a recent review (Wong 2014), discusses some published work performed with the author's students and collaborators. Financial supports from the U.S. National Institutes of Health, a Research Award from the University of Missouri-St. Louis, and Research Board Awards from the University of Missouri System are also appreciated.

The University of Missouri Bioinformatics Consortium has provided useful computational resources.

References

Adelman, J. L., A. L. Dale, M. C. Zwier et al. 2011. Simulations of the alternating access mechanism of the sodium symporter Mhp1. *Biophys. J.* 101(10):2399–2407.

Adelman, J. L. and M. Grabe. 2013. Simulating rare events using a weighted ensemble-based string method. *J. Chem. Phys.* 138(4):044105.

Andrec, M., A. K. Felts, E. Gallicchio, and R. M. Levy. 2005. Protein folding pathways from replica exchange simulations and a kinetic network model. *Proc. Natl. Acad. Sci. USA* 102(19):6801–6806.

Bairy, S. and C. F. Wong. 2011. Influence of kinetics of drug binding on EGFR signaling: A comparative study of three EGFR signaling pathway models. *Proteins Struc. Funct. Bioinformat.* 79(8):2491–2504.

Bellman, R. 1957. *Dynamic Programming*. Princeton University Press: Princeton, NJ.

Berezov, A., H. T. Zhang, M. I. Greene, and R. Murali. 2001. Disabling erbB receptors with rationally designed exocyclic mimetics of antibodies: Structure-function analysis. *J. Med. Chem.* 44(16):2565–2574.

Bolhuis, P. G., C. Dellago, P. L. Geissler, and D. Chandler. 2000. Transition path sampling: Throwing ropes over mountains in the dark. *J. Phys.: Condens. Matter* 12(8A):A147–A152.

Bowman, G. R., K. A. Beauchamp, G. Boxer, and V. S. Pande. 2009a. Progress and challenges in the automated construction of Markov state models for full protein systems. *J. Chem. Phys.* 131(12):124101.

Bowman, G. R., X. Huang, and V. S. Pande. 2009b. Using generalized ensemble simulations and Markov state models to identify conformational states. *Methods* 49(2):197–201.

Cardenas, A. E. and R. Elber. 2003a. Atomically detailed Simulations of helix formation with the stochastic difference equation. *Biophys. J.* 85(5):2919–2939.

Cardenas, A. E. and R. Elber. 2003b. Kinetics of cytochrome C folding: Atomically detailed simulations. *Proteins Struct. Funct. Genet.* 51(2):245–257.

Cerutti, D, C. F. Wong, and J. A. McCammon. 2003. Brownian dynamics simulations of ion atmospheres around polyalanine and B-DNA: Effects of biomolecular dielectric. *Biopolymers* 70(3):391–402.

Chu, J. W., B. L. Trout, and B. R. Brooks. 2003. A super-linear minimization scheme for the nudged elastic band method. *J. Chem. Phys.* 119(24):12708–12717.

Colizzi, F., R. Perozzo, L. Scapozza, M. Recanatini, and A. Cavalli. 2010. Single-molecule pulling simulations can discern active from inactive enzyme inhibitors. *J. Am. Chem. Soc.* 132(21):7361–7371.

Copeland, R. A. 2011. Conformational adaptation in drug-target interactions and residence time. *Future Med. Chem.* 3(12):1491–1501.

Copeland, R. A., D. L. Pompliano, and T. D. Meek. 2006. Drug-target residence time and its implications for lead optimization. *Nat. Rev. Drug Discov.* 5(9):730–739.

Da, L. T., F. K. Sheong, D. A. Silva, and X. Huang. 2014. Application of markov state models to simulate long timescale dynamics of biological macromolecules. *Adv. Exp. Med. Biol.* 805:29–66.

Davis, M. M., J. J. Boniface, Z. Reich et al. 1998. Ligand recognition by alpha beta T cell receptors. *Annu. Rev. Immunol.* 16:523–544.

Deng, N. J., W. Dai, and R. M. Levy. 2013. How kinetics within the unfolded state affects protein folding: An analysis based on Markov state models and an ultra-long MD trajectory. *J. Phys. Chem. B* 117(42):12787–12799.

Donovan, R. M., A. J. Sedgewick, J. R. Faeder, and D. M. Zuckerman. 2013. Efficient stochastic simulation of chemical kinetics networks using a weighted ensemble of trajectories. *J. Chem. Phys.* 139(11):115105.

Elber, R. 2007. A milestoning study of the kinetics of an allosteric transition: Atomically detailed simulations of deoxy Scapharca hemoglobin. *Biophys. J.* 92(9):L85–L87.

Elber, R. and M. Karplus. 1987. Multiple conformational states of proteins: A molecular dynamics analysis of myoglobin. *Science* 235(4786):318–321.

Elber, R. and A. West. 2010. Atomically detailed simulation of the recovery stroke in myosin by Milestoning. *Proc. Natl. Acad. Sci. USA* 107(11):5001–5005.

Ermak, D. L. and J. A. McCammon. 1978. Brownian dynamics with hydrodynamic interactions. *J. Chem. Phys.* 69:1352–1360.

Fischer, S. and M. Karplus. 1992. Conjugate peak refinement—An algorithm for finding reaction paths and accurate transition-states in systems with many degrees of freedom. *Chem. Phys. Lett.* 194(3):252–261.

Frauenfelder, H., S. G. Sligar, and P. G. Wolynes. 1991. The energy landscapes and motions of proteins. *Science* 254(5038):1598–1603.

Germain, R. N. and I. Stefanova. 1999. The dynamics of T cell receptor signaling: Complex orchestration and the key roles of tempo and cooperation. *Annu. Rev. Immunol.* 17:467–522.

Goyal, M., M. Rizzo, F. Schumacher, and C. F. Wong. 2009. Beyond thermodynamics: Drug binding kinetics could influence epidermal growth factor signaling. *J. Med. Chem.* 52(18):5582–5585.

Group, Boston Consulting. 2011. Life Sciences R&D: Changing the Innovation equation in India.

Hammes, G. G., Y. C. Chang, and T. G. Oas. 2009. Conformational selection or induced fit: A flux description of reaction mechanism. *Proc. Natl. Acad. Sci. USA* 106(33):13737–13741.

Han, W. and K. Schulten. 2013. Characterization of folding mechanisms of trp-cage and WW-domain by network analysis of simulations with a hybrid-resolution model. *J. Phys. Chem. B* 117(42):13367–13377.

Henkelman, G., B. P. Uberuaga, and H. Jonsson. 2000. A climbing image nudged elastic band method for finding saddle points and minimum energy paths. *J. Chem. Phys.* 113(22):9901–9904.

Hu, J., A. Ma, and A. R. Dinner. 2006. Bias annealing: A method for obtaining transition paths *de novo*. *J. Chem. Phys.* 125(11):114101.

Huang, Z. and C. F. Wong. 2007. A mining minima approach to exploring the docking pathways of p-nitrocatechol sulfate to YopH. *Biophys. J.* 93(12):4141–4150.

Huang, Z. and C. F. Wong. 2009a. Conformational selection of protein kinase A revealed by flexible-ligand flexible-protein docking. *J. Comput. Chem.* 30(4):631–644.

Huang, Z. and C. F. Wong. 2009b. Docking flexible peptide to flexible protein by molecular dynamics using two implicit-solvent models: An evaluation in protein kinase and phosphatase systems. *J. Phys. Chem. B* 113(43):14343–14354.

Huang, Z. and C. F. Wong. 2012a. A case study of scoring and rescoring in peptide docking. *Methods Mol. Biol.* 819:269–293.

Huang, Z. and C. F. Wong. 2012b. Simulation reveals two major docking pathways between the hexapeptide GDYMNM and the catalytic domain of the insulin receptor protein kinase. *Proteins Struc. Funct. Bioinformat.* 80(9):2275–2286.

Huang, Z., C. F. Wong, and R. A. Wheeler. 2008. Flexible protein-flexible ligand docking with disrupted velocity simulated annealing. *Proteins* 71(1):440–454.

Jimenez-Cruz, C. A. and A. E. Garcia. 2013. Reconstructing the most probable folding transition path from replica exchange molecular dynamics simulations. *J. Chem. Theory Comput.* 9(8):3750–3755.

Johnson, M. E. and G. Hummer. 2012. Characterization of a dynamic string method for the construction of transition pathways in molecular reactions. *J. Phys. Chem. B* 116(29):8573–8583.

Kapur, S. and P. Seeman. 2001. Does fast dissociation from the dopamine d(2) receptor explain the action of atypical antipsychotics?: A new hypothesis. *A. J. Psychiatry* 158(3):360–369.

Lipton, S. A. 2006. Paradigm shift in neuroprotection by NMDA receptor blockade: Memantine and beyond. *Nat. Rev. Drug Discov.* 5(2):160–170.

Lu, H., K. England, C. am Ende et al. 2009. Slow-onset inhibition of the FabI enoyl reductase from francisella tularensis: Residence time and *in vivo* activity. *ACS Chem. Biol.* 4(3):221–231.

Lu, H. and P. J. Tonge. 2008. Inhibitors of FabI, an enzyme drug target in the bacterial fatty acid biosynthesis pathway. *Acc. Chem. Res.* 41(1):11–20.

Lu, H. and P. J. Tonge. 2010. Drug-target residence time: Critical information for lead optimization. *Curr. Opin. Chem. Biol.* 14(4):467–474.

Lyons, D. S., S. A. Lieberman, J. Hampl et al. 1996. A TCR binds to antagonist ligands with lower affinities and faster dissociation rates than to agonists. *Immunity* 5(1):53–61.

MacKerell, Jr., A. D., D. Bashford, M. Bellott et al. 1998. All-atom empirical potential for molecular modeling and dynamics studies of proteins. *J. Phys. Chem. B* 102(18):3586–3616.

Maragliano, L. and E. Vanden-Eijnden. 2007. On-the-fly string method for minimum free energy paths calculation. *Chem. Phys. Lett.* 446(1–3):182–190.

Matsui, K., J. J. Boniface, P. Steffner, P. A. Reay, and M. M. Davis. 1994. Kinetics of T-cell receptor binding to peptide/I-Ek complexes: Correlation of the dissociation rate with T-cell responsiveness. *Proc. Natl. Acad. Sci. USA* 91(26):12862–12866.

Okazaki, K. I. and G. Hummer. 2013. Phosphate release coupled to rotary motion of F1-ATPase. *Proc. Natl. Acad. Sci. USA* 110(41):16468–16473.

Pan, A. C., D. Sezer, and B. Roux. 2008. Finding transition pathways using the string method with swarms of trajectories. *J. Phys. Chem. B* 112(11):3432–3440.

Peters, B., A. Heyden, A. T. Bell, and A. Chakraborty. 2004. A growing string method for determining transition states: Comparison to the nudged elastic band and string methods. *J. Chem. Phys.* 120(17):7877–7886.

Ren, W., E. Vanden-Eijnden, P. Maragakis, and E. Weinan. 2005. Transition pathways in complex systems: Application of the finite-temperature string method to the alanine dipeptide. *J. Chem. Phys.* 123(13):1–12.

Savage, P. A., J. J. Boniface, and M. M. Davis. 1999. A kinetic basis for T cell receptor repertoire selection during an immune response. *Immunity* 10(4):485–492.

Sugita, Y. and Y. Okamoto. 1999. Replica-exchange molecular dynamics method for protein folding. *Chem. Phys. Lett.* 314(1–2):141–151.

Swinney, D. C. 2004. Biochemical mechanisms of drug action: What does it take for success? *Nature Reviews Drug Discovery* 3(9):801–808.

Swinney, D. C. 2006a. Biochemical mechanisms of New Molecular Entities (NMEs) approved by United States FDA during 2001–2004: Mechanisms leading to optimal efficacy and safety. *Curr. Top. Med. Chem.* 6(5):461–478.

Swinney, D. C. 2006b. Can binding kinetics translate to a clinically differentiated drug? From theory to practice. *Lett. Drug Des. Discov.* 3(8):569–574.

Swinney, D. C. 2009. The role of binding kinetics in therapeutically useful drug action. *Curr. Opin. Drug Discov. Devel.* 12(1):31–39.

Tummino, P. J. and R. A. Copeland. 2008. Residence time of receptor-ligand complexes and its effect on biological function. *Biochemistry (Mosc).* 47(20):5481–5492.

van der Merwe, P. A. and S. J. Davis. 2003. Molecular interactions mediating T cell antigen recognition. *Annu. Rev. Immunol.* 21:659–684.

Wong, C. F. 2008. Flexible ligand-flexible protein docking in protein kinase systems. *Biochim. Biophys. Acta* 1784(1):244–251.

Wong, C. F. 2014. Molecular simulation of drug-binding kinetics. *Mol. Simul.* 40(10–11):889–903.

Wong, C. F. and S. Bairy. 2013. Rational drug design of inhibitors of protein kinases and phosphatases. *Curr. Pharm. Des.* 19(26):4739–4754.

Wu, H., D. S. Pfarr, Y. Tang et al. 2005. Ultra-potent antibodies against respiratory syncytial virus: Effects of binding kinetics and binding valence on viral neutralization. *J. Mol. Biol.* 350(1):126–144.

Yu, W., C. F. Wong, and J. Zhang. 1996. Brownian dynamics simulations of polyalanine in salt solutions. *J. Phys. Chem.* 100:15280–15289.

Zhang, R. and F. Monsma. 2009. The importance of drug-target residence time. *Curr. Opin. Drug Discov. Devel.* 12(4):488–496.

Index

A